ESSENTIAL ORTHOPAEDICS

Mary Bayonla Banks

ALLIED
HEALTH
PRESS

Essential Orthopaedics

Author: **Mary Bayonla Banks**

Allied Health Press
4164 Lakeshore Road
Burlington ON L7L 1A4
Canada
www.alliedhealthpress.com
Email: orders@arclereducation.com

ISBN: 978-1-77956-219-7

ABOUT THE AUTHOR

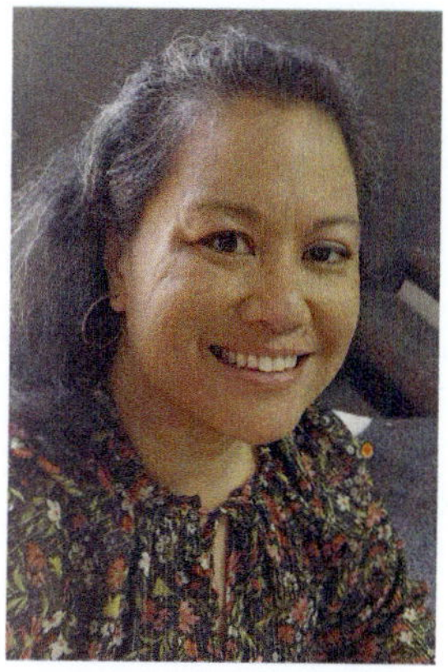

Mary Bayonla Banks is a dedicated physical therapist with a diverse background in pediatrics both school-based and outpatient, geriatrics, and orthopedics. She is also a retired secondary school athletic trainer. She currently works as a staff physical therapist in the Virginia Beach City Public School system where she works with special needs children ranging from ages 2-22 focusing on access to educational program through working on acquisition of gross motor milestones and locomotor skills, as well as attaining and maintaining independent functional mobility. She also works with the geriatric population by providing high quality outpatient orthopedic as well as aquatic physical therapy. Mary attended the Medical Campus of Virginia Commonwealth University in Richmond, VA where she earned her Doctor of Physical Therapy degree in 2004.

Word Roots, Prefixes, and Suffixes by Chapter

Chapter 1 Introduction to Fractures and Dislocations

anti-: attacks, treats condition
contra-: to go against
-cyst-: related to the bladder
-cyt(e,o)-:cell(s)
endo-: inside
extra-: outside
gen(esis)-: origin, new
hem(ato)-: blood
intra-: within

Chapter 2 Fractures in the Upper Limb

abdom-: the abdomen
arteri-: arteries
arthr-: joints
axill-,articul-: armpit region
brachi-: the arm
carp-: the wrist
clav-,cleid-: collar bone
cran-: the skull
muscul-: myo-muscle

Chapter 3 Fractures in the Lower Limb

arteri-: arteries
arthr-, articul-: joints
cardi-: the heart
myel-: spinal cord
omo-: shoulder
cort-: outer region, bark
epi-: over, above, on top
inter-: between, among

Chapter 4 Fractures of the Pelvis

ab: away from
ac: pertaining to
adren/o,: adrenal glands
angi/o: vessel (blood, lymph)
ante: before
anti: against
append/o, appendic/o: appendix
arteri/o: artery

Chapter 5 Spinal Injuries

aut-: self
brady-: slow
dia-: apart, through
epi-: above
hyper-: excessive
hypo-: insufficient
inter-: between
intra-: middle
per-: through
physio-: related to nature or physiology

Chapter 6 Peripheral Nerve and Brachial Plexus Injuries

af-: to, toward
-al: pertaining to
cerebr/o: cerebrum
crani/o: cranium, skull, helmet
dur/o: dura matter
-eal: pertaining to
epi: upon
esthesi.o: feeling, or sensation

Chapter 7 Bone and Joint Infections

arthr-: joint
chondr-: cartilage
osteo-: bone
-lysis: disintegration
-osis: disease
-tomy: incision into
carcin-: cancer
cardio-: heart

hepati-: liver

Chapter 8 Bone Tumors

Anti-: Against

Auto-: Self

Bio-: Life

Chem/o-: Chemistry

Contra-: Against

Cyt/o-: Cell

Dys-; Difficult; Abnormal

Fibr/o-: Fiber

Chapter 9 SCFE, Perthes' Disease and Other Osteochondritis

Ab-, Abs-: Away from

Ad-: Towards

Circum-: Around

Cycl-: Circle; Cycle

Dia-: Across; Through

Epi-: Upon; Outside of

Inter-: Between

Intra-: Within

Meta-:Beyond; Change

Chapter 10 Nutritional, Endocrine, Degenerative, and Autoimmune Disorders

ab-: from; away from

abdomin-: of or relating to the abdomen

aden-: of or relating to a gland

adip-: of or relating to fat or fatty tissue

aer(o)-: air, gas

ante-: describing something as positioned in front of another thing

arteri(o)-: of or pertaining to an artery

Chapter 11 Miscellaneous Conditions

arthr-: joint

chondr-: cartilage

osteo-: bone

scolio-: curved/crooked

-lysis: disintegration

-osis: disease

-tomy: incision into

meta-: beyond

Table of Contents

4 Fractures of the Pelvis 79

5 Spinal Injuries 93

6 Peripheral Nerve and Brachial Plexus Injuries 113

LIST OF FIGURES

LIST OF TABLES

LIST OF ABBREVIATIONS

AAP	American Academy of Pediatrics
AC	Adhesive Capsulitis
ACL	Anterior Cruciate Ligament
ACPA	Anti-Cyclic Citrullinated Peptide Antibodies
ACR	American College of Radiology
ACR	American College of Rheumatology
ADAMTS	A Disintegrin and Metalloproteinase with Thrombospondin Motifs
AFB	Acid-Fast Bacilli
AHO	Acute Hematogenous Osteomyelitis
AIDP	Acute Inflammatory Demyelinating Polyneuropathy
AKI	Acute Kidney Injury
ALP	Alkaline Phosphatase
AMACR	Alpha-Methyl-Acyl-Coa Racemase
AMK	Amikacin
AMPA	Anti-Modified Protein Antibodies
ANS	Autonomic Nervous System
Anti-CCP	Anti-Citrullinated Protein Antibody
anti-MAA	Anti-Malondialdehyde-Acetaldehyde Antibodies
AO/OTA	Arbeitsgemeinschaft Für Osteosynthesefragen/Orthopedic Trauma Association
AP	Anteroposterior
ASIA	American Spinal Injury Association
ATLS	Advanced Trauma Life Support
ATT	Anti-Tubercular Therapy
AVN	Avascular Necrosis
AZA	Azathioprine
BBTs	Benign Bone Tumors
BCD	Bleomycin, Cyclophosphamide, and Dactinomycin

BMD	Bone Mineral Density
BMI	Body Mass Index
BMU	Bone Multicellular Unit
BUN	Blood Urea Nitrogen
Ca^{2+}	Calcium
CAD	Coronary Artery Disease
CAM	Controlled Ankle Motion
CAP	Capreomycin
CCP	Cyclic Citrullinated Peptide
CDAI	Clinical Disease Activity Index
CDKN2A	Cyclin-Dependent Kinase Inhibitor 2A
CGRP	Calcitonin Gene-Related Peptide
CIDP	Chronic Inflammatory Demyelinating Polyneuropathy
CKD	Chronic Kidney Disease
CLIA	Chemiluminescent Immunoassay
CLPBA	Chemiluminescence Protein-Binding Assays
CMAP	Compound Muscle Action Potential
CMC	Carpometacarpal
CNS	Central Nervous System
COG	Children's Oncology Group
COX	Cyclooxygenase
CPBA	Competitive Protein-Binding Assays
CRP	C-Reactive Protein
CRPS	Complex Regional Pain Syndrome
CT	Computed Tomography
CTS	Carpal Tunnel Syndrome
CTV1	Clinical Target Volume
DALYs	Disability-Adjusted Life Years
DAS	Disease Activity Score
DCP	Dynamic Compression Plating
DEXA	Dual-Energy X-Ray Absorptiometry
DHT	Dihydrotachysterol

DIP	Distal Interphalangeal Joint
DKK1	Dickkopf-Related Protein 1
DLBCL	Diffuse Large B Cell Lymphoma
DLC	Disco-Ligamentous Complex
DMARD	Disease-Modifying Antirheumatic Drug
dRTA	Distal Renal Tubular Acidosis
DRUJ	Distal Radio-Ulnar Joint
DTR	Deep Tendon Reflexes
DXA	Dual-Energy X-Ray Absorptiometry
ECRB	Extensor Carpi Radialis Brevis
ED/EDX	Electrodiagnostic
EDB	Extensor Digitorum Brevis
EFS	Event-Free Survival
EGF	Epidermal Growth Factor
EGFR	Epidermal Growth Factor Receptor
EIA	Enzyme Immunoassay
EMA	Epithelial Membrane Antigen
EMB	Ethambutol
EMG	Electromyography
EPS	Extracellular Polymeric Substances
ESR	Erythrocyte Sedimentation Rate
EXT1	Exostine-1
FAOJ	Foot and Ankle Online Journal
FASII	Fatty Acid Synthase Type II
FAST	Focus Assessment with Sonography for Trauma
FCD	Focal Cortical Dysplasia
FCR	Flexor Carpi Radialis
FDG-PET	Fluorodeoxyglucose Positron Emission Tomography
FGF2	Fibroblast Growth Factor 2
FGF23	Fibroblast Growth Factor 23
FGFR1	Fibroblast Growth Factor Receptor 1
FHR	Familial Hypophosphatemia Rickets

FLS	Fibroblast-Like Synoviocytes
FNAC	Fine-Needle Aspiration Cytology
FQ	Fluoroquinolone
FSC	Fibroblast-Like Synovial Cells
GABA	Gamma-Aminobutyric Acid
GBS	Guillain-Barre Syndrome
GCTB	Giant Cell Tumor of Bone
GGCX	Gamma-Glutamyl Carboxylase
GM-CSF	Granulocyte-Monocyte Colony-Stimulating Factor
GTV1	Gross Tumor Volume
GTV2	Gross Target Volume
HCQ	Hydroxychloroquine
HDR	High-Dose Equivalent
Hib	*Hemophilus Influenzae* Type B
hMSC	Human Mesenchymal Stem Cells
HMSN	Hereditary Motor and Sensory Neuropathies
HPLC	High-Pressure Liquid Chromatography
HPV	Human Papillomavirus
HUPI	Hospital Universitario La Princesa Index
HZV	Herpes Zoster Virus
IE	Ifosfamide/Etoposide
IFN	Interferon
IL-6	Interleukin-6
ILD	Interstitial Lung Disease
INR	International Normalized Ratio
IOM	Institute of Medicine
IOM	Interosseous Membrane
IORT	Intraoperative Radiation Therapy
IP	Interphalangeal
JAK	Janus Kinases
JIA	Juvenile Idiopathic Arthritis

JRA	Juvenile Rheumatoid Arthritis
KAN	Kanamycin
KOH	Potassium Hydroxide
LCDCP	Limited Contact Dynamic Compression Plates
LCPD	Legg-Calvé-Perthes Disease
LDR	Low-Dose Brachytherapy
LJ	Lowenstein-Jensen
MAS	Mccune-Albright Syndrome
MCP	Metacarpophalangeal
M-CSF	Macrophage Colony-Stimulating Factor
MDR	Multidrug-Resistant
MFD	Monostotic Fibrous Dysplasia
MGIT	Mycobacteria Growth Indicator Tube
MLSB	Macrolide, Lincosamide, and Streptogramin B
MMN	Multifocal Motor Neuropathy
MMS	Mohs Micrographic Surgery
MOA	Mechanism of Action
MRI	Magnetic Resonance Imaging
MRSA	Methicillin-Resistant S. Aureus
MS	Massspectrometry
MSSA	Methicillin-Sensitive S. Aureus
mTOR	Mechanistic Target of Rapamycin
MUAP	Motor Unit Action Potential
MUS	Musculoskeletal Ultrasonography
Na^+	Sodium
NAA	Nucleic Acid Amplification
NAC	N-Acetylcysteine
NAD	Nicotinamide Adenine Dinucleotide
NCCN	National Comprehensive Cancer Network
NCCU	Neurosurgical Intensive Care Unit
NCS	Nerve Conduction Studies
NHANES	National Health and Nutrition Examination Survey

NOF	Non-Ossifying Fibroma
NP	Nanoparticle
NSAID	Nonsteroidal Anti-Inflammatory Drug
NVO	Native Vertebral Osteomyelitis
OA	Osteoarthritis
OPG	Osteoprotegerin
ORIF	Open Reduction and Internal Fixation
PAD	Peptidyl Arginine Deiminase
Pakt	Phosphorylated Protein Kinase B
PDGFR-beta	Platelet-Derived Growth Factor Receptor Beta
PET	Positron Emission Tomography
PFD	Polyostotic Fibrous Dysplasia
PGP	Pelvic Girdle Pain
Pi	Inorganic Phosphorus
PIP	Proximal Interphalangeal
PLB	Primary Lymphoma of Bone
PLC	Posterior Ligamentous Complex
PLRI	Posterolateral Rotatory Instability
PMMA	Polymethylmethacrylate
PNS	Peripheral Nervous System's
PTEN	Phosphatase and Tensin Homolog
PTH	Parathyroid Hormone
PZA	Pyrazinamide
QCT	Quantitative Computed Tomography
RA	Rheumatoid Arthritis
RADAI	Rheumatoid Arthritis Disease Activity Index
RANKL	Receptor Activator of Nuclear Factor Kappa-B Ligand
RDA	Recommended Daily Allowance
RIA	Radioimmunoassay
RIA	Reamer-Irrigator-Aspirator
rRNA	Ribosomal RNA
RT	Radiation Therapy

RT	Radiotherapy
SAPHO	Synovitis, Acne, Pustulosis, Hyperostosis and Osteitis
SBRT	Stereotactic Body Radiotherapy
SCC	Squamous Cell Carcinomas
SCFE	Slipped Capital Femoral Epiphysis
SCI	Spinal Cord Injury
SDAI	Simplified Disease Activity Index
SE	Shared Epitope
SEER	Surveillance, Epidemiology, and End Result
SHPT	Secondary Hyperparathyroidism
SLNB	Sentinel Lymph Node Biopsy
SMA	Smooth Muscle Actin
SNAP	Sensory Nerve Action Potential
SNP	Single Nucleotide Polymorphism
SNRI	Serotonin-Norepinephrine Reuptake Inhibitor
SONK	Spontaneous Osteonecrosis of the Knee
SP	Side Population
SPF	Sun Protection Factor
SSRI	Selective Serotonin Reuptake Inhibitor
SSTI	Skin and Soft-Tissue Infection
STS	Stem Cell Syndrome
SUFE	Slipped Upper Femoral Epiphysis
TB	Tuberculosis
TCA	Tricyclic Antidepressant
TCC	Total Contact Casts
TENS	Transcutaneous Electrical Nerve Stimulation
TFCC	Triangular Fibrocartilage Complex
TLICS T	horacolumbar Injury Classification and Severity Score
TmP/GFR	Tubular Reabsorption of Phosphorus per Glomerular Filtration Rate
TMP–SMX	Trimethoprim–Sulfamethoxazole
TNF	Tumor Necrosis Factor
TNM	Tumor, Node, and Metastasis

TP53	Tumor Protein 53
TRP	Total Reabsorption of Phosphorus
TSH	Thyroid-Stimulating Hormone
UL	Upper Limit
UPS	Undifferentiated Pleomorphic Sarcoma
US	Ultrasonography
USP6	Ubiquitin-Specific Peptidase 6
USPSTF	U.S. Preventive Services Task Force
VACA	Vincristine, Dactinomycin, Cyclophosphamide, and Doxorubicin
VAIA	Vincristine, Dactinomycin, Ifosfamide, and Doxorubicin
VDC	Vincristine/Doxorubicin/Cyclophosphamide
VDDR	Vitamin D Dependent Rickets
VGLL3	Vestigial-Like Family Member 3
WBC	White Blood Cell
WCC	White Cell Count
WHO	World Health Organization
XDR	Extremely Drug-Resistant
XLH	X-Linked Hypophosphatemic Rickets
ZN	Ziehl-Neelsen

PREFACE

Essential Orthopedics is a fundamental domain within medical science that focuses on diagnosing, treating, rehabilitating, and preventing disorders and injuries related to the musculoskeletal system. This includes bones, joints, ligaments, tendons, muscles, and nerves. With the rapid advancements in medical technology and a deeper understanding of the human body, the field of orthopedics has seen significant growth and evolution, catering to a wide range of conditions from fractures and dislocations to more complex diseases like osteoporosis and arthritis.

Recent research within orthopedics has been pivotal in developing innovative treatments and surgical techniques that offer improved outcomes for patients. Minimally invasive surgery, for example, has become increasingly popular due to its benefits of reduced pain, quicker recovery times, and smaller scars. Techniques such as arthroscopy, where a camera and instruments are inserted through small incisions, allow for detailed examination and treatment of joint issues with minimal disruption to surrounding tissues.

The integration of 3D printing technology in orthopedics represents another significant trend. Customized implants and prosthetics are being developed with this technology, offering patients tailored solutions that fit their unique anatomical structures. This customization can lead to better implant alignment, increased comfort, and enhanced overall functionality.

The field of regenerative medicine, including stem cell therapy and tissue engineering, aims to regenerate damaged tissues, offering promising treatments for conditions that were previously thought to be untreatable. For instance, stem cell therapy is being explored as a potential treatment for osteoarthritis, with the hope of regenerating cartilage tissue rather than simply managing symptoms.

The trend toward personalized medicine in orthopedics is gaining momentum. Considering the genetic, environmental, and lifestyle factors unique to each patient, treatments can be more effectively tailored to improve outcomes. This personalized approach is particularly relevant in the management of degenerative diseases and the choice of materials and methods used in joint replacement surgeries.

The aim of the textbook "Essential Orthopedics" is to provide a foundational and comprehensive guide to the principles and practice of orthopedics, catering primarily to medical students, orthopedic residents, and practicing physicians seeking to update their knowledge. It strives to encapsulate the vast field of orthopedic medicine by covering a broad spectrum of topics, including the diagnosis, treatment, and management of musculoskeletal disorders. This includes an in-depth examination of bone fractures, joint disorders, musculoskeletal injuries, and degenerative diseases, as well as the latest surgical and non-surgical treatment options available. The textbook is designed to facilitate a deeper understanding of the structure and function of the musculoskeletal system, enhance clinical skills, and improve patient care outcomes. Integrating theoretical knowledge with practical application, the book aims to serve as an invaluable resource for those dedicated to mastering the complexities of orthopedic medicine and delivering high-quality care to patients with musculoskeletal conditions.

Chapter 1

INTRODUCTION TO FRACTURES AND DISLOCATIONS

Contents

1.1. Introduction

The two most frequent injuries to bones and joints are dislocations and fractures. A bone dislocation occurs when a bone slips or moves out of its joint. This mostly happens as a result of trauma or the abrupt impact of a hard blow. It is typical for the ankles, knees, hips, shoulders, jaws, fingers, toes, or elbows to dislocate.

Extreme pressure causes the bone to split or shatter into small fragments. This is referred to as a fracture. Fractures are primarily caused by trauma, accidents, repetitive stress, direct pressure, and bone weakness. Children are more likely to experience fractures.

Orientation and Directional Terms

Term	Definition	Illustration
Avulsion fracture	A muscle or ligament pulls on the bone, fracturing it.	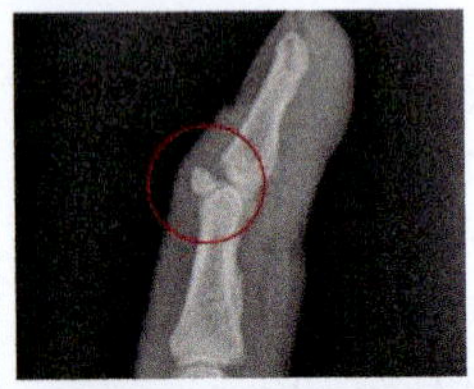
Comminuted fracture	An impact shatters the bone into many pieces.	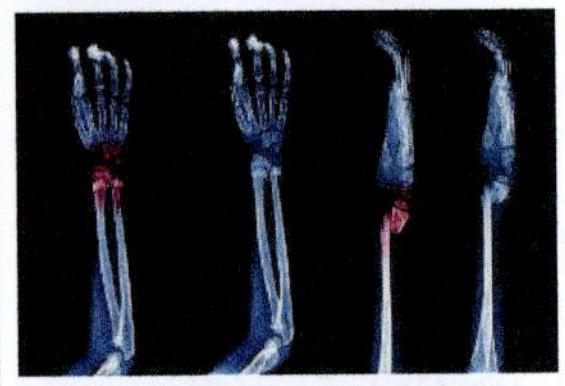
Fracture dislocation	This occurs when a joint dislocates, and one of the bones of the joint fractures.	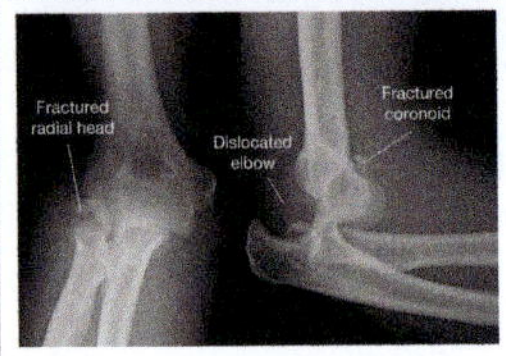
Greenstick fracture	The bone partially fractures on one side but does not completely break, as the remaining part of the bone is able to bend.	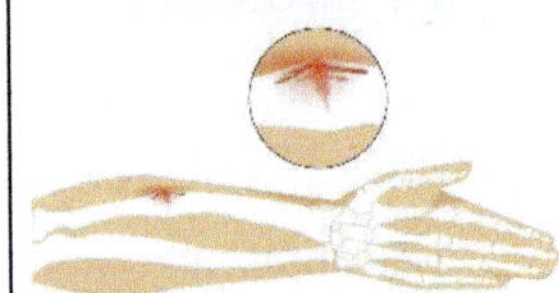
Hairline fracture	This is a thin, partial fracture of the bone.	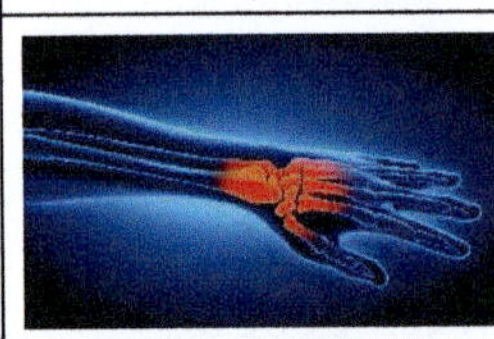
Oblique fracture	An oblique fracture is one that occurs opposite to a bone's long axis.	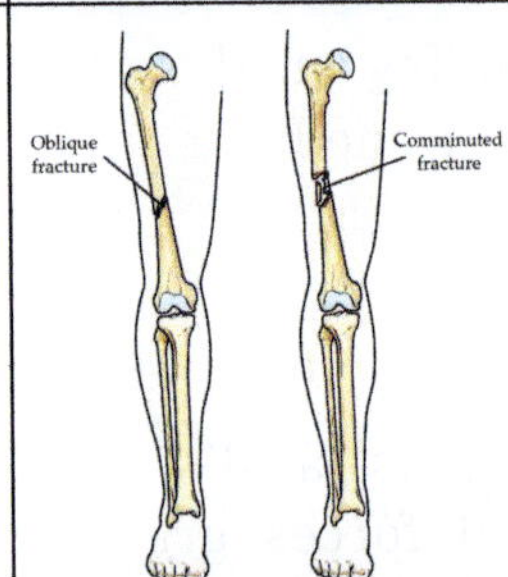
Stress fracture	Repeated stress and strain can fracture a bone, which is a common occurrence among athletes.	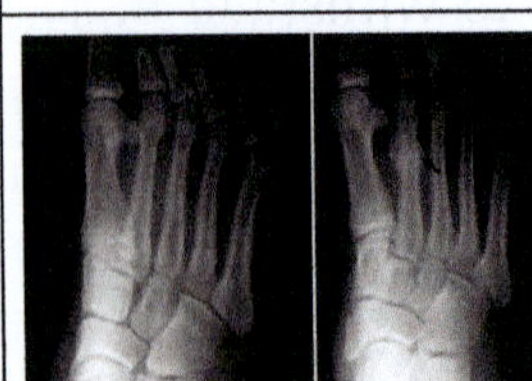

1.2. Definition of a Fracture, Types, Healing, and Treatment of Fractures

When a force applied to a bone exceeds its strength, the result is a fractured or broken bone. This weakens and fractures the bone, causing pain, loss of function, and occasionally bleeding and damage to the surrounding tissue.

Bones make up our skeleton. Connective tissue in the form of bones is strengthened by calcium (Ca^{2+}) and bone cells. Blood cells are created in the softer bone marrow, which is located in the center of bones. Our skeleton serves three primary purposes: it supports our body, permits movement, and shields our internal organs.

Different kinds of bone fractures have been documented. Depending on the force and direction, the specific bone impacted, the individual's age and overall health, and other factors, some are more severe than others. Typical bone fractures consist of:

- Wrist;
- Ankle; and
- Hip fractures (occur most often in older people).

Depending on the type of break and the patient's age and health, broken bones can heal in 4 to 8 weeks.

1.2.1. Definition

A fracture is a discontinuity caused by mechanical forces greater than the bone's capacity to withstand in a bone (or cartilage). There are several ways in which fractures can happen:

- A normal bone subjected to acute overwhelming force, usually in the setting of trauma
- Weakened bone from a focal lesion (e.g., metastasis, or bone cyst), known as pathological fractures.
- Weakened bone due to metabolic abnormalities (e.g., osteoporosis) or less frequently, genetic abnormalities (e.g., osteogenesis imperfecta). Resulting in insufficiency fractures.
- Chronic application of abnormal stresses (e.g., running), resulting in microfractures and eventually, macroscopic failure (fatigue fractures).

Together, insufficiency and fatigue fractures are often grouped together as stress fractures.

1.2.2. Types

Different types of fracture include (Figure 1.1):

- **A Closed (Simple) Fracture:** The skin has not been punctured by the broken bone.
- An open (compound) fracture occurs when a wound extends to the fracture site or when the broken bone protrudes through the skin. External bleeding and infection are more likely.
- A greenstick fracture is a tiny, thin bone crack. Children may experience this because their bones are more malleable than those of an adult.
- Hairline fractures are the most common type, which are stress fractures that usually happen in the foot or lower leg as a result of repetitive strain from running or jogging.
- **Fracture complexity:** Surrounding structures sustain damage. In addition to harming the periosteum,

which lines the inside of the bone, there could be damage to the veins, arteries, or nerves.

- A comminuted fracture is one in which the bone fragments into tiny pieces. This kind of complex fracture usually takes longer to heal.
- **Avulsion Fracture:** Tendons, a type of connective tissue, serve as the anchor between the muscles and the bone. Strong muscle contractions have the ability to separate the tendon and extract fragments of bone. The shoulder and knee joints are more susceptible to this kind of fracture.
- A compression fracture is caused by two bones pressing against each other. This type of fracture can occur in the vertebrae, the bones that make up the spine. Older individuals with osteoporosis are particularly vulnerable.

Not every fracture involves the arm or leg of the patient. Broken bones, including the skull and ribs, can result from trauma to the head, chest, spine, or pelvis.

The underlying body structure that the bone typically protects makes these fractures even more difficult to treat.

Since some of these fractures may be considered life-threatening injuries, treating them with only first-aid knowledge can be extremely challenging. Always seek emergency care if have this kind of fracture.

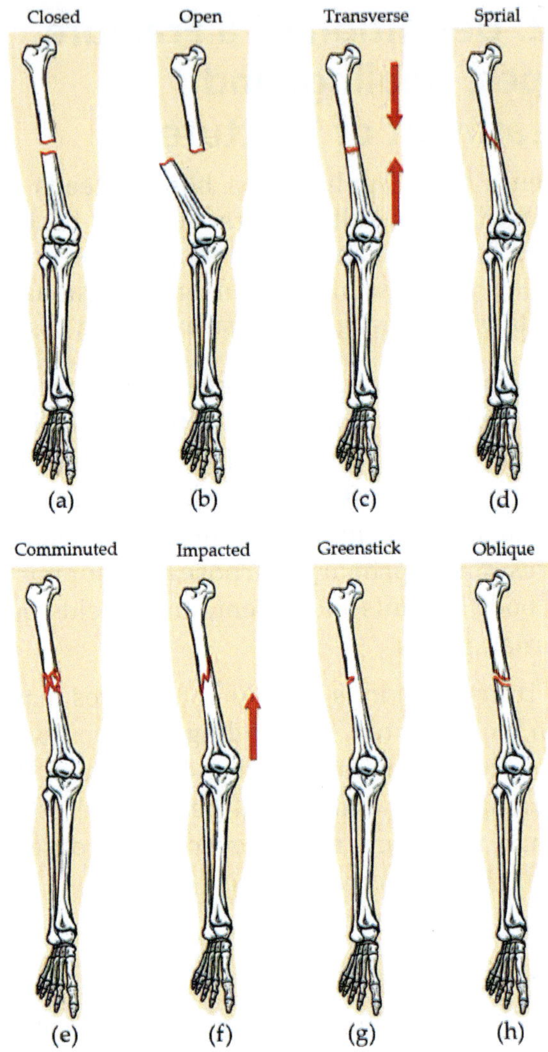

Figure 1.1. *A comparison of healthy bone with different types of fractures: (a) closed fracture; (b) open fracture; (c) transverse fracture; (d) spiral fracture; (e) comminuted fracture; (f) impacted fracture; (g) greenstick fracture; and (h) oblique fracture.*

Source: By OpenStax College – Anatomy and Physiology, Connexions, CC BY 4.0, Website: http://cnx.org/content/col11496/1.6/.

1.2.3. Healing

Bone fractures are a common injury with a challenging recovery process. Only a few tissues, including bone, can heal without leaving fibrous scars. There are two types of bone healing: primary (direct) and secondary (indirect). Bone healing is a complex process of regeneration (Figure 1.2).

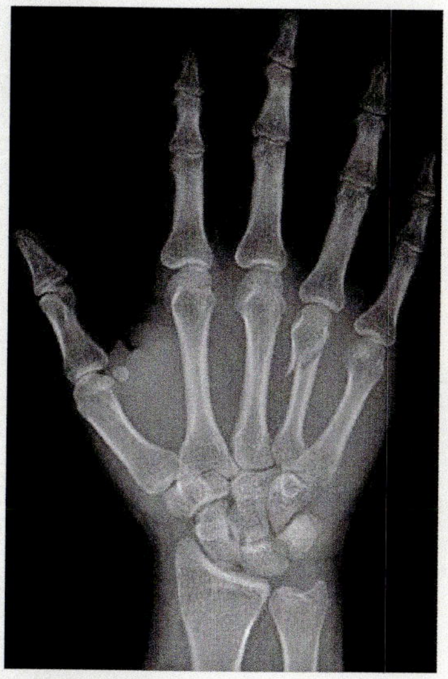

Figure 1.2. *Fracture of 4th metacarpal bone.*

Source: *By Louis Philippe Lessard/CC BY-SA (https://creativecommons.org/licenses/by-sa/4.0), https://commons.wikimedia.org/wiki/File:4th_Metacarpal_Bone_Fracture.jpg.*

When compression is used to hold the bone fragments together, direct, or primary healing takes place. No callus usually develops. The activity of osteoclasts and osteoblasts joins and heals the bony ends. Both intramembranous and endochondral bone healing are a part of indirect healing, which occurs more frequently than direct healing. Stable conditions and anatomical reduction are not necessary for indirect healing to take place. Instead, there is minimal movement and weight bearing at the fracture, which results in the formation of a soft callus and subsequent secondary bone formation. However, it should be mentioned that excessive strain or movement can cause non-union, or delayed healing, which affects 5–10% of fractures.

Indirect healing usually occurs with:

- Non-operative fracture treatment
- Operative treatments where some motion occurs at the fracture site, such as:
  - Intramedullary nailing
  - External fixation
  - Internal fixation of comminuted fractures.

1.2.4. Stages of Indirect Healing

- **Acute Inflammatory Response:** Healing requires the acute inflammatory response, which peaks in 24 hours and diminishes in 7 days. Immediately following trauma, a hematoma forms. This is made up of bone marrow cells as well as cells from peripheral and intramedullary blood. A model for callus formation is produced when the inflammatory response causes the hematoma to coagulate around the fracture ends and within the medulla. To sustain and encourage the growth of blood vessels, tumor necrosis factors like TNF-α, and interleukins like IL-1, IL-6, IL-11, and IL-18 are released.
- **Recruitment of Mesenchymal Stem Cells:** Without the attraction, multiplication, and differentiation of mesenchymal stem cells into osteogenic cells, bone regeneration is not possible. The exact origin of these cells is currently unknown.
- **Generation of Cartilaginous and Periosteal Bony Callus:** The generation of cartilaginous and

periosteal bony callus occurs after the formation of a hematoma, which is followed by the formation of a granulation tissue rich in fibrin. Endochondral formation takes place between the fracture ends and in the periosteal areas beyond. This region is less stable, leading to the development of a soft callus composed of cartilaginous tissue, providing greater stability to the fracture. Animal studies have shown that the peak of soft callus formation occurs at 7 to 9 days, characterized by high levels of type II procollagen and proteoglycan core protein extracellular markers. Simultaneously, intramembranous ossification response occurs immediately under the periosteum near the fracture ends, resulting in the formation of a hard callus. The bridging of this central hard callus creates a semi-rigid structure, allowing weight-bearing on the fracture.

- **Revascularization and Neoangiogenesis:** A sufficient blood supply is required for bone mending to take place. To allow blood vessels to migrate into the repair site, cells, and extracellular matrices must be eliminated. For this reason, angiogenic pathways, chondrocyte apoptosis, and cartilaginous degradation are crucial to this process.
- **Mineralization and Resorption of the Cartilaginous Callus:** For bone regeneration to proceed, the main soft cartilaginous callus needs to be resorbed and replaced by a hard bony callus. This stage, which includes cellular proliferation and differentiation, an increase in cellular volume, and matrix deposition, is similar to embryological bone development in certain aspects (Figure 1.3).

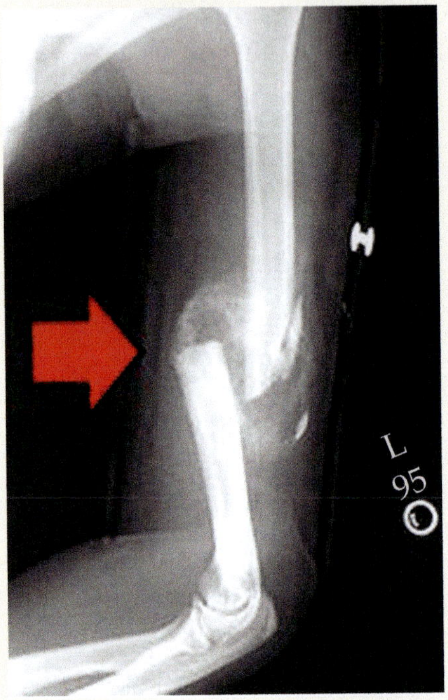

Figure 1.3. *Bone healing of a fracture by forming a callus as shown by X-ray.*

- **Bone Remodeling:** Even though the hard callus is stiff and offers support, it does not mean that the fractured area has the same characteristics as regular bone. A second phase of healing is needed, during which the hard callus is transformed into a lamellar bone structure with a central medullary cavity (Figure 1.4).

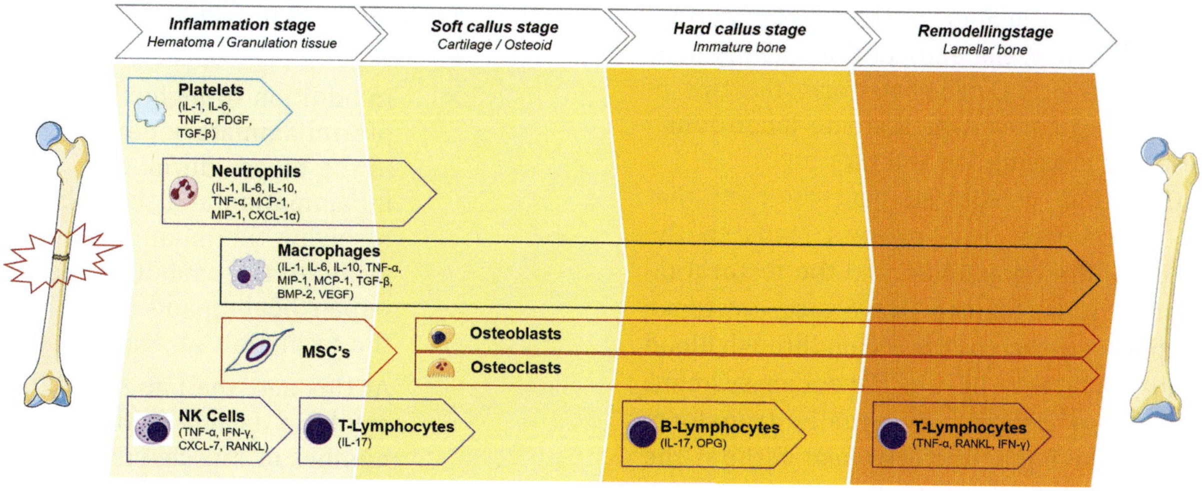

Figure 1.4. *Bone healing process.*

Source: By Khloud Shreif, creative commons attribution-ShareAlike 4.0 international, https://www.physio-pedia.com/index.php?curid=34355.

Remodeling occurs when osteoblasts deposit lamellar bone and osteoclasts resorb the hard callus. This process begins in three to four weeks, but it may take years to complete. In younger patients, remodeling may happen more rapidly (as observed in other animals). Bone remodeling is influenced by the production of electrical polarity. This process occurs when pressure is applied in a crystalline environment.

- An electropositive convex surface and an electronegative concave surface are produced when the axial loading of long bones takes place.
- This activates osteoclastic and osteoblastic activity.
- As a result, a lamellar bone structure gradually replaces the external callus. In addition, the internal callus remodels to produce a medullar cavity that resembles the diaphyseal bone.

Only in the presence of a sufficient blood supply and a progressive rise in mechanical stability can bone remodeling be effective. If not, issues like non-union could arise.

1.2.5. Direct Fracture Healing

Stable fixation and complete reduction of the fracture ends are necessary for direct healing. Therefore, it usually occurs after open reduction and internal fixation surgery rather than spontaneously.

The Haversian canals, blood vessels, and lamellar bone can all undergo direct remodeling to facilitate direct bone healing. This process can take several months or even years.

Primary healing of fractures occurs through:

- Contact healing
- Gap healing.

The goal of both procedures is to replicate the lamellar bone structure. Only when the fracture ends are compressed together and rigid fixation is applied to lessen interfragmentary strain can direct bone healing occur.

1.2.5.1. Contact Healing

When the interfragmentary strain is less than 2% and the gap between each bone end is less than 0.01 mm, a fracture can fuse together through contact healing. In these cases, cutting cones develop at the ends of the osteons near the fracture site. Osteoclasts form the tips of these cutting cones, which create longitudinal cavities by crossing the fracture line.

Over time, osteoblasts generate bone that fills the cavities. This process leads to the formation of a bony union and the restoration of the axially formed Haversian systems. Osteoblasts can access the region through blood vessels, facilitated by the Haversian systems. As bridging osteons eventually transform into lamellar bone, fractures heal without the development of a periosteal callus.

1.2.5.2. Gap Healing

The healing of gaps after a bone fracture is a unique process in which bony union and Haversian remodeling do not occur simultaneously. For gap healing to occur, the size of the gap must be less than 800 μm to 1 mm. During this period, the gap is predominantly filled with lamellar bone that is oriented perpendicular to the long axis, necessitating secondary osteonal reconstruction. Eventually, the primary bone structure is replaced by longitudinal revascularized osteons, carrying osteoprogenitor cells that mature into osteoblasts. These osteoblasts then generate lamellar bone on both sides of the gap, although the orientation of the bone makes it less robust. This process typically lasts between 3 and 8 weeks. Subsequently, a secondary remodeling phase occurs, resembling the cascade observed in contact healing with cutting cones.

1.2.6. Factors Affect Bone Healing

- Patients who smoke, have low blood sugar, or are malnourished will not experience rapid bone healing.
- Parathyroid hormones play a crucial role in bone healing as they promote osteoblast and osteoclast differentiation and proliferation.
- Aging process in which the patient will have:
  - In addition to higher levels of pro-inflammatory cytokines in the blood, chronic inflammation and the delay in resolving the inflammation to facilitate the anabolic process impair healing and result in the formation of a small callus.
  - At this age, the patient will exhibit a decline in the number of muscle stem cells, which will adversely impact the healing process.
  - There is a reduction in blood vessel density in the bone marrow compared to younger individuals, resulting in decreased vascularization and angiogenesis.
- Factors related to the fracture site:
  - Infection of the fracture site during the healing process.
  - Insufficient formation of cartilage within the fracture gap and marrow space.
  - Open, comminuted fracture and the extent of soft tissue injury also show delayed union healing.

1.2.7. Treatment of Fractures

The goal of medical care for broken bones is to ensure that the fragments of bone are correctly aligned. Broken bones heal on their own. The bone must fully regain its sensitivity, movement, and strength. Surgery or surgical traction (or both) may be required for certain complex fractures.

- **Cast Immobilization:** The most popular fracture treatment is a plaster or fiberglass cast because most broken bones heal well if they are realigned and a cast is placed to hold the broken ends in place while they heal.

- **Functional Cast or Brace:** Nearby joints can move in a restricted or controlled manner thanks to the cast or brace. This treatment is ideal for certain fractures, but not for others.
- **Traction:** The process of gently and steadily pulling a bone or bones into alignment is known as traction. It is not usually applied as a last resort.
- **External Fixation:** During this type of procedure, the surgeon drills holes above and below the fracture site to insert metal screws or pins. The screws or pins are then fastened to an external metal bar. This apparatus functions as a stabilizing frame to maintain the proper alignment of the bones during the healing process. If there is significant damage to the skin and other soft tissues surrounding the fracture, it may be necessary to wear an external fixator until the patient is well enough to undergo surgery.
- **Open Reduction and Internal Fixation:** The surgeon holds the bones together with special screws or by fastening metal plates to the outside surface of the bone after first repositioning (reducing) the broken pieces of bone into their proper alignment. Another option for holding the pieces together is to pierce the bone's center with rods.

1.2.8. Operation Procedure for Bone Fractures

Using a plaster cast is a common way to immobilize a limb. This cast is created with a gypsum preparation that solidifies upon the addition of water. The operation procedures can involve any of the following, depending on the location and severity of the fracture.

- Simple or closed fractures involve keeping the two ends of the fractured bone aligned. Once the limb is properly bandaged, wet plaster is applied. In some cases, the cast is split in half and rebandaged externally after the plaster has dried. This allows for potential swelling.
- Open or compound fractures are cleaned in the operating room to ensure no debris is left behind before setting the bone. This is important to prevent infection when a broken bone is exposed.
- Long bones, such as the femur in the thigh, can be challenging to align. Internal nailing is often used for adults in these cases. Children may require traction for a few days before a cast is applied to a broken bone. Plaster of Paris is used to immobilize the hip joint and leg once the bone ends start to heal. In other situations, pins are attached to an external frame, or "fixator," above and below the fracture. This procedure is performed under general anesthesia.

1.2.9. Complications

Even though bone fractures usually heal well with the right care, complications like these can occur.

- **Bone Heals Incorrectly:** During the healing process, bones may move or heal in the incorrect place following a fracture.
- **Bone Growth Disruption:** The normal development of a bone may be impacted if a childhood bone fracture experiences complications during the healing process. This may make a bone deformity more likely in the future.
- **Bone or Bone Marrow Infection:** In a compound fracture, the bone or bone marrow may become infected by bacteria that enter through a skin break. This could develop into a chronic infection.
- **Bone Death (Avascular Necrosis):** A bone may die if it is deprived of its vital blood supply.

1.2.9.1. Delayed Unions and Non-unions

Fractures that do not heal are known as non-unions, whereas fractures that heal more slowly are known as delayed unions.

Treatments for non-unions and delayed unions include:

- **Ultrasound Therapy:** The affected area will receive low-intensity ultrasound treatment from a medical professional. Broken bones might heal better this way.
- **Bone Graft:** If the fracture does not heal, a surgeon will implant a synthetic or natural bone to stimulate the broken bone.
- **Stem Cell Therapy:** Treatments derived from stem cells have the potential to aid in the healing of bone fractures.

1.2.10. Recovery

Fractures can heal in a few weeks to a few months, depending on the severity of the damage and how closely adhere to the doctor's instructions. Long before the fracture is strong enough to withstand the strains of regular activity, pain usually subsides. The patient might need to keep limiting the movement until the bone is strong enough for regular activity, even after the cast or brace is taken off. The patient probably lose range of motion and muscle strength in the injured area while healing. The patient can regain the normal range of motion, flexibility, and muscle strength by performing certain exercises.

1.2.11. Prevention

Numerous treatments and lifestyle modifications can lower a person's risk of bone fractures. Furthermore, a person's diet may have an impact on their fracture risk. Sufficient calcium intake is necessary for maintaining strong bones. Good sources of calcium include milk, cheese, yogurt, and dark green leafy vegetables. In order for the body to absorb calcium, vitamin D is also essential. Eggs, oily fish, and sun exposure are excellent sources of vitamin D.

Exercises involving weight-bearing can enhance bone density and muscle mass. These two factors can both lower the chance of bone fractures. Studies have indicated that individuals with osteoporosis can lower their risk of fracture by following a balanced diet and engaging in regular exercise. Additionally, during menopause, levels of estrogen, which are important for bone health, significantly decrease. This raises the risk of osteoporosis and fractures and complicates the regulation of calcium. Therefore, individuals should pay special attention to the density and strength of their bones both during and after menopause.

A fracture is a break in the structure of a bone. Fractures can occur in any bone and vary in size from small partial cracks to complete breaks.

The most common causes of fractures are physical trauma, overuse, and medical conditions such as osteoporosis. Additionally, as individuals enter late adulthood, their bones tend to weaken, increasing the likelihood of bone fractures. While the majority of fractures can heal naturally, surgery is often necessary to properly align the broken bones. These surgical interventions may involve the use of screws, plates, or external casts and splints.

1.3. Definition of Dislocation, Types, Management in General andComplications

The medical term for the displacement of bones from their normal position in a joint is a dislocation. Dislocations can occur in any joint of the body and are typically caused by trauma or sports-related injuries. It is important to never attempt to realign a dislocated joint by themselves through pushing or forcing it back.

1.3.1. Definition

At the sites where two bones meet, there are several structures holding them together. These include:

- Strong tissues called ligaments around (and sometimes inside) the joint.
- A joint capsule – a fibrous surround to the joint.
- Tendons and muscles passing around and sometimes through the joint.

Dislocations transpire when an injury engenders an impact on the joint, such as instances of falling, automobile accidents, and collisions in contact sports. Dislocations are injuries wherein the bones in a joint have been compelled apart and positioned abnormally. Smaller joints can be dislocated with less force than larger joints. Stretching the surrounding tissues that hold a joint in place can make it easier to dislocate joints that have already dislocated. Certain individuals are more vulnerable to dislocations than others. The joint's structures as well as the bones themselves may be ripped or fractured if the joint is injured and pulled apart (Figure 1.5).

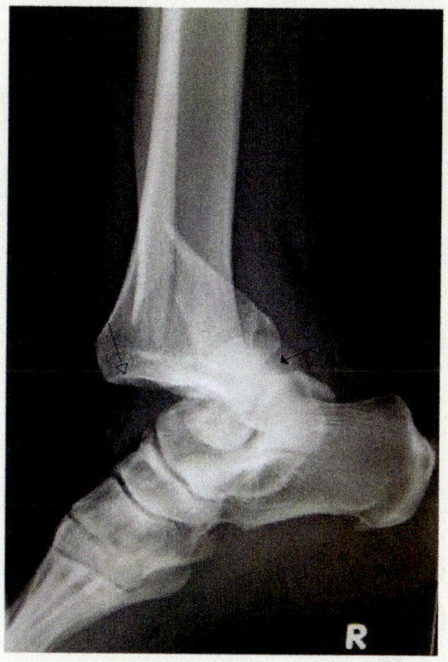

Figure 1.5. *A traumatic dislocation of the tibiotarsal joint of the ankle with a distal fibular fracture. The open arrow indicates the tibia, and the closed arrow indicates the talus.*

Source: By James Heilman, MD – Own work, CC BY-SA 3.0, https://commons.wikimedia.org/w/index.php?curid=11110496.

1.3.2. Major Types of Dislocations

The most common types of dislocations are those of the shoulder, hip, knee, and fingers. These are frequently caused by trauma or injury and necessitate immediate medical attention (Figure 1.6).

- **Dislocated Shoulder:** The humerus, which is the upper arm bone, can dislocate the shoulder when it pops out of its socket. This condition is usually caused by sudden trauma or a blow, resulting in severe pain, limited mobility, and a noticeable deformity. The initial treatment involves reducing the joint back into place, often with the use of sedation or anesthesia. Rehabilitation follows to restore flexibility and strength. In cases of recurrent dislocations, surgery may be necessary to stabilize the shoulder joint.

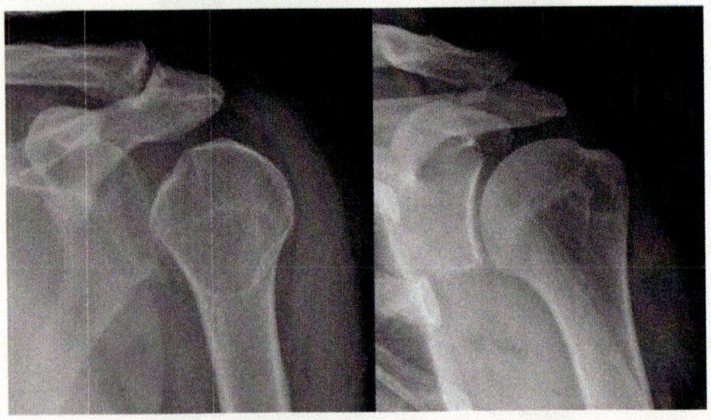

Figure 1.6. *Shoulder dislocation before (left) and after (right) being reduced.*

Source: By Hellerhoff – Own work, CC BY-SA 3.0, https://commons.wikimedia.org/w/index.php?curid=39582858.

- **Dislocated Elbow:** When the forearm bones are forced from their natural position at the elbow joint, it results in a dislocated elbow. This condition typically occurs following a traumatic injury and is accompanied by excruciating pain, edema, and immobility. Rehabilitating the elbow joint to regain strength and range of motion is a crucial part of recovery, as it ensures optimal function and helps prevent long-term issues.
- **Dislocated Hip:** A dislocated hip occurs when the femur, the femur, is forcefully removed from the hip socket. This often happens as a result of high-impact accidents or falls, causing intense pain, limited movement, and an obvious deformity. In certain cases, surgery may be necessary to stabilize the hip joint and prevent recurrence.
- **Dislocated Knee:** A dislocated knee is a severe injury that occurs when the bones in the knee joint become misaligned. This typically happens due to trauma or collisions with solid objects. This condition results in significant pain, swelling, and instability. Additional treatment, including surgery, is often necessary to address any associated ligament and cartilage damage.
- **Dislocated Ankle:** Ankle dislocations occur when the bones in the ankle joint are forcefully pushed out of their normal alignment, usually due to a traumatic injury. This condition causes intense pain, swelling, and stiffness in the ankle. Prompt medical attention is required to realign the joint and assess any potential ligament or bone damage.
- **Dislocated Wrist:** When the bones in the wrist joint are forced out of their natural position, it is known as a dislocated wrist, which often occurs due to trauma or falls. This leads to discomfort, swelling, and limited movement. Immediate medical attention is necessary to realign the wrist joint.
- **Dislocated Jaw:** A dislocated jaw refers to the dislocation of the

mandible, or lower jaw, at the temporomandibular joint. This can be caused by various factors, such as trauma or frequent mouth opening. Pain, difficulty in opening or closing the mouth, and occasionally an improper bite are the symptoms of this condition.

- **Dislocated Finger:** When the bones of a finger are forced out of their natural alignment, typically due to trauma or injury, it results in a dislocated finger. This causes swelling, pain, and deformity in the affected finger. The process of moving the bones back into alignment is known as reduction (Figure 1.7).

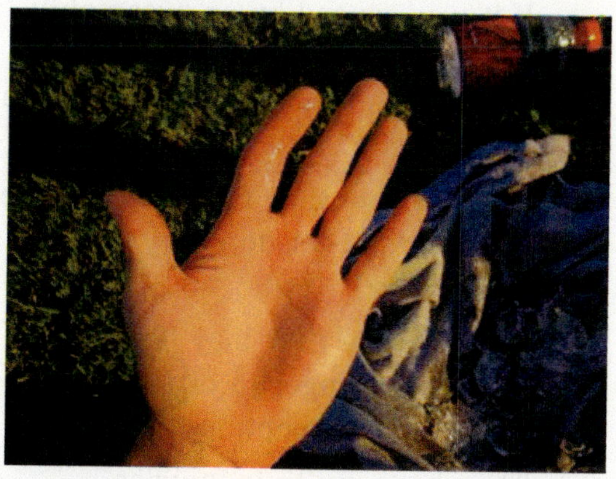

Figure 1.7. *Dislocation of the left index finger.*

Source: By Original uploader was Rbmoore at en.wikipedia – Transfered from en.wikipedia, CC BY-SA 3.0, https://commons.wikimedia.org/w/index.php?curid=3288253.

1.3.3. Rare and Specific Types of Dislocations

Jaw dislocations, hip dislocations in infants, and scapholunate dislocations of the wrist are examples of rare and specific dislocations that, due to their unique characteristics, all require specialized medical care.

- **Lunate and Perilunate Dislocation:** Dislocations of the lunate and perilunate are uncommon injuries in the wrist. A lunate dislocation occurs when the lunate bone in the wrist shifts. In a perilunate dislocation, the lunate and surrounding bones are dislocated more severely. Both conditions are caused by severe trauma. Immediate medical attention is crucial to restore alignment and prevent long-term complications.
- **Atlantoaxial Dislocation:** Atlantoaxial dislocation is an extreme and uncommon condition where the first and second cervical vertebrae misalign. This can be a congenital defect or the result of trauma. Symptoms include neck pain, neurological problems, and even paralysis. Depending on the severity, realigning the vertebrae may require surgery or conservative measures.

1.3.4. Causes of Dislocations

The most frequent cause of dislocations and other injuries to the musculoskeletal system is trauma. Trauma consists of:

- Direct force, as occurs in falls or motor vehicle accidents
- Repeated wear and tear, as occurs during daily activities or results from vibration or jerking movements
- Overuse, as may occur when athletes overtrain.

A dislocation's degree of severity is partially determined by the kind and intensity of the trauma that caused it. Certain sports can cause dislocations in certain individuals.

Dislocations are more common in specific disorders. One such condition is the rare genetic connective tissue disease known as Ehlers-Danlos syndrome, which results in extremely flexible joints. Individuals with this disorder are more prone to experiencing sprains and dislocations.

1.3.5. Symptoms of Dislocations

Bones that have become dislocated may be visibly misaligned. The joint might appear contorted or distorted. The skin surrounding a bone that protrudes abnormally may stretch and bulge.

Dislocations cause the following symptoms:

- Pain
- Swelling
- Inability to use the injured part normally
- Bruising or discoloration
- Possibly loss of feeling (numbness or abnormal sensations)

The dislocation site is painful, particularly when one attempts to use or bear weight on the injured area. Upon touch, it feels delicate. Often, the affected part—whether it be an arm, leg, hand, finger, or toe—cannot be moved normally. The area surrounding the dislocated joint may become bruised, with visible subcutaneous bleeding. Initially, the bruise appears purplish-black, but over the course of a few days as the blood is broken down and reabsorbed into the body, it gradually changes to green and yellow.

Some individuals, especially the elderly or young children, may be unable or unwilling to move the injured part due to the intense pain. In cases where a person is unable to communicate, their inability to move a body part may be the only indication of a dislocation.

1.3.6. Diagnostic Procedures for Dislocation

Diagnosis of Dislocations includes:

- A doctor's evaluation
- X-rays to identify fractures
- Sometimes magnetic resonance imaging (MRI) or computed tomography (CT)

When a sudden dislocation occurs, individuals must decide whether to visit the emergency room, schedule a doctor's appointment, or wait and observe if the pain, swelling, or other symptoms subside or improve on their own. If someone meets any of the following criteria, they should be transported to an emergency room, typically by ambulance:

- If it was caused by an automobile accident or if people are unable to use the affected body part, the issue is obviously serious.
- They believe they may have suffered a severe soft-tissue injury, such as a dislocation.
- They believe they may have a fracture (a fingertip or toe injury could be an exception).
- They have multiple injuries.
- They exhibit signs of complications, such as weakness in the affected area, loss of feeling in the affected body part, difficulty moving the affected part normally, and cold or blue skin.
- They cannot put any weight on or use the affected body part.
- An injured joint feels unstable.

People should call a doctor when;

- Although there is pain or swelling from the injury, individuals can still move the joint normally and do not believe it to be seriously broken.

- If none of the aforementioned options work and the injury appears to be minor, individuals can wait to see if the issue resolves on its own or contact a doctor. If injuries result from a serious accident, the doctor examines the following:
- To look for severe wounds and associated problems, such as an open wound, severe blood loss, nerve damage, and compartment syndrome, which can occur when the blood supply to an injured limb is cut off or restricted.

Doctors treat any injuries or complications as needed and proceed with the physical examination if any are present.

1.3.6.1. Description of the Injury

Physicians ask the patient (or a witness) to explain what transpired. Frequently, the patient is unable to accurately describe the injury or cannot recall how it happened. Doctors can identify the type of injury more accurately if they are aware of how it happened. Physicians also inquire as to which direction the joint was stressed at the time of the injury. Doctors also want to know when the pain began. If it appeared right away following the injury, a severe sprain, fracture, or dislocation could be the cause. Usually, it is a minor injury if the pain starts hours or days later. Blood flow disruption or the development of compartment syndrome could be the cause of pain if it is more severe than anticipated for the injury or if it gets worse over the course of the first few hours following the injury.

1.3.6.2. Physical Examination

The physical examination includes the following (in order of priority):

- Checking for damage to blood vessels near the injured body part
- Checking for damage to nerves near the injured part
- Checking for open wounds, joints that look misshapen, swelling, bruising, and impaired movement of the joint
- Examining and moving the injured part
- Examining the joints above and below the injured part

Doctors measure skin temperature, color, and pulse to look for indications of blood vessel damage and disturbed blood flow. A disturbed blood flow can lead to pale, cool skin, and eventually the disappearance or weakening of pulses (as in compartment syndrome). Blood pressure, which is low in patients who have lost a lot of blood, is measured by doctors.

Physicians examine the patient's ability to move their muscles normally in order to rule out nerve damage. The motor nerves, which regulate the afflicted muscles, may have been harmed if the person is unable to move them. In addition to assessing a patient's ability to feel normally through their skin, doctors also inquire about any unusual sensations the patient may be experiencing, such as tingling, numbness, or a pins-and-needles sensation. The nerves known as sensory nerves, which control skin sensation, may have been harmed if feelings are unusual or diminished.

To assess whether there are any misplaced bones and whether the area is tender, medical professionals will gently touch the injured area. Additionally, doctors look for bruises and swelling. They inquire as to whether the patient is able to move, put weight on, and use the injured area. Physicians use gentle joint movements to assess a joint's stability; however, if a fracture or dislocation is suspected, X-rays are taken beforehand to establish whether joint movement is safe. Upon moving the injured part, doctors listen for grating or crackling noises (known as crepitus). These noises could point to a break. Doctors can assess the extent of an injury by moving the afflicted joint.

The joints above and below the injured joint are also examined by doctors. Stress testing can be used to assess a damaged joint's stability. Nevertheless, stress testing is delayed until X-rays are taken to look for fractures and dislocations if these injuries are suspected. Doctors will gently move a joint in a direction that is typically perpendicular to its normal range of motion to stress it. Physicians may suspect a dislocation (or severe ligament injury) if the joint feels extremely unstable.

A local anesthetic may be injected into the injured area, or the patient may be given a painkiller, muscle relaxant, or both by mouth or injection if pain or spasms prevent them from being examined properly. Alternatively, medical professionals may immobilize the injured joint until the spasm subsides (often a few days), at which point they will assess the joint.

1.3.6.3. Tests

Imaging tests used to diagnosis dislocations and other musculoskeletal injuries include

- X-rays
- Magnetic resonance imaging (MRI)
- Computed tomography (CT)

X-rays can be used to diagnose fractures as well as dislocations. Because X-rays only display bones (and the fluid that gathers around an injured joint), they do not help identify injuries to ligaments, tendons, or muscles. To demonstrate how the bones are aligned, X-rays are typically taken from at least two different angles. To look for small fractures that could accompany a dislocation, an MRI or CT scan may be performed.

Other tests may be done to check for other injuries that may result from a dislocation:

- Angiography: X-rays or CT scans obtained after an injection of a contrast agent into the arteries to look for damaged blood vessels.
- To look for damaged nerves, use nerve conduction studies and/or electromyography (EMG) (usually performed as an outpatient procedure).

1.3.7. Immediate Care

Treating a dislocation right away includes immobilizing the affected joint, managing pain, and seeking medical assistance as soon as possible. These actions reduce the risk of further injury and enhance the likelihood of a successful reduction.

- **Immobilization/Rest:** Promptly addressing a dislocation entails immobilizing the affected joint, administering pain management, and seeking medical assistance expeditiously. These measures diminish the likelihood of further injury and enhance the potential for a successful reduction.
- **Reduction/Repositioning:** Reduction, also known as repositioning, is the process of manually or surgically realigning a dislocated joint back into its proper position. Restoring joint function and alleviating pain are crucial aspects of the treatment process for dislocations.

1.3.8. Treatment Options for Dislocation

Reduction (moving the joint into a new position), immobilization, pain control, and, in certain situations, surgery are available treatment options for dislocation.

- **Medication:** The main goals of medications for dislocations are to reduce inflammation and manage pain. Analgesics and non-steroidal anti-inflammatory medications (NSAIDs) aid in the management of pain and swelling. Muscle relaxants are prescribed in certain situations. If a wound is open, antibiotics may be administered to stop infection.
- **Surgery:** For complicated or recurring dislocations, surgery might be necessary. The goal of surgery for a dislocated joint is to repair injured tendons, ligaments, or other surrounding structures. The procedures for joint reconstruction or stabilization vary depending on the particular joint involved and the severity of the injury. Surgery may also address any related bone damage or fractures.
- **Reduction/Repositioning:** The first step in treating a dislocation is reduction, also known as repositioning, which involves realigning the displaced joint to its original position. An experienced healthcare professional can perform this manually, although it often requires sedation or anesthesia to manage pain. In some cases, surgery may be necessary to reduce the affected joint, especially for complicated or unstable dislocations. Closed reduction is a non-surgical method where the dislocated joint is manually realigned, typically without the need for surgery. On the other hand, open reduction is a surgical procedure usually reserved for complicated or severe dislocations to realign and stabilize the dislocated joint.
- **Rehabilitation:** The goal of rehabilitation is to regain strength and function in the joints. Exercises to increase muscle strength, increase range of motion, and improve joint stability are all part of customized programs. Physical therapists play a critical role in helping patients through rehabilitation by customizing exercises to fit each patient's needs and the particular joint. Effective rehabilitation promotes a person's ability to return to their regular activities by assisting with pain management, mobility restoration, and prevention of re-injury. Through physical therapy, skilled therapists create individualized treatment plans to assist patients in regaining joint strength, mobility, and function. They employ a variety of methods, such as stretches, exercises, and manual therapy, to relieve pain and increase the range of motion. To avoid joint stiffness, enhance general health, and guarantee a safe return to daily activities following a dislocation, physical therapy is essential.

1.3.9. Complications of Dislocations

Dislocations can cause more problems or complications. Serious complications are not common though. Serious complications are more likely if the skin tears, blood vessels get damaged, or nerves get damaged. Compared to fractures, dislocated joints have a higher risk of damaging blood vessels and nerves if they are not quickly put back in place. Infections, damage to blood vessels and nerves, and other problems can happen in the hours or days after the injury. Other issues, like problems with healing and joints, happen slowly over time.

- **Fractures:** It is possible that the same injury that results in a dislocation also caused a fracture. Rarely do fractures result in adjacent injured muscles swelling to the point where they reduce or obstruct blood flow to the injured limb. The limb eventually becomes cold and turns blue, and the tissues inside the limb either deteriorate or die if blood flow is not restored. This condition is referred to as compartment syndrome.
- **Blood Vessel Damage:** The blood supply to the leg may be impeded by a dislocated knee or hip. Consequently, there is a chance that the leg's tissues will not receive enough blood (ischemia) and will eventually die (necrosis). Necrosis is possible in cases of dislocated hips, especially if prompt realignment is not achieved. The hip dislocation causes the blood vessels to stretch to the femoral head, which is the top end of the femur and part of the hip joint. Due to this, the affected area of the femur does not receive sufficient blood. A dislocated knee may result in insufficient blood flow to the lower leg. If the lack of blood results in a significant amount of tissue dying, a portion of the leg may need to be amputated. The forearm may experience similar issues due to blood flow disruption caused by certain elbow injuries. It may take several hours following an injury for symptoms of disrupted blood supply to manifest.
- **Bleeding:** Internal bleeding can result from severe or traumatic dislocations, which can also damage surrounding tissues. External bleeding may result from a broken skin resulting from a dislocated bone.
- **Nerve Damage:** When a joint becomes dislocated, nerves can occasionally be strained, bruised, or crushed. A nerve can be crushed or bruised by a direct blow. More harm is done by crushing than by bruising. Depending on how severe the injury is, it can take weeks, months, or even years for it to heal on its own. Nerves are rarely torn. Nerves that have been torn may require surgical repair as they do not heal on their own. Certain nerve injuries never fully recover.
- **Infections:** When a joint dislocates, tearing of the skin can cause an infection, which can then spread to the bone and cause osteomyelitis. Osteomyelitis is extremely difficult to treat.
- **Joint Problems:** Joint surfaces, or the cartilage at the ends of the bones in a joint, can occasionally sustain damage from a dislocation. Normally, joints can move smoothly because of this resilient, smooth tissue. Osteoarthritis, a condition that causes damaged cartilage to scar and reduces joint range of

motion, is characterized by stiff joints. After a dislocation, the knee, elbow, and shoulder are especially prone to stiffness, particularly in the elderly. Additionally, the dislocation-causing injury may weaken or tear the tendons and ligaments that stabilize the joint.

To help the joint move as normally as possible and avoid stiffness, physical therapy is typically required. In many cases, surgery is necessary to replace the damaged cartilage. Following this type of operation, the cartilage is less likely to scar and, if scarring does occur, it is usually less severe. In certain cases, surgery is needed to repair torn tendons or ligaments.

1.3.10. Prevention Strategies

Joint well-being, safety measures, and injury avoidance are instances of preventative approaches that can significantly reduce the likelihood of dislocations.

- **Strengthening Exercises:** Strengthening exercises are crucial for both preventing dislocations and aiding in recovery because they strengthen the muscles surrounding the injured joint, improving stability and support. These exercises consist of functional movements and resistance training to enhance joint health, minimize the chance of re-injury, and develop strength.
- **Safety Precautions:** Dislocations are less common when safety measures are taken, such as wearing protective gear when participating in sports, using proper body mechanics when lifting heavy objects, and being cautious to avoid falls. Dislocations during daily activities can be reduced by maintaining strong, flexible muscles through regular exercise and being mindful of the surroundings.
- **Regular Check-ups:** Routine check-ups with a healthcare professional are crucial to monitor joint health, identify risk factors, and address any underlying conditions that may increase the risk of dislocations. Proactive visits help prevent potential problems and preserve joint health.

A Closer Look

First Aid for Fracture

A fracture occurs when a bone breaks and requires medical treatment. If there has been significant trauma or injury resulting in a broken bone, please contact the local emergency number.

Additionally, please call for emergency assistance if any of the following apply:

- The person is unresponsive, not breathing, or not moving. If there is no breathing or heartbeat, begin CPR.
- There is heavy bleeding.
- Even gentle pressure or movement causes pain.
- The limb or joint appears deformed.
- The bone has pierced the skin.
- The extremity of the injured arm or leg, such as a toe or finger, is numb or bluish at the tip.
- The patient suspect a bone is broken in the neck, head, or back.

If someone is exhibiting symptoms of shock, such as dizziness or rapid breathing, it is advisable to have them lie down with their head positioned lower than their body. If possible, elevate their legs.

- To stop any bleeding, apply pressure to the wound using a sterile bandage, clean cloth, or a fresh piece of clothing.
- It is important to immobilize the injured area. Do not attempt to realign or reposition any bones that may be protruding. If the patient have received training in splinting and have limited access to professional assistance, apply splints above and below the fracture sites. Use padding to provide comfort.
- To reduce swelling and alleviate pain, apply ice packs. Avoid direct contact between the ice and the skin by covering it with a cloth, towel, or other material.

1.4. Summary

- Bones constitute our skeletal framework. Connective tissue in the shape of bones is fortified by calcium and osteocytes. Hematopoietic cells are generated in the more pliable bone marrow, situated in the core of bones. Our skeletal structure serves three fundamental functions: it provides support to our physique, enables mobility, and safeguards our internal organs.
- Bone fractures are a prevalent injury with a challenging recovery process. Only a few tissues, including bone, have the ability to heal without leaving behind fibrous scars.
- The objective of medical care for fractured bones is to ensure the accurate alignment of bone fragments; broken bones have the capacity to heal on their own. The bone must have fully regained its sensitivity, movement, and strength. Surgery or surgical traction (or both) may have been required for certain complex fractures.
- Immobilizing a limb with a plaster of Paris cast is a commonly employed technique. This cast is fashioned using a gypsum preparation that solidifies upon the addition of water.
- Fractures have the ability to heal within a span of a few weeks to a few months, depending on the severity of the damage and the degree of adherence to the instructions provided by the attending physician.
- The medical term for the displacement of bones from their normal position within a joint is known as a dislocation.
- Dislocations occur as a result of an injury that imparts a forceful impact on the joint, such as falls, car accidents, and collisions in contact sports. Dislocations are injuries in which the bones within a joint are forcefully separated and positioned abnormally.
- The most prevalent types of dislocations are those affecting the shoulder, hip, knee, and fingers; these are frequently caused by traumatic incidents or injuries and necessitate immediate medical attention.
- Jaw dislocations, hip dislocations in babies, and scapholunate dislocations of the wrist are examples of rare and specific dislocations that require specialized medical care.
- Dislocated bones may appear misaligned and the joint may look twisted or deformed. The skin around the protruding bone may stretch and bulge.
- Immediate treatment involves immobilizing the affected joint, managing pain, and seeking medical help promptly. These actions reduce the risk of further harm and increase the chance of successful reduction.
- Dislocations can lead to additional complications, although serious complications are rare. They are more likely if there is skin tearing, blood vessel damage, or nerve damage.
- Maintaining joint health, taking safety precautions, and practicing injury prevention can significantly reduce the risk of dislocations.

References

1. Donal A. Wiss, (2006). *Fractures* (2nd edn.) Philadelphia: Lippincott Williams & Wilkins.
2. Dumontier, C., & Soubeyrand, M., (2014). The forearm joint. In: Bentley, G., (ed.), *European Surgical Orthopedics and Traumatology: The EFORT Textbook* (pp. 1509–1524). Springer, Berlin, Heidelberg.
3. Hunter, T. B., Peltier, L. F., & Lund, P. J., (2000). "Radiologic history exhibit." *Radio Graphics. 20*(3), 819–836. doi: 10.1148/radiographics.20.3.g00ma20819. PMID 10835130.
4. Katherine, A., (2013). *Official CPC Certification Study Guide* (p. 108). American Medical Association.
5. Noda, K., Goto, A., Murase, T., et al., (2009). Interosseous membrane of the forearm: An anatomical study of ligament attachment locations. *J. Hand. Surg. Am., 34*, 415–422. https://doi.org/10.1016/j.jhsa.2008.10.025.
6. Wiss, D. A., (2013). *Fractures* (3rd edn.) Philadelphia, PA: Lippincott Williams & Wilkins.

Chapter

FRACTURES IN THE UPPER LIMB

2

Contents

2.1. Introduction

Fractures of the upper limb can result from direct trauma or indirectly from forces acting on the limb (such as twisting injuries). The size and direction of the limb injury determine the type of fracture. The mechanism of the fracture, the location of the bone within the body, and whether or not the bone has broken through the skin on top are what characterize fractures. The severity and classification of each fracture will vary, so there is not a single treatment that works for everyone, and the healing period for upper limb fractures also varies.

Orientation and Directional Terms

Term	Definition	Illustration
Intra-articular fracture	A break that extends into the joint, such as the wrist or elbow.	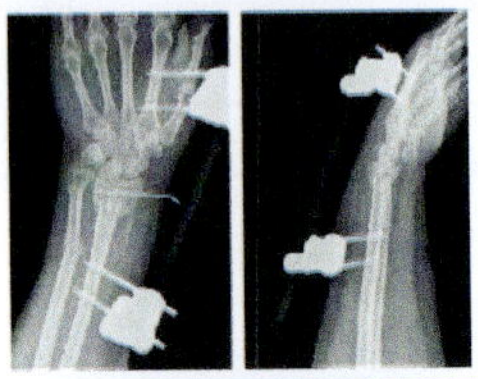
Displaced fracture	The bone breaks and is no longer straight.	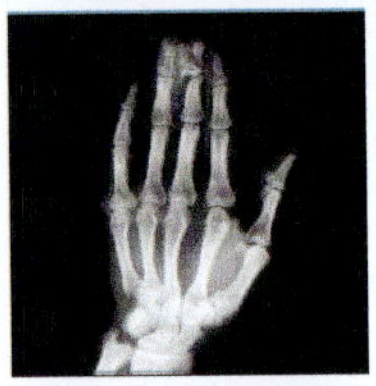
Non-displaced fracture	The bone breaks in one spot and is still straight.	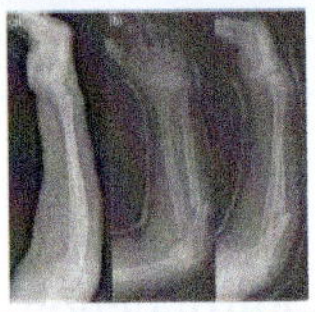
Open fracture	The bone breaks through the skin, with a significant risk of infection.	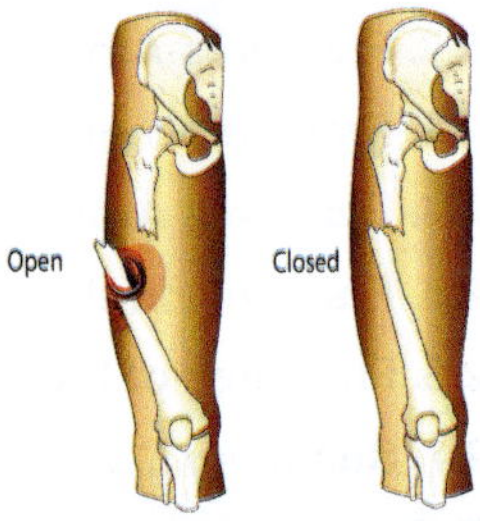
Clavicular fractures	Clavicular fractures are common and account for however, 5% (range 2.6–10%) of all fractures. They usually require minimal treatment, which relies on analgesia and a collar-and-cuff. However, in some cases, open reduction and internal fixation are required.	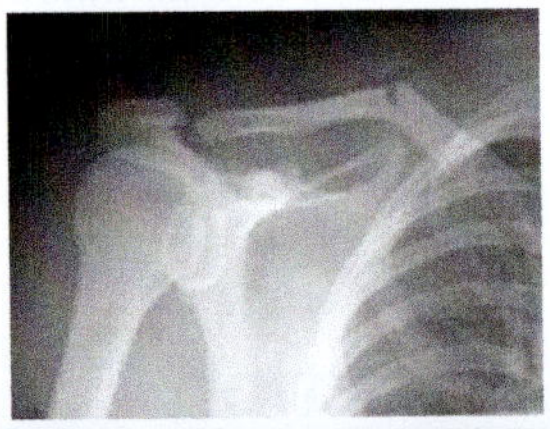
Acromion fracture	The acromion process is the lateral projection of the scapular spine that extends anteriorly. Fractures of the scapula are uncommon injuries and account for approximately 3% of all shoulder fractures, while isolated acromion fractures occur rarely and account for only 9% of all scapular fractures.	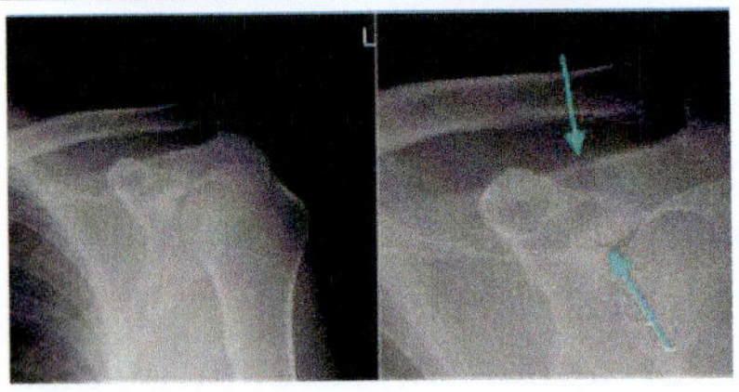

2.2. Fractures Around the Wrist

Breaking the wrist is a common injury that typically occurs when an individual trips or falls and extends their hands to protect themselves. Depending on the type and severity of the fracture, there are different treatment options for wrist fractures. The best course of action for recovering from a wrist fracture can be advised by an orthopedic surgeon.

A broken wrist typically results in immediate pain, swelling, and soreness. The injured area may also bruise or become discolored. There might also occasionally be a noticeable deformity. Get medical attention right away if in excruciating pain, have an open fracture (where the bone breaks the skin), have numbness or deformity in the wrist region, or if the fingers are discolored.

2.2.1. Types of Fractures

2.2.1.1. Distal Radius Fracture

The most frequent kind of wrist fracture is a distal radius, which frequently happens from falling on an outstretched arm.

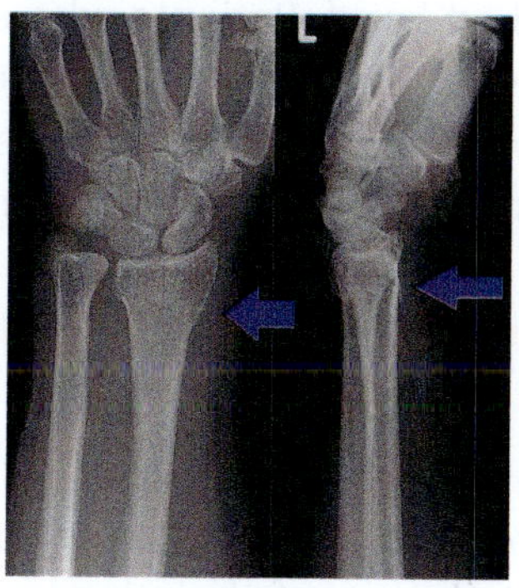

Figure 2.1. *A Colles fracture as seen on X-ray: It is a type of distal radius fracture.*

Source: By Lucien Monfils – Own work, CC BY-SA 3.0, https://commons.wikimedia.org/w/index.php?curid=4317922.

2.2.1.2. Scaphoid Fracture

The scaphoid is a bone in the wrist near the base of the thumb. It's part of two rows of small round bones. These fractures usually happen because of an injury like falling on an outstretched arm, but they can also be caused by sports or car accidents (Figure 2.2).

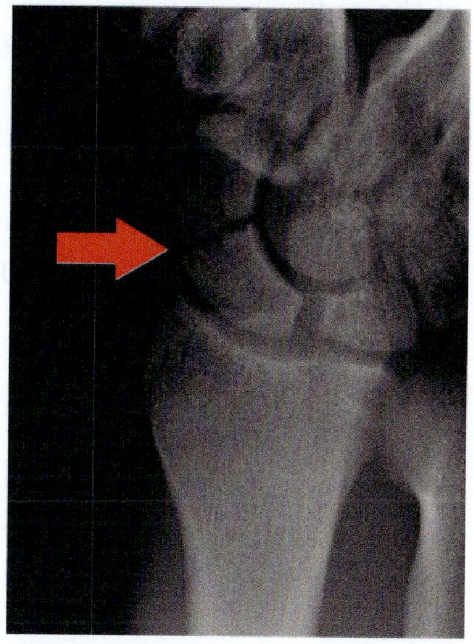

Figure 2.2. *An X-ray showing a fracture through the waist of the scaphoid.*

Source: By Gilo1969 – https://en.wikipedia.org/wiki/File:Scaphoid_waist_fracture.gif, CC BY 3.0, https://commons.wikimedia.org/w/index.php?curid=63346237.

2.2.2. Less Common Wrist Fractures

However, the wrist is a complex joint with numerous bones, making various kinds of fractures possible.

- **Barton's Fracture:** A Barton's fracture occurs when a dislocation of the radiocarpal joint, which connects the wrist to the forearm, is combined with a distal radius fracture. Similar to the diagnosis and treatment of a distal radius fracture, a Barton's fracture typically requires surgery rather than a closed reduction, which resets the fracture without surgical repair.

- **Chauffeur's Fracture (Radial Styloid Fracture):** The bulge near the base of the thumb at the end of the radius bone is called the radial styloid. The term "chauffeur's fracture" is used to describe a fracture that is typically caused by a direct blow to the radius, as early cars' hand-cranks would frequently strike the wrist. Surgery is employed as a treatment for chauffeur's fractures.
- **Ulnar Styloid Fracture:** The ulna, a smaller bone in the forearm, runs parallel to the radius. It also has a bulge known as the styloid at the end of the bone. The lump visible on the outside of the wrist is referred to as the ulnar styloid. This fracture often occurs as a result of a fall along with a distal radius fracture. Treatment for this fracture is not always necessary, especially if it is located at the styloid tip. Surgery is an option if the fracture is at the styloid base and/or if there is a risk of instability at the distal radioulnar joint, which is the small joint that connects the radius and ulna bones.
- **Other Carpal Fractures:** Scaphoid fractures account for approximately 70% of carpal bone fractures. Among the eight carpal bones, a few others are also prone to fractures:
  - The triquetrum is the second most commonly fractured carpal bone. It is often broken by a fall onto the side of the hand and is located on the ulnar side of the wrist, near the ulnar styloid.
  - The trapezium is a carpal bone situated at the base of the metacarpal bone of the index finger. Fractures of this bone can occur when the index finger is jammed or dislocated.
  - Positioned just above the radius, the lunate carpal bone is susceptible to fractures or dislocations in the event of a fall. If left untreated, lunate fractures can progress to osteonecrosis of the lunate, also known as Keinbock disease.
  - The hamate carpal bone may be impacted by fractures of the hook of hamate. These fractures are uncommon and typically occur in baseball, tennis, or racquet players when their bat or club strikes their wrist.

The majority of wrist injuries, regardless of the type of fracture, are caused by falling onto an outstretched hand. Patients who experience wrist injuries from a fall or other accident and have persistent pain should seek medical attention for diagnosis and treatment.

2.2.3. Symptoms of Lower Forearm Fractures

The wrist may be tender to touch and could appear swollen. People may experience numbness at the tip of their index finger and find it difficult to pinch their thumb and little finger together if they have damage to the median nerve. Stiffness, and/or persistent pain can be caused by a wrist fracture, especially if the broken pieces are out of place or the fracture extends into the wrist joint.

2.2.4. Diagnosis of Lower Forearm Fractures

- X-rays
- Occasionally computed tomography (CT)

People should consult a physician if they believe they may have suffered a wrist fracture. X-rays are typically used by doctors to diagnose wrist fractures. CT may be required occasionally to detect joint fractures. Through the use of computers and X-rays, CT creates a three-dimensional, and more detailed image of the injured area.

2.2.5. Treatment

Decisions on how to treat a distal radius fracture may depend on many factors, including:

- Fracture displacement (whether the broken bones shifted)
- Comminution (whether there are fractures in multiple places)
- Joint involvement
- Associated ulna fracture and injury to the median nerve
- Whether it is the dominant hand
- Occupation and activity level

In any event, a splint is applied as soon as possible after a fracture to provide comfort and manage pain. Before the fracture is put in a splint, it is reduced, or put back into its original position, if it has been displaced. Local anesthesia is used during fracture reduction, so only the painful area is sedated.

2.2.5.1. Nonsurgical Treatment

Applying a splint or cast depends on how well the distal radius fracture is positioned. It often serves as a final option until the bone has healed.

A cast is typically worn for a maximum of six weeks. Following that, a removable wrist splint will be provided for stability and comfort. Physical therapy can commence immediately after the cast is removed to restore natural strength and function to the wrists.

If the fracture has been reduced or is deemed unstable, X-rays may be taken at three and six weeks. If the fracture has not been reduced and is considered stable, X-rays may be taken less frequently. First, a displaced fracture must be realigned. A plaster splint or cast is then applied.

Local anesthesia is usually administered for the closed reduction procedure. After evaluating the fracture, the orthopedic surgeon will determine if surgery is necessary or if a cast will suffice for the next six weeks.

2.2.5.2. Surgery for Distal Radius Fractures

This choice is typically reserved for fractures that are deemed unstable or for which a cast is not a suitable treatment. Usually, an incision is made across the volar aspect of the wrist, where the pulse is palpated, to perform surgery. This allows for full access to the fracture. One or more plates and screws are utilized to stabilize the fractured parts.

In certain circumstances, to restore the anatomy, a second incision on the dorsal aspect of the wrist may be necessary. The fractured parts will be secured with plates and screws. However, if there are multiple bone fragments, fixation with plates and screws may not be feasible. In such cases, an external fixator may be used to stabilize the fracture, with or without additional wires. The majority of the hardware used with an external fixator remains outside the body.

Following the procedure, a splint will be worn for two weeks until the first follow-up appointment. At that point, the wrist splint will be removed and replaced with a removable one. It is necessary to wear the removable splint for four weeks. After the initial visit to the clinic, it will commence physical therapy to restore wrist strength and function. The removable splint can be taken off six weeks after the procedure. It is important to diligently follow the exercises recommended by the therapist and surgeon for optimal surgical recovery. For the best surgical recovery, early action is essential.

2.2.6. Recovery

Each person's recovery is unique due to the wide range of distal radius fracture types and treatment options available.

2.2.6.1. Pain Management

Most fractures cause mild discomfort for a few days to several weeks. Many patients discover that their pain can be effectively alleviated by applying ice, elevating their arm above their heart, and utilizing over-the-counter pain relievers.

To diminish pain and inflammation, the physician may have recommended taking ibuprofen and acetaminophen in combination. When both medications were taken concurrently, they proved to be significantly more effective than when taken individually. In cases of severe pain, the physician may have prescribed a medication such as an opioid for a limited duration.

Although opioids can assist in alleviating post-operative pain, it is important to note that they are narcotics and have the potential for addiction. Opioids should only be taken as directed by the physician, and discontinue their use as soon as the pain begins to subside. If, after a few days following the surgery, if pain has not started to diminish, it is advisable to consult the doctor.

2.2.6.2. Cast and Wound Care

Sometimes, the original casts are replaced when they become loose due to reduced swelling. Non-operative fractures typically have their final cast removed after approximately six weeks. It is important to keep casts and splints dry during the healing process.

When showering, using a plastic bag to cover the arm can be helpful. If the cast gets wet, it will not dry quickly and may need to be replaced. Using a hair dryer on the "cool" setting can aid in drying the cast. Surgical incisions should be kept dry and clean for a minimum of five days. The doctor will provide guidance on when to remove the bandages after the surgery.

2.2.6.3. Rehabilitation and Return to Activity

The majority of individuals are able to resume all of their previous activities. The nature of the injury, the type of care provided, and the body's response to that care all contribute to the outcome. Some individuals may experience long-term functional limitations after such injuries. Wrist stiffness is a common occurrence for almost all patients, but it typically improves and remains better for at least two years after surgery or a month or two after the cast is removed. Physical therapy usually begins a few days to weeks after surgery, or immediately after the cast is removed if deemed necessary by the doctor.

After the cast is removed or after surgery, most patients can gradually return to light activities such as swimming or lower body workouts in the gym within one to two months. Resuming light and strenuous activities may be possible three to six months after the injury.

2.2.6.4. Long-Term Outcomes

One should anticipate a minimum of one year for recovery. For the first year, some soreness with strenuous activities might be anticipated. For two years or possibly forever, patients with osteoarthritis, those over fifty, and high-energy injuries (like motorbike crashes) should expect some degree of residual stiffness or pain. But generally speaking, the stiffness is not severe enough to impair the arm's general function. Lastly, a lot of wrist fractures are caused by osteoporosis. Most people who have a wrist fracture may benefit from testing for bone weakness, particularly if they also have other risk factors for osteoporosis (e.g., advanced age). Consult the physician about osteoporosis screening.

2.3. Fractures in the Forearm

The radius and ulna are the two bones that make up the forearm. These bones can be fractured individually or in combination. Traumatic causes can lead to this condition in patients of all ages. The manner and severity of the bone fracture can vary greatly. In cases where only one bone breaks, a wrist or elbow dislocation is often present. In some instances, the bone may fracture and protrude through the skin, known as an open fracture, which requires immediate surgery. Since each type of fracture requires a different approach to care, it is crucial for the doctor to make an accurate diagnosis and provide appropriate treatment.

The forearm plays a vital role in connecting the elbow to the wrist. The shape of the forearm bones is significant as it allows for rotation. The ability of the palm to turn up and down is due to this shape. Proper alignment of the forearm bones relies on the correct movement of the wrist and elbow joints. Poor posture can impact the ability of the wrist and elbow to bend or straighten.

2.3.1. Epidemiology

With a yearly incidence of about 1 in 100 children, forearm fractures are common in the pediatric population. The age group of 5 to 14 years old accounts for approximately 34% of all cases, which is the peak incidence. Approximately 54.4% of all fractures in children under the age of 16 are diaphyseal forearm fractures. In the adult population, there is a comparatively higher incidence observed in the 25–34 age range.

The distal radius or ulna (32.9%) is the most common site of forearm fractures, while the proximal region (22.8%) is the least common location. Conversely, the diaphyseal area is typically affected by open fractures.

2.3.2. Pathophysiology

2.3.2.1. Patho-anatomy and Biomechanics

The radius, ulna, proximal and distal radioulnar joints, and secondary soft tissue stabilizers, such as the interosseous membrane (IOM) and the triangular fibrocartilage complex (TFCC), comprise the forearm unit. The radial head and proximal ulna are stabilized proximally by the annular ligament and the elbow joint capsule. The triangular fibrocartilage complex and the wrist joint capsule stabilize the ulna as it articulates with the sigmoid notch of the radius distally.

Between the ulna and the radius lies the interosseous membrane, which is composed of five parts: the dorsal oblique accessory cord, the proximal oblique cord, the accessory band, the distal oblique bundle, and the central band. Apart from providing attachment to the forearm muscles, it also offers longitudinal stability to the distal radioulnar joint.

The joint formed by the radius, ulna, and secondary soft tissue stabilizers facilitates pronation and supination movements. The primary deforming forces in forearm fractures are the biceps brachii and supinator, which assist in supination, and the pronator teres and pronator quadratus, which assist in pronation. Various movements can be performed at the distal end of the forearm, including wrist flexion, wrist extension, ulnar deviation, and radial deviation. Elbow flexion and extension occur at the ulnohumeral joint.

2.3.3. History and Physical Examination

Patients with a history of high-velocity trauma typically present at the trauma and emergency department with forearm fractures. It is imperative to exclude any additional potentially life-threatening injuries that may be associated with these fractures. The utilization of the advanced trauma life support (ATLS) protocol is recommended to conduct a comprehensive assessment, encompassing primary and secondary surveys. The cornerstone of the ATLS protocol during the initial evaluation of trauma patients is a systematic and organized primary survey. Once the patient is stabilized, the secondary survey involves obtaining a complete medical history, performing a head-to-toe examination, and conducting a local examination of the affected areas.

A thorough history, clinical examination, and relevant radiological investigations should all be employed in the diagnosis of forearm fractures. Patients typically report acute pain, swelling, localized tenderness, and an evident deformity at the site of the forearm fracture or trauma. To exclude open fractures and associated soft tissue injuries, a clinical examination should always follow the acquisition of the patient's history. To rule out any neurological injury in the affected extremity, a meticulous neurological examination of the peripheral nerves is necessary. Following evaluation, the patency of the radial and ulnar arteries should be thoroughly documented for future reference and to guide treatment decisions. Early detection of the signs and symptoms of compartment syndrome is crucial to prevent the dire consequences of tissue necrosis and ischemia.

2.3.4. Evaluation

2.3.4.1. Plain Radiography

Anteroposterior (AP) and lateral views of the forearm on plain radiographs are frequently utilized for the diagnosis of forearm fractures. When the elbow is extended and the forearm is fully supinated, a standard AP view of the forearm is obtained. In order to comprehensively assess both joints, these images should include the elbow and wrist joints. An oblique view of the forearm can aid in determining the type of fracture, such as comminuted or simple, as a lateral view may cause the ulna and radius to overlap.

Forearm fractures can often lead to injuries in the distal radio-ulnar joint (DRUJ), proximal radio-ulnar joint, and elbow dislocation. Signs of DRUJ instability may include dorsal displacement of the distal ulna, changes in ulnar variance, fractures of the base of the styloid, and widening of the DRUJ on the PA view. Fractures in the distal third radius with signs of DRUJ instability may indicate a Galeazzi fracture-dislocation. To assess associated injuries, it is recommended to utilize AP and lateral plain radiographs of the elbow, as well as posteroanterior and lateral plain radiographs of the wrist joint.

2.3.4.2. CT Scan

Only if there is a possibility of an intraarticular distal end radius fracture pattern is CT indicated. However, for the assessment of acute forearm fractures, routine CT and MRI scans are not performed.

2.3.4.3. MRI Scan

Magnetic resonance imaging (MRI) helps diagnose DRUJ injury and associated triangular fibrocartilage complex (TFCC) injury.

2.3.4.4. Classification

While there are many classification schemes for forearm fractures, only a handful are truly helpful in predicting prognosis and guiding therapy. There is no single category that encompasses all types of forearm fractures. Therefore, forearm fractures are typically described using anatomic descriptions that include the fracture pattern, degree of angulation, displacement, and associated soft tissue injuries. The Neer and Arbeitsgemeinschaft für Osteosynthesefragen/Orthopaedic Trauma Association (AO/OTA) classification is commonly used for forearm fractures. Open forearm fractures are classified using the Gustilo and Anderson classification system, as well as the Orthopaedic Trauma Association (OTA) open fracture classification system. Monteggia and Galeazzi fractures are classified using different criteria.

2.3.5. Treatment/Management

Achieving acceptable reduction, stable fixation, and bone healing, as well as enabling an early return to daily activities, preserving function, and minimizing complications, are the ultimate goals of fracture management. To achieve a favorable functional outcome in the case of a forearm fracture, it is crucial to restore length, axial and rotational alignment, and ensure proper cortical contact.

2.3.5.1. Conservative Management

Forearm fractures, such as unicortical fractures and undisplaced or minimally displaced fractures with less than 50% displacement and less than 10° of angulation, have limited indications for conservative treatment. When non-operative treatment is chosen for isolated ulna fractures, such as using a functional brace, a long-arm cast, and frequent X-ray follow-up, the success rates are very high.

2.3.5.2. Operative Management

Operative management is typically employed for treating forearm fractures, involving closed or open reduction and internal fixation. Open reduction helps achieve anatomic reduction, stable fixation, and early range of motion, enabling patients to regain their pre-injury state as soon as possible. In the pediatric population, closed reduction and internal fixation using an intramedullary nail can be performed as a minimally invasive procedure with good results. However, this approach is less ideal for adult forearm fractures due to the challenge of achieving sufficient reduction in a closed manner.

2.3.5.3. Open Reduction with Plate and Screw Fixation

The ulna and radius are fixed in the order determined by the fracture pattern and comminution in both bone forearm fractures. Restoring the length and facilitating the reduction of the other bone can be achieved by initially fixing the fracture with less comminution. If both fractures are minor, the radius should be treated first to stabilize the forearm and facilitate treating the ulna. It is usually preferred to place the plate on the volar surface. Although it offers sufficient soft tissue coverage and appropriate plate seating, it is biomechanically preferable to place the plate on the dorsal (tension) surface.

The grade of the fracture, as determined by Gustilo and Anderson's classification, determines how open fractures should be managed. After sufficient debridement in a single setting, grade 1 and 2 fractures with minimal contamination can be treated with definitive fixation. However, debridement and external fixation should be used first, followed by staged internal fixation, for grade 3 and highly contaminated wounds.

2.3.5.4. Surgical Approaches

The patient is placed in the supine position during the surgical approach for the majority of forearm fractures. The limb can be abducted onto the hand table for volar approaches in the supine position, while the limb can be adducted and internally rotated at the shoulder joint for dorsal and subcutaneous approaches. The dorsal forearm is accessible when in the prone position. It is better to use a customized strategy for the ulna and radius because a single incision will result in cross union and limit supination and pronation. Due to its close proximity to neurovascular structures, especially in the proximal third, and its surrounding muscular envelope, a surgical approach to the radius is thought to be more challenging than one to the ulna. The volar Henry approach and the dorsolateral Thompson approach are the two methods for calculating radius that are most frequently used.

The Thompson method, which utilizes the space between the extensor digitorum communis and the extensor carpi radialis brevis (ECRB), is considered to be the most effective technique for the proximal and middle thirds of the radius. The most common complication of this procedure is injury to the posterior interosseous nerve, which can be prevented or minimized by supinating the radius, allowing for safe elevation of the supinator from its insertion. The distal third of the Thompson approach is believed to be safe and relatively superficial.

A volar Henry approach constitutes an extensive method for accessing the radius. In this technique, the skin is incised along the lateral aspect of the biceps tendon to the radial styloid. The internervatory plane depends on the location of the fracture. This method offers the advantage of enhanced visualization of the proximal, middle, and distal regions of the radius. Other volar approaches to the radius include the modified FCR approach (Flexor carpi radialis) and FCR (Flexor carpi radialis), which are minor modifications to the traditional volar Henry approach. Since the ulna is subcutaneous along its entire length in the forearm, exposure and reduction of the ulna are achieved through a subcutaneous approach. The only known complication of this procedure is damage to the dorsal branches of the ulnar nerve, particularly in the distal third.

2.3.5.5. Methods of Fixation

Forearm fractures are most commonly fixed using dynamic compression and limited contact dynamic compression techniques. These techniques are primarily applied to transverse and short oblique fracture patterns, which are considered the most basic types. They provide support for primary healing and offer complete stability at the fracture site. In the case of oblique fractures, a lag screw with a neutralization plate is utilized. When the fracture is severely comminuted, bridge plating mode should be used for fixation. In addition to being a load-sharing tool, the intramedullary nail can be used to fixate fractures in the forearm. The preservation of the fracture hematoma (closed reduction) and the forearm's periosteal blood supply are the benefits of nailing.

2.3.5.6. Dynamic Compression Plate

For forearm fractures, dynamic compression plating (DCP) has long been regarded as the gold standard of care. DCP uses an eccentrically positioned screw with a congruent head-to-plate hole fit to provide axial compression. Several modes of use for the implant have been implemented, including compression, neutralization, buttress plate, and tension band. Through compression, it offers complete stability and anatomical reduction.

2.3.5.7. Limited Contact Dynamic Compression Plate

Perren and associates noted in 1990 the application of limited contact dynamic compression plates (LCDCP). The DCP and LCDCP fixation principles are extremely similar. The benefits over the DCP are as follows: (i) less periosteal compression and damage; (ii) preservation of the bone's blood supply; (iii) the wavy surface offering more area for applying bone grafts; (iv) adjusting the plate's load to apply pure tension on the plate; and (v) the avoidance of stress risers associated with implants and subsequent refracture following implant removal.

2.3.5.8. Bridging Plate

The primary application of a bridging plate is for forearm comminuted fractures. Multiple lag screws can be used to repair fractures that are minimally comminuted and have large fragments. Nonetheless, following appropriate reduction, severely comminuted fractures are repaired by bridging the proximal and distal fragments.

2.3.5.9. Intramedullary Nailing

For more than a century, the procedure of intramedullary nailing for fractures of the forearm shaft has evolved. Modern approaches to treating fractures have shifted toward biological fixation, which involves periosteal blood supply and minimal soft tissue manipulation. This method is frequently used more in children than in adults. Both open and closed techniques can be utilized for intramedullary nailing. Intramedullary nailing offers several advantages over plating: (i) preservation of soft tissues and the primary hematoma; (ii) reduced risk of infection and neurovascular injury; (iii) less invasive and cosmetic; and (iv) decreased likelihood of re-fracture.

In the past, larger V/U rods, rush pins, Steinmann pins, and Kirschner wires, all of which have small diameters, were employed. Currently, square nails, rush pins, and TENS (Titanium ElasticNail) nails are used as non-locking nails for forearm fractures. However, due to insufficient rotational and linear stability, plating is preferred over traditional non-locking nailing. To address this stability issue, a locking intramedullary nail has been recently introduced for forearm bones. Distal interlocking can be achieved without the need for fluoroscopy guidance, and it can be performed with direct visualization while providing adequate bending, axial, and rotational stability with various proximal designs. Proximal and distal locking is made possible by the ulna nail's combination of static and dynamic holes. The nails adhere to the three-point fixation principle.

Pediatric forearm fractures, segmental fractures, polytrauma, osteopenic bones, and those with poor soft tissue envelope should all be treated with intramedullary nailing. Active infections, narrow intramedullary canals, concurrent metaphyseal or epiphyseal fractures, radial head and neck fractures, ulna, and radial metaphyseal fractures that prevent appropriate locking are among the conditions that preclude nailing.

2.3.5.10. Hybrid Fixation

Hybrid fixation combines intramedullary nail fixation for one bone and plate fixation for the other, providing excellent biomechanical stability, soft tissue preservation, fewer complications, and a positive functional outcome. Compared to reversed fixation, using plate fixation for the radius and intramedullary nailing for the ulna offers superior biomechanical stability. In this combination, the plate fixation for the radius controls rotation and provides rigid fixation, while the straight nature of the ulna makes nailing easier.

2.3.5.11. Management of Galeazzi and Monteggia Fractures

The principles of management for Galeazzi fractures are similar to those for fixing simple forearm fractures. Adult Galeazzi fractures are very unstable, so it is necessary to have an open reduction and stable fixation to restore proper anatomy and function. The Volar Henry approach is frequently used for fixing these fractures, with plate fixation being the preferred method (Figure 2.3).

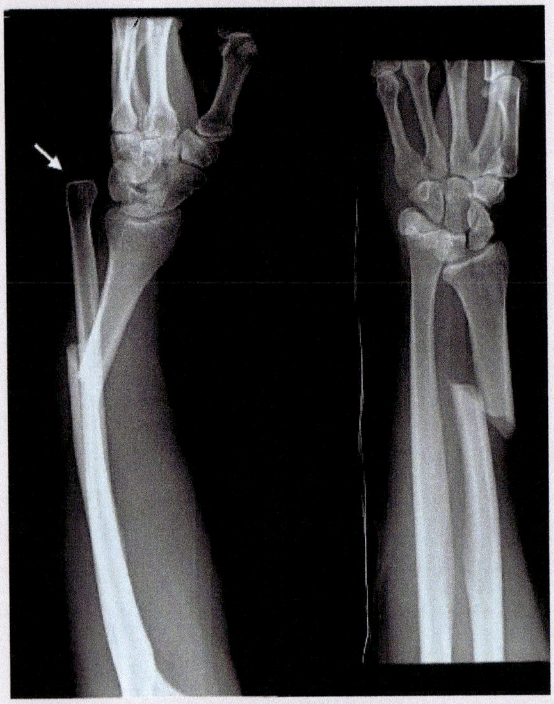

Figure 2.3. *Galeazzi facture (displaced fracture of the radius).*

Source: By Th. Zimmermann THWZ) – Own work, CC BY-SA 3.0 de, https://commons.wikimedia.org/w/index.php?curid=20683510.

The principles of managing a Monteggia fracture are two-fold: closed reduction or open reduction. The choice is contingent upon the type of fracture and the stability of the radial head. If the fracture is uncomplicated and the radial head is stable, closed reduction can be performed in an operating room with fluoroscopic guidance. However, if the radial head remains unstable post-reduction, internal fixation of the ulnar fracture is necessary, utilizing either intramedullary nailing or plating. In cases of comminuted fractures, plate and screw fixation is recommended (Figure 2.4).

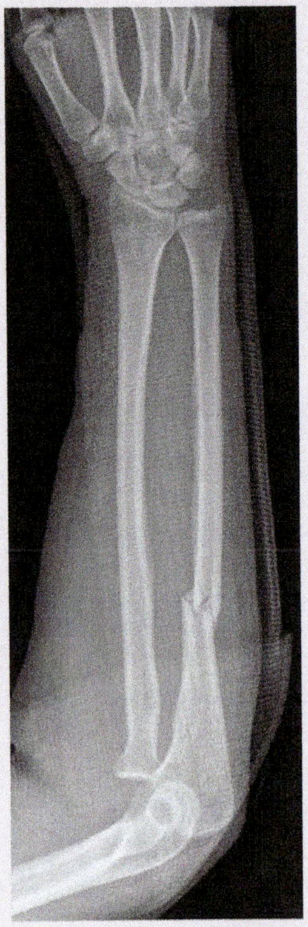

Figure 2.4. *Monteggia fracture (fracture of proximal ulna).*

Source: By Hellerhoff – Own work, CC BY-SA 4.0, https://commons.wikimedia.org/w/index.php?curid=96019136.

2.3.6. Differential Diagnosis

In addition to olecranon fractures, distal radius fractures, neuropathic osteoarthropathy, osteomyelitis, tenosynovitis, bursitis, and elbow and wrist sprains and dislocations are common differential diagnoses for forearm fractures. These conditions can be diagnosed independently through a comprehensive clinical examination and relevant radiological investigations.

2.3.7. Prognosis

The prognosis for forearm fractures is generally favorable, with union rates ranging from 95% to 98%. Several studies have reported a slightly higher union rate for radius fractures compared to ulnar fractures. When comparing plate osteosynthesis to third-generation intramedullary nail, the results are slightly better. However, the first-generation intramedullary nail performed poorly when compared to compressive plating due to its lack of rotatory stability.

The outcome of an open fracture depends on the degree and nature of the damage. Open fractures are associated with a high rate of complications such as non-union and infection, which increase the risk of morbidity and total medical expenses.

2.3.8. Complications

- **Peripheral Nerve Injuries:** Forearm fractures frequently result in neurovascular injuries, such as damage to the radial, superficial branches of the ulnar, and radial nerves. The radial and posterior interosseous nerves may sustain damage during surgical procedures.
- **Compartment Syndrome:** In the forearm, fractures, specifically fractures of the distal end of the radius, are the most frequent cause of compartment syndrome. Clinical examination and forearm compartment pressure monitoring are used to make the diagnosis. It requires immediate treatment with an early fasciotomy of the volar or dorsal compartment since it is deemed a surgical emergency. Delayed diagnosis and treatment may result in tissue ischemia and necrosis.
- **Infection:** Infection is considered the most debilitating consequence. *Staphylococcus aureus* is the most frequent microorganism responsible for infections in forearm fractures. Approximately 3% of forearm fractures treated with plate and screw fixation have an infection rate (varying from 0.8% to 6% depending on the study). Common clinical manifestations include inflammation, redness, tenderness, and a localized increase in body temperature at the infection site. Mild superficial infections can be treated with an oral antibiotic course; however, surgical debridement is the cornerstone of treatment for deep infections to prevent non-union and other complications.
- **Non-union:** It is estimated that between 2% and 10% of all forearm fractures result in non-union. The cause is complex and includes compromised bone healing biology due to infections and metabolic disorders, as well as a lack of mechanical stability (inadequate reduction or fixation construct). The non-union of forearm fractures can also be caused by fracture patterns such as comminuted fracture, open fracture, soft tissue stripping, and fracture location (distal third and middle third junction having the least blood supply). Non-union can also result from additional patient factors such as immunosuppression, diabetes, smoking, malnourishment, and steroid use.

- Non-union management principles involve removing the non-union site, opening the intramedullary canal, achieving anatomic reduction, and stabilizing the fracture. The surgical procedure aims to restore stability and function, and the use of bone grafting can promote bone formation.
- **Radioulnar Synostosis:** When treating a bone forearm fracture with a single incision, post-operative radioulnar synostosis frequently develops. It is rarely observed using distinct methodologies. The risk of synostosis is increased by bone grafting in the interosseous space. As a result, placing the bone graft on the opposing side of the interosseous space is typically advised. A head injury, soft tissue trauma, infection, and proximal third fracture are among the risk factors that can lead to the development of radioulnar synostosis. A few suggested adjuvants include indomethacin, low-dose radiation, anconeus muscle interposition, interposition fat grafting, and early range of motion exercise commencement to prevent radioulnar synostosis.
- **Refracture:** One of the less frequent outcomes following forearm fractures is refracture. Refracture is more common in patients who had an implant removed subsequent to union. When a forearm fracture is fixed with plate osteosynthesis, a stiff construct is created that results in stress shielding, decreased vascularity, osteopenia, and refracture.

2.3.9. Deterrence and Patient Education

Deterrence and patient education are crucial in managing forearm fractures. Patients who sustain forearm trauma should have their injuries assessed as soon as possible and receive the necessary care. If left untreated, these fractures can result in severe long-term disability. Additionally, inadequate management of forearm fractures may significantly restrict the rotational movements of the forearm, which can lead to limitations in day-to-day activities. Forearm fractures can be treated surgically or conservatively, but for the best functional results, appropriate rehabilitation and physical therapy are essential.

2.3.10. Enhancing Healthcare Team Outcomes

The first step in treating forearm fractures is appropriate evaluation, which necessitates a clear, focused plain radiograph of the injured area. Because of this, radiology technicians need to be skilled in obtaining the right view to prevent fractures from being overlooked. Additionally, it is important to see a hand surgeon right away to assess any related soft tissue injuries, particularly in situations where there are open fractures. Physiotherapists must be aware of the rehabilitation protocol following each case because physical therapy and rehabilitation play a critical role in achieving the best functional outcomes following fractures of this type.

2.4. Fractures Around the Elbow Joint

A fracture at the tip of the elbow is referred to as an elbow fracture. Trauma resulting from a strike to the head, impact on the elbow, or a fall on an outstretched hand can give rise to this condition.

2.4.1. Anatomy

The elbow is a joint made up of three bones:

- The humerus (upper arm bone)
- The radius (forearm bone on the thumb side)
- The ulna (forearm bone on the pinky side)

Similar to a hinge, the elbow joint allows for bending and straightening. It also plays a crucial role in forearm rotation, enabling movements such as turning the palm up or down for activities like typing or playing the piano, as well as receiving change from a cashier.

The elbow is composed of portions of three bones:

- The distal humerus, located at the lower end of the humerus, acts as a spool around which the forearm bends and straightens, forming the upper part of the elbow.
- The radial head, situated at the knobby end of the radius where it meets the elbow, slides up and down the front of the distal humerus when the arm is bent, and circles around the ulna during wrist rotation.
- The olecranon, which cups the lower end of the humerus, serves as a hinge for elbow movement. The bony point of the olecranon is easily palpable beneath the skin due to the limited tissue covering it.

The osseous structure of the elbow, along with muscles, tendons, and ligaments, holds it together. The elbow joint is crossed by three major nerves (Figure 2.5).

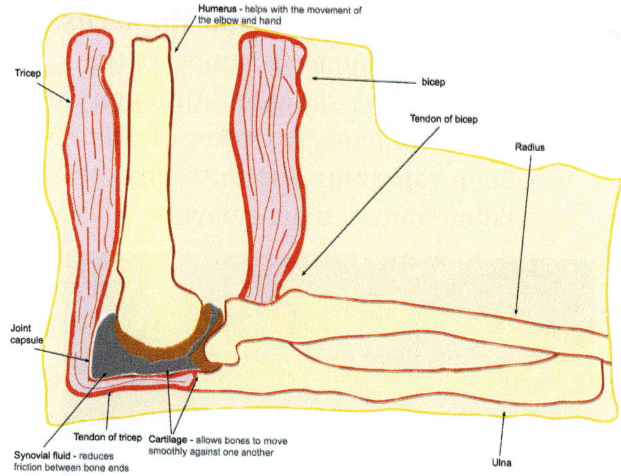

Figure 2.5. *A hand drawn image of the inside of an elbow joint with annotations in an up-close manner.*

Source: By AdamC30 – Own work, CC BY-SA 4.0, https://commons.wikimedia.org/w/index.php?curid=118283327.

2.4.2. Different Elbow Fracture Types

There are three main types of elbow fractures. These include (Figure 2.6):

- **Olecranon Fractures:** The olecranon, which is the pointy tip of the elbow, is one of the two bones that make up the forearm and is part of the ulna. Since the olecranon is not covered or shielded by muscles, it is particularly prone to breaking.
- **Fractures of the Radial Head:** The radial head is connected to the humerus, or upper arm bone. This type of fracture typically occurs when someone tries to use their arm to break a fall. As a result, the radial head presses against the humerus, causing a fracture.

- **Fractures of the Distal Humerus:** The distal humerus connects the elbow to the shoulder. Although they are uncommon, fractures of this bone can occur due to trauma or falling onto a bent elbow.

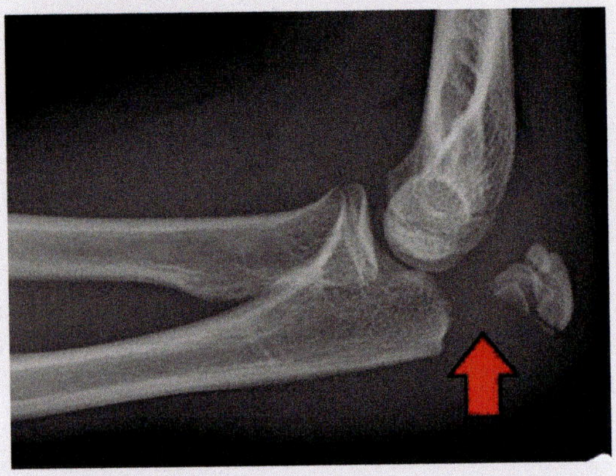

Figure 2.6. *Fracture of the olecranon.*

Source: By James Heilman, MD – Own work, CC BY-SA 4.0, https://commons.wikimedia.org/w/index.php?curid=49320713.

2.4.3. Signs and Symptoms

Elbow fractures can cause discomfort, edema, and limited range of motion. At the moment of injury, one may hear or feel a snap or pop. X-rays are initially used to confirm the injuries because visible deformity and reduced elbow range of motion may indicate that the elbow joint is dislocated or that the bones are misaligned. To obtain more information, a CT or MRI (Magnetic Resonance Imaging) scan may be required occasionally.

It is uncommon for elbow fractures to cause nerve and/or artery damage, which can cause numbness or discoloration in the arm, wrist, and hand. Although these are transient injuries, a medical practitioner has to be consulted immediately and thoroughly regarding those symptoms.

2.4.4. Treatment for Olecranon Fracture

Depending on the fracture pattern, displacement, and joint involvement, there are typically two treatments available for elbow fractures.

- **Nonsurgical Treatment:** To maintain the position of the elbow during the healing process, a splint or sling is applied. The doctor will closely monitor the fracture and schedule frequent clinic visits for X-rays. If the fracture is not displaced (out of place), the patient will gradually begin moving the elbow with the assistance of a physical therapist after a few weeks. It is important to refrain from bearing and lifting weights for a few weeks. After the cast is removed, the elbow may become extremely stiff due to the prolonged splinting period, requiring additional therapy sessions to regain range of motion. Nonsurgical treatment is rarely recommended due to this reason.
- **Surgical Treatment:** Surgical treatment is usually necessary for displaced elbow fractures, as it indicates that the bone fragments are misaligned. Orthopedic surgery may be required to realign the bones and facilitate proper healing.

Surgical treatment options may include:

- **Open Reduction and Internal Fixation (ORIF):** This procedure stabilizes and heals a broken bone. The surgeon will make an incision in the arm to realign the fractured bone. Hardware such as wires, screws, or plates will be used to keep the bones in place while they heal.

- **Total Elbow Replacement:** If there is significant joint damage, an elbow replacement may be required. This process involves replacing the injured joint, in this case the elbow, with an artificial one.
- **Radial Head Replacement:** If the radial head bone is too badly fractured to be repaired, an artificial radial head may be used instead of a complete elbow replacement. Positioned adjacent to the elbow bone, the radial head connects the two bones. It is a bulbous structure located at the end of the radius.
- **Ulnar Nerve Transposition:** A possible consequence of an elbow fracture could be an ulnar nerve injury. In such cases, surgical repositioning of the nerve may be necessary to relieve pressure on it.

2.4.5. Recovery

- **Pain Management:** Most fractures cause mild discomfort for a few days to several weeks. For many patients, the utilization of ice packs, elevation (holding the arm above the heart), and over-the-counter pain relievers is sufficient to alleviate pain. The physician may have recommended the administration of a prescription medication, such as an opioid, for a few days if the pain had been severe. It is important to note that while opioids can assist in relieving post-operative pain, opioid overdose and dependency have emerged as significant public health concerns. Therefore, opioids are typically prescribed for a brief duration. Opioids should only be utilized as directed by the physician, and discontinue their use as soon as the pain begins to subside.
- **Rehabilitation:** A strong rehabilitation program is necessary for a full recovery from an olecranon fracture, regardless of the treatment plan.
- **Recovery After Nonsurgical Treatment:** The elbow may become extremely stiff from prolonged splinting or casting, which is sometimes necessary for nonsurgical treatment. The patient might therefore require more physical therapy sessions to restore the range of motion. A physical therapist will provide the patient with exercises to help:
  - Improve range of motion
  - Decrease stiffness
  - Strengthen the muscles within the elbow

For a few weeks, the patient will be unable to lift, push, or pull anything with the injured arm. The doctor will discuss any specific restrictions.

- **Recovery After Surgical Treatment:** For a few weeks, the patient won't be able to lift, push, or pull anything with the injured arm. After surgery, the elbow might be cast or splinted for a brief period, depending on the severity of the fracture and the stability of the repair. Physical therapy will be recommended. Following surgery, patients will typically begin elbow and forearm strengthening exercises soon after, sometimes even on the same day. It is crucial that the patient diligently perform the exercises as prescribed. Only when the exercises are consistently carried out will they have a significant impact.

2.4.6. Complications of Olecranon Fractures

Some patients with olecranon fractures may experience long-term complications even after receiving successful treatment.

- **Loss of Motion:** In the majority of cases, a patient might not be able to fully regain range of motion in the injured elbow. They may be unable to fully extend or straighten their arm. Fortunately, a few degrees of straightening loss typically do not significantly affect the overall functionality of the arm. However, in rare cases where there is significant loss of motion, additional surgery, specialized bracing, or intense physical therapy may be necessary.
- **Posttraumatic Arthritis:** An olecranon fracture can lead to the development of posttraumatic arthritis in the joint. Over time, the damaged cartilage lining the joint can cause pain and stiffness. Posttraumatic arthritis is a common complication of olecranon fractures. It can manifest quickly after the fracture or take years to appear. Some patients with posttraumatic arthritis may require additional surgery for symptom relief. However, the majority of patients experience minimal pain and do not require further treatment.

2.4.7. Outcomes

While complete healing can take longer than a year, most patients can resume their regular activities in about four months. It often takes longer than the patient might think to regain arm strength. X-rays may indicate that the fracture has fully healed, but some patients still report limited range of motion. Over time, these patients typically continue to improve.

- **Questions to Ask a Doctor:** If the patient experience an olecranon fracture, here are some questions the patient may wish to ask a doctor:
  - When can I start moving my elbow?
  - How soon can I resume my normal activities?
  - What factors will prolong or delay healing?
  - If I have to have surgery, what are the benefits and risks?
  - What will my recovery be like?

2.5. Fractures in the Arm and the Shoulder

The shoulder and arm function due to the cooperation of a group of bones that compose the shoulder. The shoulder is comprised of the humerus, the clavicle (collarbone), and the scapula, also known as the shoulder blade. Within the shoulder, there are the acromioclavicular, sternoclavicular, and glenohumeral (ball and socket) joints. Fractures involving the shoulder bones can greatly restrict the range of motion and cause intense pain. Any direct impact to the shoulder, whether from a car accident, sports injury, fall, or other trauma, can lead to shoulder fractures.

2.5.1. Types of Shoulder Fractures

At least one of the three shoulder bones – the scapula, the clavicle or the humerus—is affected by a shoulder fracture. There are notable distinctions between the three types of fractures, but they can all result in shoulder pain, swelling, tenderness, and limited range of motion.

- **Clavicle Fracture:** The clavicle is a long, thin bone that starts at the base of the neck and ends at the shoulder. Clavicle fractures can occur at any age, including in the elderly. These fractures are often caused by falls, direct hits, car accidents, or contact sports such as football or hockey. Common symptoms include pain, swelling, and bruises over the clavicle area. A hematoma, or localized swelling, or a bone deformity may also cause a bump to develop over the site of injury. In most cases, patients with clavicle fractures have difficulty raising their arms.
- **Proximal Humerus Fracture:** From the elbow to the shoulder, the humerus is a long bone. A fracture at or slightly below the humeral head occurs at the top of the humerus bone, known as a proximal humerus fracture. It is common to refer to the humeral head as the ball that sits in the shoulder socket. Broken proximal humerus bones are frequent. They can occur at any age, but the risk increases as people age and develop osteoporosis (Figure 2.7).

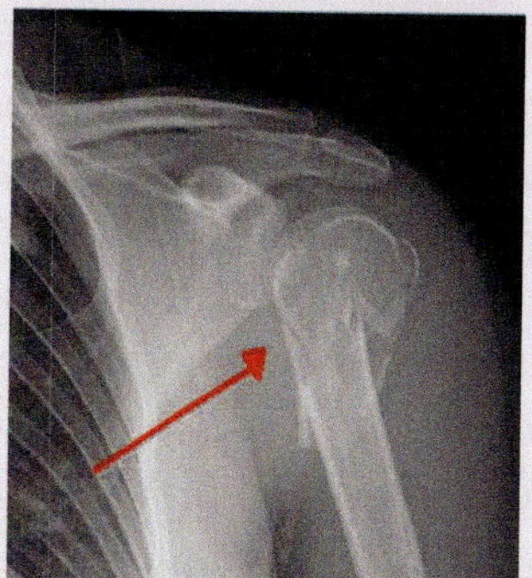

Figure 2.7. *Fracture of the proximal humerus with involvement of the greater trochanter.*

Source: By James Heilman, MD – Own work, CC BY-SA 4.0, https://commons.wikimedia.org/w/index.php?curid=49062941.

Humerus fractures come in two additional varieties. In comparison to a proximal humerus fracture, these fractures have a lesser impact on the shoulder joint.

- A fracture of the humeral shaft affects the midpoint of the humerus.
- A distal humerus fracture occurs near the elbow joint, at the lower end of the humerus.

Surgery is often not required for the treatment of a humeral fracture. The extent of displacement, involvement of the cartilage in the joint, the age and activity level of the patient, and other factors all influence the necessity of surgery.

- **Scapula Fracture:** A flat, triangular bone in the upper back is called the scapula. It provides the primary points of contact between the arm and the chest. Scapula fractures account for less than 1% of all fractures, and only 3% to 5% of shoulder fractures are caused by these injuries. The majority of men who experience scapula fractures are between the ages of 25 and

45. Traumatic incidents such as auto accidents or contact sports like football can result in scapular fractures. Patients with this type of injury often have other associated injuries, such as lung injuries, rib fractures, or nerve injuries, due to the force required to break the scapula.

- **Displaced and Non-Displaced Fractures:** The majority of shoulder fractures heal well without surgery. When the bones remain in their proper anatomical positions and are not displaced, nonsurgical treatment is an option. However, 80% of shoulder fractures are non-displaced. A shoulder fracture is considered displaced when the fragments of the broken bone are no longer in their proper anatomical position. Surgery may be necessary to realign the misplaced fractured bones so that they can heal in their proper alignments.

2.5.2. Causes of Fractures

Common causes of shoulder fractures include:

- Falling from a height, such as from a horse or during rock climbing
- Contact sports, including football
- Other traumatic events, such as motor vehicle accidents

Decreased bone mass associated with osteoporosis can increase the risk of shoulder fractures.

2.5.3. Diagnosing Shoulder Fractures

An orthopedic specialist orders advanced imaging tests to pinpoint the precise location of a shoulder fracture and assess the severity of the injury. The most recent developments in diagnostic techniques and imaging tests to check for shoulder fractures include:

- X-rays
- CT scan
- MRI
- Musculoskeletal ultrasound

2.5.4. Treatment for a Humerus Fracture

2.5.4.1. Proximal Humeral Fracture

As long as the bone fragments are not displaced, the majority of proximal humerus fractures can be treated non-operatively. Surgery is frequently performed to facilitate earlier mobility if the fragments become displaced. When deciding between nonoperative treatment and surgical fixation, additional factors are taken into consideration. During the initial two weeks of nonoperative treatment, the shoulder is often immobilized with a sling or other device. The patient will then be given weekly exercises to gradually increase the range of motion of the shoulder. X-rays of the shoulder will be taken every two weeks or every week to ensure proper healing of the fracture. In surgery, the fracture fragments are typically stabilized with plates, screws, or pins. In cases of severe fractures with prior joint degeneration, shoulder replacement may be necessary after arthroscopy. After surgery, mobilization with physical therapy begins immediately.

2.5.4.2. Humerus Shaft Fracture

Depending on the fracture pattern and any related injuries, a humerus shaft fracture may require surgery or non-surgical treatment. This includes cases of open fractures or nerve damage. Initially, a temporary splint may be used to immobilize the arm, with the elbow bent at a 90° angle.

Nonoperative treatment typically involves the use of fracture bracing, which is later replaced by a cylindrical brace called Sarmiento brace after three to four weeks. This brace supports the upper arm while allowing movement at the elbow. The doctor will provide guidance on the duration of splint or cast wear and when it can be removed. It may take several weeks to months for the broken arm to fully heal.

The goal of rehabilitation is to restore flexibility, joint range of motion, and muscle strength through gradual increases in activity levels. The success of rehabilitation depends on the patient's cooperation. Daily exercises, including strengthening and range-of-motion exercises, as directed by the physician, are essential until the muscles, ligaments, and other soft tissues regain normal function. Surgical procedures typically involve internal fixation of the fracture fragments using plates, screws, or nails. Unlike nonoperative treatment, there is no need for casts or splints. After surgery, elbow exercises can begin immediately, although shoulder exercises may need to be delayed for a few weeks depending on the fracture pattern.

2.5.5. Recovery

For a few weeks or even months following a shoulder fracture, separation, or dislocation, life can be significantly impacted. Whether treated nonsurgically or surgically, the majority of shoulder injuries necessitate a period of immobilization and then rehabilitation. After the first four to six weeks, if the injury was not severe, recovery and function return fairly quickly. However, improvements in pain, strength, and range of motion frequently last for up to a year following an injury. Shoulder exercises are typically required as part of a physical therapy program under supervision. Exercises assist the patient in regaining muscle strength, reducing stiffness, and improving range of motion.

2.6. Fractures of the Scapula

The scapula is a triangle-shaped bone that is protected by a complex network of surrounding muscles. A scapula fracture can occur as a result of high-energy, blunt trauma injuries, such as those sustained in a car accident or from a significant fall. Scapular fractures are often accompanied by other severe injuries, including damage to the head, lungs, or spinal cord, as well as fractures of the shoulder, collarbone, and ribs. Scapula fractures account for less than 1% of all fractured bones, and the vast majority of them heal without the need for surgery.

2.6.1. Etiology

In high-energy trauma situations such as car crashes, falls, and other high-impact trauma, as many as 80%–90% of all scapular fractures occur. All areas of the scapula may fracture through direct force, but fractures of the glenoid fossa and scapular neck are frequently caused by the impaction of the humeral head. Over 70% of scapular fractures are caused by motor vehicle collisions, with 52% related to drivers and 18% related to pedestrians hit by moving cars. Other reported mechanisms include electric shock and seizure because of forces on the scapula. Severe fractures of the scapula are uncommon.

2.6.2. Epidemiology

Roughly 0.4–1% of all fractures, 3% of shoulder fractures, and 5% of shoulder girdle fractures are scapular fractures. Males between the ages of 25 and 50 are more likely than females to sustain scapular fractures, which typically affect the glenoid or body.

- Body: 45%
- Glenoid Process: 35%
- Acromion: 8%
- Coracoid: 7%

2.6.3. Pathophysiology

2.6.3.1. Anatomy

The scapula serves as the attachment point for eighteen muscles that are connected to the thorax, spine, and upper extremities. In addition to the humerus and clavicle, the scapula facilitates rotational movement of the upper limb and aids in abduction and rotation at the glenohumeral joint (Figure 2.8).

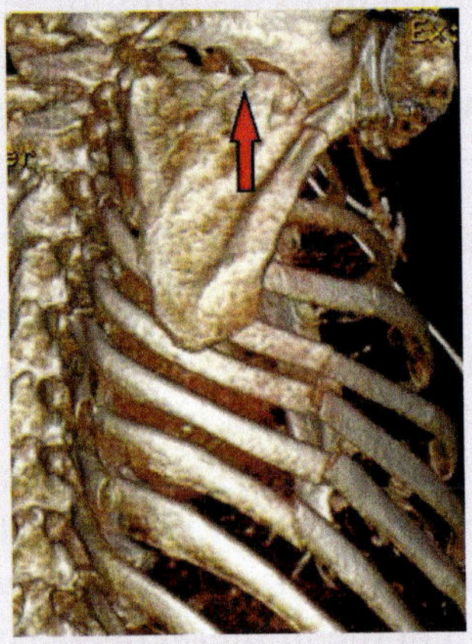

Figure 2.8. *A right-sided scapula fracture with rib fractures underneath seen on a 3D reconstruction of a CT scan.*

Source: By James Heilman, MD – Own work, CC BY-SA 4.0, https://upload.wikimedia.org/wikipedia/commons/8/8d/ScapulaFracture.png.

There are many different fracture patterns documented due to the force required to break a scapula. Fractures are categorized based on the anatomical location on the scapula. The Orthopedic Trauma Association has proposed a two-level classification system: level 1 for all trauma surgeons and level 2 for specialized shoulder surgeons. Despite the fact that this classification system is helpful for categorizing scapular fractures and determining the appropriate follow-up, no studies have found a correlation between the grading system and prognosis.

2.6.4. History and Physical Details

The most frequent mechanism is direct scapula trauma, either blunt or penetrating. The history and physical examination can provide the doctor with important details and aid in ruling out related injuries that may be fatal. This may not always be feasible in a high-energy trauma situation, contingent on the patient's mental state. It is important to conduct the physical examination of the upper extremities and shoulder in a way that permits a posterior forequarter examination. When a patient is supine in bed and has multiple injuries, this can be challenging. Asymmetry in the humeral head or shoulder displacement can be overt or covert. A comprehensive neurovascular examination of the upper extremity should be carried out after palpation and visual inspection of the bony landmarks. In 5–13% of cases, brachial plexus injuries are linked to scapula fractures. Assessing motor function can be challenging due to the pain connected to these injuries. It is wise to perform a thorough examination of the skin to check for open fractures, as open scapula fractures necessitate prompt debridement and irrigation in addition to antibiotics.

2.6.5. Evaluation

Owing to the high energy required to fracture the scapula, the majority of patients with scapula fractures also have multiple other injuries. The patient needs to be assessed as a trauma patient. Nonetheless, evaluation is necessary for certain potentially fatal injuries connected to scapular fractures. For instance, thoraco-scapular dissociations can result in potentially fatal bleeding due to disruptions of the axillary and subclavian veins.

It is important to assess scapular fractures and related trauma using diagnostic imaging. Conventional radiography frequently overlooks related injuries, even though it is adequate for evaluating the majority of scapular fractures when it includes anterior-posterior, lateral, and axillary views. Consequently, it is advised that a CT scan be done when evaluating scapular fractures. A ligamentous injury may need to be assessed with an MRI if there is a possibility that a joint is involved. Understanding the necessity of surgical intervention and appropriate management strategies can be aided by the 3D reconstruction of CT images.

2.6.6. Treatment/Management

Since more than 90% of scapular fractures are non-displaced, it is best to treat them conservatively without surgery. Fractures that have little to no displacement also tend to heal without complications. Malunion may result from scapular body fractures that have displaced, but because the scapular region has rich musculature, this may not even impair shoulder movement. However, if they are not properly realigned, displaced fractures in the glenoid or scapular processes do cause problems with shoulder mobility. As a result, although the majority of scapular fractures heal without surgery, glenoid or neck fractures necessitate the preservation of shoulder joint range of motion.

2.6.6.1. Medical Management

Following surgery or an injury, pain is a normal part of the healing process. Prescription drugs are frequently given for temporary pain relief in such cases. A wide range of drugs, including opioids, non-steroidal anti-inflammatory drugs (NSAIDs), and local anesthetics, are available to help manage pain. To reduce the need for opioids and enhance pain relief, doctors may prescribe a combination of these drugs. It is important to inform both the patient and the medical team that opioids are narcotics and can be addictive, despite their effectiveness in providing pain relief after surgery or an injury. Opioid addiction and overdose have become significant global and national public health concerns. It is crucial to strictly follow the prescribed dosage of opioids as directed by the doctor or surgeon. Opioid usage should be discontinued as soon as the patient's pain begins to diminish.

2.6.6.2. Non-surgical/Conservative Management

For the majority of scapula fractures, nonsurgical treatment with a shoulder immobilization sling is the most effective. The sling helps keep the shoulder in place while the bone heals. Typically, immobilization with a sling is maintained for six to twelve weeks to allow for proper healing. It is advised to apply ice to reduce swelling.

2.6.6.3. Surgical Management

In 90% of cases, scapular fractures heal well due to the unique muscular envelope of the scapula. However, scapular malunion can occasionally lead to serious impairments in shoulder girdle function, resulting in scapulothoracic dyskinesis, impingement syndrome, chronic pain, and cosmetic deformities. Certain types of scapular fractures that may require surgery include:

- Displaced fractures of the glenoid articular surface
- Fracture of the neck of the scapula with angulation
- Fractures of the acromion process causing impingement syndrome, where the arm bone hits against it.

2.6.6.4. Postoperative Care

- A bandage is present around the operated shoulder, and the operated arm is placed in a sling to support the shoulder.
- The application of ice to reduce pain and swelling is recommended.
- The incision is to be kept clean and

dry at all times.

- Specific instructions regarding activity and rehabilitation are to be provided to the patient.
- The patient must adhere to the exercise regimen prescribed by the physiotherapist in order to improve shoulder strength and motion and avoid stiffness. Physical therapy is necessary to restore shoulder function and strength.
- During the healing phase, the patient is asked to follow a prescribed medication schedule, maintain a healthy diet, and abstain from alcohol and tobacco use.

2.6.6.5. Risks and Complications of a Surgery

Bleeding, infection, blood clots or deep vein thrombosis, anesthesia-related side effects such as fever or nausea, nerve and blood vessel damage, stiff shoulders, fat embolism, improper healing, and the potential need for additional surgery.

2.6.7. Prognosis

It has been demonstrated that 86% of the time, conservatively managed non-operative fractures result in good to excellent functional outcomes. Studies show that although less than 1% of fractures require surgery, patients who do so have very good functional outcomes. Active and active-assisted range of motion exercises usually take six weeks for rehabilitation; strength training starts three to four months after surgery or injury. When it comes to non-operative fractures, patients can typically anticipate almost no functional deficits and good to excellent outcomes when surgical intervention is necessary.

2.6.8. Pearls and Other Issues

- Most scapular fractures are caused by a powerful force. They frequently have a connection to other injuries as a result. Associated injuries include:
  - Rib fractures
  - Hips lateral lung injuries
  - Injuries to the shoulder girdle complex
  - Neurovascular injuries
  - Suprascapular nerve injuries
  - Vertebral compression fractures
- A CT scan and radiographic imaging should be part of the evaluation.
- An orthopedic or trauma surgeon should evaluate any fractures of the scapula.

2.6.9. Enhancing Healthcare Team Outcomes

The World Health Organization has recognized interprofessional teams as crucial to providing high-quality care since 1978. Since scapular fractures usually occur in conjunction with other traumatic injuries, the necessary care is provided by highly skilled, experienced trauma teams. Trauma surgeons, orthopedic traumatologists, emergency room doctors, nurse practitioners, physician assistants, nurses, physical therapists, occupational therapists, social workers, and other specialists are frequently included in trauma teams. Higher quality care and better patient outcomes are the outcomes of effective communication and the team's use of each member's skills.

A Closer Look

Snapping Scapula Syndrome

Snapping scapula syndrome is characterized by the popping, clicking, grinding, or snapping of the bones and tissues of the shoulder blade when the arm is lifted or moved. For some individuals, this disorder is merely a minor annoyance, while for others, it can be a significant disability. The symptoms are often audible and can also be accompanied by pain. This condition is most commonly observed in young, active individuals participating in sports such as baseball, weightlifting, swimming, or in occupational settings.

The majority of cases of snapping scapula syndrome are caused by overuse of the arm, overtraining, poor posture, shoulder weakness, tumors, neck conditions, or issues with the shoulder joint. Other contributing factors include soft tissue or bone abnormalities present from birth, trauma, and inflamed bursae, which are fluid-filled sacs that provide cushioning for the muscles and bones of the shoulder blade.

As the shoulder blade moves along the chest wall, there may be grating, grinding, or snapping sounds or sensations along its edge. Occasionally, the joint may also produce popping or thumping sensations during movement. Additional symptoms include weakness or the inability to raise the arm overhead, as well as pain in the back or upper shoulder when lifting the arm or shrugging the shoulders. To confirm the diagnosis and rule out any additional damage to the spine, ribs, or shoulder blade, the doctor may order an X-ray, MRI, or CT scan, in addition to conducting a thorough physical examination and reviewing the medical history.

Non-operative measures such as physical therapy, anti-inflammatory painkillers, activity modification, rest, and steroid injections are frequently effective in treating snapping scapula syndrome. Surgery might be suggested if these treatments are ineffective at relieving the symptoms or if they worsen. When there is a bone abnormality, surgery is also the recommended course of action.

The procedure is called partial scapulectomy or scapulothoracic bursectomy. The surgeon punctures the scapulothoracic joint multiple times and inserts a tiny camera, known as an arthroscope. Using small instruments, the inflamed bursa and the upper corner of the scapula nearest the rib cage are removed. Arthroscopic surgery offers benefits such as smaller incisions, less trauma to muscles and tissues, reduced post-surgery pain, and a quicker recovery.

After surgery, patients typically wear slings for several weeks to allow the soft tissues to heal. Rehabilitation follows to regain strength, flexibility, and range of motion.

2.7. Summary

- Breaking the wrist is a common injury that typically occurs when the person trip or fall and extend the hands to protect.
- The wrist has two bones in the forearm called the radius and ulna. The radius is the bigger one. A distal radius fracture happens near the end of the radius bone, where it's more likely to break. Sometimes, the ulna bone in the forearm can also get fractured, which is called distal ulna fracture.
- The scaphoid is a carpal bone located near the base of the thumb within the wrist, forming part of two rows of small round bones. Fractures of the scaphoid are the second most common type of wrist fracture, yet they can be challenging to diagnose and manage.
- The majority of fractures have caused mild discomfort for a few days to several weeks. Numerous patients have discovered that their pain could be effectively alleviated by the application of ice, elevation of their arm above the level of their heart, and utilization of over-the-counter pain relievers.
- Between the ulna and the radius lies the interosseous membrane. It is composed of five components: the dorsal oblique accessory cord, the proximal oblique cord, the accessory band, the distal oblique bundle, and the central band. In addition to providing an attachment to the forearm muscles, it also provides longitudinal stability to the distal radioulnar joint.
- The ultimate goals of fracture management include achieving acceptable reduction, stable fixation and bone healing, early return to daily activities, preservation of function, and minimizing complications.
- In addition to fractures of the olecranon, fractures of the distal radius, neuropathic osteoarthropathy, osteomyelitis, tenosynovitis, bursitis, and sprains and dislocations of the elbow and wrist are commonly considered as differential diagnoses for forearm fractures. These conditions can be diagnosed independently through a comprehensive clinical examination and relevant radiological investigations.
- Patients who sustain forearm trauma should have their injuries assessed as soon as possible and receive the necessary care because, if left untreated, these fractures can result in severe long-term disability.
- A fracture at the tip of the elbow is referred to as an elbow fracture. Trauma resulting from a blow to the head, falling on the elbow, or falling on an extended hand can give rise to this condition.
- Elbow fractures can cause discomfort, swelling, and restricted range of motion. At the moment of injury, one might have heard or felt a snap or pop.
- Most fractures have caused mild discomfort for a few days to several weeks. For many patients, the utilization of ice packs, elevation (keeping the arm above the heart), and over-the-counter pain relievers has been sufficient to alleviate pain.
- The shoulder and arm are able to operate due to the collaboration of a collection of bones that constitute the shoulder. The humerus, the collarbone (clavicle), and the scapula, the shoulder blade, are the bones that constitute the shoulder.

- At least one of the three bones comprising the shoulder—the scapula, the clavicle, or the humerus—has been affected by a fracture. There exist notable distinctions among the three types of fractures, but all of them can lead to shoulder pain, swelling, tenderness, and limited range of motion.
- The scapula is a bone shaped like a triangle and is safeguarded by a complex network of surrounding muscles. A fracture of the scapula can occur as a result of high-energy, blunt trauma injuries, such as those sustained in a motor vehicle accident or after falling from a significant height.

References

1. Carlsen, B. T., & Moran, S. L., (2009). Thumb trauma: Bennett fractures, Rolando fractures, and ulnar collateral ligament injuries. *J. Hand. Surg. Am., 34*(5), 945-52.
2. Chung, K. C., Kotsis, S. V., & Kim, H. M., (2007). Predictors of functional outcomes after surgical treatment of distal radius fractures. *J. Hand. Surg. Am., 32*, 76–83.
3. John, M. F., David, L. S., & Peter, M. W., (2014). *Rockwood and Wilkins' Fractures in Children*. ISBN: 9781451143935
4. Matsen, F. A., (2004). *Shoulder Surgery: Principles and Procedures*. Philadelphia, PA: Saunders.
5. Mighell, M. A., Kolm, G. P., Collinge, C. A., & Frankle, M. A., (2003). Outcomes of hemiarthroplasty for fractures of the proximal humerus. *J. Shoulder Elbow Surg., 12*, 569–577.
6. William N. Levine, Louis U. Bigliani, & Guido Marra, (2013). *Fractures of the Shoulder Girdle*. New York: Marcel Dekker.
7. Ruch, D. S., & Papadonikolakis, A., (2006). Volar versus dorsal plating in the management of intra-articular distal radius fractures. *J. Hand Surg. Am., 31*, 9–16.
8. Wiss, D. A., (2013). *Fractures* (3rd edn.). Philadelphia, PA: Lippincott Williams & Wilkins.
9. Zuckerman, J. D., (2005). *Shoulder Fractures: The Practical Guide to Management*. New York: Thieme.

Chapter 3

FRACTURES IN THE LOWER LIMB

Contents

3.1. Introduction

A fracture of the lower limb, ranging from the pelvis to the feet, is referred to as a lower limb fragility fracture. It typically occurs as a result of a fall or trip. Due to the natural deterioration of our bones with age, these fractures predominantly affect individuals over the age of 60. While fractures of the femoral bone (thigh), pelvis, tibia (shin bone), knee, and foot are also common lower limb fragility fractures, hip and ankle fractures are the most prevalent. These painful injuries can significantly impair the patient's mobility and ability to live independently.

Orientation and Directional Terms

Term	Definition	Illustration
X-rays	An X-ray is a quick, painless test that captures images of the structures inside the body, particularly the bones.	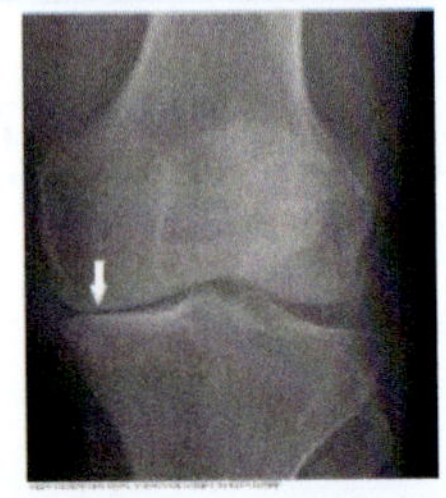
Magnetic resonance imaging (MRI) scans	Magnetic resonance imaging (MRI) is a medical imaging technique that utilizes a magnetic field and computer-generated radio waves to generate intricate images of the organs and tissues within the body.	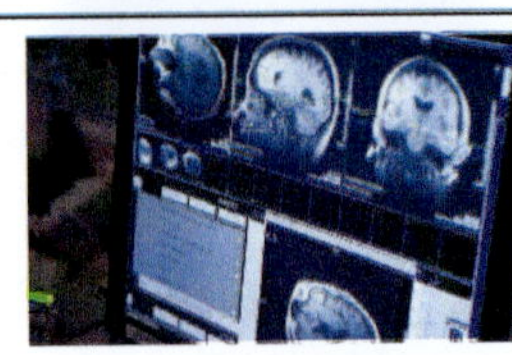
Computerized tomography (CT) scans	A computerized tomography (CT) scan combines a series of X-ray images taken from different angles around the body and uses computer processing to create cross-sectional images (slices) of the bones, blood vessels, and soft tissues inside the body.	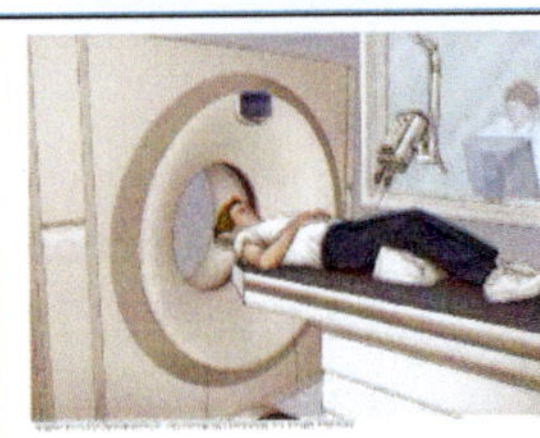
Intertrochanteric Fracture	Intertrochanteric fractures occur below the femoral neck in a broader region between the greater and lesser trochanters. The greater trochanter is the bump felt on the side of the hip. There may be two, three, or even multiple fracture fragments.	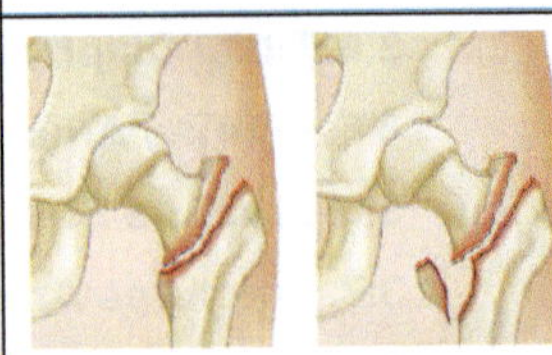
Subtrochanteric Fracture	Subtrochanteric fractures involve the upper part of the shaft of the femur, just below the hip joint.	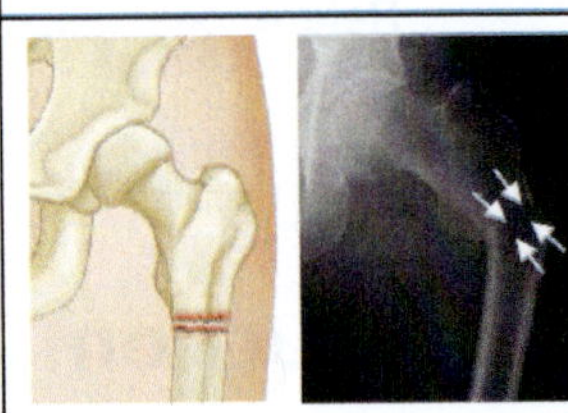

3.2. Fractures of the Foot

A fractured foot is an injury to the bone. A mere misstep or fall could lead to a fracture of the foot, as well as motor vehicle collisions. A fractured foot can exhibit varying degrees of severity. Fractures can range from minuscule breaks that penetrate the skin to minuscule fissures in the bone (e.g., fractures of the metatarsals). The precise location and extent of the fracture will determine the appropriate treatment for a fractured foot. In order to maintain proper alignment during the healing process, a severely fractured foot may require surgical intervention to implant plates, rods, or screws into the fractured bone (Figure 3.1).

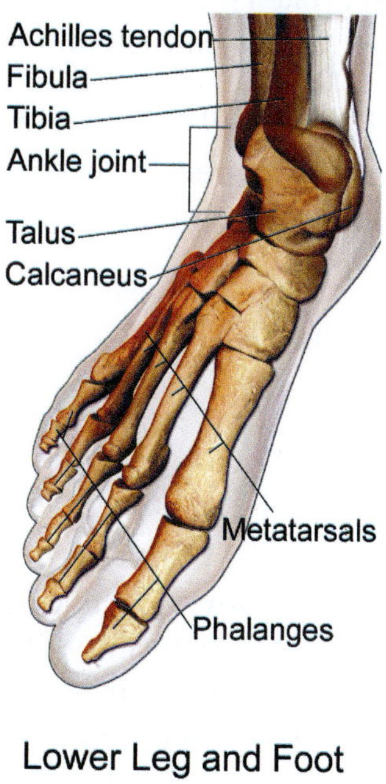

Figure 3.1. *Illustration of bones in lower leg and foot.*

Source: By BruceBlaus. When using this image in external sources, it can be cited as: Blausen.com staff (2014). "Medical gallery of Blausen Medical 2014." WikiJournal of Medicine 1(2). doi: 10.15347/wjm/2014.010. ISSN 2002-4436, Own work, CC BY 3.0, https://commons.wikimedia.org/w/index.php?curid=29849183.

3.2.1. Types of Foot Fractures

Any number of different bone breaks can be referred to as "foot fractures" when someone says they have one. Foot and ankle fractures can include metatarsal fractures, heel bone fractures, and ankle fractures. Stress fractures can also occur from overuse of the foot or ankle. It can be challenging to keep up with the variety of foot fractures that exist.

3.2.1.1. Ankle Fractures

An ankle fracture occurs when there is a break in the talus, fibula, or tibia. There are two joints in the ankle: where these three bones meet and the joint between the fibula and tibia. These factors can cause instability and should be diagnosed and treated correctly to avoid further complications. Typically, ankle fractures happen when the ankle is bearing weight and is subjected to the strain of physical activities like sports, jumping, or running.

Foot fractures can happen in a variety of settings. A few typical symptoms should be recognized. These include the inability to bear weight on the ankle, protruding bones (also referred to as a compound fracture), tenderness, pain, swelling, and bruising. An orthopedic doctor will first ask the patient about the symptoms. To assess the extent of the injury, X-rays might be required. In other situations, a CT or MRI scan will be required. The ideal course of treatment will depend on the type of fracture. Most of the time, physical therapy will be administered after the use of a cast or splint.

3.2.1.2. Heel Bone Fractures

The heel bone, or calcaneus, is located beneath the ankle joint. It is the largest tarsal bone and also forms the subtalar joint, which enables lateral movement of the hindfoot. This movement is crucial for maintaining balance, especially on uneven terrain. Fractures of the heel bone are less common and can have various causes. For instance, falling from a significant height and landing on the feet can result in this type of fracture. This impact can cause the heel to become wider and shorter when weight is applied to the foot. Fractures in the heel bone can present with several symptoms, including bruising, swelling, pain, and the inability to bear weight on the heel.

To determine the most appropriate treatment for a heel bone fracture, the symptoms will be assessed. Further evaluation of the fracture may require X-rays and CT scans. Treatment approaches vary depending on the type and severity of the fracture. Options may include surgical procedures, physical therapy, and the use of braces or casts (Figure 3.2).

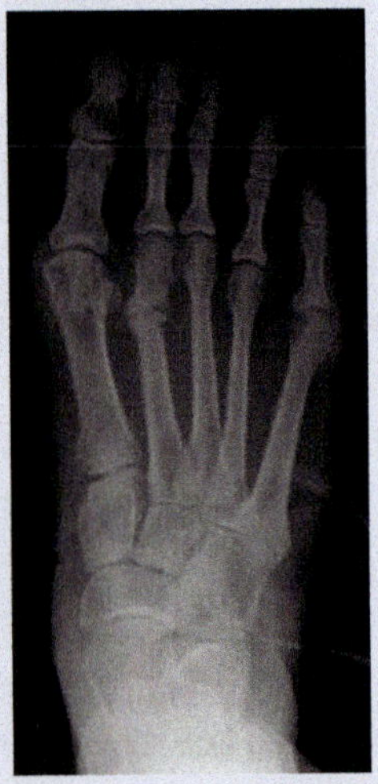

Figure 3.2. *Stress fracture of the second metatarsal bone (below the knuckles of the second toe).*

Source: By Personalo at English Wikipedia, CC BY-SA 3.0, https://commons.wikimedia.org/w/index.php?curid=50136438.

3.2.1.3. Metatarsal Fractures

The five metatarsal bones on each foot join the toes to the ankle. They provide support to the foot and contribute to improved balance during standing or walking.

These fractures are common, with football players being particularly vulnerable to them. Fractures can occur from falls, being kicked or stepped on, or sudden twisting of the foot. Overuse of the bones can also lead to stress fractures, which are small cracks in the bone.

At the site of the injury, there may be a cracking sound. Symptoms include pain, tenderness, swelling, and bruising. Weight-bearing may be difficult, and movement may be limited. In some cases, the pain may subside within an hour or two.

3.2.2. Symptoms

A person with broken foot may experience some of the following signs and symptoms:

- Immediate, throbbing pain
- Pain that increases with activity and decreases with rest
- Swelling
- Bruising
- Tenderness
- Deformity
- Difficulty in walking or bearing weight

When to See a Doctor*:* Consult a physician if there is a noticeable deformity, if self-care is ineffective in reducing the pain and swelling, or if the symptoms worsen over time. Consult a physician if the injury makes it difficult to walk.

3.2.3. Causes

The most common causes of a broken foot include:

- **Car Accidents:** The common crushing injuries sustained in auto accidents can result in breaks that need to be surgically repaired.

- **Falls:** Tripping and falling can break bones in the feet, as can landing on the feet after jumping down from just a slight height.
- **Impact from a Heavy Weight:** Dropping something heavy on the foot is a common cause of fractures.
- **Missteps:** Sometimes just putting the foot down wrong can result in a broken bone. A toe can get broken from stubbing the toes on furniture.
- **Overuse:** The weight-bearing bones in the feet are prone to stress fractures. Running long distances is one type of overuse or repetitive force that can eventually cause these tiny cracks. However, they can also occur when a bone that has been weakened by an illness like osteoporosis is used normally.

3.2.4. Diagnosis

During the physical examination, the physician will examine the tender spots in the foot. The exact location of the pain can help identify its source. They may also move the foot in various ways to assess the range of motion. Additionally, the patient may be asked to walk a short distance so that the doctor can evaluate the gait.

3.2.4.1. Imaging Tests

The following imaging tests may be recommended by the doctor if the symptoms indicate a possible break or fracture.

- **X-rays:** Most foot fractures can be seen in X-ray images. To minimize overlap between the bone images, the technician may need to take X-rays from different angles. Stress fractures may not be visible on X-rays until the healing process has begun.
- **Bone Scan:** A small amount of radioactive material will be injected into a vein by a technician to perform a bone scan. The radioactive material attracts to the areas of the bones that have been damaged, particularly in the case of stress fractures. Damaged areas, including stress fractures, appear as bright spots in the resulting image.
- **Computerized Tomography (CT) Scans:** CT scans produce cross-sectional images of the internal structures of the body by combining X-rays taken from various angles. CT scans provide more information about the bone and the surrounding soft tissues, which can help the doctor determine the most appropriate course of action.
- **Magnetic Resonance Imaging (MRI):** By using a strong magnetic field and radio waves, detailed images of the ligaments that hold the foot and ankle together can be created. This imaging technique can detect fractures that may not be visible on X-rays and can provide visualization of both bones and ligaments.

3.2.5. Treatment

Depending on the broken bone and the extent of the damage, there are different treatment options for a broken foot.

- **Medications:** An over-the-counter pain reliever like acetaminophen (Tylenol, among others) might be suggested by the doctor.
- **Therapy:** The patient will likely need to retrain their stiff foot muscles and ligaments after the

bone has healed. The patient learns exercises to increase the strength and flexibility from a physical therapist.

Surgical and Other Procedures:

- **Reduction:** If the fracture is displaced, or the two ends are not aligned, the doctor may need to perform reduction surgery to move the broken pieces back into place. The patient might require a muscle relaxant, sedative, or even a general anesthetic prior to this procedure, depending on how much pain and swelling they are experiencing.
- **Immobilization:** In order for a fractured bone to mend, its ends need to be immobilized. This usually necessitates a cast. For minor foot fractures, a boot, shoe, or detachable brace with a stiff sole is needed. A piece of gauze is typically placed between a fractured toe and its neighboring toe.
- **Surgery:** An orthopedic surgeon may occasionally need to use screws, plates, or pins to keep the bones in the right positions while they heal. If these materials are painful or conspicuous, they may be removed once the fracture has healed.

3.2.6. Risk Factors

The patient may be at higher risk of a broken foot or ankle if they are:

- **Engaging in High-impact Sports:** Participating in sports such as football, basketball, gymnastics, tennis, and soccer, which involve stresses, hard hits, and twisting movements, can lead to foot fractures.
- **Using Improper Technique or Sports Equipment:** Using defective equipment, such as worn-out or ill-fitting shoes, can cause stress fractures and falls. Foot injuries can also occur due to improper training methods, such as skipping warm-ups and stretching exercises.
- **Abruptly Increasing Activity Level:** Suddenly increasing the frequency or duration of workouts, regardless of training level, can elevate the risk of stress fractures.
- **Working in Specific Occupations:** Certain work environments, like construction sites, pose the risk of falling from heights or having heavy objects fall on the foot.
- **Maintaining a messy or dimly lit house**: Moving around in a cluttered or poorly lit home increases the chances of foot injuries and falls.
- **Having Certain Conditions:** Osteoporosis, a condition characterized by decreased bone density, heightens the risk of foot bone injuries.

3.2.7. Complications

Complications of a broken foot are uncommon but may include:

- **Arthritis:** Years later, arthritis may result from fractures that penetrate a joint. See the doctor for an assessment if the foot pain persists after a break.
- **Osteomyelitis:** If the patient has an open fracture, which is a fracture where one end of the bone shows

through the skin, bacteria that cause infection may come into contact with the bone.

- **Nerve or Blood Vessel Damage:** Foot trauma can cause damage to nearby blood vessels and nerves, occasionally even rupturing them. if experience any numbness or circulation issues, get medical help right away. A bone may die and collapse as a result of inadequate blood flow.

3.2.8. Prevention

These basic sports and safety tips may help prevent a broken foot:

- **Wear Appropriate Footwear:** on rugged terrain, wear hiking shoes. If required, wear steel-toed boots in the workplace. Select athletic footwear that is appropriate for the sport.
- **Regularly Replace Athletic Shoes:** Throw away sneakers as soon as the tread or heel becomes worn down, or if there is uneven wear. If the patient run, change the shoes every 300 to 400 miles.
- **Start Slowly:** This applies to a new fitness program and each individual workout.
- **Cross-Train:** Stress fractures can be avoided by alternating the activities. Alternate cycling or swimming with running.
- **Strengthen the Bones:** Foods high in calcium, such as milk, yogurt, and cheese, are incredibly beneficial to the health. Supplementing with vitamin D can also be beneficial.
- **Use Night Lights:** Many broken toes are the result of walking in the dark.
- **Declutter the House:** Keeping clutter off the floor can help to avoid trips and falls.

3.3. Injuries Around the Ankle

Sports injuries are frequently associated with ankle injuries. However, turning the ankle and hurting it doesn't require to be an athlete or even a weekend warrior. A painful and incapacitating sprain can result from something as simple as walking on an uneven surface. Anyone at any age can sustain an ankle injury. However, compared to women over 30, who have higher rates than men, men between the ages of 15 and 24 have higher rates of ankle sprains. During athletic activity, ankle sprains occur in half of cases. In the U.S., 25,000 people suffer ankle sprains on a daily basis. Additionally, more than a million people seek care in emergency rooms annually due to ankle injuries. The most frequent injuries to the ankle are sprains and fractures, which affect the bones and ligaments of the ankle. However, a tendon can also be torn or strained.

3.3.1. The Different Types of Ankle Sprains

It is beneficial to review fundamental aspects of the ankle in order to comprehend ankle injuries. The ankle is made up of the fibula, talus, and tibia, three major bones, as well as ligaments and tendons that help with movement. Together, these components in the joint not only help to move but also keep things stable. Any small shifts in the ankle can cause trouble. Strains, sprains, and fractures are the most commonly encountered ankle injuries.

While ankle injuries can arise from nearly any activity, they most frequently occur from sports and fitness activities, tripping or falling, and twisting the ankle during any activity. The symptoms of a strain, sprain, or fracture can be similar, thereby making it challenging to differentiate between them without a medical examination.

- **Ankle Strains:** A strained muscle or tendon is the thick tissue that connects a muscle to a bone. It can be torn or stretched, and strains can range from minor to severe, potentially causing tears.
- **Ankle Sprains:** Injury to the ankle ligaments can result in three types of sprains: Grade I, Grade II, and Grade III. Physicians assign a grade to each injury severity, with Grade I being the least severe and Grade III being the most severe.
- **Ankle Fractures:** Ankle fractures can vary in severity, from minor breaks in one bone that do not hinder walking, to major fractures that may require surgery and months of non-weight bearing. Ligaments can also be damaged as a result of a fracture.

3.3.2. Severity of Ankle Sprains

- **First Degree:** There is minimal swelling and no instability, with the ligaments holding the ankle's bones together stretched but not torn. In a few weeks, the patient should be back playing sports.
- **Second Degree:** The ankle typically swells quickly due to partial tears in the ligaments. It might take three to six weeks for this sprain to heal completely. There is some instability, and walking and bearing weight frequently cause pain.
- **Third Degree:** This type of ligament tear is more severe and takes six to twelve months to heal completely. Severe pain, bruising, and swelling are frequently present (Figure 3.3).

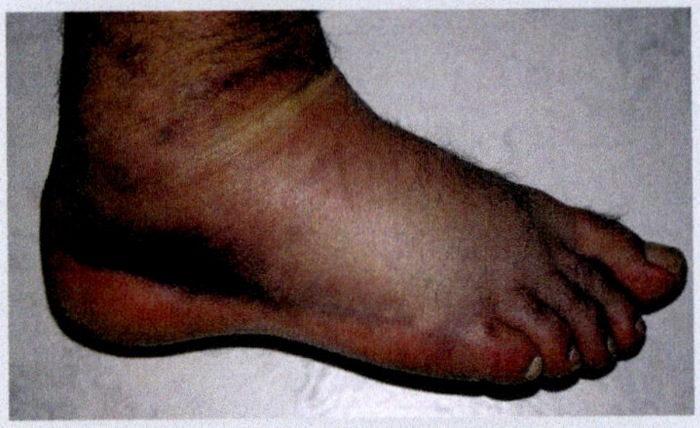

Figure 3.3. *Right foot, 3rd degree sprain. One day after injury.*

Source: By Usien – Own work, CC BY-SA 3.0, https://commons.wikimedia.org/w/index.php?curid=14795567.

3.3.3. Symptoms of Ankle Injuries

The symptoms of each ankle issue are unique, but when it comes to the ankle, many of the symptoms are similar. Ankle pain is the first sign of a problem; it usually manifests suddenly and severely. Second, bruising, swelling, and the inability to walk or bear weight on the injured joint are common symptoms of ankle injuries. Third, there's a chance that the ankle will feel hard, sensitive, or even malformed. The patient might experience weakness or intermittent ankle pain if the problem is at a lower level. In addition, an increase in the height of the foot's arch may be a sign of instability, which could be problematic. An ankle problem may be indicated by a snapping sensation.

3.3.4. Treatments for Ankle Injuries

Treatment for ankle injuries can vary depending on the problem. After evaluating the situation, doctors will recommend a course of action. Use RICE, or rest, ice, compression, and elevation, to treat minor injuries. Most of the time, the patient won't require a cast or splint; instead, they just need to take some days off of weight bearing on the ankle before strengthening and stretching it.

3.3.4.1. Treatment of Fractures

There are two types of fracture treatment: surgical and nonsurgical. If only one bone is broken and the ankle is stable and the other bones are in their proper places, the doctor may be able to treat the break without the need for surgery by immobilizing the ankle. Usually, the physician will accomplish this by applying a cast or a brace that doubles as a splint. Surgery will be used to treat the fracture if the ankle is unstable. A metal plate and screws are frequently used to stabilize the ankle and hold the bones in place. After surgery, the ankle is first protected with a cast, then a splint until the swelling subsides.

The healing process of the bones typically takes at least six weeks. In order for the bones to heal in the right alignment, the doctor will likely advise to avoid bearing any weight on the ankle during that period. After a fracture has completely healed, ligaments and tendons may require additional time to heal. After an ankle fracture, full pain-free motion and strength recovery can take up to two years, although most people are back to their regular routine in three to four months. When the doctor says it's safe to begin moving the ankle, physical therapy may be required to help with gait training, balance, strengthening, and mobility movements. The therapist will create a program to follow at home so that the patient can resume the prior level of normal function. It might take several months to get back to normal, limp-free walking.

3.3.4.2. Treatment of Sprains

The severity of the injury determines how a sprain is treated. Three grades are assigned: mild, moderate, and severe. Generally speaking, surgery is not a recommended course of action unless the damage is severe, affects more than just the ligaments, or other treatments are ineffective. The RICE method is used to treat mild sprains, or grade 1, for a few days until the pain and swelling go down. The patient won't require a cast or splint for a mild sprain. As long as the patient can handle it, the doctor will advise to apply weight to the ankle as soon as possible—within one to three days—and will also recommend range-of-motion, stretching, and strengthening exercises (Figure 3.4).

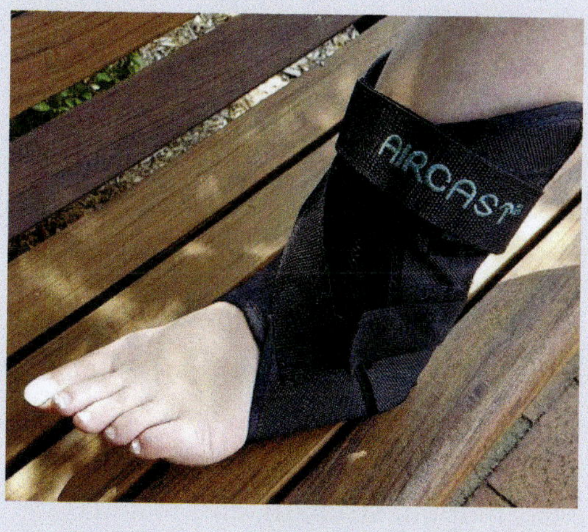

Figure 3.4. *A brace offering moderate support and compression for a grade I ankle sprain.*

Source: By Whoisjohngalt, CC BY-SA 4.0, https://commons.wikimedia.org/w/index.php?curid=50191948.

If the doctor diagnoses the sprain as grade 2, or moderate, they will still apply the RICE protocol but give the injury more time to heal. The ankle may also be immobilized by the physician using a boot or splint. Exercises to increase the range of motion and then to strengthen and stretch the ankle will be given to you. To help regain complete use of the ankle, the doctor might also recommend physical therapy.

A grade 3 sprain, also known as a severe rip or rupture of a ligament, requires a lot more time to heal. The joint is immobilized as part of the treatment, and then physical therapy is administered for a longer duration to improve strength, range of motion, and flexibility. On rare occasions, surgery to repair the torn ligaments may be considered, particularly if the sprain does not heal within a reasonable amount of time. The first course of treatment for a sprain usually consists of protecting and resting the ankle for approximately a week until the swelling subsides. After that, the patient should exercise for one to two weeks to regain the strength, flexibility, and range of motion. It may take a few more weeks or months to progressively resume the regular activities while you're still working out.

3.3.4.3. Treatment of Tendon Injuries

Options for treating tendon injuries are similar to options for treating sprains. They include:

- Immobilization using a cast or splint
- Oral or injected anti-inflammatory drugs to reduce pain
- Physical therapy for range of motion, strength, and balance
- A brace to provide support during activities
- Surgery is performed to repair the tendon or tendons, and sometimes to repair the supporting structures of the foot.

3.4. Tibial Diaphyseal Fractures

Breaks to the tibia are common injuries. The tibia is more susceptible to open injuries due to its subcutaneous nature. The musculature surrounding the lower leg is divided into four compartments by fascial tissue. Many fibula fractures occur alongside tibia fractures (Figure 3.5).

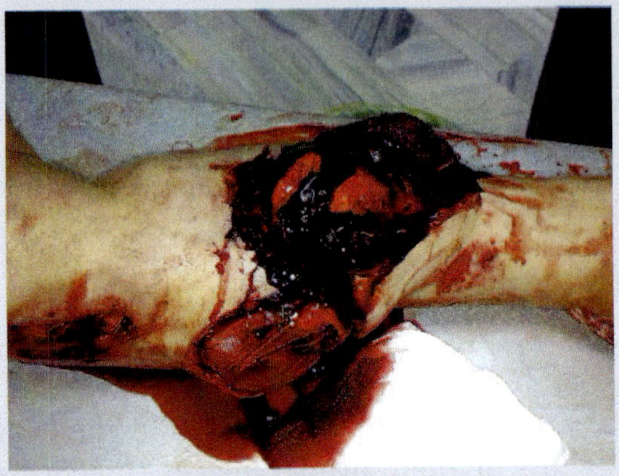

Figure 3.5. *Open fracture of the shaft of the tibia.*

Source: By Armin – Own work, Public Domain, https://commons.wikimedia.org/w/index.php?curid=25767473.

3.4.1. Cause

The most common cause of tibial shaft fractures is a high-energy collision, such as a car or motorcycle accident. These types of situations can result in a comminuted fracture, which breaks the bone into multiple pieces. Lower-energy injuries that can lead to tibial shaft fractures are often related to sports, such as collisions with other players or falls while skiing. These fractures, which typically result in an oblique or spiral fracture, are usually caused by a twisting force.

3.4.2. Symptoms

Symptoms of a tibial shaft fracture typically include immediate and severe pain. Other symptoms may include:

- Inability to walk or bear weight on the leg
- Deformity or instability of the leg
- Bone "tenting" over the skin at the fracture site or bone protruding through a break in the skin
- Occasional loss of feeling in the foot

3.4.3. Evaluation

Imaging: AP and lateral radiographs of the tibia are recommended, as well as imaging of the ankle and knee joints above and below. CT scans are not always necessary for tibial shaft fractures. However, intra-articular injuries that extend into the tibial plateau or plafond are often assessed using a CT scan. Basic labs (CBC, BMP, and PT/INR if applicable), as well as an EKG and chest radiograph, should be included in the medical evaluation of every surgical patient.

For older patients with presumptive or confirmed heart disease, a preoperative cardiology assessment may be beneficial. The tibia can be formally classified using the AO/OTA (Arbeitsgemeinschaft für Osteosynthesefragen/Orthopedic Trauma Association) classification system. The tibial shaft represents bone segment 4. Fractures are classified as C-complex, B-wedge, or A-simple. The AO/OTA classification system also has additional subclassifications based on the location and presence of associated fibula fractures. This classification is used more frequently in research. Fractures can also be classified descriptively, as open or closed, and by location (transverse, oblique, spiral, or comminuted) or position (proximal, mid-shaft, or distal).

3.4.4. Treatment/Management

The use of early antibiotics is the most crucial factor in lowering the infection rate. It is recommended to apply a temporary splint and perform bedside debridement.

Acceptable Alignment:

- <5° of varus/valgus
- <10°
- >50% cortical apposition
- <1 cm of shortening
- <5–10 rotational deformity

Acceptable alignment occurs when the fracture lies within the previously mentioned acceptable alignment ranges. A closed reduction can be employed to achieve satisfactory alignment in fractures with moderate displacement. Patients who receive long leg casting should also consider nonoperative management (Figure 3.6).

Operative:

- **Intramedullary Rod:** It is the most frequently used method of treatment for tibial diaphyseal fractures and is preferred for closed fractures and low-grade open fractures.

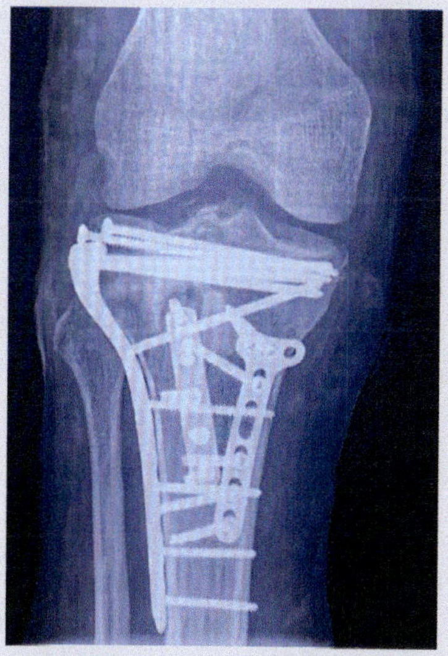

Figure 3.6. *Repair of a tibial plateau fracture.*

Source: By Ryanaparent – Own work, CC BY-SA 4.0, https://commons.wikimedia.org/w/index.php?curid=104925633.

- **Open Reduction Internal Fixation:** It can be used to treat tibial fractures, although it is more frequently used when the fracture does not respond well to intramedullary fixation or extends into the articular surface.
- **External Fixation:** It is beneficial

for severe edema or extensive soft tissue injury. An external fixator is used as a temporary procedure until internal fixation can be achieved.

- **Debridement and Irrigation:** Thes are necessary for any open wounds.
- **Fasciotomies:** It should be carried out if compartment syndrome is a clinical concern. Compartment pressures can be measured with a Stryker monitor, particularly in sedated patients.

3.4.5. Prognosis

Research indicates that many patients experience a decline in function after a tibial fracture, which gradually improves over the course of six to twelve months. The functional score may not return to baseline after five years. Functional scores at the 12-year follow-up following intramedullary nailing may indicate subjective leg swelling (33%) or persistent knee pain (73%).

3.4.6. Complications

Pain that is out of proportion or that hurts when stretched passively is the first and most sensitive sign of compartment syndrome. While many of the other symptoms may not appear immediately, the other classic signs include palpable swelling, pallor, pulselessness, and paresthesias. The signs and symptoms of compartment syndrome in children include increased agitation, anxiety, and an increasing need for medication.

- **Malunion:** Ankle and apex anterior (procurvatum) deformities are particularly prone to malalignment in proximal tibia fractures.
  Nonunion: Usually indicated by a fracture not healing on radiographs after six months or by the fracture not healing without surgery. The most frequent side effect following intramedullary nail insertion is anterior knee pain.

3.4.7. Differential Diagnosis

- **Hematoma:** Lower leg trauma can result in swelling even in the absence of a fracture.
- **Compartment Syndrome:** Lower leg trauma can result in swelling even in the absence of a fracture.

3.4.8. Postoperative and Rehabilitation Care

Examining the suggested weight-bearing status for the injury is crucial. Patients who undergo non-operative treatment, are in an external fixator, or have comminuted fracture patterns may find it difficult to bear weight, whereas patients with more straightforward fracture patterns that are fixed with intramedullary fixation may be able to do so as long as they are able. Patients should receive assistance with physical and occupational therapy to aid in their recovery. Patients receiving non-operative care in a cast should be closely monitored in the office to ensure that there is no loss of reduction. If loss of reduction is observed during follow-up, the cast may need to be adjusted, or the fracture may need to be reduced while under anesthesia.

3.4.9. Consultations

In cases of intense trauma, such as car crashes and trauma, the trauma team member evaluating the patient should be on the lookout for additional injuries. For skin grafting or flap coverage, plastic surgery might be required, depending on the degree of soft tissue loss or damage. Patients who have suffered a tibial shaft fracture may require comorbidity management both before and after surgery. Depending on the patient's comorbidities, this multidisciplinary care team may consist of orthopedics, geriatrics, internal medicine, trauma surgery, anesthesia, pharmacists, and any other subspecialty that may be helpful.

3.4.10. Enhancing Healthcare Team Outcomes

The emergency room will see the majority of patients who have fractures to the tibial shaft. A proper history, physical examination, and sufficient imaging should be promptly conducted. Patients who have open wounds or who may have compartment syndrome should be evaluated immediately, following triage guidelines. Antibiotics should be initiated even before imaging if there is visible bone or a known open fracture, in order to help reduce the risk of infection. Provisional splinting and bedside debridement of gross contamination are also necessary. After surgery, antibiotic therapy can be continued.

All members of the healthcare team must be aware of the signs and symptoms associated with compartment syndrome. Both closed and open tibia fractures, as well as times before or after surgery, can result in compartment syndrome. The circumferential nature of casts means that even slightly displaced fractures treated with a cast may represent or worsen overnight. Floor nurses must be alert to any signs of increasing pain in patients who initially presented with mild swelling. Ice should be applied to the injury and the affected extremity should be elevated in all patients with tibial shaft fractures.

3.5. Injuries Around the Knee

The knee joint is a complex structure that functions like a door hinge, enabling individuals to flex and extend their legs for activities such as sitting, squatting, jumping, and running.

There are four parts to the knee:

- Bones;
- Cartilage;
- Ligaments; and
- Tendons.

The femur is located at the top of the knee joint, while the tibia is found at the bottom. The patella covers the area where the femur and tibia meet. Cartilage is the tissue that provides cushioning to the bones in the knee joint, allowing ligaments to move smoothly over the bones and protecting them from impact. The knee joint is held together and stabilized by four ligaments that act like ropes. Tendons connect the muscles that support the knee joint to the bones in the upper and lower leg. There are various types of knee injuries, with the following list identifying 10 of the most common ones.

- **Fractures:** A fracture can occur in any of the bones in or near the knee. The patella is the most frequently broken bone in a joint. Knee fractures are most commonly caused by high impact trauma, such as falls or auto accidents. A simple trip or incorrect step can cause a knee fracture in someone with underlying osteoporosis.
- **Anterior Cruciate Ligament (ACL) Injuries:** It is responsible for providing crucial stability to the knee joint. It runs diagonally down the front of the joint. ACL injuries can be quite serious and often require surgical intervention. These injuries are categorized into three grades, ranging from one to three. A grade 3 tear indicates a complete rupture of the ACL, while a grade 1 sprain represents a more moderate injury. ACL injuries are commonly

observed in athletes participating in contact sports such as football or soccer. However, there are other causes for this injury apart from contact sports. An ACL tear can occur due to sudden changes in motion direction or incorrect landing after a jump.

- **Dislocation:** When the knee bones are misaligned and improperly positioned, the knee can become dislocated. During a knee dislocation, one or more bones may become detached. Structural abnormalities or traumatic events such as collisions, falls, and contact sports can lead to knee dislocation.
- **Meniscal Tears:** When someone mentions a meniscal tear, they are typically referring to a tear in the cartilage of the knee. The menisci are two rubbery cartilage wedges located between the thigh and tibia. These cartilage fragments are prone to tearing during sports activities. Aging can also contribute to a gradual tearing of the menisci. A degenerative meniscus tear occurs when the meniscus tears naturally due to aging. An abrupt meniscus tear may be accompanied by a popping sensation in the knee. In the days following the initial injury, pain, swelling, and tightness may increase.
- **Bursitis:** Bursitis is another condition that can affect the knee. Bursae are small sacs filled with fluid that act as cushions for the knee joints, allowing ligaments and tendons to glide smoothly. When these sacs are overworked or repeatedly compressed, such as during kneeling, they can become inflamed and swollen, leading to bursitis. Most cases of bursitis can be managed with self-care measures and are not severe. However, in some cases, antibiotic therapy or aspiration, which involves removing fluid with a needle, may be necessary.
- **Tendonitis:** Patellar tendinitis is the term used to describe inflammation or tendinitis of the knee. In this case, the tendon that connects the tibia to the patella becomes injured. The patellar tendon works together with the front of the thigh to allow for knee extension and facilitate activities such as running and jumping. Tendonitis is frequently seen in athletes who engage in frequent jumping. However, tendinitis can occur in any physically active individual.
- **Tendon Tears:** Tendon tears are a common occurrence, particularly in the patellar tendon of the knee. Athletes or individuals in their middle age who engage in regular physical activity may experience tendon tears or overstretching. Additionally, a tear in the tendon can result from a direct impact, such as a fall or blow.
- **Collateral Ligament Injuries:** Collateral ligament injuries are often seen in athletes, especially those involved in contact sports. These ligaments connect the thigh bone to the shin bone and can be torn due to direct impacts or collisions with other players or objects.

- **Iliotibial Band Syndrome:** A common condition among long-distance runners is iliotibial band syndrome. It is caused by friction between the outside of the knee joint and the iliotibial band, which is located on the outside of the knee. Initially, the pain is mild, but it can worsen over time, leading the runner to take a break from running in order to allow the iliotibial band to heal.
- **Posterior Cruciate Ligament Injuries:** The posterior cruciate ligament is located at the back of the knee. It is one of the many ligaments that connect the tibia and femur. This ligament prevents excessive backward movement of the tibia. Injuries to the posterior cruciate ligament usually occur when the knee is bent and subjected to strong force. Such force is typically experienced in cases of severe falls onto a bent knee or accidents involving the knee while it is bent.

3.5.1. Knee Injury Signs and Symptoms

Pain and swelling in the knee are two indicators that something is wrong with the knee. It is possible that the patient will experience difficulty moving the joint. The leg may feel locked up, tight, or as though it is catching when they bend and straighten it. It is extremely concerning if they hear the knee pop and then give out when it hits something. Something tearing could be the source of this popping sound. After a knee injury, the patient might feel as though the ligaments are unstable and cannot stand firmly on the leg. The patient might feel as though their knee is giving out.

3.5.2. Diagnosis of Knee Injuries

The physician will assess and inquire about the symptoms. They may apply light pressure around the patella to check for fluid in the knee joint. Additionally, the doctor will ask the patient to explain how and where they hurt themselves, as well as the nature of their pain. To check for any damage to the patient's knee ligaments or soft tissues, the doctor might ask them to stand, sit, or lie down. The patient's leg will be moved into various positions and their knee will be bent and straightened. The physician will refer the patient to an orthopedic surgeon (a physician with expertise in bone, tendon, and ligament surgery) if they think the patient needs surgery.

The patient may need to have some other tests too.

- An X-ray or CT scan – this can be used to check for arthritis or a fractured bone.
- An MRI scan – this may help to show up damage to the cartilage or soft tissues of the knee after an injury.
- Knee aspiration – The doctor may remove a sample of fluid from the knee.
- Knee arthroscopy – The surgeon might use a telescope coupled with a tiny camera to peer inside the knee. This may assist in demonstrating the presence of meniscus, cartilage, or ligament damage. The knee injury may be treated concurrently by the physician.

3.5.3. Knee Injury Treatment

If the level of pain in the knee is not excessive, it could be due to overexertion rather than an injury. The standard treatment for this type of pain is rest, ice, compression, and elevation (RICE). If this technique helps alleviate the symptoms and the patient returns to normal, they may not need to consult a doctor. However, it is crucial for them to seek medical attention if they experience severe pain, swelling, bruising, or instability. Ignoring the issue could lead to worsening of the condition, potentially turning a minor sprain into a tear. One of the initial steps in the healing process is to stabilize the injured knee.

The doctor will likely recommend using a brace to restrict movement of the knee joint, which will aid in proper healing, especially in the case of bone fractures. Additionally, crutches may be prescribed to prevent weight-bearing on the injured leg.

1. **Physical Therapy:** The physical therapy program will consist of a series of stretches and exercises over a few weeks to help regain the function of the knee joint. These exercises will also work to strengthen the muscles around the joint.

2. **Surgical Treatment:** In some instances, surgery may be necessary to fully restore function to the knee injury when physical therapy and other treatments are unsuccessful. Certain injuries, like a completely torn ligament, may require surgical intervention as they cannot heal on their own. Many knee surgeries can be minimally invasive and performed using arthroscopic techniques with small incisions and miniature tools. In more severe cases, the surgeon may need to make a larger incision to repair the injury.

3.5.4. Injury Prevention

The following tips may help prevent common knee injuries:

- Warm up by walking and stretching gently before and after playing sports.
- Keep the leg muscles strong by using stairs, riding a stationary bicycle, or working out with weights.
- Avoid sudden changes in the intensity of exercise.
- Replace worn-out shoes. Choose ones that fit properly and provide good traction.
- Maintain a healthy weight to avoid added pressure on the knees.
- Always wear a seatbelt.
- Use knee guards in sports where knees could get injured.

It is crucial to have strong and flexible leg muscles to prevent knee injuries. Seeking immediate medical attention for any knee injuries is important to ensure accurate diagnosis and proper treatment. It is also beneficial to keep the supporting leg muscles strong and practice injury prevention to maintain knee health throughout life.

3.6. Fracture Shaft of Femur

The longest and strongest bone in the body is the femur, which is found in the thigh. The femur is extremely strong, so breaking it typically requires a significant amount of force. For example, car crashes are the leading cause of femur fractures. The femoral shaft, which is the long and straight portion of the femur, is prone to fractures. A fracture along this length of bone is referred to as a femoral shaft fracture. Surgery is almost always necessary for this type of leg fracture to heal.

3.6.1. Types of Femoral Shaft Fractures

Classification systems are used by doctors to describe fractures to each other. The severity of femur fractures is determined based on:

- The location of the fracture (the femoral shaft is segmented into three sections: distal, middle, and proximal).
- The pattern of the fracture (for example, the bone can break in different directions, such as crosswise, lengthwise, or in the middle)
- Whether the skin and muscle over the bone is torn by the injury

The most common types of femoral shaft fractures include:

- **Transverse Fracture:** The break in this kind of fracture is across the femoral shaft in a straight, horizontal line.
- **Oblique Fracture:** An angled line across the shaft characterizes an oblique fracture.
- **Spiral Fracture:** The fracture line bears resemblance to the stripes on a candy cane, encircling the shaft. This type of fracture is induced by a twisting force applied to the thigh.
- **Comminuted Fracture**: A comminuted fracture is one in which the bone has fractured into three or more fragments. The quantity of bone pieces typically matches the force required to shatter the bone.

3.6.2. Cause

A high-energy collision is typically the cause of femoral shaft fractures in young individuals. Auto accidents and motorbike crashes are the most frequent causes of femoral shaft fractures. In addition to gunshot wounds and falls from heights, being struck by a car while walking is also a common cause. A femoral shaft fracture can occur from a lower-force incident in an older person with weaker bones, such as a fall from standing.

3.6.3. Symptoms

A femoral shaft fracture usually results in immediate and severe pain. The injured leg may appear deformed, shorter than the other leg, and no longer straight. Weight-bearing on the affected leg will not be possible.

3.6.4. Diagnosis for Femoral Shaft Fractures

A thorough physical examination is crucial when evaluating these injuries, as important nerves and blood vessels are located near this bone and can be damaged during a fracture. In cases where blood vessels are injured, immediate surgical intervention may be required. The doctor will carefully examine for any open wounds near the injury, as these typically require surgical treatment. In some cases, the bone may protrude through the skin, forming a "tent." If left untreated, this can lead to skin necrosis or the bone cutting through the skin. X-rays are utilized to assess the placement and extent of the fracture. This aids in guiding doctors and patients in making well-informed treatment decisions. Typically, multiple X-rays are taken to display the pattern of the injury. If the fracture extends toward the hip or knee joint, a CT scan is frequently requested to assist in treatment and surgical planning. Occasionally, an MRI is requested for minor fractures or to assist in diagnosing stress fractures that do not appear on regular X-rays.

3.6.5. Non-Surgical Femoral Shaft Fracture Treatment

Adult femur shaft fractures are rarely treated non-operatively. The majority require surgery for proper healing. Children under the age of five may receive braces or casts as treatment. Regular follow-up care, including physical examinations and X-rays, is crucial to ensure proper healing and maintenance of the fracture's position if non-operative care is chosen. Surgery may be necessary in cases of a single fall, persistent noncompliance with bracing or casting, or early walking against medical advice that causes bone displacement.

Without surgery, it may take three to four months for this bone to heal, depending on health and the nature of the injury. Approximately six weeks after the bone has sufficiently healed to prevent displacement with motion, physical therapy is initiated to improve the range of motion in the hips and knees.

3.6.6. Surgical Treatment for Femoral Shaft Fractures

Femoral shaft fractures should be promptly treated by surgeons. However, there are instances when patients are too ill or unstable to undergo surgery, necessitating a postponement of the procedure. The preferred methods for fixing the femur are intramedullary nails or metal plates and screws.

The most popular approach is the insertion of an intramedullary nail through a small incision at the hip or knee. This technique often allows for immediate weight bearing and boasts an exceptionally high success rate. Alternatively, plates and screws can be used, although they require larger incisions and do not permit immediate weight bearing. These are typically employed in adults who have undergone total hip or knee replacements, rendering intramedullary nailing impractical, or in children with open growth plates. Surgery typically lasts one to two hours, and most patients are required to stay overnight.

In certain cases, some patients may require external fixation prior to definitive surgical treatment. This is necessary when there is severe injury to the muscles, nerves, or arteries, or when there is significant contamination from dirt, rocks, or grass. During this procedure, small incisions are made in the bone to insert metal pins, which are then connected to bars to provide stability. After additional procedures to cleanse the wound or heal skin injuries, the external fixator can be removed, and plates, intramedullary nails, or screws and plates can be inserted.

3.6.7. Surgical Complications

Complications can arise from any surgical procedure, regardless of size, with the risk of infection being a major concern. Larger and more contaminated wounds pose a higher risk. Administering antibiotics before surgery can help reduce this risk. There is also a risk of damage to blood vessels and nerves, which can be minimized by having a skilled surgeon involved. Patients with femur fractures are at risk of developing blood clots that can travel to the lungs, potentially leading to serious complications or death. Failure to comply with blood thinning medication can have fatal consequences. In some cases, bones may not heal properly, necessitating additional surgery, often due to patient noncompliance, diabetes, or the use of nicotine products like smoking or chewing tobacco.

3.6.8. Recovery

Typically, it takes 3 to 6 months for femoral shaft fractures to fully heal, with some cases lasting even longer, especially if the fracture was compound, comminuted, or if the patient is a tobacco user.

- **Pain Management:** After undergoing surgery or experiencing an injury, pain is a customary component of the healing process. The physician and nursing staff will endeavor to alleviate the patient's discomfort in order to expedite their recovery. Following surgery or an injury, prescription medications are frequently administered for temporary pain relief. There exist numerous pharmaceutical options to assist in managing pain, including muscle relaxants, opioids, gabapentinoids, acetaminophen, nonsteroidal anti-inflammatory drugs (NSAIDs), and topical analgesics. To minimize the necessity for opioids and facilitate pain control, the doctor may combine these medications. Certain analgesics may have adverse effects that impede the patient's ability to operate a vehicle or perform other tasks. The patient and their doctor will discuss the potential side effects of the pain medications.
- **Weight Bearing:** Early in the healing process, many doctors recommend leg movement. To avoid issues, it is critical to adhere to the doctor's instructions regarding the amount of weight the patient put on the injured leg. After surgery, doctors may occasionally permit patients to bear as much weight as possible on the affected leg. However, the patient might not be able to fully extend the leg weight until the fracture has begun to heal. The patient should carefully follow the doctor's instructions. When patient first start walking, the patient will most likely need assistance from a walker or crutches.
- **Physical Therapy:** Exercises during the healing process are important because the injured area is likely to lose muscle strength. Normal joint motion, flexibility, and muscle strength can all be restored with the aid of physical therapy. It can also assist in controlling the post-operative pain. The patient will probably start learning specific exercises from a physical therapist while the patient is still in the hospital. The therapist will also teach how to use a walker or crutches.

3.6.9. Outcomes

The majority of individuals who experience femoral shaft fractures recover successfully and can resume their usual activities and functions. By six weeks, patients typically feel very comfortable, but they should wait around three months before engaging in more strenuous activities like manual labor, skiing, and motocross to prevent re-injury, hardware issues, or failed healing. If problems arise, revision surgery may be necessary. Occasionally, metal hardware may cause irritation to muscles and tendons, which can be alleviated by removing it approximately one-year post-surgery.

3.7. Fractures Around the Hip

Hip fractures are common. Each year, more than 3,00,000 people in the US experience a hip fracture.

3.7.1. Symptoms

Signs and symptoms of a hip fracture include:

- Inability to get up from a fall or to walk
- Severe pain in the hip or groin
- Inability to put weight on the leg on the side of the injured hip
- Bruising and swelling in and around the hip area
- Shorter leg on the side of the injured hip
- Outward turning of the leg on the side of the injured hip

3.7.2. Causes

Hip fractures can happen to anyone at any age due to a severe impact, like a car crash. A fall from a standing height is the most common cause of hip fractures in older adults. Merely standing on one leg and twisting can result in a hip fracture in a person with extremely weak bones.

3.7.3. Different Types of Hip Fracture

The most common types of hip fractures are:

- **Femoral Neck Fracture**: A femoral neck fracture can occur anywhere between one and two inches away from the hip joint. These fractures can be associated with osteoporosis and are common in the elderly. Due to the fracture's typical interruption of blood supply to the head of the femur, which forms the hip joint, complications may arise.
- **Intertrochanteric Hip Fracture:** An intertrochanteric hip fracture occurs between three and four inches away from the hip joint. This type of fracture may be easier to repair as it does not disrupt the bone's blood supply (Figure 3.7).

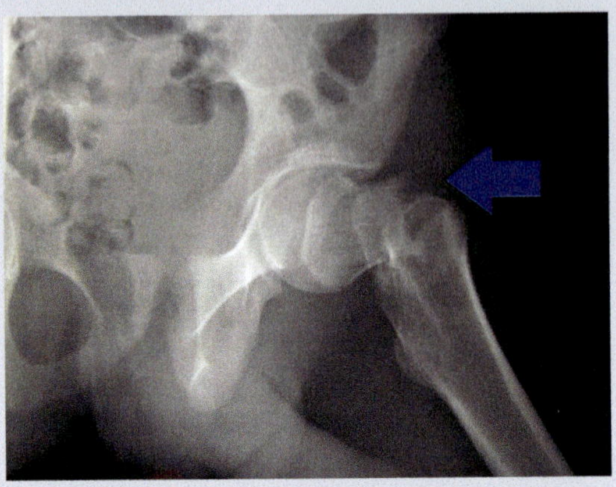

Figure 3.7. *X-ray image of the hip, with the top of the femur broken.*

Source: By Booyabazooka – This is a photograph of an X-ray., CC BY-SA 3.0, https://commons.wikimedia.org/w/index.php?curid=806028.

These two groups account for approximately 90% of hip fractures, with each group having a similar number of cases. Diagnosing a different type of fracture called stress fracture of the hip can be more challenging. This type of fracture is a small crack in the femur that may not affect the entire bone. Stress fractures can occur due to overuse or repetitive motion. The symptoms of this injury can be mistaken for those of a muscle strain or tendinitis.

3.7.4. Risk Factors

There are several factors that can increase the risk of hip fractures.

- **Patient's Age and Sex:** As individuals age, their bone density and muscle mass typically decline. Older adults may experience issues with vision and balance, which predispose them to a higher risk of falls. Women are more likely to sustain hip fractures compared to men, as women experience a faster decrease in bone density due to the decrease in estrogen levels during menopause. It is important to note that men can also develop dangerously low levels of bone density (Figure 3.8).

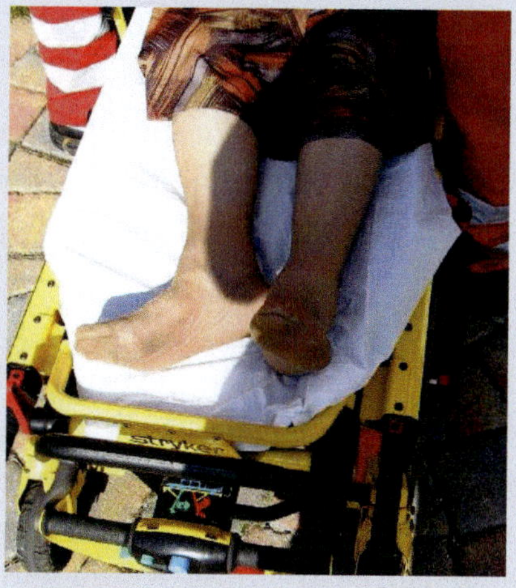

Figure 3.8. *The affected extremity is often shortened and unnaturally externally rotated compared to the unaffected leg.*

Source: By DocP at German Wikipedia – Self-photographed, CC BY-SA 3.0 de, https://commons.wikimedia.org/w/index.php?curid=39746622.

- **Medical Conditions:** The risk of hip fracture can be increased if the patient have:
  - **Osteoporosis:** This disorder weakens and increases the risk of bone fractures.
  - **Thyroid issues:** Fragile bones may result from an overactive thyroid.
  - **Intestinal disorders:** Weakened bones can also result from conditions that decrease the absorption of calcium and vitamin D.
  - **Balance issues:** Peripheral neuropathy, Parkinson's disease, and stroke can all raise the chance of falling. Low blood pressure or blood sugar levels can also increase the chance of falling.
- **Certain Medications:** Long-term use of cortisone medications, such as prednisone, can weaken bones. Dizziness is a side effect of certain medications and combinations of medications that can increase the risk of falling. The medications most commonly associated with falls are sedatives, antipsychotics, and sleep aids.
- **Nutritional Problems:** Inadequate intake of calcium and vitamin D during youth can decrease peak bone mass and elevate the chances of fractures as one ages. It is crucial to ensure sufficient calcium and vitamin D consumption in later years to help sustain bone density. Additionally, being underweight can also heighten the risk of bone deterioration.
- **Lifestyle Choices:** Weakened bones and muscles from not getting regular weight-bearing exercise, such as walking, increase the risk of fractures and falls. Both alcohol and tobacco can impede the regular processes that build and maintain bone, potentially resulting in bone loss.

3.7.5. Hip Fracture Treatment

Surgery is the typical treatment for a hip fracture, which may involve reinforcing the hip with metal implants or complete replacement. The aim is to alleviate pain and restore the ability to engage in everyday activities. The specific surgical approach chosen will depend on the following:

- Patient's age, overall health, and medical history

- The type of fracture(s) identified and the precise location(s)
- Patient's tolerance for specific medications, procedures, or therapies
- Patient's goals and expectations
- Patient's opinions and preferences

Following hip surgery, patients generally require a period of hospitalization prior to proceeding with their rehabilitation either at home or in a rehabilitation facility (Figure 3.9).

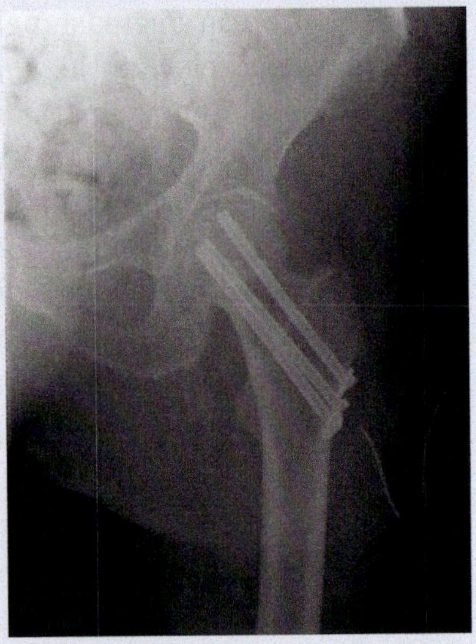

Figure 3.9. *Fracture treated with cannulated screws.*

Source: By Chris-martin, CC BY-SA 3.0, https://commons.wikimedia.org/w/index.php?curid=806170.

3.7.6. Complications

Following hip surgery, patients typically require a period of hospitalization prior to commencing their rehabilitation either at home or in a specialized rehabilitation facility.

In cases where hip fractures have resulted in prolonged immobility, potential complications may include:

- Formation of blood clots in the lower extremities or lungs
- Bedsores
- Occurrence of pneumonia
- Progressive loss of muscle mass, thereby heightening the risk of falls and subsequent injuries
- Mortality

3.7.7. Prevention

Early in adulthood, adopting a healthy lifestyle increases peak bone mass and lowers the chance of developing osteoporosis later in life. Adopting the same measures at any age could potentially reduce falls and enhance general health.

To avoid falls and to maintain healthy bone:

- Ensure an adequate intake of calcium and vitamin D. Generally, individuals aged 50 and above should consume 1,200 mg of calcium and 600 IU of vitamin D daily.
- Engage in exercise to strengthen the bones and improve balance. Weight-bearing exercises such as walking help maintain optimal bone density. Exercise also enhances overall strength, reducing the risk of falls. Given that balance tends to decline with age, it is crucial to include balance training to minimize the risk of falls.
- Steer clear of smoking and binge drinking. The use of alcohol and tobacco can lower bone density. Overindulging in alcohol consumption can also cause balance problems and raise the chance of falling.
- Examine the house for any risks.

Throw rugs should be removed, electrical cords should be secured against the wall, and any potential tripping hazards should be cleared out. Ensure that every room and hallway has sufficient lighting.

- Regularly check eyes. Have your eyes examined every two years, or more frequently if the patient has diabetes or another eye condition.
- Consider using a walker, cane, or walking stick. If the patient have difficulty maintaining stability while walking, consult an occupational therapist or healthcare professional. These devices may provide assistance.

A Closer Look

Role of Osteoporosis and Aging in Geriatric Fractures

The femoral neck undergoes alterations with aging that increase the risk of fracture. Age-related increases in cortical bone porosity are also observed, with porosity rising from 4% in young, healthy patients to nearly 50% in elderly patients. Moreover, as individuals age, the number of microcracks in cortical bone significantly increases. These microcracks develop gradually. Generally, women experience a faster accumulation of these microcracks compared to men. Additionally, the nonenzymatic cross-linking of collagen within the bone can also negatively impact its integrity. These changes in the material properties of bone, including decreased strength, elasticity, and fracture toughness (the energy required to cause a fracture), make low-energy fractures more likely. Elasticity is defined as the maximum stress in a load to failure test. Furthermore, as people age, the cortex of the femoral neck expands, resulting in cortical bone thinning due to greater endosteal expansion than periosteal expansion. Cortical thinning is particularly prominent in the superior aspect of the femoral neck, as it is more susceptible to fractures. This is because it bears less load compared to the inferior regions of the femoral neck.

3.8. Summary

- A fractured foot is a bone injury. An inadvertent misstep or fall could lead to a fractured foot, as well as motor vehicle collisions.
- Foot and ankle fractures can include metatarsal fractures, calcaneus fractures, and ankle fractures. Stress fractures can also occur from overuse of the foot or ankle. It can be challenging to keep up with the various types of foot fractures that exist.
- The physician will examine the tender areas of the foot during the physical examination. The precise location of the pain can aid in identifying its origin.
- Ankle injuries are often linked to sports-related injuries. However, twisting and injuring the ankle does not require the person to be an athlete or even a weekend warrior.
- The ankle is composed of the fibula, talus, and tibia, three major bones, as well as various ligaments and tendons that facilitate movement. Collectively, these components in the joint not only enable movement but also provide stability. Even minor displacements to any part of the ankle have the potential to cause harm. Strains, sprains, and fractures are the most common ankle injuries.
- Ankle discomfort is the initial indication of an issue; it typically presents abruptly and severely. Secondly, discoloration, inflammation, and the incapacity to ambulate or support weight on the affected joint are prevalent symptoms of ankle injuries. Thirdly, there is a possibility that the ankle will feel rigid, sensitive, or even deformed. Weakness or intermittent ankle discomfort may have been experienced if the issue had been at a lower level.
- Fractures to the tibia are common occurrences. The tibia is particularly susceptible to open injuries due to its location beneath the skin. The musculature surrounding the lower leg is divided into four compartments, which are separated by fascial tissue.
- The primary etiology of tibial shaft fractures is a high-impact collision, such as a motor vehicle or motorcycle accident. Such circumstances have the potential to give rise to a comminuted fracture, wherein the bone is fragmented into multiple pieces.
- The utilization of antibiotics in the early stages is the utmost pivotal element in reducing the rate of infection. It is strongly advised to administer a provisional splint and perform a debridement at the bedside.
- The knee joint is an intricate framework that operates akin to a door hinge, allowing individuals to flex and extend their legs for activities such as sitting, squatting, jumping, and running.
- Discomfort and inflammation in the knee are two indications that something has gone awry with the knee. The patient might have encountered difficulty in moving the joint.
- The femur, situated in the thigh region, is the longest and most robust bone in the human body. It possesses exceptional strength, making it highly resistant to fractures that necessitate a significant amount of force. Notably, motor vehicle accidents are the primary cause of femur fractures.

- The femoral shaft, which denotes the elongated and straight segment of the femur, is susceptible to fractures along its length, commonly referred to as femoral shaft fractures. Surgical intervention is almost always imperative to facilitate the healing process of such a broken leg.
- A hip fracture is a fracture in the femur or upper part of the femur. The majority of hip fractures occur in elderly patients whose osteoporosis has weakened their bones.

References

1. Bachmann, L. M., Kolb, E., Koller, M. T., Steurer, J., & Ter, R. G., (2003). Accuracy of Ottawa ankle rules to exclude fractures of the ankle and mid-foot: Systematic review. *BMJ, 326*(7386), 417.
2. Bauer, M., Bergströ, M., B., Hembor, G., A., & Sandegård, J., (1985). Malleolar fractures: Nonoperative versus operative treatment a controlled study. *Clinical Orthopedics and Related Research, 199*, 17–27.
3. Bernstein, J., (2003). *Musculoskeletal Medicine* (p. 242). Rosemont, IL; American Academy of Orthopedic Surgeons.
4. Beynnon, B. D., Murphy, D. F., & Alosa, D. M., (2002). Predictive factors for lateral ankle sprains: A literature review. *Journal of Athletic Training, 37*(4), 376.
5. Doherty, C., Delahunt, E., Caulfield, B., Hertel, J., Ryan, J., & Bleakley, C., (2014). The incidence and prevalence of ankle sprain injury: A systematic review and meta-analysis of prospective epidemiological studies. *Sports Medicine, 44*(1), 123–140.
6. Fong, D. T., Hong, Y., Chan, L. K., Yung, P. S., & Chan, K. M., (2007). A systematic review on ankle injury and ankle sprain in sports. *Sports Medicine, 37*(1), 73–94.
7. Hubbard, T. J., & Hicks-Little, C. A., (2008). Ankle ligament healing after an acute ankle sprain: An evidence-based approach. *Journal of Athletic Training, 43*(5), 523–529.
8. Alexander Senk, Kersten L. Schwanz, Dean Wundrach, Katherine Weir, Sima C. Patel, and Michael V. Nguyen. *Ankle and Foot Neuropathies & Entrapments.* PM& R Knowledge Now. Available from: https://now.aapmr.org/ankle-and-foot-neuropathies-entrapments/ (accessed on 20 March 2024).
9. Lacerda, D., Pacheco, D., Rocha, A. T., Diniz, P., Pedro, I., & Pinto, F. G., (2022). Current concept review: State of acute lateral ankle injury classification systems. *The Journal of Foot and Ankle Surgery, 62*(1), 197–203.
10. Larkins, L. W., Baker, R. T., & Baker, J. G., (2020). Physical examination of the ankle: A review of the original orthopedic special test description and scientific validity of common tests for ankle examination. *Archives of Rehabilitation Research and Clinical Translation, 2*(3), 100072.
11. Marc, A. M., (2023). *Talofibular Ligament Injury* [Internet]. Background, Epidemiology, Functional Anatomy. Medscape. Available from: https://emedicine.medscape.com/article/86396-overview (accessed on 20 March 2024).
12. McKay, G. D., Goldie, P. A., Payne, W. R., & Oakes, B. W., (2001). Ankle injuries in basketball: Injury rate and risk factors. *British Journal of Sports Medicine, 35*(2), 103–108.
13. Melanson, S. W., & Shuman, V. L., (2022). Acute ankle sprain. In: *StatPearls*. Treasure Island (FL): Stat Pearls Publishing.

14. Norkus, S. A., & Floyd, R. T., (2001). The anatomy and mechanisms of syndesmotic ankle sprains. *Journal of Athletic Training, 36*(1), 68.

15. Rhon, D. I., Fraser, J. J., Sorensen, J., Greenlee, T. A., Jain, T., & Cook, C. E., (2021). Delayed rehabilitation is associated with recurrence and higher medical care use after ankle sprain injuries in the United States military health system. *J. Orthop. Sports Phys. Ther., 51*(12), 619–627. doi: 10.2519/jospt.2021.10730.

16. Roos, K. G., Kerr, Z. Y., Mauntel, T. C., Djoko, A., Dompier, T. P., & Wikstrom, E. A., (2017). The epidemiology of lateral ligament complex ankle sprains in National Collegiate Athletic Association Sports. *The American Journal of Sports Medicine*, *45*(1), 201–209. https://doi.org/10.1177/0363546516660980.

17. Soboroff, S. H., Pappius, E. M., & Komaroff, A. L., (1984). Benefits, risks, and costs of alternative approaches to the evaluation and treatment of severe ankle sprain. *Clinical Orthopedics and Related Research*, (183), 160–168.

18. Yeung, M. S., Chan, K. M., So, C. H., & Yuan, W. Y., (1994). An epidemiological survey on ankle sprain. *British Journal of Sports Medicine*, *28*(2), 112–116. https://doi.org/10.1136/bjsm.28.2.112

Chapter 4

FRACTURES OF THE PELVIS

Contents

4.1. Introduction

The pelvis is a complex of bones in the shape of a basin that, according to human anatomy, connects the trunk to the legs, balances, and supports the trunk, and houses and supports the internal sex organs, the intestines, and the bladder. The pelvis is made up of paired hipbones that are joined in front at the pubic symphysis and in the back by the sacrum. Each hipbone is composed of three bones: the pubis, which is in front, the ischium, which is behind and below where the weight falls when sitting, and the ilium, which is shaped like a blade and located above and to either side. Early in adulthood, all three come together at a triangular suture in the acetabulum, the cup-shaped socket where the head of the femur (thighbone) joins the hip. In females, the ring formed by the pelvis serves as the birth canal. The muscles that move the legs, hips, and trunk as well as balance and support the trunk are attached to the pelvis. The human infant's pelvis is nonsupportive and narrow. The child's pelvis widens and tilts as they start to walk, the lumbar curve of the lower back develops, and the sacrum descends deeper into its articulation with the ilia.

The pelvis is positioned horizontally, and the ilium is long and somewhat spoon-shaped. When a person stands upright, their center of gravity is above their midsection, and their weight is distributed from the spinal column to the thigh, knee, and foot through the pelvis. The ileum broadens backward in a fan shape, forming a deep sciatic notch posteriorly. The anterior superior iliac spine, located on the upper front edge of the iliac blade, is closer to the hip joint. The ischium is shorter, and a bone strut called the arcuate eminence has developed on the ilium diagonally from the hip joint, contributing to lateral balance in upright posture. These are some of the morphological differences from apes. The pelvis of the extinct mammal *Australopithecus africanus* is unmistakably that of a hominin (of human ancestry) from over 2 million years ago. The pelvises of *Homo erectus* and all subsequent extinct hominins, including Neanderthals, were completely modern.

The pelvis differs significantly between the sexes, reflecting the need for the female to provide a sufficient birth canal for a fetus with a large head. The female pelvis differs from the male pelvis in that the pubic symphysis is short, with the pubic bones forming a broad angle with one another. The sacrum is short, broad, and only slightly curved, while the coccyx is movable. Additionally, the acetabula is farther apart. The birth canal is rounded and capacious. It is only during puberty that these disparities take on adult proportions. For both males and females, the age at death can be estimated based on wear patterns on the pubic symphyses.

Limb-girdle muscular dystrophy affects the pelvis. Over time, the voluntary muscles surrounding the shoulder and pelvic regions weaken. Pelvic girdle pain (PGP) is a condition that can arise during pregnancy due to increased instability in the pelvic joints. While full recovery may take years, PGP usually resolves on its own in the weeks or months after childbirth.

Orientation and Directional Terms

Term	Definition	Illustration
Pelvic bone	The pelvic skeleton is formed posteriorly (in the area of the back) by the sacrum and the coccyx, and laterally and anteriorly (forward and to the sides) by a pair of hip bones.	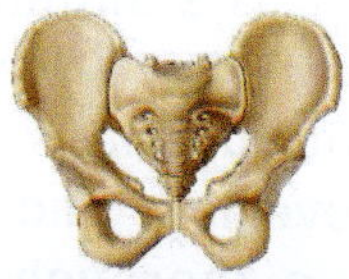
Pelvic cavity	The pelvic cavity is a body cavity that is bounded by the bones of the pelvis and primarily contains reproductive organs and the rectum.	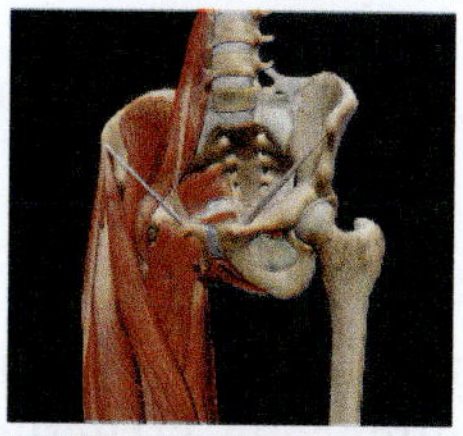
Pelvic floor	The pelvic floor has two inherently conflicting functions: one is to close the pelvic and abdominal cavities and bear the load of the visceral organs, while the other is to control the openings of the rectum and urogenital organs that pierce the pelvic floor and weaken it.	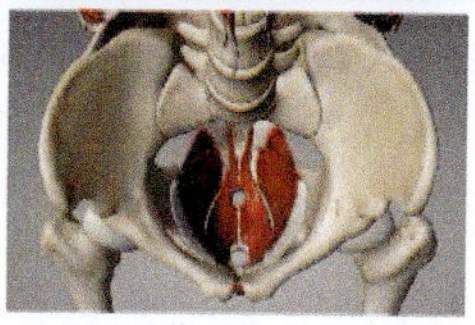
Levator ani	The levator ani is a broad, thin muscle group, situated on either side of the pelvis. It is formed from three muscle components: the pubococcygeus, the iliococcygeus, and the puborectalis.	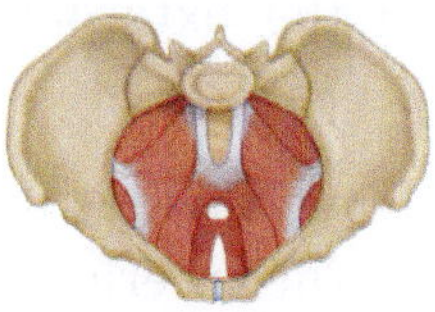
Coccygeus muscle	The coccygeus muscle, also known as the ischiococcygeus, is a muscle of the pelvic floor. It is located posterior to the levator ani and anterior to the sacrospinous ligament.	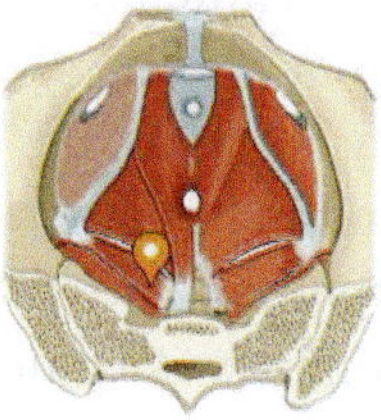

4.2. Structure and Function

The pelvis serves multiple functions, primarily providing structural support and stability for activities such as standing, walking, and running. Each unique structure within the pelvis allows for specific functions that contribute to the overall movement and stability of the body. Therefore, a thorough understanding of each individual structure is essential in comprehending the pelvis's overall functions.

4.2.1. The Bony Pelvis

From a load-bearing standpoint, the bony pelvis serves numerous structural purposes. The way the ligaments and bones in the pelvis are arranged enables the pelvis to support an individual's weight above it, stabilize them, and enable them to sit and stand while their inferior legs move. In addition to protecting the pelvic and abdominopelvic viscera, the bony structure acts as an anchor for various muscles and other tissues, including the external reproductive organs.

The bony pelvis is divided into an anterior and posterior part. The anterior portion, known as the pelvic girdle, includes the pubis, ischium, and ilium. It is connected to the pelvic spine at the back, which is made up of the coccyx and sacrum. The pubic bone, ischial bone, and iliac bone come together on each side to form the innominate bones, with one on the right and one on the left. The two innominate bones create a pelvic ring structure, with stability provided by strong ligaments. Displacement can only occur if the ring is disrupted in two places. Most neurovascular structures are located at the back of the pelvis.

Four pelvic joints are composed of the pelvic bones. Two sacroiliac joints are connected to the sacrum, one symphysis pubis is located anteriorly, and one sacrococcygeal joint is located posteriorly. The sacrococcygeal joint is a hinge joint that connects the coccyx and sacrum. The sacroiliac joints are the strongest joints in the body. There is cartilage between the cartilaginous joints that form the symphysis pubis. The slightly movable joint that connects the sacrum and coccyx is known as the sacrococcygeal symphysis. As individuals age, this joint typically deteriorates. Between the two ischial tuberosities, there is a line that divides the area into two triangles. The term "urogenital triangle" refers to the anterior triangle, while the term "anal triangle" refers to the posterior triangle. In males, the penis is located in the anterior triangle, while the anus is located in the posterior triangle in both genders.

There are four types of coccyx:

- **Type I:** This coccyx is curved anteriorly with its apex turned downwards.
- **Type II:** This coccyx has a deeper curvature with its apex turned forward.
- **Type III:** This coccyx is angled sharply forward.
- **Type IV:** This coccyx is subluxated at the sacrococcygeal joint.

4.2.2. The Pelvic Cavity

The pelvic cavity is the area that lies between the pelvic bones. The abdominal and pelvic cavities are connected superiorly. The Pelvic Floor borders the pelvic cavity inferiorly. The greater and lesser pelvises are the two sections that make up the pelvic cavity. The greater pelvis is also known as the false pelvis because it is a component of the abdomen. The lesser pelvis is also referred to as the true pelvis since it is a component of the pelvis. The posterior region contains the coccyx and sacrum. The rectum, internal reproductive organs, pelvic colon, and urinary bladder are all housed inside the pelvic cavity. Other internal tissues and structures found in the pelvic cavity include muscles, arteries, veins, nerves, and the pelvic connective tissue.

4.2.3. The Pelvic Floor

The lowermost layer of muscle in the pelvic cavity is known as the pelvic floor. It separates the perineum, which is located below the pelvic floor, from the superior pelvic cavity. It provides support for the visceral organs and acts as a boundary between the abdominal cavity and the pelvis. Additionally, it plays a role in controlling the opening of the urogenital and rectal canals. The pelvic floor supports various structures including the rectum, anus, pelvic colon, female vagina, uterus, and female urinary bladder. Through tonic contractions, it also functions as an anal sphincter and bladder sphincter. The muscle fibers of the pelvic floor help prevent incontinence by sphinctering the urethra and rectum. These muscles relax to facilitate urination and defecation. Moreover, the pelvic floor aids in maintaining intra-abdominal pressure during activities such as coughing or lifting heavy objects.

The pelvic floor is composed of the urogenital triangle, the urogenital diaphragm, and the pelvic diaphragm:

- **Urogenital Triangle:** It is innervated by the pudendal nerve and consists of the external anal sphincter, the superficial transverse perineal, the Ischiocavernosus, and the Bulbospongiosus muscles.
- **Urogenital Diaphragm:** This which includes the Compressor urethra and the Ureterovaginal sphincter, is also innervated by the pudendal nerve.
- **Pelvic Diaphragm:** On the other hand, is innervated by sacral nerve roots S3 through S5 and is comprised of the levator ani, the coccygeus, the piriformis, and the obturator internus.

4.2.4. The Perineum

The urogenital hiatus and the rectal hiatus are two openings in the pelvic floor. The female urethra and vagina are located in the urogenital hiatus, while the anal canal is located in the rectal hiatus. The perineal body is situated at the urogenital and rectal hiatuses. The perineum, which is a diamond-shaped region, extends from the male scrotum to the vagina in females and from the anus to both.

4.3. Types of Pelvic Fracture

Since the pelvis is composed of a ring of bones, a forceful injury to one area of the structure may result in a corresponding fracture at another location. Depending on the orientation and intensity of the trauma, there are a few common patterns (Figure 4.1).

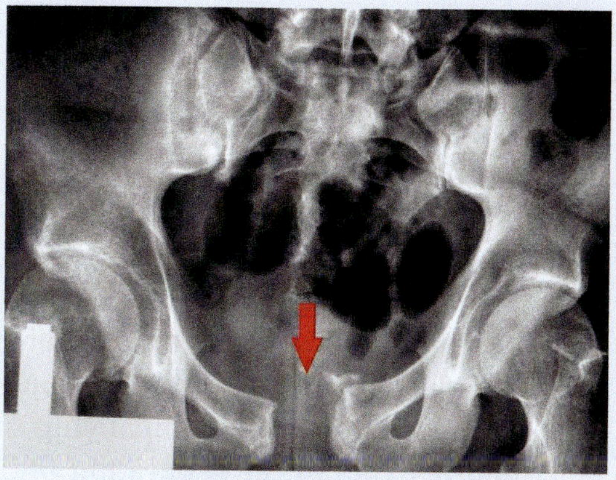

Figure 4.1. *Post-traumatic open book pelvis fracture and significant diastasis in the symphysis pubis.*

Source: By © Nevit Dilmen, CC BY-SA 3.0, https://commons.wikimedia.org/w/index.php?curid=11808703.

4.3.1. Stable and Unstable Fractures

Differentiating pelvic fractures into stable and unstable fractures may be the most crucial classification scheme. Most fractures of the pelvis are stable:

- **Stable Fracture:** The ring has maintained its shape because the fractured bones are still correctly aligned. Typically, a single fracture affects just one bone.

Common fracture patterns include:

- Breaks across the top of one ilium;
- Cracks to the pubic ramus on one side;
- Cracks in the sacrum.

The remaining bones in each of these situations are sound and will maintain the integrity of the pelvic bony ring. Other forms of stable pelvic fractures are pelvic stress fractures, which are hairline cracks that do not extend completely across the bone, and pelvic avulsion fractures, in which a piece of bone is broken off due to the pull of a muscle.

- **Unstable Fracture:** This typically occurs when the ends of the broken bones separate and there are two or more breaks in the pelvic ring. Since this type of fracture is more likely to occur following a high-impact injury, there may also be accompanying injuries. Due to the separation of the broken bones, the bleeding from these injuries is significantly more extensive compared to stable fractures. They may also cause actual harm to the internal organs.

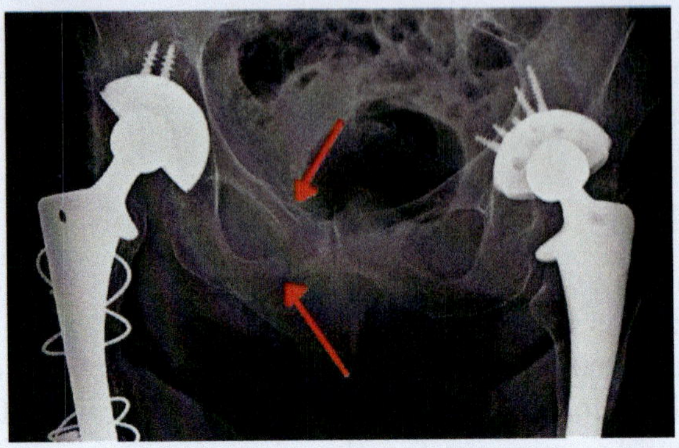

Figure 4.2. *Fractures of the superior (in two places) and inferior pubic rami on the person's right, in a person who has had prior hip replacements.*

Source: By James Heilman, MD – Own work, CC BY-SA 4.0, https://commons.wikimedia.org/w/index.php?curid=49061288.

Several common patterns of unstable fractures exist. These include "open book" fractures, which happen when a strong force from the front breaks the pelvis both in the front and back (as in a major car accident), and lateral (or sideways) force fractures, which often involve fractures in the sacroiliac and pubic rami joints and occasionally affect the hip socket as well (Figure 4.2).

4.3.2. Open and Closed Fractures

Pelvic fractures can be categorized as either stable or unstable, and can also be classified as either open or closed. Open fractures involve injuries to the skin, making the broken bones visible, while closed fractures do not break the skin. Open fractures are considered more severe as they are susceptible to infection, which can easily reach the wound and potentially worsen contamination from the initial injury.

4.4. Causes of Pelvic Fractures

Major pelvic fractures are caused by major trauma such as:

- Road traffic accidents;
- Crush injuries (for example, being run over by a car or rolled on by a horse);
- Falls from a height.

High-speed or high-force injuries can result in pelvic fractures, which are frequently unstable and require immediate hospital care. After falls or trips, less severe fractures involving undisplaced fractures can happen, especially if the bones are "thin" (osteoporosis). Because they often have "thinner" bones and are occasionally more likely to fall, elderly people are more likely to suffer from painful but stable fractures.

4.4.1. Causes of Pelvic Avulsion Fractures

A pelvic avulsion fracture occurs when a muscle tendon separates from the bone, taking a small piece of the bone with it. The front of the ilium, where one of the large quadriceps muscles attaches, or the bottom of the ischium, where the major hamstring muscles are attached, are the most common sites for this type of fracture. Sports that involve sudden stops and accelerations are the primary cause of these fractures, particularly in younger athletes who are still growing and developing.

Examples are:

- Hurdling;
- Sprinting;
- Long-jumping;
- Football (particularly miskicks that hit the ground).

A pelvic avulsion fracture may also be caused by a car accident.

4.4.2. Causes of Pelvic Stress Fractures

Repetitive stresses to the bone, usually from sports, can result in pelvic stress fractures. These fractures typically do not require cessation of exercise, but they often affect the pubic bone and cause pain that worsens with physical activity. The highest risk of stress fractures is found in sports such as running and jumping, which involve repeated impact. Stress fractures frequently occur in individuals who suddenly increase their training distance or intensity, including those who are inactive and begin exercising. They are uncommon in the pelvis, although more common in women and those with 'thinning' of the bones (osteoporosis).

4.5. Symptoms

Significant trauma can cause significant fractures of the pelvis in any person. Seniors with "thinner" bones (osteoporosis) are more likely to experience less severe, stable fractures. Adolescent athletes are especially susceptible to avulsion fractures. Although stress fractures more frequently affect sites other than the pelvis, they are commonly observed in runners.

4.5.1. Symptoms of Stable Pelvic Fractures

A stable pelvic fracture typically causes pain in the hip or groin, which worsens when the hip is moved or when walking. Despite the discomfort, some patients may still be able to walk. Keeping one hip or knee bent may provide some relief for the pain.

Other symptoms will vary with the severity of the fracture. They may include:

- Pain and tenderness in the groin, hip, lower back, buttock, or pelvis;
- Bruising and swelling over the pelvic bones;

- Numbness or tingling in the genital area or in the upper thighs;
- Pain may also be present on sitting or straining.

There might be obvious evidence of bleeding. There are various locations on the skin where bleeding can appear, some of which are more likely to be seen than others. They include:

- Bruising over the pelvic bones themselves;
- Bruising or a tender lump in the groin or on the perineum;
- Bruising in the small of the back;
- Vaginal bleeding in women and bruising to the scrotum in men;
- Blood in the urine or coming from the back passage.
- *Note:* Even in patients who are initially walking around, a significant trauma such as a car accident increases the likelihood of a serious pelvic fracture. Following a major accident, it is critical to keep survivors warm and motionless until emergency services arrive. This could prevent deadly bleeding and even save lives.

4.5.2. Symptoms of Unstable Pelvic Fractures

4.5.2.1. Major and Unstable Pelvic Fractures

Major and unstable pelvic fractures are likely to result in significant blood loss, sufficient to produce life-threatening symptoms or even death, as well as excruciating pain. Pain may be experienced in the back, groin, pelvis, stomach (abdomen), or down the legs.

Due to their size and abundant blood supply, the pelvic bones bleed profusely and take a long time to stop when fractured. Blood pressure will drop suddenly due to this amount of blood loss, even though the blood may not be visible because it is inside the stomach. Those who are affected will appear pale, clammy, and extremely ill—possibly even unconscious.

4.5.2.2. Pelvic Avulsion Fractures

Pelvic avulsion fractures most commonly occur in young, active athletes who are still growing. Symptoms typically include sudden pain during a powerful movement, often felt in the bottom, buttock crease, or front of the hip. Weakness and pain may follow when performing movements that involve the affected tendon and muscle. Bruising and swelling are common.

4.5.2.3. Pelvic Stress Fractures

One of the mildest types of stable fractures is stress fractures, which are caused by a tiny crack in the bone that does not go through completely. Pelvic stress fractures can be difficult to detect because the pain can be elusive. The most common symptom is a dull pain that is initially hard to pinpoint. With more exercise, this might get better, but eventually, it might get worse.

4.6. Evaluation

Abdominal and pelvic computed tomography (CT) scans provide optimal visualization of pelvic anatomy and allow for assessment of intraperitoneal, retroperitoneal, or pelvic bleeding. Furthermore, a CT scan can confirm hip dislocation and aid in determining the presence or absence of an associated acetabular fracture. Conversely, anteroposterior (AP) pelvic radiograph serves as the most effective screening test for pelvic fractures, detecting approximately 90% of pelvic injuries. While routine CT scans of the abdomen and pelvis are typically performed for most trauma patients, AP pelvic radiographs should be considered as a rapid diagnostic method for hemodynamically unstable patients, facilitating prompt initiation of treatment. As part of the Focus Assessment with Sonography for Trauma (FAST) examination, the pelvis should also be evaluated to identify the source of intraperitoneal bleeding and potentially detect pelvic injuries. In patients with suspected urethral tear, retrograde urethrography may be performed, such as in men presenting with blood at the urethral meatus or women who, despite cautious attempts, are unable to undergo Foley catheter placement, or those with a vaginal tear or palpable fragments adjacent to the urethra.

Individuals presenting with hematuria in the setting of an intact urethra (e.g., suspected of having a urinary bladder injury) should undergo cystography. Pelvic angiography can be used to identify hidden or apparent injuries, enable embolization of any injured arteries, and aid in visualization before manipulative reduction if a patient is still bleeding after receiving sufficient intravenous fluid replacement and pelvic stabilization.

4.7. Fractured Pelvis Treatment and Surgery

Depending on the stability of the broken bone and whether the fracture is displaced or not, treatment for pelvic fractures can involve either non-surgical or surgical methods. Surgery is typically necessary for severe pelvic fractures.

4.7.1. Non-Surgical Treatment

For stable, non-displaced fractures of the pelvis, it is recommended to pursue nonsurgical treatment. These include specific fractures of the iliac wing, isolated fractures of the sacrum, fractures of the isolated pubic ramus, and avulsion fractures. Non-operative treatment is also typically administered to elderly patients with insufficiency fractures. To ensure proper healing and maintenance of the fracture's correct alignment, regular follow-up care, including physical examinations and X-rays, is crucial if non-operative care is chosen. If the patient have diabetes, it is imperative to reduce or cease smoking and maintain strict control over blood sugar levels to facilitate the recovery process. Surgery may be necessary in cases of a single fall or persistent disregard for medical advice regarding early ambulation.

While some fractures do not require immediate weight bearing, others do. Patients will need walkers or crutches as gait aids. Without surgery, this bone may take three to four months to heal, depending on health and the nature of the injury. About six weeks after the bone has sufficiently healed to prevent displacement with motion, physical therapy is initiated to improve the range of motion in the hips and knees. For two to six weeks, the majority of patients will be put on a blood thinner to prevent clots.

4.7.2. Surgical Treatment

Surgery is necessary for an unstable fractured pelvis. These pelvic fractures are best treated as soon as possible by surgeons. However, the surgery must wait until the patients are given the all-clear by the general surgeons to undergo surgery because a significant number of them have additional injuries. In some cases, a patient may be too ill or unstable to undergo surgery, resulting in a postponement of several days. There are various surgical techniques and types of pelvic fracture surgery available to treat hip socket fractures, as they can occur in different ways. The most suitable approach for each pattern of injuries will be determined by the surgeon. Typically, plates and screws are used to secure these fractures. A combination of large and small incisions is made to treat these injuries. The surgery usually takes one to three hours. After the surgery, the majority of patients remain in the hospital for a few days.

4.8. Complications

Any surgery, regardless of size, can have complications. Surgical repair for a pelvic fracture carries several common risks that are listed below:

- Significantly larger and more contaminated traumatic wounds carry a higher risk of infection. Administering an antibiotic dose before surgery can minimize this risk.
- Neural or vascular damage can develop following pelvic fracture surgery. With care from an experienced surgeon, this risk can be minimized.
- After surgery, blood clots may form in the legs. If left untreated, these blood clots may break off and enter the lungs, potentially resulting in fatalities and significant bleeding issues. It is important to properly administer blood-thinning drugs, as they can be fatal if taken improperly. In some cases, additional surgery may be required if the bone does not heal. Factors such as diabetes, patient noncompliance, or nicotine use (such as smoking and chewing tobacco) are typically associated with this.
- Sexual dysfunction is a complication of surgery for pelvic fractures, as these injuries are unique. Approximately 30% of patients experience sexual dysfunction, which may include painful sex for women and erectile dysfunction for men. It is crucial to inform the surgeon about these symptoms in order to receive the appropriate referral and care.

4.9. Recovery After Pelvic Fracture Surgery

It usually takes 4–6 months for most people to heal from a broken pelvis. Patients can resume their previous activities and function if anatomic alignment was achieved during surgery and no complications arise. Patients feel reasonably at ease after six weeks. It takes approximately four months to fully release them to activities like manual labor, motocross, and skiing. Re-fracture, hardware breakage, or nonunion can occur from an aggressive return to activity too soon. Revision surgery is necessary in these circumstances. The hardware used during surgery may cause pain to patients. Six to twelve months after surgery, some of these screws may be extracted.

4.9.1. Pain Management

After undergoing surgery, there will be some discomfort. This is a customary phase of the recovery process. The surgeon and nursing staff will endeavor to alleviate the discomfort so that the patient can expedite the healing from the surgery. Following the procedure, medications are frequently prescribed to provide temporary relief from pain. A wide array of medications, including opioids, non-steroidal anti-inflammatory drugs (NSAIDs), and local anesthetics, are available to assist in managing pain. To minimize the necessity for opioids and enhance pain relief, the doctor may combine these medications.

While opioids can alleviate post-operative pain, they are still classified as narcotics and have the potential to be habit-forming. In the United States, opioid addiction and overdose have emerged as significant public health concerns. Opioids should only be used as prescribed by the physician, and the patient should discontinue their use as soon as the pain begins to diminish. If, after a few days following the surgery, the patient's pain has not started to subside, please consult the doctor.

4.9.2. Early Movement

The doctor will usually recommend early movement. As soon as possible following surgery, the majority of patients start walking, albeit with weight-bearing restrictions, and engaging in foot and leg exercises.

4.9.3. Physical Therapy

The patient can improve the range of motion and flexibility in the hips by performing specific exercises. Additionally, enhance the ability to carry out daily tasks by incorporating additional exercises that will help to gain strength and endurance.

4.9.4. Blood Clot Prevention

Despite the encouragement of early movement, the post-operative mobility will still be somewhat restricted. To mitigate the risk of blood clots forming in the deep veins of the legs and pelvis, the doctor may prescribe an anticoagulant, also known as a blood thinner.

4.9.5. Weightbearing

For a period of time, the doctor might advise to utilize a walker or crutches. After three months, or once the bones have completely healed, the patient can typically resume full weight bearing. It is possible that the patient may need to rely on a cane or other walking assistance for an extended duration.

A Closer Look

History and Physical of Pelvis Fracture

A comprehensive trauma evaluation is necessary because injuries to the pelvis indicate a high-energy mechanism of injury. According to the guidelines of the American College of Surgeons, every patient should undergo regular evaluations, such as the advanced trauma life support protocol, to assess for potentially fatal injuries, regardless of whether they are hip-related. Pelvic ring fractures are often associated with axial or appendicular spine trauma. The spine and extremities should also be examined to check for limb length disparities and evident angular or rotational deformities. An initial neurological examination is essential for appropriate management and monitoring, as pelvic injuries may involve neurovascular structures that traverse the pelvis.

Even in closed fractures, concurrent blood loss is common, so medical professionals should closely monitor the hemodynamic status of patients with pelvic fractures. Intraabdominal bleeding occurs in up to 40% of cases, but these injuries can also result in intrathoracic, retroperitoneal, or compartmental bleeding. Bleeding within the pelvis, typically caused by shearing of the venous plexus, can result in hemorrhages containing up to 4L of blood. An arterial injury to the superior gluteal artery due to posterior pelvic fractures is a surgical emergency. Evaluation of soft-tissue injuries can provide further insight into the extent of the patient's injuries. It is particularly important to check for any perineum lacerations, such as the rectum or vagina, as this would indicate a severe injury and fractures potentially contaminated by urine, stool, or other environmental contaminants.

The L5 or S1 nerve roots are frequently affected by neurological injuries caused by pelvic fractures. In addition to a sacral fracture, there may also be an injury to the S2–S5 sacral nerve roots, which can result in sexual dysfunction and bowel or bladder incontinence.

4.10. Summary

- The pelvis serves multiple functions, primarily providing structural support and stability for activities such as standing, walking, and running.
- The osseous pelvis is partitioned into a preceding and subsequent segment. The preceding segment, recognized as the pelvic girdle, encompasses the pubis, ischium, and ilium. It is connected to the pelvic spine at the posterior, which is composed of the coccyx and sacrum.
- The pelvic cavity is the region that is situated between the pelvic bones. The abdominal and pelvic cavities are connected in a superior manner. The Pelvic Floor delineates the pelvic cavity in an inferior direction. The greater and lesser pelvises constitute the two divisions that comprise the pelvic cavity.
- The deepest layer of muscle in the actual pelvic cavity is referred to as the pelvic floor. It separates the perineum, which is situated below the pelvic floor, from the superior pelvic cavity. It provides support for the weight of the visceral organs and acts as a boundary between the abdominal cavity and the pelvis.
- The urogenital hiatus and the rectal hiatus are two apertures in the pelvic floor. The female urethra and vagina are situated within the urogenital hiatus. The anal canal is situated within the rectal hiatus.
- Differentiating pelvic fractures into stable and unstable fractures may be the most crucial classification scheme.
- Pelvic fractures can be classified as either stable or unstable, and can also be categorized as either open or closed. Open fractures involve injuries to the skin, thereby rendering the broken bones visible, while closed fractures do not rupture the skin.
- High-speed or high-force injuries can lead to pelvic fractures, which are frequently unstable and necessitate immediate hospital care.
- A pelvic avulsion fracture occurs when a muscle tendon becomes detached from the bone, carrying a small fragment of the bone along with it. The most common sites for this type of fracture are the anterior aspect of the ilium, where one of the major quadriceps muscles attaches, or the inferior aspect of the ischium, where the large hamstring muscles are attached.
- Repetitive stresses to the bone, usually from sports, result in pelvic stress fractures.
- Significant trauma can result in substantial fractures of the pelvis in any individual. Elderly individuals with "thinner" bones (osteoporosis) are more prone to experiencing less severe, stable fractures. Adolescent athletes are particularly vulnerable to avulsion fractures. Although stress fractures more commonly affect areas other than the pelvis, they are frequently observed in runners.
- Abdominal and pelvic computed tomography (CT) scans provide the most comprehensive view of pelvic anatomy and allow for the assessment of any intraperitoneal, retroperitoneal, or pelvic bleeding.

- Based on the stability of the fractured bone and the presence of displacement, the management of pelvic fractures may encompass either non-operative or operative approaches. Surgical intervention is generally indicated for severe pelvic fractures.
- It usually takes 4–6 months for most people to heal from a broken pelvis. Patients can resume their previous activities and function if anatomic alignment was achieved during surgery and no complications arise.

References

1. Coccolini, F., Stahel, P. F., Montori, G., et al., (2017). Pelvic trauma: WSES classification and guidelines. *World J. Emerg. Surg., 12*, 5. doi: 10.1186/s13017-017-0117-6. eCollection 2017.
2. Dallimore, J., Jules, B., Jon, D., McClellan, C. M., Harvey, P., James, C., & James, W., (2015). *Treatment: Limbs and Back*. Oxford University Press. http://dx.doi.org/10.1093/med/9780199688418.003.0014.
3. Dallimore, J., Jules, B., Jon, D., McClellan, C. M., Harvey, P., James, C., & James, W., (2018). *Treatment: Limbs and Back*. Oxford University Press. http://dx.doi.org/10.1093/med/9780199688418.003.0014_update_001.
4. Davis, D. D., Foris, L. A., Kane, S. M., & Waseem, M., (2021). Pelvic fracture. *StatPearls* [Internet]. Treasure Island, FL: StatPearls Publishing. https://www.ncbi.nlm.nih.gov/books/NBK430734/ (accessed on 20 March 2024).
5. Filler, A. G., (2018). In: Meghan, E. L., Nasa, F., & Kevin, C. C., (eds.), *Piriformis Syndrome and Other Nerve Entrapments of the Posterior Pelvis*. Oxford University Press. http://dx.doi.org/10.1093/med/9780190617127.003.0011.
6. OrthoInfo. *Pelvic Fractures*. https://orthoinfo.aaos.org/en/diseases--conditions/pelvic-fractures/ (accessed on 20 March 2024).
7. Parikh, R. A., & David, M. W., (2018). In: Lowell, K. S., Bulent, A., & Abdulrahman, M., (eds.), *Proximal Arterial Occlusion During Treatment of Pelvic High-Flow Arteriovenous Malformations*. Oxford University Press. http://dx.doi.org/10.1093/med/9780199986071.003.0029.
8. Ribbans, B., & Cathy, S., (2013). *Injuries to the Foot*. Oxford University Press. http://dx.doi.org/10.1093/med/9780199533909.003.0033.
9. Sabri, O., & Martin, B., (2016). *Management of Limb and Pelvic Injuries*. Oxford University Press. http://dx.doi.org/10.1093/med/9780199600830.003.0336.
10. Soles, G. L. S., & Ferguson, T. A., (2012). Fragility fractures of the pelvis. *Current Review of Musculoskeletal Medicine*, *5*(3), 222–228. https://www.ncbi.nlm.nih.gov/pmc/articles/PMC3535080/#!po=1.85185 (accessed on 20 March 2024).
11. Speed, C., Jae, R., & Fares, H., (2013). *Injuries to the Pelvis, Hip, and Thigh*. Oxford University Press. http://dx.doi.org/10.1093/med/9780199533909.003.0027.
12. Stacey, V., (2013). *Major Trauma*. Oxford University Press. http://dx.doi.org/10.1093/med/9780199592777.003.0004.
13. Wolman, R., (2011). *Sports Injuries in the Pelvic Region*. Oxford University Press. http://dx.doi.org/10.1093/med/9780199550647.003.007015.

Chapter 5

SPINAL INJURIES

Contents

5.1. Introduction

Damage to the spinal cord, a substantial bundle of nerve fibers that connects the brain to nearly every other nerve in the body, results in a spinal cord injury (SCI). These injuries can range from minor and treatable to severe and irreversible. The spinal cord is one of the two components of the central nervous system (CNS). It functions like a multilane freeway, facilitating the flow of information to and from the brain. The other component of the CNS is the nervous system, which contains channels for incoming and outgoing information to the brain.

The spinal nerves, resembling on-ramps, branch out from the spinal cord and connect to various parts of the body. These nerves transmit nerve signals, acting as vehicles on this expressway. Spinal cord injuries, similar to lane closures on a freeway, can disrupt the flow of nerve signals. However, unlike an actual expressway, there are no detours in the spinal cord. Consequently, the traffic utilizing the blocked lanes is unable to reach its destination. If the damage is significant enough, the closure may be irreversible. This is what leads to paralysis and other symptoms associated with severe SCI injuries.

Orientation and Directional Terms

Term	Definition	Illustration
Facet	A structure of the vertebra is located at the back of the spine. A facet moves with the facet of the neighboring vertebra to form a facet joint. This joint allows motion in the back or along the spinal column. Each vertebra has two superior (above) and two inferior (below) facets.	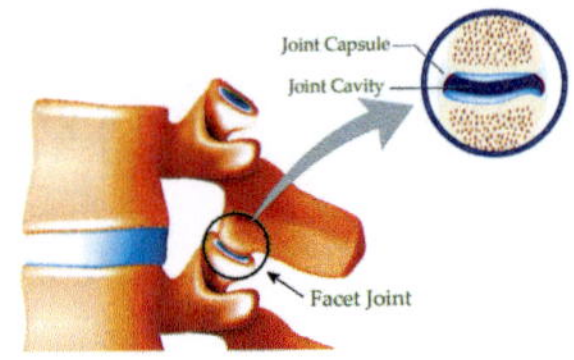
Intervertebral disc	The structure located between each spinal vertebra acts as a cushion or shock absorber for the spine. The disc has a thick outer layer called the annulus fibrosus, which surrounds an inner gel-like substance called the nucleus pulposus.	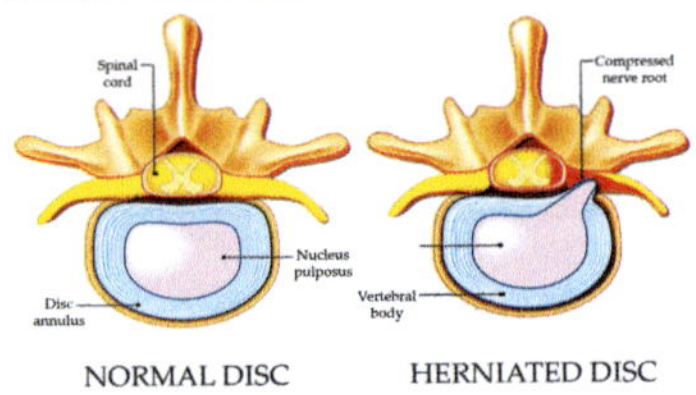
Lamina	Part of a vertebra that forms the arched covering or roof of the spinal canal. Each vertebra has two laminae that connect the pedicles on each side of the spine to the spinous processes in the middle of the spine.	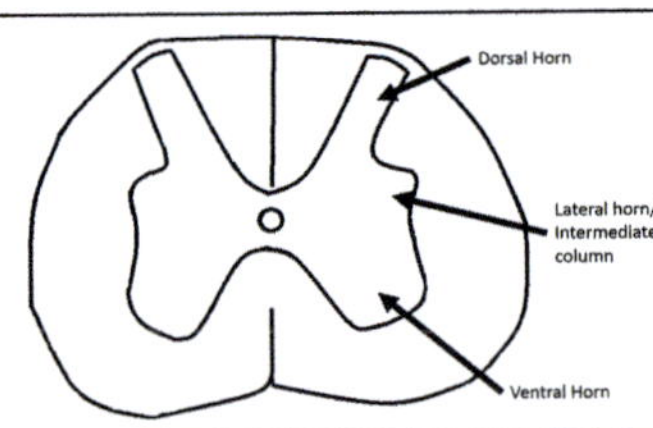
Nerve root	The beginning or foundation of a nerve that is located at the spinal cord and passes through the spinal foramen.	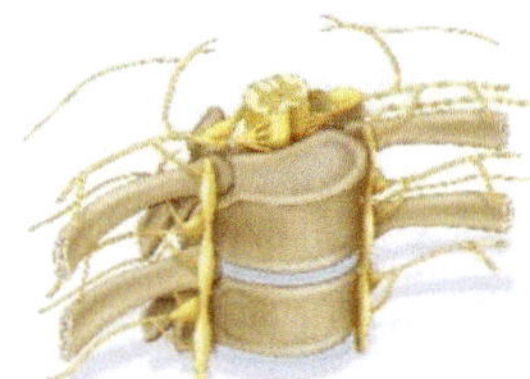
Thoracic spine	The thoracic spine is the middle portion of the spine located between the cervical and lumbar spinal regions. It is comprised of twelve vertebrae, known as T1 to T12. The rib cage is connected to the thoracic spine.	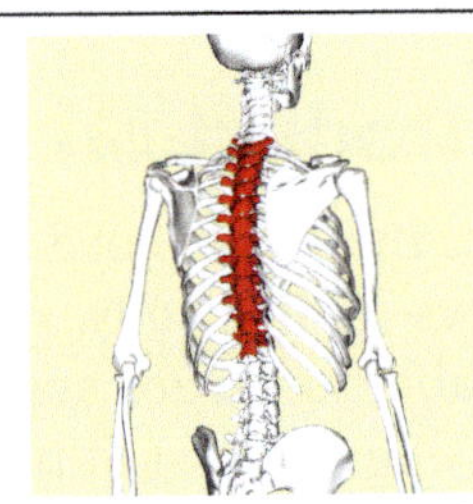

5.2. Structure and Functions of the Spinal Column

A component of the CNS is the spinal cord. It is a long, pipe-like structure that passes through the vertebral column of the backbone and emerges from the medulla oblongata, a region of the brain made up of a group of nerve fibers.

It is divided into two roots (ventral and dorsal), which are made up of nerve fibers that unite to form the spinal nerves.

5.2.1. Spinal Cord Anatomy

The spinal cord is typically 40 cm long and 2 cm wide in adults. It creates a crucial connection between the body and the brain.

The spinal cord is divided into five different parts.

- Sacral cord;
- Lumbar cord;
- Thoracic cord;
- Cervical cord; and
- Coccygeal.

Every segment of the spinal cord contains multiple spinal nerves. There are twelve thoracic, five sacral, eight pairs of cervical, and five lumbar nerves, and one coccygeal spinal nerve.

As it sends sensory signals via afferent fibers from every part of the body to the CNS, it carries out the basic processing of information. The uniform distribution of gray and white matter makes up nerve tissue. The ventral horn projects axons that carry motor neurons, which in turn cause distinct reflexes in the smooth muscles and the skeletal system carrying nerve fibers (Figure 5.1).

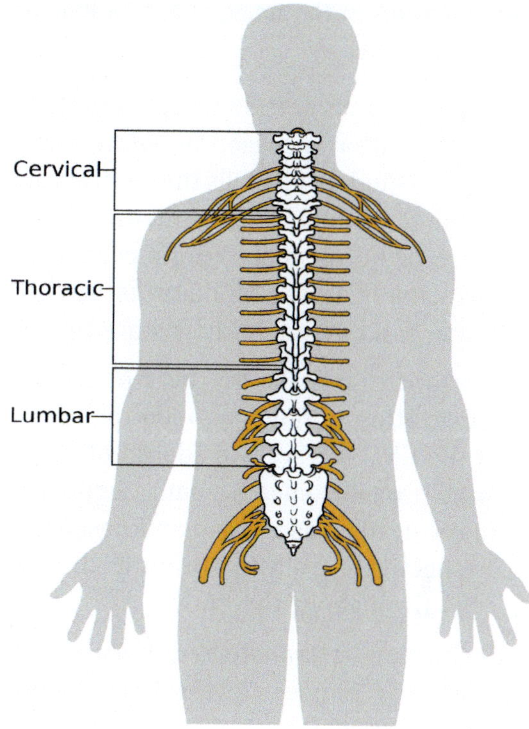

Figure 5.1. *Diagram of the spinal cord showing segments.*

Source: By Cancer Research UK uploader, CC BY-SA 4.0, https://upload.wikimedia.org/wikipedia/commons/thumb/4/48/Diagram_of_the_spinal_cord_CRUK_046.svg/603px-Diagram_of_the_spinal_cord_CRUK_046.svg.png.

Additionally, the spinal cord assists in blocking the autonomic regulation of visceral functions, which are controlled by neurons with descending axons. It is a delicate area that suffers greatly from traumatic injuries. Comprehending the physiology of the spinal cord facilitates the identification and selection of therapeutic approaches for disorders and impairments pertaining to the spinal cord.

5.2.2. Structure of Spinal Cord

Encased within the vertebral column, the spinal cord runs from the skull through a hollow space. Different regions of the vertebral column give rise to spinal nerves, which are named based on their location in the neck, chest, pelvic, and abdominal regions.

Spinal cord cross-section reveals a butterfly-shaped gray matter encircled by white matter. Cerebrospinal fluid, or CSF, fills the central canal, which is the focal point of gray matter. Its four projections, or horns, make up its core, which is primarily made up of CNS neurons and cells. Two ventral and two dorsal horns are present.

The axons that make up the white matter allow information to flow between the various levels of the CNS. A tract is made up of several axons that transmit specific data. Signals are sent and received by ascending and descending tracts, respectively, from the brain to different nerve cells throughout the body.

Information is transferred between the spinal cord and the rest of the body through the spinal nerves, which serve as intermediaries. The spine contains 31 pairs of nerves.

Three layers of meninges surround the spinal cord and spinal nerve roots that are called:

- Dura mater;
- Arachnoid mater; and
- Pia mater.

The dura mater is composed of periosteal and meningeal layers. There exists an epidural gap between these two layers. The subarachnoid space lies between the pia mater and the arachnoid mater, containing cerebrospinal fluid.

5.2.3. Spinal Cord Nerves

There are thirty-one nerves in the group of spinal nerves. The dorsal sensory root and the ventral motor root connect these nerves to the spinal cord. Sensory root fibers transport sensation impulses to the spinal cord, while motor roots carry impulses from the spinal cord.

Certain areas of the body, called dermatomes, have corresponding skin regions. The spinal nerves transmit and receive messages to and from these areas.

The spinal cord nerves can be grouped as follows (Figure 5.2):

- **Cervical Nerves:** A cervical injury is to the neck. The cervical spine gives rise to 8 cervical nerves (C1–C8).

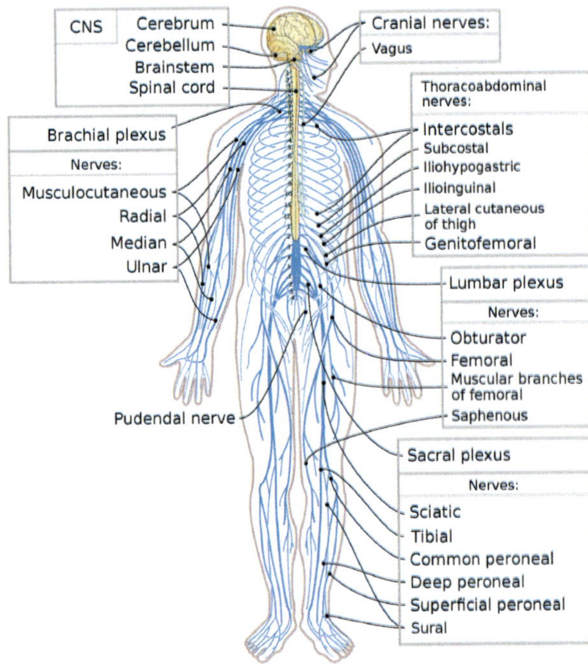

Figure 5.2. *The spinal cord (in yellow) connects the brain to nerves throughout the body.*

Source: By Medium69, Jmarchn – File:Nervous system diagram.png, CC BY-SA 4.0, https://commons.wikimedia.org/w/index.php?curid=36395693.

- **Thoracic Nerves:** The term "thoracic" refers to the chest area. There are a total of 12 thoracic nerves that originate from the thoracic spine, specifically from T1 to T12.
- **Lumbar Nerves:** "Lumbar" refers to the area of the lower back. The

lumbar spine gives rise to 5 lumbar nerves (L1–L5).

- **Sacral Nerves:** "Sacral" pertains to the sacrum, which is a bony plate located at the base of the vertebral column. The sacral bone is the source of 5 sacral nerves (S1–S5).
- **Coccygeal Nerves:** "Coccygeal" refers to the tailbone. The coccygeal bone is where one nerve exits.

5.2.4. Function of Spinal Cord

Important functions of spinal cord are mentioned below:

- Forms a connecting link between the brain and the PNS;
- Provides structural support and builds a body posture;
- Facilitates flexible movements;
- Myelin present in the white matter acts as an electrical insulation;
- Communicates messages from the brain to different parts of the body;
- Coordinates reflexes;
- The sensory information is received from receptors and then transmitted to the brain for processing.

5.3. Mechanisms of Injury and Concepts

Most frequently, spinal cord injuries result from compression caused by fractured vertebrae, masses like epidural hematomas or abscesses, or direct trauma to the spinal cord. Less frequently, blood flow disruption, inflammatory reactions, metabolic disorders, or exposure to toxins can cause spinal cord injuries.

5.3.1. Primary Injury

SCI occurs as a result of an initial insult, such as mechanical forces, known as primary injury. The most common primary injury mechanism is direct impact, with persistent compression often caused by bony fragments in fracture-dislocation injuries. In contrast, hyperextension injuries typically result in less frequent impact, combined with transient compression. Another mechanism is distraction injury, which involves the stretch and tear of the spinal cord in its axial plane when two adjacent vertebrae are pulled apart. Lastly, laceration/transection injury occurs due to sharp bone fragments, severe dislocations, and missile injuries.

5.3.2. Secondary Injury

Secondary injury is a complex biological process that starts shortly after the initial primary injury and can last for weeks or even months. It is divided into two phases – the acute phase, which occurs after the spinal cord injury and involves vascular damage, ionic imbalances, free-radical formation, inflammation, and excitotoxicity. The subacute phase follows, which includes demyelination of surviving axons, Wallerian degeneration, matrix remodeling, and the development of a glial scar.

5.3.3. Immune Response Spinal Cord Injury

Depending on the time point and immune cell condition after SCI, neuroinflammation may have either advantageous or harmful effects. Inflammatory events occurring within the first three days after a stroke involve the attraction of resident microglia, astrocytes, and blood-borne neutrophils to the site of injury. The second stage, which takes place approximately three days after the initial damage, includes the recruitment of B- and T-lymphocytes, as well as macrophages, to the injury site. Antigen-presenting cells activate CD4+ helper T cells, which subsequently release cytokines that stimulate B cells to produce and release antibodies. This process exacerbates neuroinflammation and leads to tissue destruction. Acute SCI is characterized by a more robust neuroinflammatory response.

The subacute and chronic phases of ongoing inflammation can persist throughout a patient's life. The composition and phenotype of inflammatory cells vary depending on the stage of inflammation and the signals present in the injury microenvironment. T cells, B cells, and microglia/macrophages can adopt either a pro- or anti-inflammatory pro-regenerative phenotype. Below the site of injury, motor and sensory functions are lost due to disruption of the nerve axons that traverse spinal cord tracts. The patterns of disability vary depending on the extent of the damage and the spinal tracts involved.

Within the anterior portion of the spinal cord, the spinothalamic tracts can be found. These tracts are responsible for transmitting temperature and pain signals. When damage occurs to these tracts, the opposite side of the body loses the ability to feel pain and temperature. On the lateral aspects of the spinal cord, the corticospinal tracts are located. These tracts are responsible for managing motor function through their nerve axons. Injuries to these tracts can result in paralysis or weakness in the same side of the body.

The axons from the cervical spine that go to the upper extremities are situated near the center of the spinal cord, while those that go to the lower extremities are found on the periphery. The dorsal columns, located in the posterior region of the spinal cord, store information related to vibratory, proprioceptive, and tactile sensations. Damage to these tracts can lead to contralateral loss of tactile, proprioceptive, and vibratory sensation.

5.4. Specific Types of Fractures and Incomplete Cord Injury Syndromes

Since spinal cord injuries are inherently the result of trauma, the initial assessment and presentation will take place in an emergency response environment. A pulmonary evaluation is part of the initial assessment to identify lung damage or loss of ventilation. During this preliminary assessment, signs of hemorrhage and neurogenic shock are also examined. Lastly, and perhaps most importantly for physical therapy, a neurological assessment is performed, which includes testing perineal function, deep tendon reflexes (DTR), sensory evaluation, and motor function.

An international standard neurological assessment has been established by the ASIA (American Spinal Injury Association) that can be used to categorize the lesion based on a particular cord syndrome. This covers sensory and motor assessment. An impairment scale that shows the severity of the lesion is also included.

5.4.1. Specific Types of Spinal Fractures

Spinal fractures can be of several different kinds, including compression, burst, flexion-distraction, and fracture-dislocation. The physician may also refer to a fracture as stable, unstable, minor, or major.

5.4.1.1. Compression Fracture

Patients with osteoporosis or those whose bones have been compromised by other illnesses, such as bone cancer, are vulnerable to this type of fracture. A sudden, high force may exceed the bone's capacity to withstand, as the vertebrae can only endure a certain amount of pressure. Consequently, a vertebral fracture may occur. One type of compression fracture is known as a wedge fracture, which transpires when a portion of the vertebra, typically the anterior (front) part, collapses under stress and assumes the shape of a wedge (Figure 5.3).

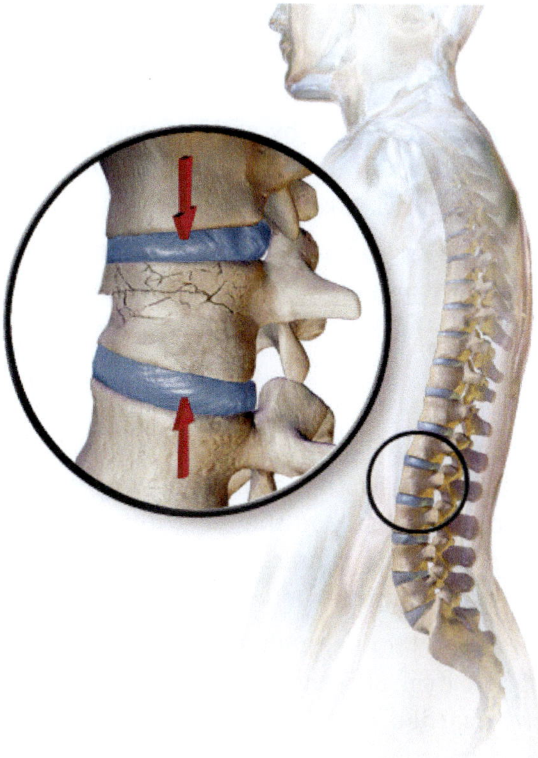

Figure 5.3. *Vertebral compression fracture.*

Source: *Blausen.com staff (2014). "Medical gallery of Blausen Medical 2014". WikiJournal of Medicine* ***1*** *(2). DOI:10.15347/wjm/2014.010. ISSN 2002-4436.*

5.4.1.2. Burst Fracture

The cause of burst fractures is severe trauma, such as an automobile mishap. They arise from the application of tremendous force, effectively crushing the vertebra. In contrast to compression fractures, more than one vertebral body is broken. A burst fracture involves multiple fractures to the vertebra. Because the vertebra is completely crushed, there is a risk of bony fragments spreading and injuring the spinal cord. Compared to compression fractures, burst fractures are more serious (Figure 5.4).

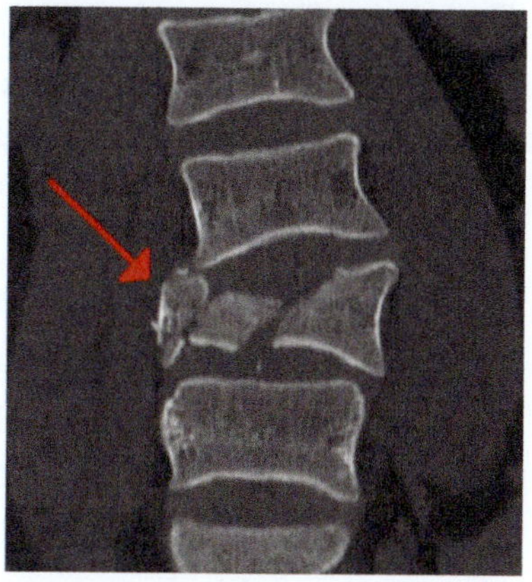

Figure 5.4. *A burst fracture of L4 as seen on CT.*

Source: By James Heilman, MD – Own work, CC BY-SA 4.0, https://commons.wikimedia.org/w/index.php?curid=49062931.

5.4.1.3. Flexion-Distraction Fractures

A flexion-distraction fracture can occur in a car accident when the body is forced forward, causing excessive stress on the spine and potentially leading to a vertebra or vertebrae breaking. This type of fracture typically involves damage to the posterior and middle columns of the spine. An illustration of a flexion-distraction fracture is provided in Figure 5.5.

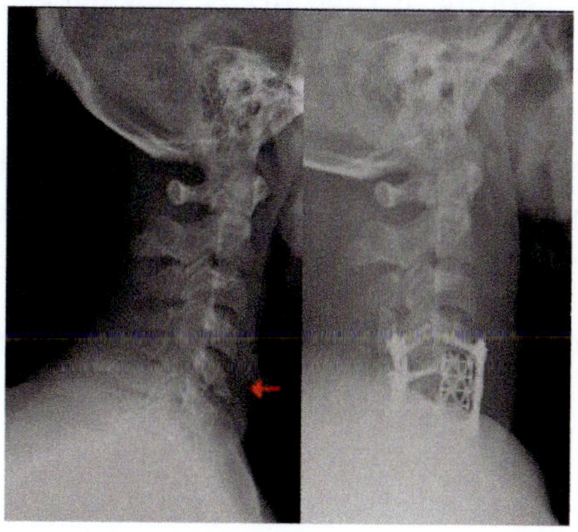

Figure 5.5. *Fracture of the cervical spine treated with metal fixation.*

Source: By Moquito 17 at the English-language Wikipedia, CC BY-SA 3.0, https://commons.wikimedia.org/w/index.php?curid=7940879.

5.4.1.4. Fracture-Dislocation

A fracture-dislocation is present in cases where one or more of the aforementioned fractures are accompanied by a significant movement of the vertebrae. The three-column concept is typically involved in these fractures, which severely destabilize the spine.

5.4.1.5. Stable and Unstable Fractures

- Neurologic (nerve) issues or spinal deformities are not caused by stable fractures. Even with a stable fracture, the spine can still support and distribute weight fairly well, although not as effectively as it would without a fracture.
- On the other hand, it is difficult for the spine to support and distribute weight when there are unstable fractures. Unstable fractures can worsen and may require additional treatment, potentially leading to spinal deformity.

5.4.1.6. Major and Minor Fractures

- A minor fracture is defined as a break in one or more posterior (back) vertebral segments, which are not as crucial to the stability of the spinal column as they are to the stability of the fractured segment. The spinous process and the facet joints, also referred to as the articular processes, are examples of the posterior elements. It is usually not too serious if the patient fracture this portion of the vertebrae.
- A major fracture occurs when there is a break in the lamina, pedicles, or vertebral body. Because the vertebral body supports a great deal of weight and distributes the force of the movements, fractures to it are regarded as major. If it is broken, the vertebrae may not line up properly, which could cause major issues. Breaking the pedicles or lamina is risky as there is a greater chance of nerve damage. In addition, the lamina and pedicles offer a great deal of the support the spine needs to remain stable. If they break, the back might become unsteady.

5.4.2. One Method to Classify Thoracic and/or Lumbar Spinal Fractures

The Denis Classification method is used by medical professionals to categorize spinal fractures in the lumbar, thoracic, or thoracolumbar regions of the spine. According to this method, the lateral (side) spine is divided into three sections – the back, middle, and front.

The Denis classification – the three-column concept is as follows:

- **Anterior (Front) Column:** The anterior region refers to the portion of the vertebra that faces inward toward the body. It includes the front portion of the vertebral body and intervertebral disc. The anterior column also includes the anterior longitudinal ligament, which is located on the front of the spine.
- **Middle Column:** This column plays a crucial role in spinal stability. It consists of the intervertebral disc and the rear portion of the vertebral body. The middle column also includes the posterior longitudinal ligament, which is located on the back of the spinal body. If there is a fracture in the middle column along with the anterior or posterior

columns, there is a higher risk of nerve damage and spinal instability. On the other hand, if the middle column remains intact, there is a greater chance of having a stable fracture.

- **Posterior (Back) Column:** It is composed of every vertebral segment on the back. It includes the pedicles, lamina, facet joints, and spinous process—the bony portion of the spine that can feel when run the finger up it.

The three-column concept simplifies the visualization of spinal fracture severity and extent. It also helps in understanding the different levels of stability in fractures. For example, a fracture that only affects the front column (such as a wedge fracture) may still provide enough stability for weight bearing. Fractures that affect both the front and middle columns usually result in instability.

5.4.3. Spinal Cord Injury

Spinal cord injuries can be classified into various types, with doctors typically categorizing them as either complete or incomplete injuries. A complete injury occurs when an individual loses all sensation and movement below the site of the spinal cord injury (Figure 5.6).

Even after experiencing an incomplete spinal cord injury, individuals may retain some sensation or motor function in the affected areas. The location of the injury also determines its type. The spinal cord is divided into four sections:

- Cervical spine (vertebrae C1 through C7, which contain a total of eight cervical nerve roots);
- Thoracic spine (vertebrae T1 through T12);
- Lumbar spine (vertebrae L1 through L5); and
- Sacral spine (vertebrae S1 through S5).

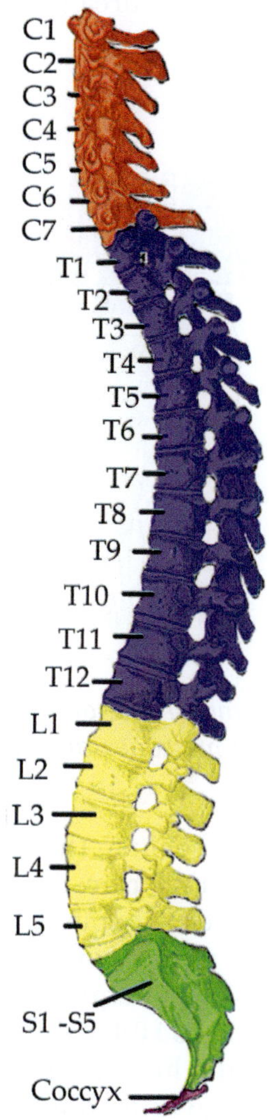

Figure 5.6. *The effects of injury depend on the level along the spinal column.*

Source: By Henry Vandyke Carter - Henry, G., (1918). Anatomy of the Human Body. Bartleby.com: Gray's Anatomy, Plate 111altered by User:Uwe Gille and User:delldot, Public Domain, https://commons.wikimedia.org/w/index.php?curid=46472029.

Different body parts are under the control of each of the four sections. In the majority of cases, individuals with a spinal cord injury will experience loss of sensation and control in the limbs below the affected area (Figure 5.7).

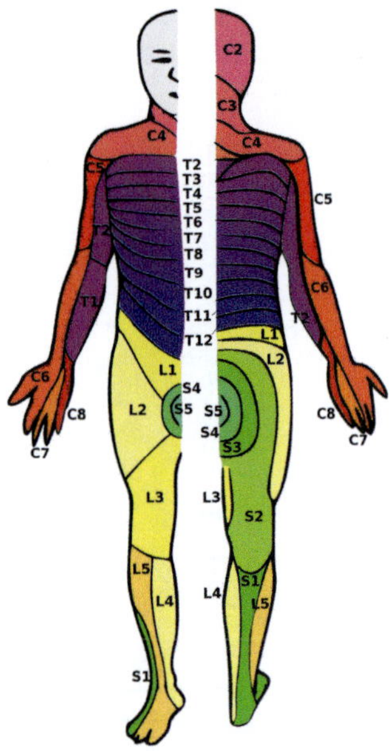

Figure 5.7. *A dermatome is an area of the skin that sends sensory messages to a specific spinal nerve.*

Source: By Ralf Stephan (mailto:ralf@ark.in-berlin.de) – altered from File:Dermatoms.svg. Colors changed, a couple corrections. Original **source:** http://www.ark.in-berlin.de/senszonen.svgz (https://web.archive.org/web/20080525104214/www.ark.in-berlin.de/neuropics.html), Public Domain, https://commons.wikimedia.org/w/index.php?curid=46154280.

5.4.3.1. Cervical Spinal Injury

The cervical spine is the upper part of the spine that contains the vertebrae of the neck. Cervical spine injuries are typically the most severe kind because they are located closest to the brain and can affect most of the body. Tetraplegia, also known as quadriplegia, is a common result of cervical spine injuries. It is characterized by complete or partial paralysis of the torso and all four limbs.

5.4.3.2. Thoracic Spinal Injury

The thoracic spine comprises the upper and middle regions of the back. An injury to the thoracic spine often affects the muscles of the lower back, legs, and abdomen. A thoracic spine injury can result in paraplegia, which is the paralysis of portions of the trunk and legs. Despite being paraplegic, individuals can still use their hands and arms.

5.4.3.3. Lumbar Spinal Injury

In the spine, the lumbar region is the lowest major segment. Due to their increased weight support compared to other regions of the spine, the vertebrae in this section of the spine are larger. An injury to the lumbar spine may cause partial loss of function in the hips and legs, but the upper limbs are typically still under control. With braces on or in a wheelchair, some people with injuries to their lumbar spines may be able to walk.

5.4.3.4. Sacral Spinal Injury

The region directly above the tailbone is called the sacral spine. This region of the spinal cord gives rise to the nerves that control the backs of the thighs, the groin, and the hips. A sacral spine injury may result in partial hip and leg function loss. Additionally, it might impair bowel and bladder control. Still, many people who have suffered a sacral spine injury are able to walk.

5.5. Management

The temporary or permanent loss of normal spinal motor, sensory, and autonomic function is known as a spinal cord injury (SCI), and it can be extremely devastating for many reasons. Individuals with spinal cord injuries (SCI) have severe psychological aftereffects and physical dependence, which means that caring for these patients necessitates intensive medical, rehabilitative, and social services. These resources are expensive; in the US, it is estimated that each patient will spend between $3,75,000–$1,149,000 in the first year following their injury, and a 25-year-old tetraplegic patient will spend approximately $5,100,000 in their lifetime. Major trauma is the leading cause of death for people under 50 in the United Kingdom, and survivors may have lifelong disabilities. An estimated 1,200 individuals in the UK suffer from traumatic spinal cord injuries each year, and approximately 40,000 people live with long-term disabilities as a result of SCI, though some charities think the number may be higher. The spinal cord is damaged in about 14% of spinal fractures, of which 50% are incomplete. Half of these will walk upon discharge if handled properly. Thus, it is imperative to provide appropriate initial care, which should focus on maintaining spinal cord function while preventing further complications.

5.5.1. Acute Management

Trauma care begins even before a patient arrives at the hospital. Traumatic spinal cord injuries can occur in up to 25% of cases following the initial insult during handling, extraction, or transportation. Prioritizing spinal immobilization in patients whose injury mechanism is consistent with spinal trauma is associated with improved outcomes. The standard method for spinal protection is the use of a rigid spinal board to maintain alignment of the rest of the spine, along with three-point immobilization of the cervical spine using blocks, collars, and tape. While these safety measures are necessary to prevent further spinal injuries, they can lead to complications such as pressure sores, aspiration, elevated intracranial pressure, and interference with the initial evaluation. The removal of immobilizing devices should be done as soon as it is safe to do so.

Patients with spinal cord injuries (SCI) can also have concurrent head injuries in as many as 25–50% of cases, and up to 57% of SCI patients may have concurrent spinal fractures or other injuries. The presence of associated injuries is important to consider when discussing SCI. Managing other potentially life-threatening injuries in the presence of suspected SCI can be challenging, especially when establishing a secure airway or managing hypotension exacerbated by neurogenic shock. Secondary damage to the spinal cord can also occur as a result of other injuries that cause hypoxia and hypotension. To prevent overlooking spinal cord injuries and other potentially life-threatening injuries, all trauma patients should be evaluated and treated according to the Advanced Trauma and Life Support (ATLS) protocol. While maintaining spinal alignment is crucial, injuries that pose an immediate threat to life should take precedence.

Individuals who have suffered spinal cord injuries may exhibit systemic symptoms. Patients who may need ventilation may experience respiratory difficulties due to diaphragmatic innervation being affected by cervical lesions in the C3–C5 region. Due to paralytic ileus and decreased tone of the gastroesophageal sphincter, these patients are also susceptible to regurgitation and pulmonary aspiration; however, this risk can be mitigated by using a nasogastric tube to decompress the stomach. Neurogenic shock is another common phenomenon observed in up to 20% of patients with high spinal cord injuries. This phenomenon can result in bradycardia, unopposed vagal tone, decreased systemic vascular resistance, and profound hypotension. This is frequently misdiagnosed as hemorrhagic shock brought on by internal bleeding in cases of severe trauma. But fluid-resistant hypotension in neurogenic shock frequently occurs, so inotropic/vasopressor support might be a better course of action. Urinary catheterization can help evaluate fluid balance when pelvic fractures are not present. This is particularly true for patients who are at risk of urine retention and have a denervated bladder. The focus can shift to evaluating the spine after injuries that pose a threat to life or limb have been treated while spinal immobilization is maintained. The patient needs to be properly imaged and assessed for any spinal injuries. An American Spinal Injury Association (ASIA) chart should be filled out after a neurological examination, which should include an assessment of anal tone.

Patients with acute spinal cord injury (SCI) frequently arrive with spinal shock, an acute condition of reduced spinal function characterized by complete loss of all sensorimotor abilities caudal to the site of injury. Neurogenic shock and spinal shock are not the same thing. Neurogenic shock refers to circulatory collapse as previously discussed, whereas spinal shock describes decreased spinal cord function after an acute insult to the cord. Since spinal shock is a temporary condition, a second neurological examination performed a few days after the initial injury is essential to ascertain the actual extent of spinal cord damage.

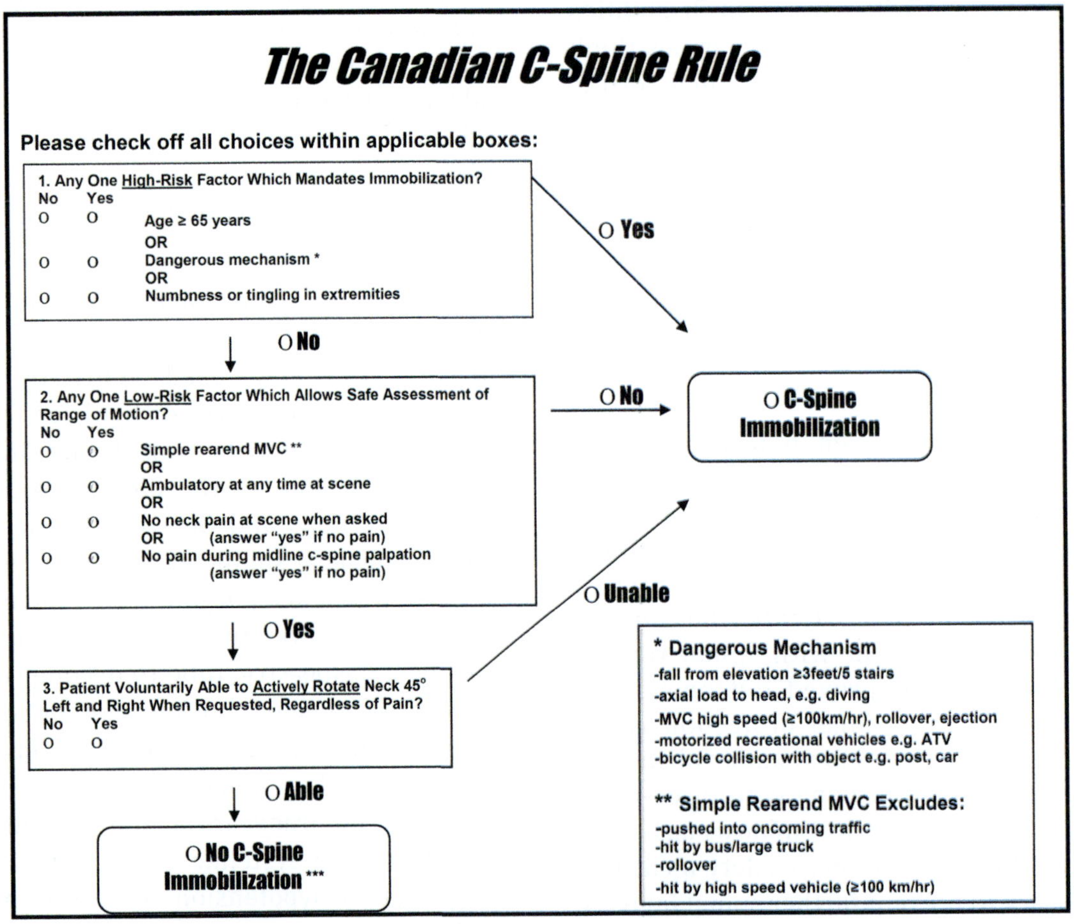

Figure 5.8. *Canadian C-spine rule. [GCS: Glasgow coma scale].*

Source: Vaillancourt, C., Charette, M., Kasaboski, A., Maloney, J., Wells, G. A., & Stiell, I. G., (2011). Evaluation of the safety of C-spine clearance by paramedics: design and methodology. BMC Emerg Med., 11, 1. doi: 10.1186/1471-227X-11-1.

Depending on the location of the suspected injury, adult patients with distracting injuries, spinal pain, limb weakness/paraesthesia, priapism, confusion, or altered consciousness may require an X-ray of the thoracolumbar spine or a computed tomography (CT) of the cervical spine. If the X-ray results are inconclusive, additional CT scanning of the thoracolumbar spine is necessary. For adult patients who do not meet the aforementioned risk factors but are still suspected of having C spine injuries, the Canadian C-spine rule should be applied. Patients with high-risk factors such as paraesthesia in the upper or lower limbs, a risky mechanism of injury, or who are older than 65, require a CT scan of the C-spine. If the patient can rotate their neck 45° to the left and right and only low-risk factors are present, there is no need for additional immobilization or imaging. Patients who have no radiological abnormalities on their X-ray or CT scan and no clinical evidence of spinal pain or neurological deficit may have their spines "cleared" and their immobilization devices removed. In patients under 16 years old with a strong suspicion of C spine injury, an MRI scan is the preferred imaging modality, as determined by the Canadian C-spine rule and clinical assessment. Before clearing the spine, a senior radiologist should review any CT and MRI scans (Figure 5.8).

5.5.2. Timing of Surgery

It is crucial to comprehend that spinal cord damage in traumatic brain injury (SCI) arises from secondary injuries that occur during the early acute phase (minutes to hours) and subacute phase (days to weeks). The primary pathophysiologic alterations responsible for secondary spinal cord injury during the acute phase encompass vasogenic edema, microvessel vasospasm, inflammation, failure of sodium ion pumps, and free radicals. The primary processes causing cellular damage during the subacute phase are macrophage activity, apoptosis, and microglial stimulation.

The data seems to support early surgical intervention to reduce morbidity, length of stay, and medical expenses. If performed promptly enough, it may even enhance neurological recovery. Unfortunately, in a survey involving 2,000 neurosurgeons, 80% of them endorsed early surgery, but less than half believed it was feasible to operate within 24 hours. The primary challenge was the scarcity of supplies for weekend or overnight surgeries. Importantly, if patients received treatment at a trauma center, there was a 33% decrease in long-term paralysis.

5.5.3. Non-Surgical Management

The decision of whether or not to proceed with surgery in cases of spinal trauma is a complex one. In addition to possessing the necessary tools and expertise, patient factors such as suitability for surgery and the presence of any additional injuries that may pose a risk to life or limb must be considered. Non-operative treatment may be beneficial when there is well-established neurological impairment and instability, as well as when the spine is stable and there are no neurological issues. However, prolonged immobility increases the risk of complications such as pneumonia, deep vein thrombosis, and pressure sores.

Scoring systems are used to assess spinal fracture patterns in the thoracolumbar and sub-axial cervical regions. The Thoracolumbar Injury Classification and Severity Score (TLICS) is used for the thoracolumbar region, while the Sub-axial Injury Classification and Severity Scale (SLIC) is used for the sub-axial cervical region. These scoring systems take into account the integrity of the disco-ligamentous complex (DLC)/posterior ligamentous complex (PLC), the morphology of the fracture, and the neurological status. Generally, scores below 4 can be managed conservatively, scores above 4 indicate a preference for surgical intervention, and a score of 4 is typically based on the surgeon's individual preference. These scoring systems have demonstrated good reliability among different observers and when predicting which patients can be managed non-operatively.

Spinal orthoses can be used to improve acute pain and enable early ambulation in cases where the score is less than 4. Before being released, standing X-rays should be taken to check for occult ligamentous injuries, stability, and alignment. When there is no neurological deficit or PLC injury, non-operative management of compression or burst fractures in the thoracolumbar region is typically utilized. Transverse and spinous process fractures also usually do not require surgery. There are three types of cervical injuries: sub-axial (C3–C7), C1, and C2 injuries. Rigid collars can be used to treat C2 dens fractures type 1 and 3 and simple C1 injuries with an intact transverse alar ligament; however, individual patient factors must be taken into account for the risk of non-union with C2 dens fractures. The SLIC scoring system should be taken into account when choosing between operative and non-operative sub-axial injury management.

5.5.4. Rehabilitation

Physical therapy, skill-building exercises, and counseling are all incorporated into rehabilitation programs for individuals with spinal cord injuries (SCI) to improve their independence and quality of life, as well as to offer social and emotional support. The rehabilitation team may consist of social workers, occupational and physical therapists, recreational therapists, rehabilitation nurses, rehabilitation psychologists, vocational counselors, nutritionists, case workers, and other specialists. The team is typically led by a physician with expertise in physical medicine and rehabilitation.

Regaining leg and arm strength, as well as communication skills, are typically the main goals of the first stage of rehabilitation following an injury. Adaptive or supportive devices can help people with spinal cord injuries (SCI) become more mobile and enhance their quality of life. The individual may require braces, a wheelchair, electrical stimulators, assisted walking training, neural prosthetics (assistive devices that stimulate the nerves to restore lost functions), computer adaptations, and other computer-assisted technology, depending on the severity of the injury. Additionally, communication skills like typing, writing, and using the phone can be improved with the aid of adaptive devices.

- Physical therapy includes exercise programs geared toward strengthening muscles.
- Occupational therapy aids in the restoration of fine motor skills, especially those required to carry out activities of daily living such as eating, using the restroom, getting in and out of bed, and maintaining personal hygiene. Additionally, occupational therapy may include teaching the patient coping mechanisms for autonomic dysreflexia, neurogenic pain, and spasticity.
- Identification of fundamental job skills, as well as mental and physical capacities that can support paid employment, are all part of vocational rehabilitation. Through this process, the individual and their team can establish a user-friendly workspace, identify suitable locations for the workspace, and determine any assistive technology that may be required.

- Engaging in educational training can help individuals acquire skills for a new career that is not solely dependent on physical capabilities. It is recommended for individuals with SCI to participate in activities that promote satisfaction and self-esteem, such as educational courses, pursuing hobbies, joining special interest groups, and attending family and community events.
- Recreation therapy encourages people with SCI to engage in sports, the arts, or other leisure activities that they can enjoy with their increased mobility. This can help individuals lead balanced lives with opportunities for social interaction and self-expression.

5.6. Complications

A spinal cord injury can cause complications and changes to daily functioning. These may include:

- **Loss of the Ability to Control One's Bowels and Bladder:** Individuals who have spinal cord injuries may need to learn how to void when they don't feel the urge to.
- **Loss of Muscular Tone:** When a person's arms or legs are immobile, their muscles may atrophy and weaken. It's also possible for the person's physical fitness to decline.
- **Spasms in the Muscles:** A spinal cord injury may occasionally result in spasticity or involuntary movements.
- **Nerve Pain:** Studies indicate that long-term nerve pain is experienced by over two-thirds of individuals with spinal cord injuries. Parts of the body with residual sensation or areas with little to no feeling may be affected by the pain.
- **Skin Injuries and Sores:** People who are unable to perceive specific parts of their body might not be aware of cuts, burns, or other injuries they have sustained there. They will need to regularly inspect their nails and skin for injuries to help prevent infections and other complications.
- **Lung Issues:** A person may not be able to adequately clear their lungs following a spinal cord injury if they are unable to cough or breathe. They are more likely to contract pneumonia as a result of this difficulty.
- **Blood Clots:** Individuals with low blood pressure are at a higher risk of experiencing swelling and blood clots.
- **Stroke and Cardiac Arrest:** Certain spinal cord injuries carry the risk of a sudden and dangerously elevated blood pressure spike. This condition, known as autonomic dysreflexia, can lead to seizures, myocardial infarction, and stroke.
- **Obesity Risk:** Individuals who are unable to walk or move as they once did may spend more time being sedentary. This change in lifestyle can result in weight gain or obesity, as well as related diseases such as type 2 diabetes and heart disease.
- **Sexual Function Changes:** Spinal cord injuries can diminish or eliminate the ability to achieve an erection or feel sexually aroused. Additionally, they may make orgasms difficult or impossible.

- **Infertility:** Spinal cord injuries can sometimes prevent males from ejaculating and make it difficult for women to conceive.
- **Impact on Mental Health:** Spinal cord injuries have been found to have a negative impact on mental health, with many individuals experiencing high rates of depression according to research findings.

A spinal cord injury may result in challenging and permanent side effects. However, many of these issues can be managed with the assistance of medical professionals, such as physicians and rehabilitation therapists.

A Closer Look

Prognosis

The outlook for individuals with a spinal cord injury is directly affected by the severity and completeness of the neurologic damage and any related impairments. Complete lesions of the spinal cord, indicated by AIS Grade A with no Zone of Partial Preservation, make full recovery of neurological function unlikely. In these cases, the outcome is dependent on the effectiveness of rehabilitation in maximizing any remaining function. Surgical intervention may help prevent further damage in cases of progressive spinal cord lesions, potentially leading to some improvement in overall neurologic status. The functional expectations and prognosis following a spinal cord injury vary based on individual factors.

- Neurological level of spinal cord injury;
- Severity of spinal cord injury (complete vs. incomplete, AIS impairment scale);
- Patient-specific factors:
  - Age, health, and pre-morbid fitness/function;
  - Past medical history/co-morbidities;
  - Associated injuries;
  - Secondary complications;
  - Motivation and psychosocial well-being.

There is little chance of accurately predicting clinical outcomes after a spinal cord injury based on an early examination. At 72 hours to 1 week after injury, the ability to retain sacral sensation at the S4–S5 dermatome, particularly pinprick, is thought to be the most significant predictor of a better outcome and useful recovery; 75% of people with sacral sparing are able to walk again. The prognosis for walking if injured is best for patients with Brown-Sequard or Cervical Central Cord Syndrome. It is more difficult to predict the ability to walk at the time of injury, but estimates show that very few patients with ASIA A lesions at the time of injury ultimately ambulate with or without assistance, 30% to 45% of patients with ASIA B lesions ambulate for at least short distances, and most patients with ASIA C and D lesions become community ambulators.

After sustaining a spinal injury, most individuals experience a recovery of one level of motor function within 72 hours, based on their original classification. The majority of functional improvement occurs within the first six months. For example, someone with C6 tetraplegia at the time of the injury may progress to C7 tetraplegia three to six months later. It is widely recognized that individuals with incomplete spinal cord injuries can continue to make useful recoveries for up to two years following the injury. In some cases, recovery may occur at a slower pace over an extended period, particularly for incomplete tetraplegics. Around 50% of patients initially diagnosed with ASIA B or C Lesions show improvement within the first few months, advancing by one ASIA level (e.g., from ASIA B to ASIA C, or from ASIA C to ASIA D). In comparison, 90% of individuals with an incomplete spinal cord injury experience some recovery of motor function in their upper limbs, compared to only 70%–85% of those with complete injuries.

A high risk of subsequent complications, mental health issues, financial insecurity, and social isolation are just a few of the major challenges to overall well-being that come with spinal cord injuries, a serious and pervasive health issue that can cause widespread impairment. Older age at the time of injury, health issues, cognitive impairments, low self-efficacy or control perceptions, and a lack of social support all predict low social participation and more challenges with reintegrating into the community after release. Even though employment rates following spinal cord injuries are generally low, those who were injured at a younger age and with less severe injuries have better employment outcomes and a higher level of functional independence.

5.7. Summary

- The spinal cord is typically 40 centimeters in length and 2 centimeters in width in adults. It establishes a vital connection between the body and the brain.
- Enclosed within the vertebral column, the spinal cord extended from the skull through a hollow space. Various regions of the vertebral column have given rise to spinal nerves, which were named based on their location in the neck, chest, pelvic, and abdominal regions.
- There exist thirty-one nerves within the cluster of spinal nerves. The dorsal sensory root and the ventral motor root establish the connection between these nerves and the spinal cord. Sensation impulses are conveyed to the spinal cord through the sensory root fibers. Conversely, impulses from the spinal cord are conveyed by the motor roots.
- Spinal cord injuries most commonly arise from compression resulting from fractured vertebrae, masses such as epidural hematomas or abscesses, or direct trauma to the spinal cord. Less frequently, spinal cord injuries can be caused by disruption of blood flow, inflammatory reactions, metabolic disorders, or exposure to toxins.
- Depending on the time point and immune cell condition following spinal cord injury, neuroinflammation can have either beneficial or detrimental effects. Inflammatory events within the first three days after a stroke involve attracting resident microglia and astrocytes, as well as blood-borne neutrophils, to the site of injury.
- A pulmonary assessment is conducted as part of the initial evaluation to identify any lung damage or ventilation loss. During this preliminary assessment, signs of hemorrhage and neurogenic shock are also examined.
- Spinal fractures can take on various forms, including compression, burst, flexion-distraction, and fracture-dislocation. The physician may also classify a fracture as stable, unstable, minor, or major.
- The Denis Classification method is utilized by medical professionals to categorize a spinal fracture in the lumbar, thoracic, or thoracolumbar regions of the spine. This method divides the lateral (side) spine into three sections: the posterior, middle, and anterior.
- The temporary or permanent loss of normal spinal motor, sensory, and autonomic function is known as a spinal cord injury (SCI), and it can have devastating consequences for numerous reasons. Examples of how SCI often occurs unexpectedly include a motorcycle operator who experiences paralysis due to a road traffic accident, a gymnast who fractures their neck and is left wheelchair-bound for life, or a rugby player who sustains a cervical spine injury during a scrum.
- Rehabilitation programs for individuals with spinal cord injuries (SCI) encompass the integration of physical therapy, skill-building exercises, and counseling. These interventions aim to enhance their independence and quality of life, while also providing social and emotional support.

References

1. Cho, T. A., (2015). Spinal cord functional anatomy. *Continuum (Minneap Minn), 21*(1 Spinal Cord Disorders), 13–35. doi: 10.1212/01.CON.0000461082.25876.4a
2. Doran, G. T., (1981). There's a S.M.A.R.T. Way to write management's goals and objectives. *Management Review, 70*, 35, 36. https://community.mis.temple.edu/mis0855002fall2015/files/2015/10/S.M.A.R.T-Way-Management-Review.pdf (accessed on 20 March 2024).
3. Harvey, L., (2008). *Management of Spinal Cord Injuries: A Guide for Physiotherapists.* Elsevier Health Sciences.
4. Khazaeipour, Z., et al., (2015). *Depression Following Spinal Cord Injury: Its Relationship to Demographic and Socioeconomic Indicators.* https://www.ncbi.nlm.nih.gov/pmc/articles/PMC4568096/ (accessed on 20 March 2024).
5. McDonald, J. W., & Sadowsky, C., (2002). Spinal cord injury. *The Lancet, 359*(9304), 417–425.
6. Moreno-Duarte, I., et al., (2014). *Targeted Therapies Using Electrical and Magnetic Neural Stimulation for the Treatment of Chronic Pain in Spinal Cord Injury.* https://www.sciencedirect.com/science/article/abs/pii/S1053811913005995?via%3Dihub (accessed on 20 March 2024).
7. Nógrádi, A., & Vrbová, G., (n.d.). *Anatomy and Physiology of the Spinal Cord.* https://www.ncbi.nlm.nih.gov/books/NBK6229/ (accessed on 20 March 2024).
8. Wade, D. T., (2009). Goal setting in rehabilitation: An overview of what, why and how. *Clinical Rehabilitation, 23*(4), 291–295. https://doi.org/10.1177/02692155091035519.
9. Waters, R. L., Adkins, R., Yakura, J., et al., (1994). Prediction of ambulatory performance based on motor scores derived from standards of the American Spinal Injury Association. *Arch. Phys. Med., Rehabil., 75*, 756–760.
10. Waters, R. L., Adkins, R. H., Yakura, J. S., et al., (1994). Motor and sensory recovery following incomplete tetraplegia. *Arch. Phys. Med. Rehabil., 75*, 306–311.
11. Waters, R. L., Adkins, R. H., Yakura, J. S., et al., (1994). Motor and sensory recovery following incomplete paraplegia. *Arch. Phys. Med. Rehabil., 75*, 67–72.
12. Wolfe, D. L., & Hsieh, J. T. C., (2006). Rehabilitation practice and associated outcomes following spinal cord injuries. In: Eng, J. J., Teasell, R. W., Miller, W. C., et al., (eds.), *Spinal Cord Injury Rehabilitation Evidence* (pp. 3.1–3.44). Vancouver.

Chapter 6

PERIPHERAL NERVE AND BRACHIAL PLEXUS INJURIES

Contents

6.1. Introduction

Peripheral nerve injuries and brachial plexus injuries refer to damage to the group of nerves that supply the hands and arms. These injuries can be caused by peripheral tumors, trauma, or birth-related palsies. The brachial plexus, a network of nerves that extends from the cervical spinal cord in the neck to the hand, arm, and shoulder, is responsible for both sensory and motor functions of the upper extremities. Damage to one or more of these nerves can result in varying degrees of weakness, paralysis, and numbness in the upper extremities.

Nerve injuries can occur in different forms, including pulling, stretching, tearing, or compression. Patients with temporary nerve injuries often regain most, if not all, of their ability to function independently with the help of occupational therapy and time. However, more severe nerve damage may require a combination of occupational therapy and surgery for optimal recovery (Figure 6.1).

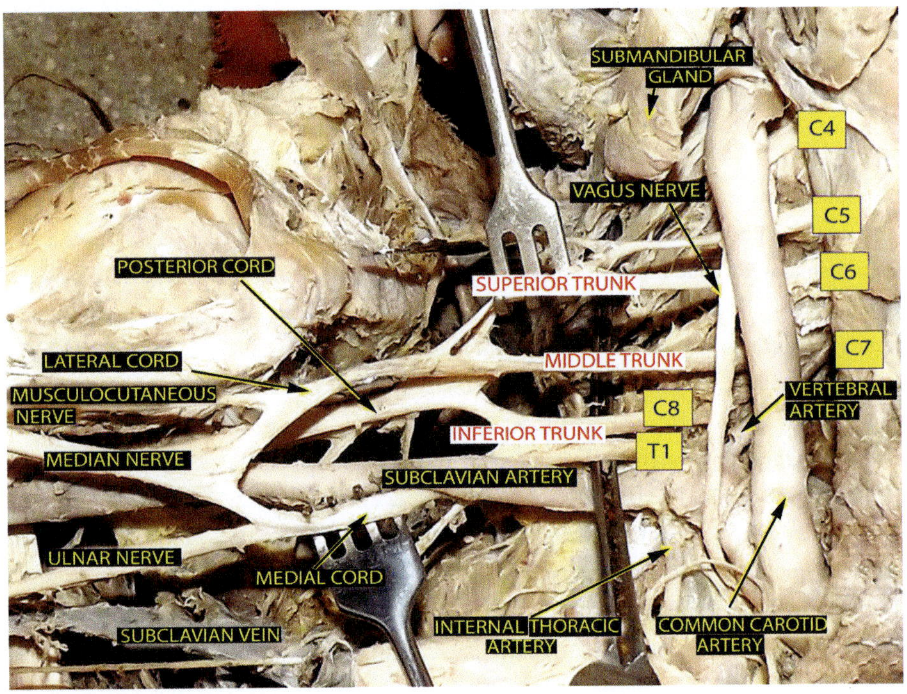

Figure 6.1. *The brachial plexus is a network of nerves running from the cervical spinal cord in the neck to the shoulder, arm, and hand.*

Orientation and Directional Terms

Term	Definition	Illustration
Cranial nerves	Cranial nerves consist of 12 pairs that emerge from the brain. Examples of cranial nerves include optic and olfactory, among others.	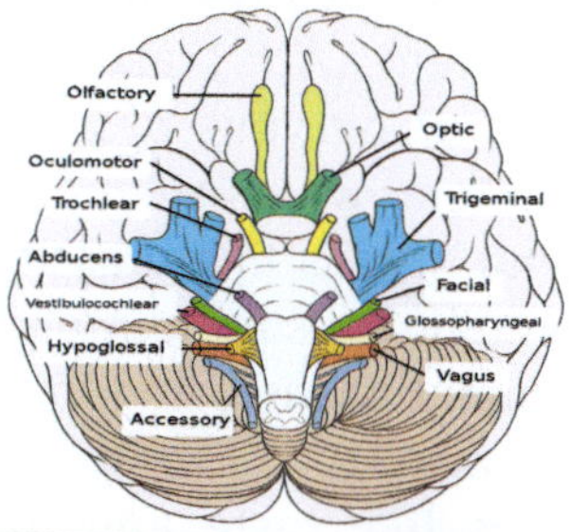
Spinal nerves	Spinal nerves have their point of emergence as the spinal cord. There are 31 pairs of spinal nerves. They emerge from the spinal cord into dorsal and ventral roots. At the junction of these two roots, the sensory fibers continue into the dorsal root, and the motor fibers into the ventral root.	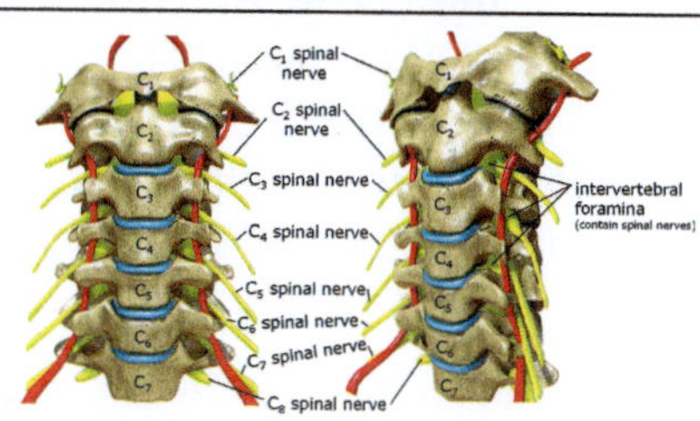
Sympathetic nervous system	The sympathetic nervous system consists of nerves arising from the spinal cord between the neck and waist region. It prepares the body for violent actions against abnormal conditions and is generally stimulated by adrenaline.	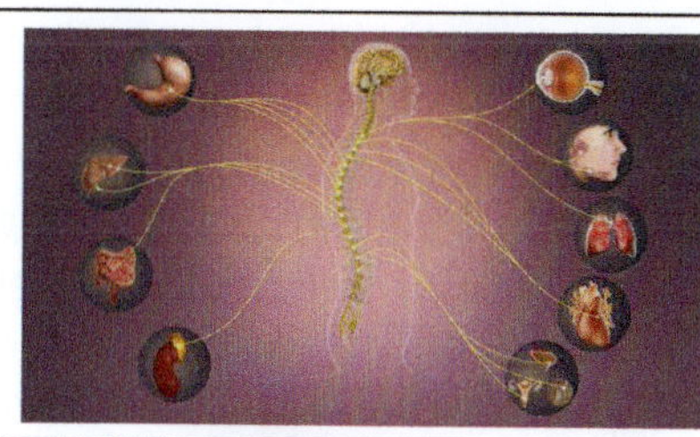
Parasympathetic nervous system	The parasympathetic nervous system is located anteriorly in the head andw neck and posteriorly in the sacral region. It is primarily involved in restoring normal conditions after intense activity.	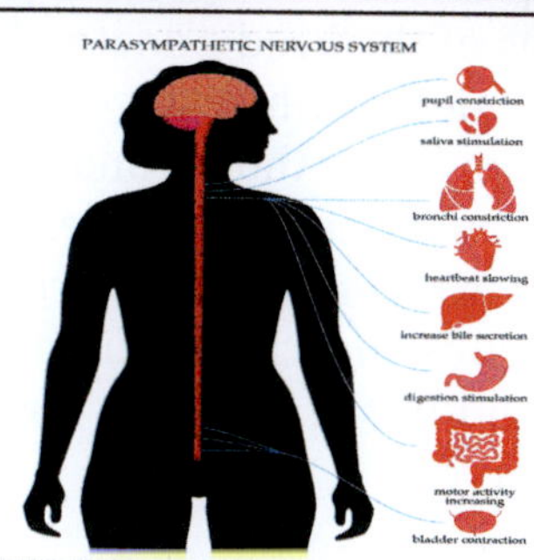
Lumbosacral plexus	Divides and recombines nerve fibers that go to the legs and feet.	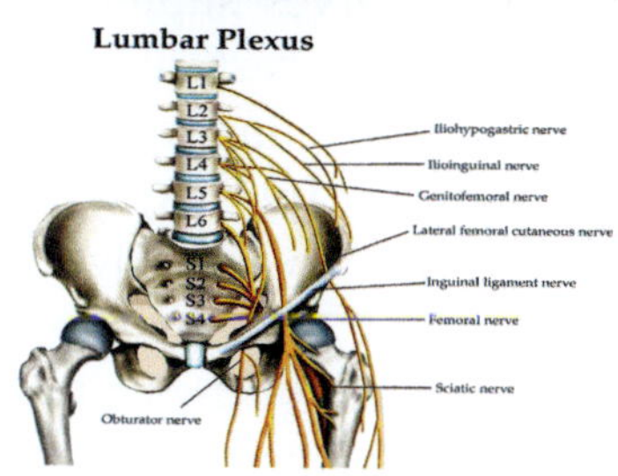

6.2. Structure of a Peripheral Nerve

The somatic nervous system and the autonomic nervous system (ANS) are two subtypes of the peripheral nervous system. The somatic nervous system, which relays signals from the brain to end organs like muscles, is controlled voluntarily. The sensory nervous system, which is a component of the somatic nervous system, sends messages to the brain and spinal cord from senses like taste and touch, including both fine and coarse touch. The ANS is a "self-regulating" system that affects the operation of organs that are not under conscious control, like the heart rate or digestive system.

6.2.1. Somatic Nervous System

The somatic nervous system is composed of numerous nerves that perform both somatic and sensory functions, as well as the somatosensory and sensory nervous systems. Cranial nerves in the head and neck transmit somatosensory information. With a few notable exceptions, the twelve cranial nerves—ten of which emerge from the brainstem—primarily regulate the operations of the head's anatomical structures. The vagus nerve, which receives sensory data from organs in the thorax and abdomen, is one special type of cranial nerve. The accessory nerve, which innervates the sternocleidomastoid and trapezius muscles—neither of which are solely found in the head—is the other distinct cranial nerve.

The spinal nerves supply somatosensory information to the rest of the body. These originate from the spinal cord. They typically begin as a network (plexus) of interconnected nerve roots that eventually organize into individual nerves. These nerves manage the functions of the rest of the body. Humans have 31 pairs of spinal nerves: 1 coccygeal, 8 cervical, 12 thoracic, 5 lumbar, and 5 sacral. The names of these nerves are determined by the spinal vertebrata next to which their nerve roots are located. The spinal nerve roots emerge in the cervical region above the corresponding vertebrae (i.e., spinal nerve C1) is the nerve root that runs between the skull and the first cervical vertebrae. The spinal nerve roots emerge below the corresponding vertebrae from the thoracic to the coccygeal regions. However, an issue arises when naming the spinal nerve root between C7 and T1 (spinal nerve root C8). The spinal nerve roots pass through the dural sac and descend as the cauda equina below the level of L2 in the lumbar and sacral regions.

6.2.1.1. Cervical Spinal Nerves (C1–C4)

Numerous nerves that supply the neck and back of the head are produced by the splitting and recombining of the first four cervical spinal nerves, C1 through C4. The suboccipital nerve, or spinal nerve C1, innervates the muscles at the base of the skull with motor function. Many of the neck's nerves, which provide both motor and sensory control, are made up of C2 and C3. The greater occipital nerve, which supplies feeling to the back of the head, the lesser occipital nerve, which supplies feeling to the region behind the ears, and the greater and lesser auricular nerves are among them. The phrenic nerve, which emerges from nerve roots C3, C4, and C5, is a nerve vital to human survival. It gives the thoracic diaphragm the supplies it needs to breathe. Spontaneous breathing is not possible if the spinal cord is transected above C3.

6.2.1.2. Brachial Plexus (C5–T1)

The brachial plexus, also known as the plexus brachialis, is a complex network of nerves that interweave, merge, and diverge to form the nerves that innervate the upper back and upper limbs. It consists of the last four cervical spinal nerves, C5 through C8, and the first thoracic spinal nerve, T1. Despite its intricate appearance, the brachial plexus follows a highly organized and consistent pattern, with minimal variation among individuals.

6.2.1.3. Lumbosacral Plexus (L1–Co1)

The lumbosacral plexus (L1–Co1) comprises the anterior divisions of the lumbar, sacral, and coccygeal nerves, with the first lumbar nerve often connected to a branch from the twelfth thoracic nerve. For descriptive purposes, the lumbosacral plexus is typically divided into three sections (Figure 6.2).

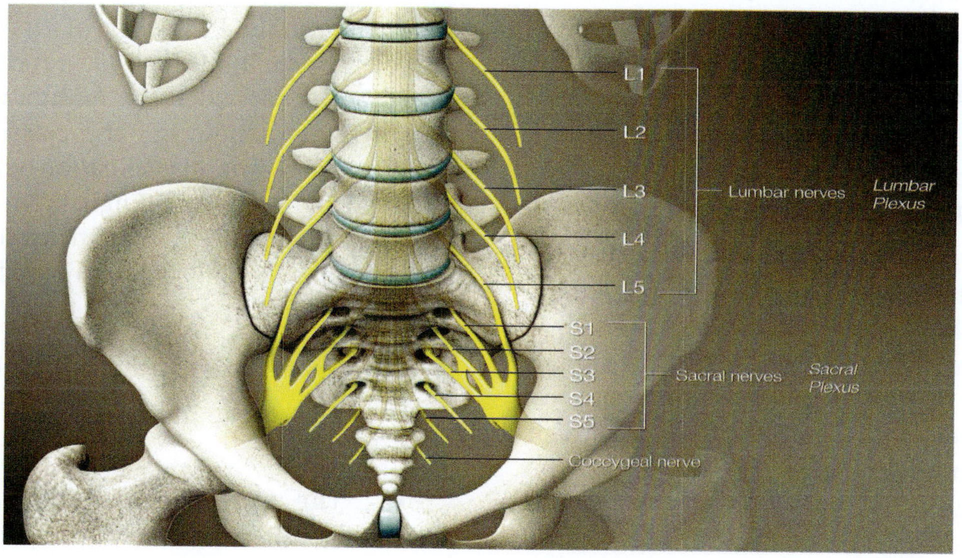

Figure 6.2. *3D medical animation still shot of lumbosacral plexus.*

Source: By https://www.scientificanimations.com – https://www.scientificanimations.com/wiki-images/, CC BY-SA 4.0, https://commons.wikimedia.org/w/index.php?curid=88600117.

6.2.2. Autonomic Nervous System (ANS)

Involuntary reactions are managed by the autonomic nervous system (ANS) to maintain physiological balance. Organs with smooth muscle, such as the heart, bladder, and other cardiac, exocrine, and endocrine-related organs, are connected to the brain and spinal cord of the central nervous system (CNS) through ganglionic neurons. Pupil constriction and dilation as well as salivation are the two most prominent physiological effects of autonomic activity. Although it is always active, the ANS is either parasympathetic or sympathetic. Different types of neurotransmitters may be released depending on the circumstances, where one state may overshadow the other.

6.2.2.1. Sympathetic Nervous System

The sympathetic nervous system is responsible for responding to mental stress or physical danger, commonly known as the "fight or flight" response. During this response, neurotransmitters like norepinephrine and epinephrine are released, which increase heart rate and blood flow to muscles while slowing down non-essential functions like digestion. The sympathetic system operates independently, allowing specific parts of the body to be activated while others remain relaxed.

6.2.2.2. Parasympathetic Nervous System

On the other hand, the parasympathetic nervous system promotes a restful and digestive state in the body. It primarily uses acetylcholine as its neurotransmitter. When the parasympathetic system is dominant, activities such as salivation and digestion increase, while heart rate and other sympathetic responses decrease. Unlike the sympathetic system, humans have voluntary control over certain functions in the parasympathetic system, such as urination and defecation.

6.2.2.3. Enteric Nervous System

The enteric nervous system is a lesser-known branch of the ANS. It is located only in the vicinity of the digestive tract. This system is capable of receiving and responding to signals from the rest of the body, but it only permits local control without input from the sympathetic or parasympathetic branches. The enteric system manages numerous gastrointestinal system-related processes.

6.3. Response of a Nerve to Injury

After an injury, the neuron degenerates and disintegrates. The amount of time needed varies depending on the size and myelination of the nerve, as well as in sensory and motor fibers. Primary or retrograde degeneration is the change that happens proximally to the injury, whereas secondary or antegrade degeneration (also known as Wallerian degeneration) occurs distally from the injury. Distal degeneration shows up as the removal of dead tissue, emptying the tube, and getting it ready for the axonal buds to sprout. On the other hand, proximally occurring changes help the neuron recover and get ready to grow and regenerate. These alterations transpire for fifteen to thirty days. The greater the recovery and return of function, the less disruptive the situation. The degree of disruption determines the degree of recovery and function return.

6.4. Classification of Nerve Injury

6.4.1. Seddon Classification

Seddon (Nuffield Professor of Orthopaedics) studied approximately 460 nerve cases in Oxford and established the foundation for our current understanding of the classification of nerve injuries. The classification was initially proposed by Seddon in English (in brackets), but Henry Cohen, a renowned neurologist at the time, suggested using Greek to avoid confusion (Figure 6.3).

- *Neurapraxia* (transient block).
- This is the mildest type of nerve injury.
- The prognosis is favorable, and complete recovery is expected as long as the insult is promptly removed.
- There is myelin sheath degeneration that is localized.
- *Axonotmesis* (lesion in continuity)
- This is a more severe injury than neurapraxia.
- Axons are completely severed, and the nerve fiber's ability to conduct signals outside of the injured area is lost.
- The prognosis is still favorable and recovery can be accomplished if the insult is removed promptly.
- Supporting structures (Schwann tubes, endoneurium, and perineurium) are preserved.

- *Neurotmesis* (division of a nerve).
- This is the most severe form of nerve injury.
- If the nerve is completely transected, there is no possibility of recovery. In such cases, surgery is the sole option.
- The recovery can be unpredictable.
- Histologically, every vital component is destroyed, but there can be disruptions without any noticeable loss of continuity.

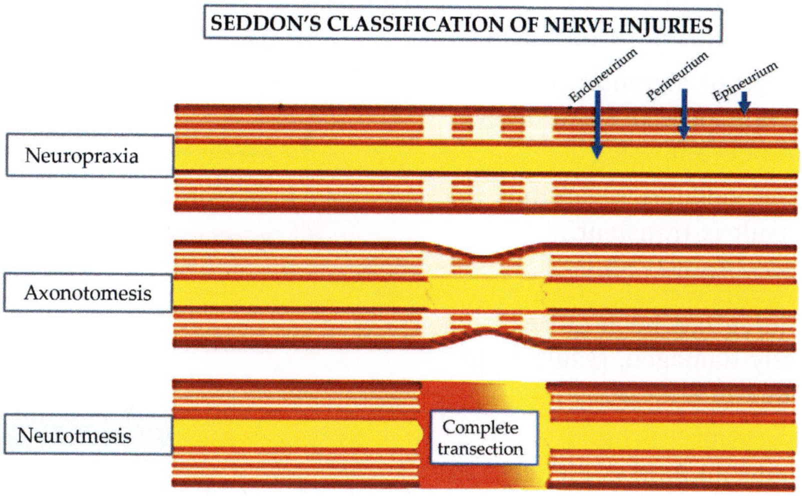

Figure 6.3. *Seddon's classification. The image shows the three types of nerve injuries in increasing severity from top to bottom.*

Source: By Davplast – File:Nerve_injuries_Armenian.jpg, CC BY-SA 4.0, https://commons.wikimedia.org/w/index.php?curid=73037258.

6.4.2. Sunderland Classification

The usage of Greek in academic writing did not sit well with Sunderland, the former Melbourne University anatomy professor and later dean. Sunderland predicted that Greek would be incomprehensible to doctors of today. Instead, he suggested a numbered classification (I–V) based on the increasing involvement of the different nerve sheaths. This classification was derived from a thorough analysis of the peripheral nerve anatomy and a lengthy examination of 300 cases of peripheral nerve damage. Sunderland mentioned that type I is comparable to neurapraxia, but he did not state that type I and neurotmesis are comparable to each other.

The disruption of nerve sheaths increases with the severity of nerve injuries (III to V), potentially leading to cross-wiring of the regenerating axons. This cross-wiring may cause incorrect muscle firing and a misinterpretation of the signals that the nerve is sending to the brain.

6.4.3. Lundborg Classification

To help us understand the wide range of clinical behaviors in seemingly benign insults to the nerves, another giant in nerve surgery, Lundborg, proposed the concept of physiological conduction block:

- Type A:
  - The intraneural circulatory arrest is a result of the insult;
  - This type of metabolic block does not cause any pathology to the nerve fibers;
  - It is immediately reversible, as the insult is transient.
- Type B:
  - The nerve has been more severely damaged, resulting in intraneural edema;
  - The pressure of the endoneurial fluid is higher;
  - It is reversible within days or weeks (after removal of the insult).

6.4.4. Birch and Bonney Classification

In the United Kingdom, Birch and Bonney proposed a practical distinction between non-degenerative and degenerative nerve lesions, significantly advancing our understanding of nerve injuries. In the latter case, the nerve fiber undergoes Wallerian degeneration.

6.4.5. Mixed Injury

It is important to note that nerve injuries are often mixed, and the severity of the lesion can vary from segment to segment. While many pioneers in nerve surgery made this observation, Mackinnon and Dellon were the ones to coin this crucial concept as "VI" according to Sunderland" (Figure 6.4).

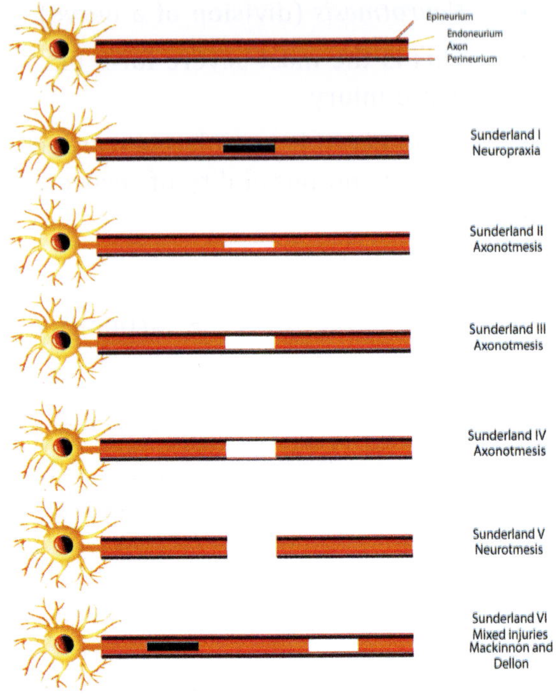

Figure 6.4. *Classification of nerve injury.*

Source: Lopes, B., Sousa, P., Alvites, R., Branquinho, M., Sousa, A. C., Mendonça, C., Atayde, L. M., Luís, A. L., Varejão, A. S. P., & Maurício, A. C., (2022). Peripheral nerve injury treatments and advances: One health perspective. International Journal of Molecular Sciences, 23(2), 918. https://doi.org/10.3390/ijms23020918.

6.5. Clinical Symptoms, Signs, and Tests Useful in Diagnosis

The body as a whole receives messages from the brain and spinal cord via peripheral nerves. They assist in functions such as sensing cold feet and activating the body's walking muscles. Axons, which are the fibers that make up peripheral nerves, are protected by surrounding tissues. Nerves in the periphery are delicate and susceptible to injury. A nerve injury can compromise the brain's ability to communicate with muscles and organs. Damage to the peripheral nerves is referred to as peripheral neuropathy. In the case of a peripheral nerve injury, it is crucial to seek medical attention as soon as possible. Timely diagnosis and treatment can prevent complications and irreversible damage.

6.5.1. Mechanisms of Injury for Peripheral Nerves

Peripheral nerve injuries can occur via a variety of ways. Most frequently, these injuries result from three mechanisms: stretches, cuts, and compressions.

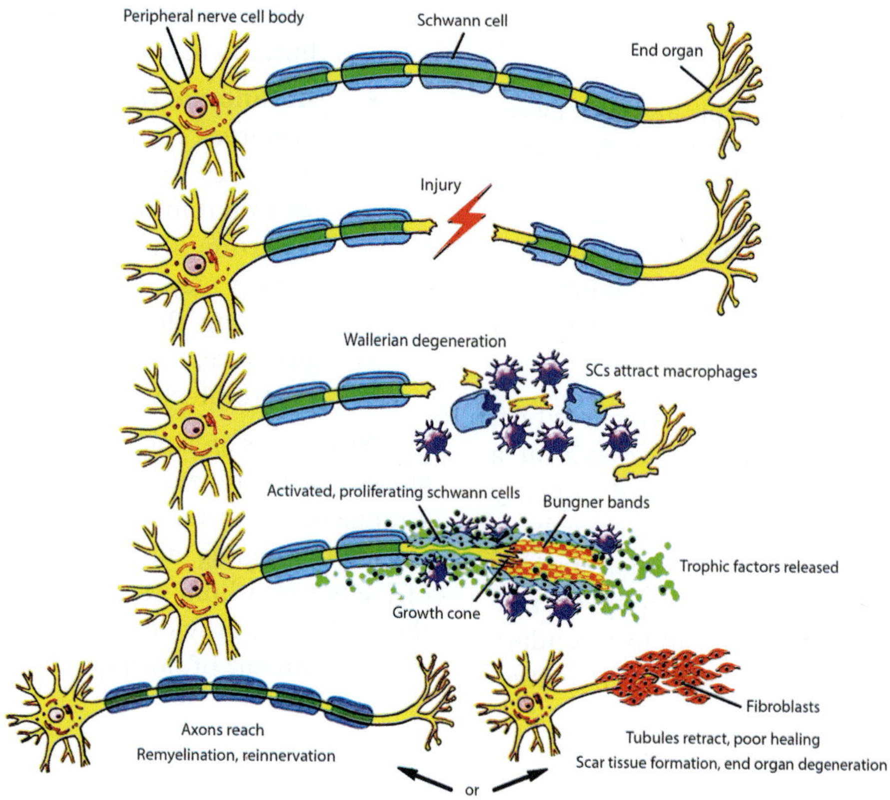

Figure 6.5. *Visual representation of peripheral nerve injury mechanisms.*

Source: Juckett, L., Saffari, T. M., Ormseth, B., Senger, J. L., & Moore, A. M., (2022). The effect of electrical stimulation on nerve regeneration following peripheral nerve injury. Biomolecules, 12(12), 1856. https://doi.org/10.3390/biom12121856.

Among these three, sprains are the most frequent, followed by cuts, and finally compressions.

Additionally, peripheral nerve injuries may be caused by radiation, electricity, injections, crush injuries, cold injuries, and intra- and extra-neural pathologies (Figure 6.5).

Peripheral nerves are elastic, so if the traction force exceeds the nerves' elasticity, stretch-related injuries may occur. In cases where the traction force surpasses the nerves' stretching capacity, a complete tear may result. However, it is more common for this type of injury to maintain nerve continuity.

6.5.1.1. Lacerations

Lacerations are the second most common type of peripheral nerve injuries. In this mechanism of injury, a sharp object partially or completely severs a nerve. Broken glass, metal fragments, knives, and similar objects are the most frequent sources of cuts.

6.5.1.2. Compression

Compression nerve injuries typically affect large-caliber nerves that pass over bony structures or between rigid surfaces. Sharp compression, such as chronic compression injuries (e.g., Saturday Night Palsy), can cause these injuries. Compression injuries can be classified into two main subcategories, including carpal tunnel syndrome (CTS).

Although the nerve fibers remain intact, compression nerve injuries can result in a complete loss of both motor and sensory function. These types of injuries have been associated with two pathological mechanisms: ischemia and mechanical compression. Mechanical compression can lead to secondary ischemia, which can impair the microcirculation of nerves.

6.5.2. Symptoms

The patient's daily activities may be severely limited by mild to moderate symptoms following a peripheral nerve injury. The symptoms the patient experience will often depend on which nerve fibers are damaged:

- **Motor Nerves:** These nerves control the muscles involved in walking, talking, and gripping objects. Damage to these nerves can result in muscle weakness, excruciating cramping, and uncontrollable twitching.
- **Sensory Nerves:** These nerves transmit information about touch, temperature, and pain. Symptoms may include tingling or numbness in the hands or feet. Difficulties with walking, maintaining balance with closed eyes, feeling pain or temperature changes, or fastening buttons may arise.
- **Autonomic Nerves:** This group of nerves regulates involuntary activities such as breathing, heart and thyroid function, and food digestion. Dysfunction in these nerves may manifest as profuse sweating, fluctuations in blood pressure, intolerance to heat, and gastrointestinal issues.

Numerous peripheral nerve injuries can affect multiple types of nerve fibers, resulting in a range of symptoms. If the patient experience weakness, tingling, numbness, or complete loss of feeling in a limb, it is important to consult the healthcare provider to determine the cause. Early treatment of peripheral nerve injuries is crucial.

6.5.3. Causes

Peripheral nerves can be damaged in several ways:

- Accidents, falls, or sports-related injuries can cause nerves to stretch, compress, crush, or cut.
- Diseases such as carpal tunnel syndrome (CTS), diabetes, and Guillain-Barre syndrome.
- Autoimmune conditions like lupus, rheumatoid arthritis, and Sjogren's syndrome. Tumors, hormone abnormalities, and artery narrowing are additional causes.

6.5.4. Diagnosis

In addition to reviewing the patient's medical history and inquiring about any accidents or previous surgeries, the physician will also discuss the symptoms with the patient. Furthermore, a neurological and physical examination will be conducted by the doctor. If the neurological examination reveals signs of nerve injury, the doctor may recommend diagnostic tests such as the following:

- **Electromyography (EMG):** This involves inserting a thin-tipped electrode into the muscle to record electrical activity during and after muscle contraction. Muscle atrophy may indicate nerve damage.
- **Nerve Conduction Study:** This test measures the efficiency of electrical signals traveling through nerves by placing electrodes at two different locations on the body.
- **Magnetic Resonance Imaging (MRI):** It uses radio waves and a magnetic field to produce detailed images of areas affected by nerve injury.
- **Ultrasound:** Similar to MRIs, ultrasound uses high-frequency sound waves to create precise images of the region affected by nerve damage.

6.6. Electrodiagnosis

A wide range of conditions that harm and impair the nerves of the peripheral nervous system in various ways are collectively referred to as peripheral neuropathy, also known as peripheral polyneuropathy. Electrodiagnostic (EDX) testing can assist the clinician in determining the etiology, severity, and prognosis of the disorder, as well as in determining the presence of peripheral neuropathy. When a patient presents with symptoms of peripheral neuropathy, a comprehensive history, physical examination, and EDX testing are all essential components of the evaluation and treatment process. Peripheral neuropathies are associated with numerous medical conditions, although peripheral polyneuropathies are frequently observed in patients with diabetes mellitus or excessive alcohol consumption. Certain peripheral polyneuropathies, such as Charcot-Marie-Tooth, may be inherited, while others can be acquired, such as those caused by diabetes mellitus, amyloidosis, HIV, or cis-platinum chemotherapy. The majority of peripheral polyneuropathies are characterized by paresthesias, numbness, or pain in the hands or feet, or in the distal extremities. While many have a more insidious onset, some can manifest acutely. Patients may report stumbling over their feet or experiencing difficulty with fine motor tasks, which could be indicative of disease progression and increasing weakness. Acquired polyneuropathies typically present as burning or tingling sensations, while inherited polyneuropathies can manifest with ataxia and muscle cramping.

The etiology can be determined and treatment direction can be guided with the help of EDX testing. Thus, it is imperative to obtain a comprehensive medical history that encompasses prescription drugs, dietary habits, social and occupational history, as well as family history. Peripheral polyneuropathies can arise as a result of exposure to heavy metal toxins, certain medications such as vincristine and amiodarone, or a significant medical history of hypothyroidism or vitamin B12 deficiency. Patients with a family history of hereditary motor and sensory neuropathies (HMSN) such as Charcot-Marie-Tooth Type 1 disease (HMSNI) or Refsum's disease (HMSNIV) may indicate a hereditary cause for the neuropathy. Peripheral neuropathy symptoms can also manifest in autoimmune-mediated disorders such as acute inflammatory demyelinating polyneuropathy (AIDP) or chronic inflammatory demyelinating polyneuropathy (CIDP), as well as infectious diseases like HIV and Lyme disease.

The physical examination can assist in determining the characteristics and cause of peripheral neuropathy. Patients with diabetic peripheral neuropathy often experience numbness in their hands and feet in a "stocking-glove" distribution. Musculoskeletal deformities, cataracts, and deafness may indicate a hereditary cause. Reduced sensitivity to light touch or vibration may indicate predominant sensory neuropathy, while distal muscle weakness and decreased deep tendon reflexes (DTR) may indicate predominant motor neuropathy. For example, a patient receiving dapsone therapy may exhibit weakness and abnormal DTRs, along with EDX findings primarily indicative of axonal motor neuropathy. Patients who have received high doses of cis-platinum therapy may still have strong muscles and DTR, but they may also experience abnormal sensations and other side effects such as GI distress and ototoxicity. EDX testing often reveals the presence of primarily axonal sensory neuropathy in cases of cis-platinum peripheral neuropathy.

6.6.1. Anatomy and Physiology

The specific etiology of each common peripheral neuropathy determines its pathophysiology. For example, ETOH-related peripheral neuropathy may be caused by starvation or direct nerve injury. Multifocal motor neuropathy (MMN), an immune-mediated condition, leads to asymmetric inflammatory demyelination and remyelination.

HIV-related neuropathies can be classified into different categories and present in various ways depending on the affected nerves. Mononeuropathy multiplex, for instance, manifests at all stages of HIV infection due to different etiologies. Thrombosis of the vasa nervorum is often the underlying cause, resulting in multiple lesions in different nerves and primarily causing axonal loss with relative myelin sparing. Autonomic neuropathy can also occur in HIV patients when there is damage to the nerves controlling autonomic processes such as blood pressure, heart rate, or bowel and bladder emptying.

It is important to note that small fiber neuropathies cannot be detected through EDX testing, as this type of testing is limited to Type I fibers. However, if a patient presents with typical symptoms of peripheral neuropathy and normal EDX testing results, these tests can help guide the clinician towards a diagnosis of small fiber neuropathy. Additional tests such as autonomic reflex testing or a skin biopsy may be necessary for confirmation. Small fiber neuropathies are often associated with conditions such as diabetes, HIV, and amyloidosis.

6.6.2. Indications

The clinician may use EDX testing to determine whether a peripheral neuropathy may be present when a patient presents with symptoms such as paresthesias, pain, or weakness in more than one extremity that cannot be explained by a focal mononeuropathy, such as a nerve entrapment neuropathy. Specific risk factors for peripheral nerve damage, such as toxic, metabolic, hereditary, microangiopathic, or autoimmune exposures or disorders, are usually identified through a comprehensive history and physical examination. Based on the common EDX features of the disease, EDX testing may also aid in narrowing the differential diagnosis.

6.6.3. Contraindications

There are few situations in which nerve conduction studies (NCS) and electromyography (EMG) needle testing are completely prohibited. In patients with implanted cardiac pacemakers and defibrillators, doctors may choose to postpone necessary EDX testing due to concerns about potential harm to the device. Numerous investigations have shown that pacemakers equipped with bipolar sensing do not exhibit electromagnetic interference activity. However, two studies examining repetitive nerve stimulation and unipolar pacemaker sensing did find some evidence of interference activity. The majority of contemporary pacemakers use bipolar sensing, and repetitive nerve stimulation studies are not commonly performed in most nerve conduction studies for peripheral neuropathy.

It is widely recognized that NCS typically does not pose a risk to pacemakers with current bipolar implants. However, it is advised to avoid direct stimulation in the area immediately in front of or near the device. In the case of implanted defibrillators and pacemakers with unipolar sensing, it is crucial to follow the instructions provided by the device manufacturers and seek the opinion of the patient's cardiologist. It is also possible to conduct the EDX study after deactivating the device and monitor the patients through telemetry. Patients with external cardiac pacemakers should not undergo NCS as the wires may be more electrically sensitive. Additionally, it is recommended to avoid stimulating over a central line as it may stimulate the heart.

Individuals with severe bleeding disorders should not undergo needle EMG. However, patients on anticoagulation may still be candidates with close monitoring to ensure appropriate bleeding control. It is not always necessary to keep anticoagulant or antiplatelet medications on hand. When patients have low platelet counts or an international normalized ratio (INR) that is higher than the recommended range, clinicians should proceed with caution. Never insert needles into areas where there is an active soft tissue infection.

6.6.4. Equipment

The equipment listed below is a general guideline and is not meant to be an all-inclusive list:

- Electrodiagnostic machine with a stimulator;
- Surface electrodes (wire ring, disposable or standard bar);
- Ultrasound gel;
- Needle electrodes;
- Alcohol prep pads;
- 4×4 gauze;
- Adhesive bandages.

6.6.5. Personnel

For EDX testing, a physiatrist or neurologist with subspecialization in neurodiagnostic studies is consulted. Sometimes, a specially trained technician will gather the nerve conduction studies and electromyographic results, which the specialist can read and interpret after the examination. This is not advised, though, as the doctor may need to modify and adapt the examination in real-time, depending on the patient's unique presentation or specific test results.

6.6.6. Preparation

Prior to the examination day, patients should be informed about the components of the test. On the day of the exam, they should be instructed to take their prescriptions and eat as usual. Before the exam, patients should bathe or clean their skin, and they should refrain from applying any lotions or creams to their extremities. In order to facilitate better access to the proximal musculature on the day of the examination, the patient may be instructed to change into a loosely fitting gown or dress. It is important to pay attention to both the room temperature and the temperature of the limbs, as cool limbs can cause waveform changes that could result in an incorrect diagnosis. A drop in body temperature can momentarily alter the protein structure of sodium channels, delaying the opening and closing of the channels. This can artificially increase or decrease the amplitude and conduction velocity. Generalized cooling of limbs may result in prolonged latency and decreased conduction velocity with a normal amplitude, while focal cooling of the extremities can cause delayed latency, decreased conduction velocity, and abnormally high amplitude. The clinician should take note of these effects and repeat the examination after adjusting the room's thermostat and warming the extremities with heat packs for a few minutes.

6.6.7. Technique or Treatment

The purpose of the EDX study is to evaluate the pattern and severity of peripheral neuropathy, as well as to confirm its existence. EMG testing and nerve conduction studies (NCS) are two types of EDX testing. The planning of an EDX study begins with a thorough physical examination and history taking. Instead of using a standardized approach, the study design should be tailored to the patient's unique presentation. For example, certain vasculitic neuropathies, chronic inflammatory demyelinating polyradiculopathy, and occasionally diabetes mellitus may initially exhibit abnormalities in the upper limbs. In such cases, the clinician may choose to customize the tests accordingly. It is recommended to perform sensory and motor nerve conduction studies, as well as needle EMG testing, on at least one upper and lower extremity, with testing in both proximal and distal muscles. However, most tests actually involve at least three limbs. Since longer nerves are typically affected first, it is advisable to proceed with nerve conduction studies and EMGs from distal to proximal in order to evaluate the longer nerves before the shorter ones.

Motor conduction in one lower extremity is typically the initial point for nerve conduction studies, which also encompass standard Peroneal and Tibial motor studies and their F-wave responses. The Tibialis Anterior muscle may be utilized in peroneal motor studies if motor responses are absent when recording over the usual distal muscles, such as the extensor digitorum brevis (EDB) muscles. If necessary, tibial motor studies can be conducted at the Soleus muscle, which is closer to the bone. A symmetry test should be performed on the opposite limb. When comparing side by side, amplitude differences exceeding 50% would be deemed abnormal. Although it can be examined, the soleus H reflex often does not contribute to the study and is absent in polyneuropathies where the ankle reflex is absent. A sensory response in the lower extremity, such as from the Sural or Superficial Peroneal nerves, should be obtained by the clinician following the completion of motor studies in the lower extremities. Due to frequently very small amplitude responses in polyneuropathies, averaging might be necessary.

An upper extremity test is conducted after the studies on the lower extremities. One option is to select the Ulnar motor and sensory nerve conduction study in the non-dominant hand. If there is concurrent entrapment neuropathy at the wrist, it is less likely to be affected. Since the radial sensory response is much less frequently involved in entrapment neuropathy, one may also choose to utilize it. When sensory responses are absent in the lower extremities but present in the upper extremities due to severe polyneuropathies, the clinician may decide to test both upper extremities to determine symmetry when sensory responses in the lower extremities are absent.

Prior to conducting the EMG study, the muscle is examined for any abnormal spontaneous muscle fiber activity while at rest. Additionally,

Motor Unit Action Potentials (MUAP) can be measured when the muscles are voluntarily contracting. Similar procedures are applied to EMG testing in polyneuropathy, which involves sampling the proximal and distal muscles of at least one upper and lower extremity. Muscle samples are continuously collected until a negative proximal muscle is identified. The anterior tibialis muscle is particularly useful as it is typically not atrophic and only mildly affected. However, the intrinsic foot muscles are not evaluated during the EMG due to their frequent pain and difficulty in activation, which poses challenges for MUAP assessment. Some degree of atrophy is common in certain healthy older adults, especially in the EDB muscle.

6.6.8. Complications

Both nerve conduction studies and EMG needle exams rarely carry a significant risk of complications. The tested nerves are typically not harmed in any way, either temporarily or permanently, by electrical stimulation. The insertion of the needle during the EMG carries some risk, as does any needle stick procedure. However, this risk can be reduced with appropriate antiseptic and pressure techniques. The electrical stimulation NCS studies are uncomfortable for most patients but bearable. A patient may occasionally find the examination intolerable because of the uncomfortable "shock" feeling, the needle exam, or, extremely infrequently, a vasovagal episode. The patient has the option to reschedule the exam for a later time or take breaks during it. Usually, these issues can be avoided by informing patients in advance of what to expect and advising them not to eat or drink right before the exam.

6.6.9. Clinical Significance

Peripheral neuropathy can be investigated using EDX testing to determine its cause, degree, prognosis, and potential courses of treatment. Although there is frequent overlap, it can distinguish between the following primary neuropathy characteristics: axonal, demyelinating, sensory, motor, multifocal, or diffuse.

Prolonged distal latency, slowed conduction velocity, and prolonged F-wave latency are classic findings in nerve conduction studies (NCS) for demyelinating injuries. Demyelination typically occurs at multiple locations along a nerve, leading to conduction blocks or slowed conduction velocities in the propagation of nerve action potentials. Abnormal temporal dispersion, also known as abnormal dispersion of arrival times of nerve action potentials at the recording site, is caused by non-uniform patterns of slowed conduction velocity. Conduction block, defined as the blockage of numerous axons over a short segment of nerve, is most commonly observed at entrapment sites in mononeuropathies, such as peroneal neuropathy at the knee or CTS. Focal conduction block in peripheral neuropathies may indicate focal demyelination at a site unaffected by entrapment. It is also important to note that slowed conduction can result from reversible metabolic issues that do not damage myelin.

Although conduction block and aberrant temporal dispersion are more common in acquired demyelinating peripheral neuropathy than in hereditary demyelinating peripheral neuropathy, they may still indicate demyelinating injury. In Charcot-Marie-Tooth type 1 neuropathy, which progresses slowly and causes uniform changes to myelin along nerve fibers, the compound muscle action potential (CMAP) amplitude does not significantly decrease between distal and proximal stimulation sites. As a result, conduction velocity is diffusely slowed down without aberrant temporal dispersion.

Weakness may manifest approximately one month after an upper respiratory or gastrointestinal ailment or vaccination in patients with AIDP, which includes a common variant known as Guillain-Barre syndrome (GBS). This is likely due to a viral attack on the myelin and Schwann cells. Early EDX testing may yield relatively normal results, but abnormal F-waves. Subsequent EDX testing may reveal motor demyelinating neuropathy rather than sensory neuropathy, with evidence of temporal dispersion and conduction block. Recognizing this illness can help guide treatment, such as promptly initiating IV immunoglobulins. It is important to note that other GBS variants, such as axonal motor and sensorimotor variants, present with different EDX characteristics.

Reduced sensory nerve action potential/compound muscle action potential (SNAP/CMAP) amplitude is observed in axonal injury NCS findings, along with near-normal distal latency and conduction velocity. It is also noteworthy that mild axonal damage may develop as peripheral neuropathy that is primarily demyelinating worsens. Axonal polyneuropathies can primarily manifest as motor or sensory predominant patterns, though mixed patterns are also possible. EDX testing in Acute Intermittent Porphyria frequently shows axonal degeneration with secondary demyelination in motor nerves more than sensory nerves. A sensory predominant axonal neuropathy is the traditional association between Friedreich's ataxia and it.

To determine whether an axon loss lesion is chronic, needle EMG is utilized. EMG testing ought to evaluate motor unit action potential (MUAP) activity during voluntary activity as well as spontaneous activity while at rest. Positive sharp waves and fibrillations, which would not be present in a demyelinating-type polyneuropathy, indicate denervation from axonal loss.

Abnormal spontaneous activity with amplitudes less than 50 μV is indicative of a chronic denervation that progresses gradually. Determining the recruitment, as well as the amplitude and complexity of the MUAP, can aid in determining the time course. The needle electrode records from approximately three to five MUAPs at low activation levels, which can be useful in determining the MUAP recruitment pattern. Motor unit loss is supported by the observation of multiple MUAPs discharging at frequencies higher than 20 Hz. It is also possible to check MUAP waveforms for increased amplitude. In neuropathies that progress slowly and are typically inherited, there will be a noticeable decrease in recruitment, a very high amplitude (approximately 5 to 10 times normal), and minimal complexity. Moderately decreased recruitment and moderately increased MUAP amplitude and complexity can be observed in axonal peripheral neuropathies with ongoing denervation. Up to 10% of the motor units in healthy people have increased MUAP complexity; hence, a clinician should not rely solely on the presence of this characteristic to make a diagnosis.

The presence of EDX evidence supporting a multifocal (segmental) disease pattern, as opposed to a diffuse (uniform) disease pattern, forms the basis of another significant classification scheme. A multifocal-type peripheral neuropathy affects one or more nerves in an asymmetric patchy distribution, whereas a patient with diffuse polyneuropathy presents with peripheral neuropathy that affects most nerves in a length-dependent manner. Contrary to porphyria and vasculitis, which more frequently exhibit multifocal axonal neuropathies, heavy metal toxins and drugs like alcohol usually manifest as diffuse axonal mixed sensorimotor polyneuropathy. Guillain-Barre syndrome is characterized by a multifocal demyelinating motor greater than sensory neuropathy, while

Charcot-Marie-Tooth Type I (HMSN-I) presents as a diffuse demyelinating mixed sensorimotor polyneuropathy. Diabetic neuropathy is a common cause of polyneuropathy, which is a widespread condition. Patients typically experience numbness and incapacitating dysesthesias in their lower extremities. Physical examination results show diminished two-point discrimination and symmetric vibratory sensation in the lower extremities. As the condition progresses, it gradually moves closer to the starting point. EDX results usually reveal a consistent mixed axonal and demyelinating sensorimotor polyneuropathy. Similar EDX findings are observed in patients with chronic renal failure, as well as in all patients requiring dialysis.

6.6.10. Enhancing Healthcare Team Outcomes

Regardless of specialization, peripheral polyneuropathies can occur in a variety of clinical contexts and result in severe morbidity for patients due to the pain, weakness, and deformity associated with them. According to some estimates, the prevalence of this condition is between 1% and 7% in the general population, with higher rates observed in patients over 50. It is crucial for internists, pediatricians, physiatrists, and neurologists to recognize the symptoms and risk factors associated with peripheral neuropathies. Additionally, they should be aware that EDX testing can provide valuable insights for diagnosis and treatment planning.

The primary care physician or referring physician should ideally conduct a comprehensive history, covering past medical history, surgeries, medications, diet, recreational drug or alcohol use, exposure to work-related hazards, and family history. This information can assist the electrodiagnostician in making an accurate diagnosis. The referring physician and the physician performing the EDX testing should engage in a candid conversation as part of an interprofessional approach to patient care. Prior to the EDX testing, discussing relevant history, physical examination findings, and laboratory results can help narrow down the differential diagnosis and guide the planning of NCV and EMG studies. In some cases, a cerebrospinal fluid (CSF) analysis or nerve biopsy may be warranted to further investigate and aid in the diagnosis and treatment plan.

6.7. Management

Nerve injury can be caused by a variety of trauma types and is a major contributor to functional morbidity. Neural death from trauma is a significant clinical issue because nerve trauma is the most frequent type of nervous system trauma seen in clinical practice. Many medications used to treat pain from nerve damage were first developed as anticonvulsants and antidepressants, so pharmacists should be knowledgeable about the indications for which each medication is prescribed as well as the appropriate dosage for that specific condition. The severity of the injury is a key indicator of both potential symptoms and potential recovery.

6.7.1. Mechanisms of Traumatic Nerve Injury

A number of conditions can cause nerve damage, including mechanical trauma, crush injuries (like those seen in fractures, hematomas, and compartment syndrome), penetrating traumas (like stab wound lacerations and surgical incisions), and stretch injuries (nerves can stretch 10% to 20% before becoming structurally damaged).

6.7.2. Nerve Repair and Regeneration

In the central nervous system (CNS), damaged areas of nerves are replaced by intact areas through a process called plasticity. Damaged nerves do not heal themselves. The peripheral nervous system's (PNS) nerves, on the other hand, make an effort to regenerate and reinnervate themselves. Peripheral nerves can undergo segmental remyelination, Wallerian degeneration, or axonal degeneration in response to damage or illness. Axonal degeneration is more commonly observed in metabolic and toxic nerve disorders like diabetes mellitus and renal failure, whereas segmental demyelination and Wallerian degeneration are repair mechanisms relevant to traumatic nerve injury. For PNS neurons to regenerate successfully, a variety of internal and external factors are necessary. Depending on the kind of damage, different nerve regeneration techniques apply. Remyelination is the method used to heal Grade I injuries; collateral axon sprouting and proximal-to-distal nerve regeneration are used to heal greater-grade injuries. The emergence of new axons from the shafts of preexisting axons is known as collateral axonal sprouting.

6.7.3. Treatment of Nerve Injuries

The treatment of nerve injuries can be traced back to William A. Hammond, who served as the surgeon general of the U.S. Army during the American Civil War. The objectives of treatment include restoring function to the injured nerve, enhancing quality of life, and reducing neuropathic pain. It is crucial to address both the nerve damage and any external sources of injury. In the early stages of severe pain syndrome, the most pressing issue is the development of axonal sprouting and neuroma formation due to nerve injury. Nerve pain is characterized by dysesthesias and a burning sensation, resulting from a combination of somatosensory, cognitive, and emotional changes. Treating this type of pain, which is typically neuropathic, can be challenging. Specific drugs designed for neuropathic pain management are necessary in treating severe pain syndrome. However, only about 70% of patients receive adequate care, highlighting the need for more effective approaches such as combination therapy for certain individuals. A common strategy is to use short-acting drugs to alleviate symptoms until longer-acting drugs, such as antidepressants or antiepileptics, take effect. In cases of refractory pain, an additional antidepressant or antiepileptic with a different mechanism of action may be required. Narcotics should only be used for more intense pain management.

6.7.4. Pharmacologic Therapy

A variety of agents may be used to treat nerve pain:

- **Analgesics:** Although they provide immediate and temporary pain relief, analgesics generally have limited efficacy. Opioids, tramadol, and nonsteroidal anti-inflammatory drugs (NSAIDs) are examples of analgesics. However, dosages are limited due to toxicity and adverse effects. Opioid analgesia is dose-dependent and correlated with serum levels. Anesthetics and topical medications such as capsaicin also possess analgesic properties. Nevertheless, the use of capsaicin is not recommended due to its inconsistent pain-reducing ability and potential to exacerbate pain.
- **Antidepressants:** These are highly effective in reducing pain, but their use is restricted due to associated side effects. Tricyclic antidepressants (TCAs), selective serotonin reuptake inhibitors (SSRIs), and serotonin-norepinephrine reuptake inhibitors (SNRIs) are particularly effective in this regard. TCA use is linked to anticholinergic side effects such as

dry mouth, constipation, orthostatic hypotension, and dizziness. Patients taking SSRIs and SNRIs may also experience diarrhea, dry mouth, somnolence, and sexual dysfunction.

- **Anticonvulsants:** These are utilized in the treatment of neuropathic pain due to the pathophysiological similarities between neuropathy and epilepsy. Changes in the expression of genes encoding sodium (Na)+ and calcium $(Ca)^{2+}$ channels lead to alterations in the distribution and composition of these channels. Similar to epileptic hyperexcitability, injured neurons exhibit abnormal biophysical characteristics and abnormal accumulation of Na+ channels in nociceptors and sensory nerves, resulting in high-frequency ectopic firing.

Chemically related to TCAs, carbamazepine was the first anticonvulsant to be investigated for the relief of neuropathic pain. Na channel blockers such as carbamazepine and phenytoin prevent high-frequency ectopic discharges, which explains their effectiveness in preventing seizures and neuropathic pain. This blocking activity is higher than lidocaine's ability to block Na channels. Compared to phenytoin, carbamazepine is more effective in the treatment of nerve pain.

Wind-up in spinal dorsal horn neurons can be induced by plateau potentials that are calcium-dependent. When C-fibers are repeatedly activated, neurons exhibit a progressive increase in responsiveness known as wind-up. Antiepileptic medications that target high-voltage activated Ca channels, such as lamotrigine, oxcarbazepine, and gabapentin, are beneficial in the treatment of nerve pain. Although it does not bind to gamma-aminobutyric acid (GABA) receptors or interfere with GABA uptake or metabolism, gabapentin was initially developed as a GABA analog. The precise mechanism is unknown, but gabapentin acts through alpha-2-delta type Ca^{2+} channels. Gabapentin has demonstrated the most pronounced analgesic effect in several trials when it comes to treating neuropathic pain. The dosage typically starts at 300 mg daily and can be increased by 300 mg every day until the patient experiences dose-limiting side effects or achieves an adequate analgesic response. Effective dosages range from three divided doses of 900–3,600 mg per day. The most common side effects of gabapentin include mild to moderate dizziness, somnolence, ataxia, and confusion. In general, gabapentin is well tolerated.

Pregabalin does not impact GABA receptors and shares a MOA resembling that of gabapentin. Pregabalin has an analgesic effect that is noticeable during the first week of treatment. The recommended daily dosage for this medication is 150–600 mg, taken orally in two or three divided doses. Peripheral edema, somnolence, and dizziness are the most frequent side effects of pregabalin, which is generally well tolerated. Over 98% of the medication that is eliminated through renal excretion stays in the urine unaltered.

When treating neuropathic pain in patients with a history of cardiovascular disease, glaucoma, or urinary retention, gabapentin, and pregabalin are especially helpful.

Lamotrigine inhibits glutamate release by blocking sodium channels. While its use is less established than that of carbamazepine, gabapentin, or pregabalin, it has a relatively good potential to modulate and control neuropathic pain.

Recently, L-carnitine and N-acetylcysteine (NAC), two neuroprotective pharmacologic factors, have drawn the attention of researchers. Perhaps as a result of their antioxidant qualities, both have been demonstrated to be secure and efficient neuroprotective agents.

Regenerative genes are simultaneously transcriptionally triggered by the signaling of cell death. The fate of the nerve cell is ultimately determined by the ratio of genes involved in cell death to those involved in regeneration.

Neuronal death is assumed to be caused by both mitochondrial dysregulation and blocking entry into the cell cycle. Since reactive oxygen species appear to be necessary for these processes, antioxidants like L-carnitine and NAC may be appealing as neuroprotective drugs.

6.7.5. Nonpharmacologic Therapy

For certain patients, transcutaneous electrical nerve stimulation may be able to reduce pain. In certain patients, endoneurial edema linked to peripheral nerve injury may be reduced with antivirals and steroids. Research on the treatment of nerve injuries focuses on neuroprotection. There is a therapeutic window for neuroprotection because neuroprotective therapies halt cell death, which is a gradual process. The neuroprotective growth factors were the first class of drugs to be studied; however, their clinical use was limited for two main reasons: (i) the need for different growth factor cocktails required for each type of nerve, since different neuronal subpopulations respond differently to different neurotrophic factors; and (ii) the limiting side effects associated with these drugs.

6.7.6. Surgical Treatment

Restoring the injured nerve, maximizing the number of axons that grow back through the site of injury, and increasing the percentage of axons that grow back to their intended targets are the three primary objectives of surgical treatment. The extent of nerve damage, the location and viability of the damaged nerve, the patient's age and health, the potential for partial restoration of function through surgery, and the balance between benefits, risks, expenses, and lost productivity will all determine the most suitable surgical approach that will facilitate the greatest axon regeneration.

6.7.7. Future Developments

In terms of future developments, research is currently focused on addressing the root cause of pain in addition to managing the symptoms, with the aim of improving pain management in cases of nerve injury. One approach to minimize nerve damage or promote the regeneration of damaged axons is to emulate the organism's natural response. While surgical techniques have advanced, the functional outcome of nerve injury still remains unsatisfactory.

6.8. Pathomechanics of Paralytic Deformities and Clinical Signs

The range of tasks that our hands can accomplish is immense. They give us the flexibility, dexterity, and ability to execute both fine and gross motor movements. The stability and mobility provided by the skeleton, muscles, and nerves enable the application of the exact amount of pressure required to hold an object.

The ability to use one's hands well is essential for job performance. Intrinsic muscle impairment affects the skills necessary for independence and participation in a variety of physical activities, resulting in decreased handgrip strength and characteristic deformities that negatively impact quality of life.

6.8.1. Etiology

Impairment can result from intrinsic palsy or intrinsic contracture of the hand. Trauma is often the primary cause of intrinsic contracture, typically linked to metacarpal fractures or conditions such as compartment syndrome. Intrinsic contractures lead to adhesion formation and fibrosis in the muscles and tendons of the hand. Other causes include neurologic conditions, rheumatoid arthritis, osteoarthritis, and arthrogryposis.

Intrinsic palsy is most commonly caused by traumatic injury to the ulnar nerve. Additional causes include compartment syndrome, rheumatoid diseases, entrapment of the nerve along its path in the arm (compression neuropathy), Leprosy (Hansen disease), rheumatoid arthritis, Charcot-Marie-Tooth disease, prolonged immobilization, and failure to splint a crush-injured hand using intrinsic plus posture.

6.8.2. Epidemiology

The most common cause of intrinsic palsy and intrinsic contractures is trauma. Nerve damage can occur from single ulnar or median nerve injuries, or from a combination of the two. In young, active patients, nerve injuries are a major cause of morbidity, leading to sensory and motor sequelae. Men are more likely than women to have hand deformities with a traumatized etiology. A combined injury is present in about 22% of nerve injuries involving the volar forearm. The most prevalent entrapment neuropathy is CTS, which affects 1 to 3 people out of every 1,000 person-years. With a reported incidence of 25–28 cases per 1,00,000 person-years, compressive neuropathy of the ulnar nerve is the second most common entrapment neuropathy after CTS.

6.8.3. Pathophysiology

The intrinsic muscles of the hand are divided into five groups:

- Thenar eminence muscles;
- Hypothenar eminence muscles;
- Lumbrical muscles;
- Dorsal interosseous muscles; and
- Volar interosseous muscles.

The most common cause of the intrinsic plus hand is spasticity in the intrinsic muscles, which causes the interphalangeal joints to extend and the metacarpophalangeal (MCP) joints to flex. Nevertheless, extrinsic muscle weakness (flexor digitorum superficialis and profundus or extensor digitorum communis) may also be the cause. The loss of intrinsic muscle action, which results in the loss of MCP flexion and interphalangeal extension—which are more noticeable in the fourth and fifth fingers—causes the intrinsic minus hand.

6.8.4. History and Physical Details

6.8.4.1. Intrinsic Muscles Palsy

Intrinsic muscle palsy is primarily caused by dysfunction of the ulnar nerve. There are two categories of ulnar nerve injuries: low and high injuries. Damage to the lower ulnar nerve occurs when it is farther away from the motor branches of the flexor digitorum profundus and flexor carpi ulnaris. The volar aspect sensibility of the fifth and fourth fingers of the hand is reduced. If the injury happens close to the dorsal ulnar sensory nerve, the dorsal aspect of these fingers also loses its sensibility. Paralysis affects all of the interosseous muscles, two ulnar lumbricals, the adductor pollicis, the hypothenar muscles, and the deep head of the flexor pollicis brevis. The MCP hyperextension and interphalangeal joint flexion of the fourth and fifth fingers (Duchenne sign) are caused by the loss of intrinsic muscle contraction, which also impairs MCP joint flexion and interphalangeal joint extension. This position is known as the intrinsic minus or claw posture. It is also referred to as the benediction sign and is more visible when the patient is asked to spread their fingers. The integrity of the flexor and extensor extrinsic muscles is necessary for the development of this position. Injuries to the ulnar half of the flexor digitorum profundus muscle resulting from high ulnar flexions therefore cause less severe defects.

Pinch and grip strength are lost between 60% and 80% of the time due to intrinsic weakness. In patients with adductor pollicis weakness, performing a pinch with the thumb pulp against the second finger pulp causes excessive flexor pollicis longus contraction, resulting in excessive thumb interphalangeal flexion, also known as the Froment sign. If there is MCP joint laxity, the thumb's MCP joint exhibits hyperextension, which is referred to as Jeanne's sign. Weakness in the first interosseous muscle causes the second finger to exhibit proximal interphalangeal joint hyperflexion (>90°), known as the Mannerfelt sign.

The Andre-Thomas sign, characterized by the patient assuming a wrist-flexing position to achieve better MCP extension by increasing the pull on the extensor digitorum communis, is another indicator of interosseous weakness. However, this posture ultimately exacerbates the deformity by increasing MCP extension. The loss of adduction (palmar interosseous) and abduction (dorsal interosseous) of the fingers is observed. In third palmar interosseous palsy, the fifth finger is abducted due to an unopposed extensor digiti minimi pull, known as Wartenberg's sign. When the palm is flat on a table, third finger impairment in its ability to move is observed in cases of second and third dorsal interosseous palsy, referred to as Pitres-Testut's sign/Egawa's sign. In more severe cases, atrophy of the hypothenar and interosseous muscles, along with a flattened palmar metacarpal arch, can be observed, known as Masse's sign.

6.8.4.2. Median Nerve Injuries

High and low injuries are alternative terms for median nerve injuries. The volar extrinsic muscles affected by the high median nerve cause the hand to supinate and deviate towards the ulna. A small group of intrinsic hand muscles, including the superficial head of the flexor pollicis brevis, the abductor pollicis brevis, the opponens pollicis, and two radial lumbricals, are also innervated by the median nerve. The innervated ulnar interosseous muscles cause weak flexion of the MCP joints when this muscle group is paralyzed. Paralysis of the flexor digitorum profundus and flexor digitorum superficialis prevents flexion of the interphalangeal joints of the thumb, second finger, and third finger combined. The abductor pollicis brevis and opponens pollicis are paralyzed, resulting in impaired thumb opposition and the thumb lying in the same plane as the metacarpals. The benediction sign is a distinctive posture that worsens when the patient is asked to clench their fist. In severe cases, the thenar eminence begins to atrophy.

Extrinsic muscle function is preserved in cases of low median nerve injury. Due to the lack of flexion at the MCP joints, the patient's second and third fingers lag behind their ring and little fingers when attempting to make a fist. However, the thumb is also in the same plane as the palm and exhibits poor opposition.

6.8.4.3. Intrinsic Contractures of the Hand

The intrinsic muscles of the hand extend the interphalangeal (IP) joints and flex the MCP joints. The examiner can passively flex the proximal interphalangeal joint and passively extend the patient's MCP joints without encountering any resistance or limitations in movement when there is appropriate balance between the intrinsic and extrinsic musculature and normal muscle tone. The maneuver known as the "intrinsic tightness test," was originally published in 1948 by Sterling Bunnell. This test is considered positive when the force required to flex the proximal interphalangeal joint is greater when the MCP joint is passively extended compared to its flexion, indicating contracture of the intrinsic muscles. This occurs because the intrinsic muscles are located dorsal to the axis of the proximal interphalangeal joint and volar to the axis of rotation of the MCP joint. The intrinsic muscles are thus tightened by MCP joint hyperextension. Conversely, contracture of the extrinsic extensor is indicated when the force required to flex the MCP joint increases the interphalangeal joint flexion. It is important to consider the presence of lateral band adhesions, as they may cause restricted flexion of the interphalangeal joint in both flexion and extension of the metacarpophalangeal joint. Individuals with intrinsic contractures often express concerns about hand weakness and may struggle to hold large objects.

6.8.5. Evaluation

A comprehensive physical examination is imperative for making an accurate diagnosis. During the assessment, special attention should be given to the patient's hand posture, range of motion, and signs of muscle atrophy.

Placing the patient's ulnar side hand on the examination table allows for the evaluation of the first dorsal interosseous muscle. The examiner applies resistance while instructing the patient to abduct the second finger. Simultaneously comparing the strength of both hands provides a more sensitive assessment. The patient is asked to abduct all fingers against resistance to evaluate the strength of the second to fourth dorsal interosseous muscles. Measuring the strength of the volar interosseous muscles involves placing a piece of paper between the patient's extended and adducted fingers and asking them to hold it while the examiner attempts to pull it away.

Bunnell's test is used to assess the presence of intrinsic muscle tightness by comparing the range of motion and force required to passively flex the proximal interphalangeal joints while the MCP joints are passively extended and flexed. This test also helps determine whether tightness is caused by interphalangeal capsule adhesions or extrinsic muscle contracture.

To evaluate the abductor digiti minimi, instruct the patient to abduct their fifth finger against resistance. By extending the MCP joint and the interphalangeal joints while the examiner resists at the base of the proximal interphalangeal joint, the flexor digiti minimi brevis can be assessed. To evaluate the opponens digiti minimi, instruct the patient to pinch their thumb from pulp to pulp. To assess the abductor pollicis brevis, ask the patient to abduct their first finger against resistance. The opposition to the fifth finger serves as an indicator of the opponens pollicis. To assess the adductor pollicis, instruct the patient to pinch a piece of paper between their thumb and second finger. Thumb MCP flexion against resistance is used to assess the flexor pollicis brevis.

The most common mechanisms of ulnar nerve injury include contusions, sprains, and lacerations. It is crucial to differentiate between neurotmesis, which requires surgical intervention, neuropraxia, and axonotmesis, which can be managed non-surgically. EDX tests are a valuable tool for assessing the extent of damage. However, the time elapsed between the injury and the evaluation can impact the conclusions drawn from these tests. It is generally recommended to delay the performance of an EDX study until approximately three to four weeks after the injury, allowing for two weeks of Wallerian degeneration. Early testing can provide significant information as follows:

- Finding the location of the injury is aided by studies conducted during the first week of recovery.

- Studying for 1–2 weeks can assist in determining if the lesion is fully healed or still in progress.
- Studies lasting three to four weeks provide the most diagnostic data. They facilitate the distinction between neuropraxia and axonotmesis or neurotmesis.
- 3–4 month studies help to determine if there are signs of reinnervation.

MRIs and high-resolution ultrasounds are helpful diagnostic instruments. They are capable of precisely identifying perilesional scar tissue, neuromas, and any discontinuity in the nerve.

6.8.6. Differential Diagnosis

It is important to conduct a thorough investigation into the traumatic or systemic event that caused intrinsic tightness or ulnar nerve paralysis. Additional hand disabling conditions consist of:

- High ulnar nerve injuries – neuropathy;
- Anterior interosseous nerve compressive neuropathy;
- Parsonage-Turner syndrome;
- Brachial plexus neuritis;
- Carpal tunnel syndrome (CTS);
- Pronator syndrome;
- Forearm Volkmann contracture;
- Dupuytren contracture.

Individuals diagnosed with complete ulnar nerve palsy should not have any intrinsic motor function in ulnar nerve-innervated muscles. The presence of clinical findings associated with incomplete palsy in patients with a proven complete ulnar nerve injury suggests the presence of anomalous anastomoses (Martin-Gruber) between the anterior interosseous nerve and ulnar nerve, which occurs in 15% of the population.

6.9. Formation of Brachial Plexus

The skin and upper limb musculature are supplied by the brachial plexus, which is a network of nerve fibers. It originates at the base of the neck, passes through the axilla, and extends throughout the entire upper limb. The plexus is formed by the combination of the first thoracic spinal nerve, T1, and the anterior rami (divisions) of the cervical spinal nerves C5, C6, C7, and C8.

6.9.1. Structure

There are six divisions (three anterior and three posterior), three cords, five branches, three trunks, and five roots that make up the brachial plexus. The plexus has multiple branches that emerge at different points along its length, including five terminal branches and a large number of pre-terminal or collateral branches such as the long thoracic nerve, the thoracodorsal nerve, and the subscapular nerve. In cadaver dissections, the M or W formed by the musculocutaneous nerve, lateral cord, median nerve, medial cord, and ulnar nerve is a frequently used structure to identify a portion of the brachial plexus.

6.9.1.1. Roots

The five roots of the spinal nerves are their five anterior primary rami, which remain after supplying the neck muscles with their segmental supply. The brachial plexus emerges at five stages: C5, C6, C7, C8, and T1. The middle trunk is formed by C7, the lower trunk is established by C8 and T1, and the upper trunk is formed by the merger of C5 and C6. In certain instances, prefixed or postfixed formations involve C4 or T2, respectively. The dorsal scapular nerve, which originates in the superior trunk, innervates the rhomboid muscles responsible for retracting and rotating the scapula downward. The subclavian nerve, originating from both C5 and C6, innervates the subclavius muscle involved in raising the first ribs during breathing. The long thoracic nerve has its origins in C5, C6, and C7. This nerve innervates the serratus anterior muscle, which draws the scapula laterally and is the main muscle involved in pushing and reaching forward.

6.9.1.2. Trunks

These roots merge to form the trunks:

- "Superior" or "upper" (C5–C6);
- "Middle" (C7);
- "Inferior" or "lower" (C8–T1).

6.9.1.3. Divisions

Each trunk then splits in two, to form six divisions:

- Anterior divisions of the upper, middle, and lower trunks;
- Posterior divisions of the upper, middle, and lower trunks;
- The anterior divisions are superficial to the posterior divisions when viewing the body in its anatomical position.

6.9.1.4. Cords

The three cords, or large fiber bundles, are formed when these six divisions come together. The location of the cords in relation to the axillary artery determines their names (Figure 6.6):

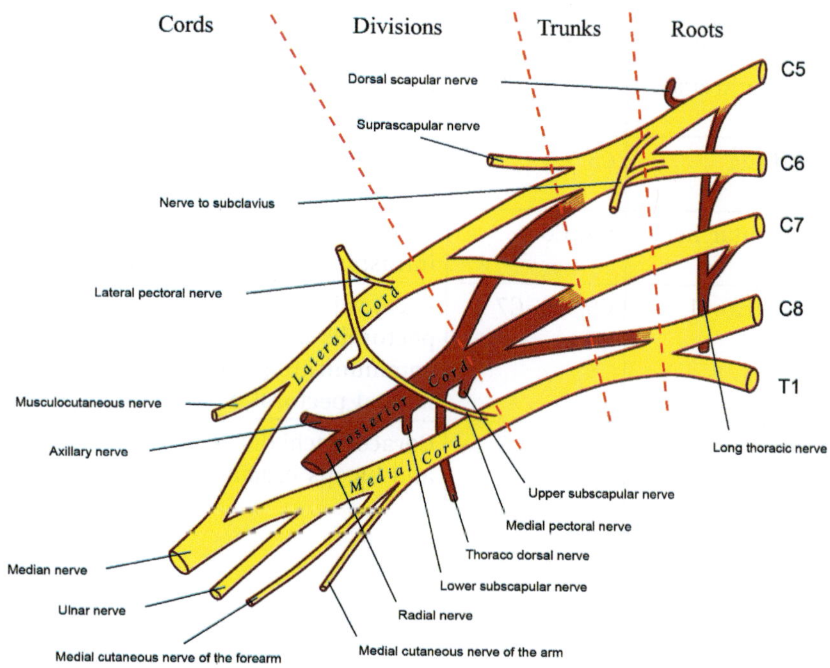

Figure 6.6. *Anatomical illustration of the brachial plexus.*

Source: Vara, G., Tuzzato, G., Bianchi, G., Miceli, M., Spinardi, L., Golfieri, R., Rinaldi, R., & Facchini, G., (2022). Clinical application of diffusion tensor imaging for a brachial plexus injury. Diagnostics, 12(7), 1687. https://doi.org/10.3390/diagnostics12071687.

- **Posterior Cord:** It is formed by the three posterior divisions of the trunks (C5–C8, T1).
- **Lateral Cord:** The lateral cord is formed by the anterior divisions of the upper and middle trunks (C5–C7).
- **Medial Cord:** It is simply a continuation of the anterior division of the lower trunk (C8, T1).

6.9.2. Branches

The branches are mentioned in the list below. A small number of branches (shown in italics) originate directly from earlier structures, but the majority of branches grow from the cords. The five branches on the left are regarded as terminal. These include the radial nerve, the ulnar nerve, the median nerve, the musculocutaneous nerve, and the axillary nerve. The median nerve and the musculocutaneous nerve have a strong connection since they both emerge from the lateral cord. Even more evidence linking the two nerves is the musculocutaneous nerve's branching off to the median nerve. Although there have been a few documented variations in the branching pattern, these are extremely uncommon (Table 6.1).

Table 6.1. *Branches of Brachial Plexus**

From	Nerve	Roots	Muscles	Cutaneous
Roots	Dorsal scapular nerve	*C4*, **C5**	Rhomboid muscles and levator scapulae	–
Roots	Long thoracic nerve	**C5**, **C6**, C7	Serratus anterior	–
Roots	Branch to phrenic nerve	**C3**, **C4**, **C5**	Diaphragm	–
Upper trunk	Nerve to the subclavius	*C5*, **C6**	Subclavius muscle	–
Upper trunk	Suprascapular nerve	**C5**, C6	Supraspinatus and infraspinatus	–
Lateral cord	Lateral pectoral nerve	C5, **C6**, C7	Pectoralis major and pectoralis minor (by communicating with the medial pectoral nerve)	–
Lateral cord	Musculocutaneous nerve	C5, C6, C7	Coracobrachialis, brachialis, and biceps brachii	The lateral cutaneous nerve of the forearm becomes innervated, supplying the skin of the anterolateral forearm and the elbow joint.
Lateral cord	Lateral root of the median nerve	*C5*, C6, C7	Fibers to the median nerve (see below)	–
Posterior cord	Upper subscapular nerve	C5, C6	Subscapularis (upper part)	–

Posterior cord	Thoracodorsal nerve (middle subscapular nerve)	C6, **C7**, C8	Latissimus dorsi	–
Posterior cord	Lower subscapular nerve	C5, C6	Subscapularis (lower part) and teres major	–
Posterior cord	Axillary nerve	**C5**, C6	Anterior branch: deltoid and a small area of overlying skin. Posterior branch: teres minor and deltoid muscles.	The posterior branch becomes the superior lateral cutaneous nerve of the arm. It innervates the skin of the lateral shoulder and arm, including the shoulder joint.
Posterior cord	Radial nerve	C5, C6, C7, C8, T1	Triceps brachii, supinator, anconeus, the extensor muscles of the forearm, and brachioradialis	The skin of the posterior arm and posterior forearm is innervated by the posterior cutaneous nerve of the arm and the posterior cutaneous nerve of the forearm, respectively. Additionally, the superficial branch of the radial nerve supplies the back of the hand, including the web of skin between the thumb and index finger.
Medial cord	Medial pectoral nerve	C8, T1	Pectoralis major and pectoralis minor	–
Medial cord	Medial root of the median nerve	C8, T1	All of the flexors in the forearm, except for the flexor carpi ulnaris and that part of the flexor digitorum profundus that supplies the 2nd and 3rd digits, as well as the 1st and 2nd lumbrical muscles, are supplied by a recurrent thenar branch that innervates the muscles of the thenar eminence.	Portions of the hand not served by the ulnar or radial nerves include the skin of the palmar side of the thumb, the index and middle fingers, half of the ring finger, and the nail bed of these fingers.
Medial cord	Medial cutaneous nerve of the arm	C8, T1	–	Front and medial skin of the arm.

Medial cord	Medial cutaneous nerve of the forearm	C8, T1	–	Medial skin of the forearm.
Medial cord	Ulnar nerve	C7, C8, T1 (C7 because it supplies to the Flexor carpi ulnaris)	Flexor carpi ulnaris, the medial two bellies of flexor digitorum profundus, the intrinsic hand muscles, except the thenar muscles and the two lateral lumbricals of the hand which are served by the median nerve.	The skin of the medial side of the hand and medial one-and-a-half fingers on the palmar side and medial two-and-a-half fingers on the dorsal side.

****Bold** indicates the primary spinal root component of the nerve. Italics indicate spinal roots that frequently, but not always, contribute to the nerve.*

Source: https://en.wikipedia.org/wiki/Brachial_plexus.

6.9.3. Function

The skin and muscles of the arms receive nerve supply from the brachial plexus, except for the muscles of the trapezius (supplied by the spinal accessory nerve) and a region of skin near the axilla (supplied by the intercostobrachial nerve). By connecting the plexus roots, gray rami communicantes allow the brachial plexus to communicate with the sympathetic trunk.

6.10. Different Injuries of Brachial Plexus

The classification of brachial plexus injuries is determined by the degree of the injury and how the nerves are harmed.

6.10.1. Brachial Plexus Neuropraxia (Stretch)

Neuropraxia is the term used to describe when nerves are stretched to the point of injury. This injury can happen in two main ways: traction or compression. A compression injury occurs when the head rotates, compressing the brachial plexus nerve root. The most prevalent type of compression neuropraxia usually affects older adults. When a nerve is pulled, usually downward, traction neuropraxia develops. Although this injury is more common in adolescents and young adults, it is less common than compression neuropraxia. These injuries are sometimes called brachial plexus "burners" or "stingers," depending on whether a burning or stinging sensation is the primary complaint. They may also have an electric shock-like sensation.

6.10.2. Brachial Plexus Rupture

A strong stretch that causes the nerve to tear, either completely or partially, results in a brachial plexus rupture. Compared to neuropraxia, this injury is more serious. Ruptures can render some muscles useless and result in weakness in the hand, arm, or shoulder. Severe pain is another possible side effect of these injuries. Surgery is frequently an option for treating these injuries, depending on the rupture's location and severity.

6.10.3. Brachial Plexus Neuroma

Scar tissue can occasionally develop when nerve tissue is damaged, such as from a cut sustained during surgery, as the nerve tries to mend itself. One of the brachial plexus nerves may become painfully knotted as a result of this neuroma-like scar tissue. One of the surgical treatments for brachial plexus neuromas is the excision of the damaged nerve tissue. To stop another neuroma from developing, the surgeon then either caps the nerve or joins it to another nerve.

6.10.4. Brachial Neuritis

Brachial neuritis, also known as Parsonage-Turner syndrome, is an uncommon and gradually worsening condition that affects the brachial plexus nerves. This syndrome presents with acute, sharp pain in the upper arms and shoulders, which then progresses to weakness, muscle atrophy, and eventual loss of sensation. While it can also impact the diaphragm and legs, this syndrome primarily affects the arm and shoulder. The exact cause of brachial neuritis is unknown, but it may be associated with an autoimmune reaction triggered by an injury, infection, childbirth, or other factors.

6.10.5. Brachial Plexus Avulsion

A complete separation of the nerve root from the spinal cord results in a brachial plexus avulsion. Trauma, such as being involved in an automobile or motorcycle accident, is typically the cause of this injury. Avulsions can cause significant pain, sometimes even more than ruptures. Avulsions can lead to permanent weakness, paralysis, and loss of sensation because reattaching the root to the spinal cord is difficult, if not impossible.

6.11. Signs, Symptoms, Diagnosis, and Management of Brachial Plexus

The upper extremities are innervated by the nerves that branch off of the brachial plexus, so damage to this structure can be extremely problematic. The affected area of the plexus determines the clinical signs and symptoms, which typically lead to anesthesia or paralysis. The spectrum of symptoms includes partial upper limb weakness and temporary nerve dysfunction. Owing to variations in the brachial plexus' anatomy, diagnosing these injuries can be difficult.

6.11.1. Mechanism of Injury

Traction brought on by vigorous movements and strong impacts are the primary causes of brachial plexus palsies. Brachial plexus injury can result from inflammation, tumors, or injuries to the shoulder, among other causes. Despite no visible damage, the uncommon Parsonage-Turner Syndrome results in brachial plexus inflammation and incapacitating symptoms. However, brachial plexus lesions are generally categorized as obstetric or traumatic. A mechanical injury involving shoulder dystocia during a challenging childbirth may result in obstetric injuries. Excessive stretching of the neck during birthing can cause an inferior trunk or an injury to the upper brachial plexus, respectively. About one brachial plexus injury occurs for every 1,000 live births.

Penetrating or sports-related injuries, falls, injuries sustained at work, radiation therapy, and iatrogenic causes (i.e., brachial plexus block, shoulder surgery, and initial rib resection) can also lead to such injuries. However, traction injuries are the most frequent type of injury mechanism, as the neck and shoulder are forced apart.

6.11.2. Causes of Brachial Plexus Injuries

6.11.2.1. Brachial Plexus Injury at Birth (Obstetric Brachial Plexus Injury)

During birth, the brachial plexus nerves in the shoulder of an infant are susceptible to injury. Brachial plexus injuries during childbirth are relatively common, occurring in one to two births out of every 1,000. Babies of diabetic mothers and larger babies delivered vaginally with difficulty are particularly vulnerable to this type of injury. Large babies may have a higher risk of experiencing brachial plexus injuries during childbirth. Injuries to the brachial plexus nerves can occur if the baby's head is extended beyond the shoulder. Babies born in the breech position, where their bottom end emerges first, and those with abnormally prolonged labors can also be at risk for brachial plexus injuries. Shoulder dystocia, which is when the shoulder becomes momentarily lodged under the pubis during childbirth, can cause brachial plexus injury.

Brachial plexus injury at birth generally takes one of two forms:

- **Erb's Palsy:** A common injury to the upper brachial plexus that results in loss of motion and numbness around the shoulder, as well as an inability to raise the arm, flex the elbow, or bring objects to the mouth.
- **Klumpke's Palsy:** A less frequent injury to the lower brachial plexus that results in loss of sensation and/or movement in the hand and wrist, including the inability to move fingers.

The severity of these injuries can vary greatly. With physical and occupational therapy, the majority of children who suffer birth injuries to the brachial plexus will regain all or most of their normal function. However, some children may recover without intervention. For a smaller group, surgery may be necessary to achieve optimal function. Prompt diagnosis and treatment can significantly improve long-term outcomes.

6.11.2.2. Causes of Brachial Plexus Injuries in Adults

In adults, brachial plexus injuries have a range of causes, including:

- **Blunt Trauma:** Such as falls or motor vehicle accidents.
- **Athletic Injuries:** Especially from contact sports like football.
- **Gunshot Wounds:** A bullet tears through or close to the nerves.
- **Medical Trauma:** This occurs when a nerve is cut during a surgical procedure, damaged by an injection, or affected by the positioning of the body during surgery.
- **Cancer:** A tumor invades the brachial plexus.
- **Radiation Therapy:** Radiation treatment in the area damages the nerves.

6.11.3. Brachial Plexus Injury Symptoms

The symptoms are determined by the location and severity of the injuries along the length of the brachial plexus. Injuries to the shoulder occur when the nerves in the neck, which are rooted higher up on the spinal cord, are damaged. Damage to the nerves that originate lower in the brachial plexus affects the arm, wrist, and hand.

Typical signs of injuries to the brachial plexus include:

- Numbness or loss of feeling in the hand or arm;
- Inability to control or move the shoulder, arm, wrist or hand;
- An arm that hangs limply;
- Burning, stinging or severe and

sudden pain in the shoulder or arm.

The severity and type of brachial plexus injury can determine how severe the pain is, as well as whether it is short-term or long-term. For instance, a simple stretched nerve may cause pain for approximately a week, while a ruptured nerve can result in severe and chronic pain that may require physical therapy or even surgical intervention.

6.11.4. Diagnosis

Individuals who have suffered injuries to the brachial plexus should be assessed and treated as soon as possible; this is typically within six to seven months after the injury. The likelihood of a muscle functioning normally in the future decreases as the muscle is left without nerve input for a longer period of time. This remains true even if the muscle eventually regains its nerve signals. The specific timing of seeking medical attention will depend on the nature and location of the injury.

6.11.4.1. Physical Examination

A thorough examination will be conducted by the doctor to diagnose any suspected brachial plexus injuries and rule out any accompanying conditions. They will assess each group of nerves regulated by the brachial plexus to determine the precise location and extent of the nerve damage (Figure 6.7).

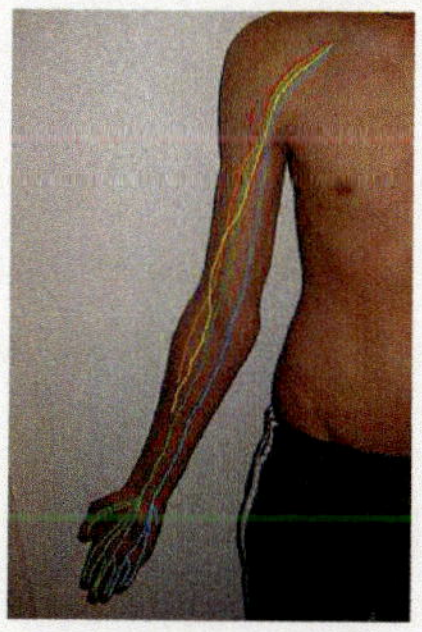

Figure 6.7. *The anterior view of the five brachial plexus nerves on the human arm.*

Axillary, Median, Musculocutaneous, Radial, Ulnar

Source: By Kinstudent – Own work, CC BY-SA 3.0, https://commons.wikimedia.org/w/index.php?curid=24622160.

The doctor will be able to identify possible sites of nerve injury with the help of the pattern by which nerves from the brachial plexus control different muscles of the arm and hand. The physician will assess every group of nerves that the brachial plexus regulates.

Moreover, certain patients exhibit particular indicators that help locate the nerve injury:

- Signs that indicate the injury is close to the spinal cord include drooping of the eyelid, narrowing of the pupils, and Horner's syndrome, which prevents the face from sweating.
- Damage further away from the spinal cord is indicated by a shooting pain that feels similar to a nerve when the physician taps along the afflicted nerves (Tinel's sign). An indication that the injury is healing on its own is if the Tinel's sign gradually moves down the arm toward the hand.

The doctor will check the range of motion and stability in the arm and shoulder during the physical examination.

6.11.4.2. Imaging Tests

Radiology images. Dense structures, such as bone, can be clearly seen in X-ray images. To rule out related fractures, X-rays of the arm, shoulder, chest, and neck are taken.

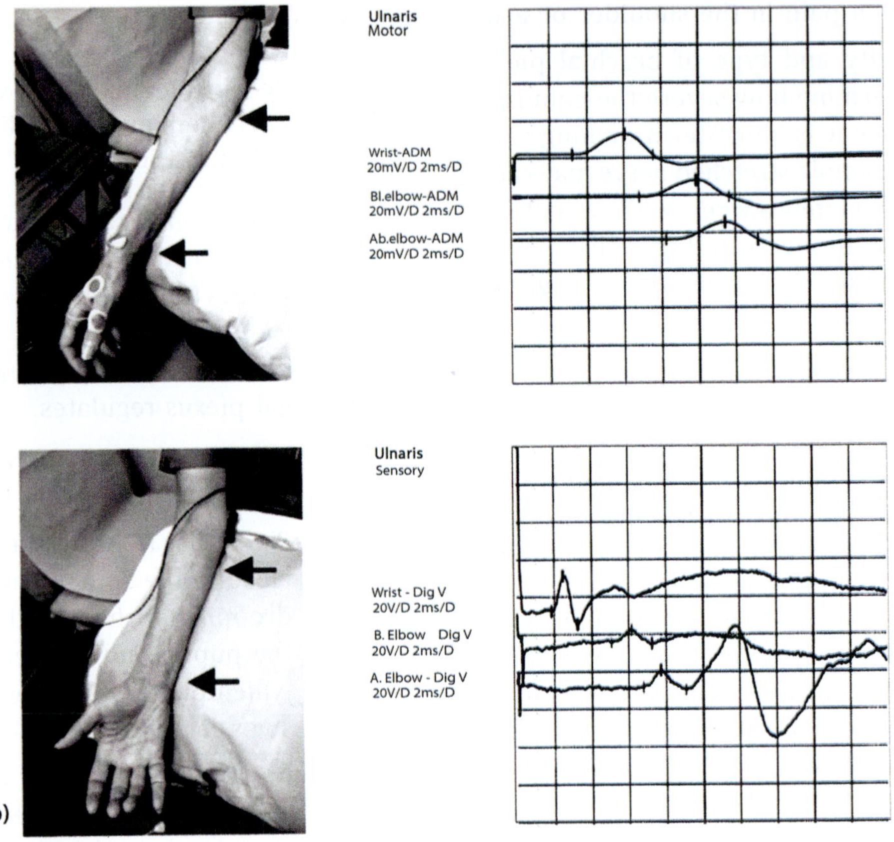

Figure 6.8. *Nerve conduction studies measure the signals traveling in the nerves of your arm and hand.*

Source: *Richards, J., Gechev, A., Alexander, J., Macedo, L., May, K. A., & Lindley, S. B., (2021). The effect of local cooling at the elbow on nerve conduction velocity and motor unit behavior: An exploration of a novel neurological assessment. Sensors, 21(20), 6703. https://doi.org/10.3390/s21206703.*

X-rays of the chest are taken to check for lung injuries and rib fractures. The doctor may consider pulmonary function testing with the assistance of a pulmonologist if the patient are unable to take a full, deep breath during the chest X-ray in order to rule out damage to the nerves that regulate deep breathing (Figure 6.8).

6.11.4.3. CT Scan (Computerized Tomography)

The most accurate test for identifying spinal nerve avulsion (pull out) injuries is thought to be a CT scan. To enhance the visibility of the injury on the CT scan, contrast dye is injected around the spinal cord in the neck. Usually, CT is done three to four weeks following the injury to give any possible blood clots around the nerve root time to dissolve. Additionally, some facilities might perform magnetic resonance imaging (MRI) scans in addition to or instead of CT scans. Studies using electrodiagnosis are also conducted. These examinations quantify muscle signals and nerve conduction. They can locate the nerve injury, characterize its severity, and determine the rate of nerve recovery, making them crucial evaluation tools. Three to four weeks after the injury, a baseline EDX examination is conducted. This makes it possible to identify any potential nerve degeneration. To determine whether the nerves are healing, EDX studies are conducted again two to three months after the first study and then regularly thereafter.

6.11.5. Nonsurgical Treatment

Many brachial plexus injuries, especially those that are mild, heal on their own over a few weeks to months without the need for surgery. Self-healing nerve injuries typically result in better functional outcomes. The doctor may decide to postpone procedures and simply monitor the injury if they believe there is a good chance it will heal without surgery. While the nerve healing process takes time, the doctor might recommend physical therapy to prevent joint and muscle stiffness.

6.11.6. Surgical Treatment

When the nerves are unable to heal on their own or have not healed enough to allow the arm and hand to regain the necessary function, surgery is usually recommended. It is important to remember that depending on the severity of the injury, even surgery may not be able to fully restore function to the arm or hand.

6.11.6.1. Considerations

- **Recuperation:** The physician must establish reasonable expectations and goals for the surgical course of care. Nerves recover gradually. Following surgery, there is often a long recovery period that requires a strong commitment to an extensive rehabilitation program in order to regain physical abilities. This should be taken into account when deciding whether to proceed with surgery.
- **Candidates for Surgery:** Although many patients find that brachial plexus surgery helps them regain function, there are certain conditions that make a patient ineligible for surgery, chief among them being irrational expectations. Additional elements consist of:
  - Having joint stiffness and contractures;
  - Advanced age;
  - Additional injuries or medical conditions;
  - Having a traumatic brain injury or spinal cord injury.

The doctor will discuss with the patient whether the patient are a candidate for surgery:

1. Complications:
   - It is possible that the surgical wound may become infected or that the desired movement may not be restored by the treatment. In either of these cases, additional surgery may be required.
   - Any major reconstructive surgery carries additional risks for patients with pre-existing medical conditions, such as blood clots, heart attacks, strokes, chronic pain, and even death.
2. **Surgical Procedures:** Depending on the nature of the injury and the amount of time that has passed since the injury, several surgical techniques are used to treat nerve injury. The surgeon typically makes an incision just above the collarbone, close to the neck. The surgeon might have to make another incision at the front of the shoulder if the damage goes down the brachial plexus. Surgeons frequently

use tiny, specialized instruments and powerful microscopes to reconnect or repair nerves.

3. **Nerve Repair:** The two torn edges of a severed nerve are reattached by the surgeon during this procedure. When a sharp injury, like a knife wound, tears a nerve, nerve repair is usually done right away.
   - **Transplant of Nerves:** A healthy nerve from another area of the body is sewn in between the two ends of a ruptured nerve during a procedure known as nerve grafting. The damaged ends are supported as they heal and fuse back together by the transplanted nerve, which functions as a scaffold. Nerve grafting can only be done when there is a functional nerve stump at the spinal cord to conduct a nerve signal. The transplanted nerve is intended to direct nerve regrowth to power the paralyzed muscles.
   - **Transfer of Nerves:** In cases where there are no viable nerve stumps in the neck to which nerve grafts can be attached, a nerve transfer procedure is performed. A healthy donor nerve is chopped and reattached to the damaged nerve during this procedure to send a signal to a paralyzed muscle. The healthy nerve is frequently located closer to the injured muscle. In other situations, the damaged nerve of the brachial plexus is linked to the healthy nerve.
4. **Muscle and Tendon Transfers:** Individuals who postpone their initial medical appointment for over a year following their injury typically experience unfavorable results from nerve reconstruction or repair surgeries. Surgery aimed at reconstructing the muscle (free-functioning muscle transfer) or tendon (tendon transfer) is more effective in managing these patients. To restore a particular motion or motor function, a tendon transfer procedure involves cutting and sewing the tendon of a functioning muscle into the tendon of a nonfunctioning muscle. A muscle from one area of the body is transferred to the injured area, along with its tendon, artery, vein, and nerve, in a free-functioning muscle transfer. To restore motion or motor function, each of these structures is linked to the corresponding structures in the injured area.

6.11.7. Recovery and Rehabilitation

Patients may not see results for several months following a brachial plexus injury due to the slow rate of nerve regeneration, which occurs at a rate of about 1 mm per day. The key to healing and rehabilitation is maintaining a positive outlook and receiving support from loved ones, friends, and medical professionals. Occupational therapists provide guidance to patients on how to perform everyday tasks such as eating and grooming using the unaffected arm during the healing period.

Specific exercises are employed in physical therapy to prevent contractures, atrophy, or stiffness in the shoulder, elbow, wrist, and fingers. To provide support to the weak arm and joints, a physical therapist may recommend assistive technology such as supportive bracing or splinting. Compression sleeves and gloves can be used to manage swelling in the affected arm and prevent pain and joint contractures.

To manage pain, various methods including assistive devices, counseling, and medication can be utilized. Additionally, patients will need to learn effective coping mechanisms to adapt their daily activities and work to accommodate a potentially less functional arm or hand.

6.11.8. Future Developments

Despite the fact that brachial plexus injuries can be fatal and challenging to treat, a team approach to care has significantly improved patient function. While the restoration of some function to the arm is a significant advancement, current technology is unable to return patients with a flail limb to their preinjury state. Newer methods of nerve transfer or repair, as well as new drugs or materials to support and stimulate healthy nerve regeneration, are potential advancements in the treatment of these injuries in the future.

A Closer Look

Erb's Palsy (Brachial Plexus Birth Palsy)

One type of brachial plexus palsy is Erb's palsy. It bears the name of Wilhelm Erb, one of the physicians who initially described this ailment. All of the nerves in the arm originate from a network called the brachial plexus, which is located near the neck. These nerves are responsible for the movement and sensation of the shoulder, arm, hand, and fingers. Brachial plexus birth palsy leads to weakness and loss of motion in the arm. Palsy refers to weakness. Approximately one or two out of every 1,000 babies develop birth palsy related to the brachial plexus. It often occurs when an infant's neck is stretched to the side during a difficult birth. Maternal diabetes, high birth weight, and prolonged labor are associated with this condition. The majority of newborns with brachial plexus birth palsy will regain sensation and movement in the affected arm. Physical therapy is an essential part of the treatment. Parents and guardians must play an active role in helping their child regain maximum function in the injured arm.

- **Anatomy:** As the nerves for the arm, hand, and fingers exit the spinal cord and pass between the neck bones, they come together to form the brachial plexus. From there, this network of nerves extends behind the collarbone and branches out into the arm.
- **Description:** The upper brachial plexus nerves are affected in the majority of cases of brachial plexus birth palsy. This condition is commonly referred to as Erb's palsy. The baby may have limited shoulder movement but still be able to move their fingers. Less common forms of brachial plexus birth palsy, such as Klumpke's palsy and total plexus palsy, may involve the participation of other nerves.

In general, there are four types of nerve injuries:

- Neurapraxia;
- Neuroma;
- Rupture; and
- Avulsion.

All of these could happen to the same baby at the same moment. While loss of feeling and partial or total paralysis are the same symptoms of all four types of nerve injury, there are differences in the likelihood of recovery. Treatment choices and the extent of potential recovery are influenced by the severity of the injury.

1. **Neurapraxia:** A stretch injury that "shocks," but does not tear the nerve is the most common type. This is called neurapraxia.

   Normally, these injuries heal on their own, usually within 3 months.

   Neurapraxia can occur in adults as well as infants. For example, when it occurs in football players who are injured during play, it is referred to as a "burner" or "stinger."
2. **Neuroma:** Scar tissue may arise from a stretch injury that compromises some of the nerve fibers. The remaining healthy nerve may be compressed by the scar tissue. This

condition is referred to as a neuroma. Some, but not complete, recovery usually occurs.

3. **Rupture:** A ruptured or torn-apart nerve from a stretch injury will not heal by itself. A rupture occurs when there is a rip in the nerve. By splicing (joining together) the injured nerve with a nerve graft taken from another area of the child's body, a rupture may be repaired.
4. **Avulsion:** The tearing of a nerve from the spinal cord results in an avulsion. An avulsion from the spinal cord cannot be healed, in contrast to a ruptured nerve. When a detached nerve is replaced with a nerve from another muscle, it may be possible to partially restore arm function in certain situations.
5. **Cause:** Brachial plexus birth palsies in newborns may occur:
   - When the baby is large, the delivery is breech, or the labor is prolonged, or during a difficult delivery.
   - Additionally, when a difficult birth occurs and the person assisting with the delivery needs to expedite the process and apply force to extract the baby from the birth canal, it can stretch the baby's neck on one side and potentially harm the surrounding nerves.

It is worth noting that babies delivered by Caesarean section (C-section) and babies without any risk factors may also develop brachial plexus birth palsy.

Symptoms: Symptoms of brachial plexus birth palsy may include:

- Weakness in one arm;
- Loss of feeling in the arm;
- Partial or total paralysis of the arm.

Doctor Examination: Based on the physical examination and arm weakness, a pediatrician is typically the one to diagnose brachial plexus birth palsy. The physician attending to the child may prescribe an X-ray, ultrasound, or other imaging test, such as a magnetic resonance imaging (MRI) scan, to determine whether the neck and shoulder bones and joints have sustained any damage. The shoulder's development and growth may be impacted by the nerve injury. To find out if the upper arm muscle receives any nerve signals, the doctor might also perform certain tests. These examinations could involve nerve conduction studies (NCS) or electromyograms (EMGs).

Treatment: The majority of infants with brachial plexus birth palsy recover on their own, but the child's physician will check in with them again to make sure the nerves are healing. Nerves grow and heal very slowly; full recovery can take up to two years.

- **Nonsurgical Treatment:** Erb's palsy is primarily treated with daily physical therapy. Parents must actively assist in maintaining the limber joints and fit functioning muscles in their infant because they are unable to move the affected arm on their own. The physician or physical therapist for the child will show how to perform exercises with the infant to maintain the health of their arm. From approximately three weeks of age, a baby starts receiving daily physical therapy and range-of-motion exercises as often as possible during the day. The hand, wrist, elbow, and shoulder ranges of motion will all be preserved by the exercises. This will stop joint contracture, a condition where the joint becomes permanently stiff.

- **Surgical Treatment:** To improve the prognosis, the child's physician might recommend nerve surgery if there is no improvement within the first three to six months.
- **Microsurgery:** Powerful microscopes and tiny, specialized instruments are frequently used by surgeons when performing microsurgeries. Generally, nerve surgery is not beneficial for older infants and does not fully restore normal function.
- **Nerve Graft:** Ruptures can be repaired, depending on the nature of the nerve injury. In some cases, a nerve graft taken from another area of the child's body is used to splice or join the damaged nerve.
- **Nerve Transfer:** Occasionally, it may be possible to restore some function to the arm by using a nerve from another muscle as a donor.

Nerves heal very slowly, so it can take months or even years for the muscles in the lower arm and hand to receive nerve repairs made at the neck. After surgery, the baby's physician or physical therapist will provide with at-home rehabilitation exercises to help regain strength and range of motion.

Other Procedures: Other surgical options for treating brachial plexus birth palsy may include:

- **Joint Contracture Release:** This procedure involves releasing stiff soft tissues surrounding the elbow and shoulder joints to increase the range of motion.
- **Tendon Transfer:** In this procedure, a functional tendon is relocated from its original position in the body and attached in the shoulder region to improve the ability to raise the arm.
- **Joint Reduction:** Tighter and thicker tissues surrounding joints can lead to dislocation, especially in the shoulder. In certain cases, surgery is necessary to realign the joint, which is referred to as a reduction.
- **Osteotomy:** This surgical technique involves realigning the bones and joints of the affected limb to optimize function.
- **Outcomes:** Many children who experience brachial plexus injuries will always have some degree of weakness in their fingers, hands, shoulders, or arms. Additional surgical procedures that may enhance function can be considered in the future. As the child develops, the physician will discuss the various options for care and provide a recommendation based on the child's unique circumstances.

Living with Erb's Palsy

The afflicted arm is notably smaller than the unaffected arm in certain children because nerves influence growth. The child's affected arm will still grow, but it will do so more slowly and with a more pronounced size difference as the child gets older. Children can easily adapt to changes in their environment. Be encouraging and supportive, and keep attention on all that child is capable of. This will compensate for any functional deficits and assist the child in forming a positive sense of self-worth. With a physical difference like brachial plexus birth palsy, many children go on to lead productive lives, engaging in regular sports and activities.

6.12. Summary

- The somatic nervous system is comprised of numerous nerves that carry out both somatic and sensory functions, in addition to the somatosensory and sensory nervous systems. Cranial nerves located in the head and neck region transmit somatosensory information.
- Involuntary reactions are regulated by the autonomic nervous system (ANS) in order to maintain physiological equilibrium. Organs containing smooth muscle, such as the heart, bladder, and other cardiac, exocrine, and endocrine-related organs, are connected to the brain and spinal cord of the central nervous system (CNS) via ganglionic neurons.
- Following an injury, the neuron undergoes degeneration and disintegration. The duration required varies depending on the size and myelination of the nerve, as well as in sensory and motor fibers.
- In order to enhance our comprehension of the broad spectrum of clinical behaviors observed in apparently benign insults to the nerves, Lundborg, another prominent figure in the field of nerve surgery, put forth the notion of a physiological conduction block.
- Peripheral nerve damages can arise through various means. The most common mechanisms leading to peripheral nerve injuries are stretches, incisions, and compressions. Among these three, sprains are the most prevalent, followed by incisions, and ultimately compressions. Additionally, peripheral nerve injuries can be induced by radiation, electricity, injections, crush injuries, cold injuries, as well as intra- and extra-neural pathologies.
- Furthermore, apart from reviewing the medical history and inquiring about any accidents or previous surgeries, the physician will also engage in a discussion regarding the symptoms. Moreover, a neurological and physical examination will be conducted by the doctor.
- A wide range of conditions that harm and malfunction the peripheral nervous system's nerves in various ways are collectively referred to as peripheral neuropathy, also known as peripheral polyneuropathy.
- The healthcare provider may utilize electrodiagnostic (EDX) testing to ascertain whether a peripheral neuropathy may have been present when a patient presented with symptoms such as paresthesias, pain, or weakness in multiple extremities that could not be accounted for by a focal mononeuropathy, such as a nerve entrapment neuropathy.
- The objective of the electrodiagnostic study is to assess the pattern and severity of peripheral neuropathy in addition to confirming its existence. Electromyography (EMG) testing and nerve conduction studies (NCS) are two forms of electrodiagnostic (EDX) testing.
- Many conditions can cause nerve damage, including mechanical trauma, crush injuries (like those seen in fractures, hematomas, and compartment syndrome), penetrating traumas (like stab wound lacerations and surgical incisions), and stretch injuries (nerves can stretch 10% to 20% before becoming structurally damaged).
- The stability and mobility provided by the skeletal structure, muscular system, and nervous system enable the application of the precise amount of pressure necessary to grasp an object.

- The skin and upper limb musculature are innervated by the brachial plexus, an intricate network of nerve fibers. It originated at the base of the neck, traversed through the axilla, and subsequently extended throughout the entire upper limb. The first thoracic spinal nerve, T1, and the anterior rami (divisions) of the cervical spinal nerves C5, C6, C7, and C8 combined to form the plexus.
- The classification of brachial plexus injuries is determined by the degree of the injury and how the nerves are harmed.
- The upper extremities are innervated by the nerves that emanate from the brachial plexus, thus injury to this structure can be exceedingly troublesome. The impacted region of the plexus determines the clinical indications and manifestations, which commonly result in anesthesia or paralysis. The range of symptoms encompasses partial weakness of the upper limb and transient dysfunction of the nerves.

References

1. Burnett, M. G., & Zager, E. L., (2004). Pathophysiology of peripheral nerve injury: A brief review. *Neurosurgical Focus, 16*(5), 1–7.
2. Campbell, W. W., (2008). Evaluation and management of peripheral nerve injury. *Clinical Neurophysiology, 119*(9), 1951–1965.
3. James, S. W., (2008). *Neurobioscitifity*, McGraw-Hill Professional. ISBN 978-0-07-149623-0.
4. Johns Hopkins Medicine, *Peripheral Nerve Injury.* Available from https://www.hopkinsmedicine.org/health/conditions-and-diseases/peripheral-nerve-injury (accessed on 20 March 2024).
5. Magee, D. J., & Manske, R. C., (2020). *Orthopedic Physical Assessment* (7th edn.). St. Louis: Elsevier.
6. Saladin, K., (2024). *Anatomy & Physiology: The Unity of Form and Function* (10th edn., p. 1076). New York, NY: McGraw Hill. ISBN 9781266041846.

Chapter 7

BONE AND JOINT INFECTIONS

Contents

7.1. Introduction

Infections of the bones and joints result in severe morbidity and present challenging management issues. They can lead to discharging wounds, chronic pain, acute sepsis with bone and joint destruction, and irreversible disability. Infections of the bones and joints, especially those involving medical devices, will place additional strain on healthcare resources as the population ages. Well-coordinated multidisciplinary collaboration is crucial for efficient management.

Orientation and Directional Terms

Term	Definition	Illustration
Osteoblasts	Osteoblasts are large cuboidal cells that comprise about 4%–6% of the total bone cells. These cells synthesize and mineralize bone during bone synthesis and remodeling. They form a closely packed sheet-like surface on the bone. They are formed through the differentiation of osteogenic cells. Osteoblasts produce various cellular products, including alkaline phosphatase, growth factors, collagenase, and collagen fibers.	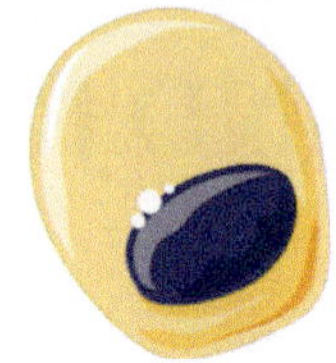
Osteoclast	Osteoclasts are large multinucleated cells that break down bone tissues. Bones are dynamic tissues that undergo constant remodeling to withstand the stress and requirements of our body. Osteoclasts are phagocytic cells that are derived from the macrophage-monocyte cell lineage.	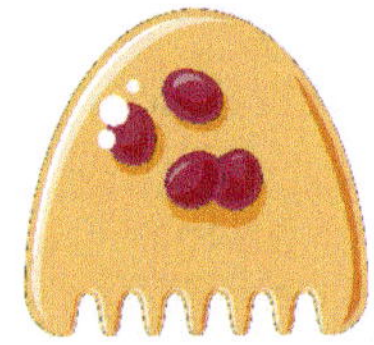
Fossa	A fossa is a depression or hollow, usually in a bone, such as the hypophyseal fossa, the depression in the sphenoid bone.	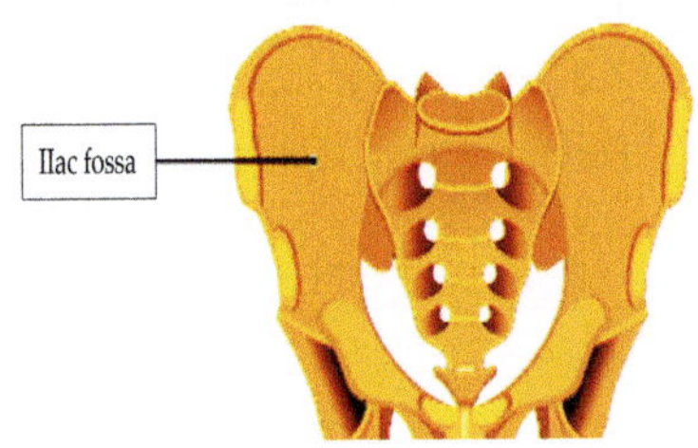
Diaphysis	The long, relatively straight main body of a long bone is referred to as the diaphysis. It is the region of primary ossification and is also known as the shaft.	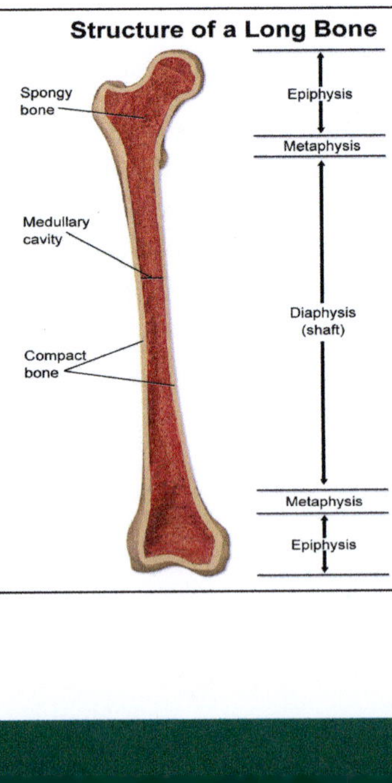

7.2. Nonspecific Bone and Joint Infections

Pathogens can enter bones and joints directly through inoculation from a contiguous focus of infection or through the bloodstream (haematogenous route). Acute hemorrhagic infections most commonly affect children and the elderly. The presence of foreign material such as dead bone or implanted devices greatly reduces the amount of foreign material needed to cause an infection. Normal skin commensals, such as coagulase-negative *Staphylococcus* species, can also become significant pathogens when foreign or non-viable material is present. Microorganisms adhere to the inert surface because it provides protection against the immune system, blood supply, and antibiotics. Certain organisms, including *Staphylococcus* species, can produce extracellular polymeric substances (EPS).

Microorganisms embedded in EPS form a biofilm on inert surfaces. They can regulate growth and adapt to their environment by up- and down-regulating gene expression through mutual communication. Biofilm formation is an essential mechanism for bacterial survival in chronic bone and joint infections. Even with prolonged antimicrobial therapy, a chronically established bone and joint infection may persist, change, or recur. Biofilm significantly affects surgical and antibiotic management, as well as diagnostics.

7.2.1. Osteomyelitis

Osteomyelitis is the term used to describe a bone infection. It is an inflammatory process, either acute or chronic, that affects the bone and its supporting structures as a result of pyogenic organism infection, which can be caused by bacteria, fungi, or mycobacteria. It is interesting to note that animal fossils found in archaeological excavations had evidence of bone infection, indicating that this is a relatively ancient illness. Over time, several terms were used to characterize infected bone before Nelaton coined the term osteomyelitis in 1844. Before the discovery of penicillin in the 1940s, the primary surgical treatments for osteomyelitis included extensive debridement, saucerization, and wound packing. After that, the affected area was left to heal intentionally, which increased the risk of sepsis. The mortality rates from osteomyelitis, including staphylococcal osteomyelitis, have significantly decreased since antibiotics became available (Figure 7.1).

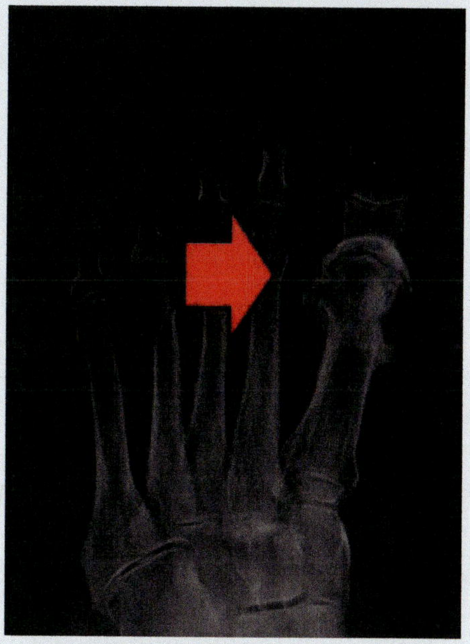

Figure 7.1. *Osteomyelitis of the 1st toe.*

Source: By James Heilman, MD – Own work, CC BY-SA 4.0, https://commons.wikimedia.org/w/index.php?curid=49086925.

7.2.1.1. Etiology

Bone that is healthy and intact resists infection. Bone sites are exposed to microorganisms, making the bone vulnerable to disease in the presence of a significant bacterial inoculum, trauma, ischemia, or foreign bodies. *Staphylococcus aureus* is one of the bacteria that attaches itself to the bone by expressing adhesins, which are receptors for laminin, collagen, fibronectin, and bone sialoglycoprotein, among other elements of the bone matrix. The role of the fibronectin-binding adhesin in the attachment of bacteria to surgically implanted devices in bone was recently discovered. *S. aureus* also expresses a collagen-binding adhesin that allows it to attach to bone cartilage. It is noteworthy that *S. aureus* can endure inside cells once it is taken up by osteoblasts in culture. Certain bacteria form a biofilm layer of defense around themselves and the surfaces beneath them. The ability of certain bacteria to survive intracellularly, adhere to bone and surgically implanted devices, and exhibit phenotypic resistance to antibiotic therapy may contribute to the persistence of bone infections and the high failure rates of shorter courses of antimicrobial therapy.

7.2.1.2. Epidemiology

Although the exact prevalence of osteomyelitis in the US is largely unknown, reports suggest that it may be as high as 1 in 675 hospital admissions or roughly 50,000 cases annually. According to other research, there are 21.8 cases of osteomyelitis overall for every 1,00,000 person-years. For unclear reasons, the incidence was higher in men; however, as people age, the incidence rises, mostly as a result of comorbid conditions like diabetes mellitus and peripheral vascular disease. More accessible sensitive imaging tests, like bone scintigraphy and magnetic resonance imaging (MRI), have also increased diagnostic precision and enhanced infection characterization.

7.2.1.3. Pathophysiology

The hematogenous route of infection can infect bone by direct inoculation from trauma or surgery, contiguous spread from surrounding tissue and joints, or bacteremic seeding of bone from a distant source of infection. Compared to adults, children are more likely to experience hematogenous osteomyelitis, and long bones are typically impacted. Hematogenous osteomyelitis primarily affects the vertebrae in adults. In younger adults, contiguous osteomyelitis usually results from trauma and associated surgery; in older adults, infection is usually associated with decubitus ulcers and infected joint arthroplasties. Diabetes mellitus is usually present when osteomyelitis linked to vascular insufficiency arises.

Osteomyelitis in diabetic patients is typically caused by a reduced blood supply to the lower extremities, which impedes skin healing and local immunity, thus facilitating the spread of infection. To make matters more complicated, sensory neuropathy in the context of diabetes mellitus increases the risk of developing skin ulcers at pressure and trauma points. Contiguous osteomyelitis is a common condition that arises in bedridden or severely disabled patients who are prone to pressure-related skin ulcerations, particularly in the heel, hips, buttocks, and sacrum. Polymicrobial flora from the skin and gastrointestinal tract usually colonize these ulcers, making it possible for a soft tissue infection to spread swiftly to the underlying bone. Additional causes of contiguous osteomyelitis include soft tissue and trauma that results in infected, exposed skin. When orthopedic hardware is placed, bone reconstructive surgery is performed, or there is an open fracture, osteomyelitis due to direct bacterial inoculation may develop.

7.2.1.4. Histopathology

The areas of the bone with good blood flow but few phagocytes, known as the metaphyzes, are commonly infected in cases of hematogenous osteomyelitis affecting the long bones. Blood supply enters the long bones at the mid-shaft and then branches out to both ends of the metaphysis. Reduced blood flow in these areas allows for the buildup of bacteria, leading to infection. Phagocytes release enzymes that break down bone in response to the infection, causing inflammation and the formation of pus. If left untreated, the pus can push through the bone to the outer layer known as the periosteum, cutting off blood flow and resulting in bone death. The dead bone fragments, called sequestra, may contain pus, and new bone formation known as involucrum can partially encase them. Drainage from a sequestrum can create a sinus tract.

In acute osteomyelitis, the main histopathological findings include microorganisms, congested or thrombosed blood vessels, and infiltrates of neutrophils. Conversely, chronic osteomyelitis is characterized by necrotic bone, a predominance of mononuclear cells, replacement of osteoclast resorbed bone by granulation, and fibrous tissue leading to bone loss and the formation of sinus tracts. Native vertebral osteomyelitis (NVO) usually results from a hematogenous infection affecting two adjacent vertebral endplates, which can be attributed to the segmental arteries bifurcating to supply two adjacent endplates of contiguous vertebrae. The spread of spondylodiscitis from a urinary tract focus, especially in older men, may be explained by venous drainage from Batson's plexus.

The histopathological results, not the length of illness, are used to classify osteomyelitis as acute or chronic. Acute osteomyelitis is defined as an infection that occurs before sequestra formation and typically manifests two weeks after the disease first appears. Sequestra can develop quickly in certain circumstances, such as vertebral osteomyelitis, and slowly in others, such as when it is associated with prosthetic devices or open fractures. The infection is considered chronic when necrotic bone and sequestra begin to form. There are two main classification systems for osteomyelitis. The first was created by Lew and Waldvogel, while the second was created by Cierny and Mader. Lew and Waldvogel categorized osteomyelitis based on the mechanism of infection (hematogenous or contiguous) and the duration of the illness (acute or chronic). Another level of classification is determined by whether contiguous infection is associated with vascular insufficiency.

The Cierny and Mader system provides guidance for managing patients. This system classifies osteomyelitis based on the patient's health status and anatomical stage.

The categories and corresponding anatomic types are as follows:

- **Stage 1:** Disease confined to the medullary of the bone.
- **Stage 2:** Superficial disease.
- **Stage 3:** Localized spread.
- **Stage 4:** Diffuse disease.

The local and systemic factors which define host health status are as follows:

- **A:** Normal host.
- **Bs:** Host with systemic compromising factors.
- **Bl:** Host with local compromising factors.
- **Bsl:** Host with both local and systemic compromising factors.
- **C:** Host for whom treatment of the osteomyelitis is worse than the disease itself.

Systemic host compromise can be caused by immunodeficiency diseases, diabetes mellitus, renal and hepatic failure, neoplasms, chronic hypoxia, and malnutrition. Tobacco use, major and small vessel disease, arteritis, peripheral neuropathy, chronic lymphedema, and venous stasis are local factors that compromise the host's health status.

7.2.1.5. History and Physical

The etiology determines how osteomyelitis manifests clinically. Adult diagnosis can occasionally be challenging and call for a high index of suspicion. A thorough medical history and physical examination are essential components of the initial assessment. Patients with endocarditis, trauma, open fractures, intravenous drug use, bacteremia, or other underlying conditions are at a higher risk of developing osteomyelitis. Additionally, patients with peripheral vascular disease, peripheral neuropathy, orthopedic hardware, or chronic poorly healing wounds are more susceptible. Acute osteomyelitis typically presents within two weeks, although it can also develop gradually over a few days. Local symptoms at the infection site may include erythema, swelling, and warmth. Patients may experience dull pain with or without movement, as well as constitutional symptoms such as chills or fever. Some patients may present subacutely with generalized malaise, mild pain lasting for several weeks, and minimal fever or other constitutional symptoms. Septic arthritis can also occur as a symptom of acute osteomyelitis, particularly when the bone metaphyzes are located within the contaminated joint capsule. Osteomyelitis of the proximal radius, humerus, and femur can be further complicated by septic arthritis of the elbow, shoulder, and hip joints, respectively. In cases where a patient has endocarditis, bacteremia, elevated inflammatory markers (CRP, ESR), fever, or new or worsening neck or back pain, it is important to consider native vertebral osteomyelitis (NVO).

The symptoms of chronic osteomyelitis typically take longer to manifest—more than two weeks. Similar to acute osteomyelitis, patients may also exhibit erythema, pain, and swelling at the infection site; however, fever and other constitutional symptoms are less frequent. Patients should be suspected of having osteomyelitis if they have large or deep ulcers that do not heal after several weeks of appropriate therapy, especially if they have diabetes or are otherwise incapacitated. The main goals of a physical examination should be to evaluate peripheral vasculature, sensory function, and potential infection foci. One important finding in vertebral osteomyelitis may be tenderness to palpation over the vertebral bone. When a blunt, sterile instrument can be used to probe an ulcer all the way to the bone, it is strongly suggestive of osteomyelitis. When used in conjunction with the patient's pretest probability for osteomyelitis, the probe to bone test serves as a screening tool to ascertain whether further diagnostic testing, such as radiographic imaging or bone biopsy, is necessary before initiating treatment.

7.2.1.6. Evaluation

Although they are typically not specific to osteomyelitis, laboratory results can provide valuable information in the evaluation of the condition. Leukocytosis, an increase in ESR, and C-reactive protein (CRP) may or may not be present. The CRP level can be utilized to monitor treatment progress as it correlates with the clinical response to therapy. Blood cultures may yield positive results, especially in cases of hematogenous osteomyelitis affecting the pubis, clavicle, or vertebrae. Radiographic imaging assessment is crucial when osteomyelitis is suspected in a patient. Technetium-99 bone scintigraphy, magnetic resonance imaging (MRI), and plain radiographs are the most beneficial investigations in terms of clinical utility. Although a plain radiograph is typically the initial imaging modality of choice, osteomyelitis-related findings may not become apparent for up to 14 days. However, they are used to rule out alternative hypotheses for the symptoms, such as osteoporotic fractures or metastasis. Soft tissue edema, osteopenia, osteolysis, bone loss, and nonspecific periosteal reaction are commonly observed. Plain radiographs only show lytic lesions after 50–75% of the bone matrix has been lost, so they are not a useful modality for identifying early bone disease. In rare cases, a child who has been experiencing pain for months without a fever may be diagnosed with Brodie's abscess, which presents as a well-circumscribed lytic lesion.

MRI has the highest combined sensitivity and specificity (78% to 90% and 60% to 90%, respectively) of all the imaging modalities currently in use for diagnosing osteomyelitis. Although it can identify early bone infection three to five days after the disease starts, its application is restricted when surgical hardware is present. If symptoms have been present for at least a week, a negative result on an MRI is sufficient to rule out the disease because of its high negative predictive value. While it aids in distinguishing between an abscess, necrotic tissue, and phlegmon, intravenous contrast does not enhance disease detection. While its specificity is very low, nuclear imaging has a high sensitivity for identifying early signs of bone disease. It is especially helpful if using an MRI is restricted by metal hardware. Tagged white blood cell scans and three-phase technetium-99 bone scans are the two most often utilized modalities.

Obtaining a bone biopsy, whether through an open procedure or a percutaneous method, is crucial for accurately diagnosing osteomyelitis, determining the cause of the infection, and obtaining susceptibility data necessary for effective antibiotic treatment. Superficial wound cultures or samples from needle punctures should not be relied upon for diagnosis, as they do not provide accurate results compared to bone biopsies. In cases where patients have positive blood cultures and evidence of osteomyelitis on imaging studies, a bone biopsy may not be as helpful. If possible, an open bone biopsy is preferred over a percutaneous biopsy. It is not always necessary to stop antibiotics before a bone biopsy, as cultures often yield positive results regardless due to the nature of bone infections. When performing a percutaneous biopsy, it is important to ensure the skin is intact to avoid sampling errors. Guided imaging techniques such as fluoroscopy or CT scans are recommended for accuracy. Whenever possible, a percutaneous biopsy should be conducted before starting antibiotic treatment to increase the likelihood of positive microbiological results. It is typically recommended to collect two samples during the biopsy procedure, one for histopathological analysis and the other for culture and gram staining.

7.2.1.7. Treatment/Management

Whereas osteomyelitis brought on by direct inoculation or contiguous spread is typically polymicrobial or monomicrobial, hematogenous osteomyelitis is predominantly monomicrobial. The age of the patient determines which pathogens are most prevalent in osteomyelitis. *Staphylococcus aureus* is the most frequent cause of both acute and chronic hematogenous osteomyelitis in adults and children. *Staphylococcus aureus* that is resistant to antibiotics is being isolated from osteomyelitis patients more frequently (called MRSA). According to certain studies, more than one-third of all staphylococcal isolates were MRSA. Additional common pathogens include enterococci, beta-hemolytic streptococcus, coagulase-negative staphylococcus, and anaerobic and aerobic gram-negative bacteria (*Peptostreptococcus, Clostridium species, Bacteroides,* and *Pseudomonas* species, among others).

It is important to consider immunocompromised patients and less common pathogens in the appropriate epidemiological context. These pathogens include Candida species; fungi such as *Blastomyces, Coccidiodes, Cryptococcus*, and *Aspergillus;* nontuberculous mycobacteria (such as Mycobacterium avium intracellulare and Bacille Calmette-Guerin, which can complicate intravesical therapy for bladder cancer); and *Mycobacterium tuberculosis*, which can spread from the lungs to the spine. *Actinomyces* and *Sporothrix* infections typically occur after traumatic inoculation. While *Brucella* and *Salmonella* are associated with spinal infections, *S. aureus* and *Salmonella* are linked to hematogenous osteomyelitis in sickle cell disease. *Pasteurella multocida* or *Eikenella corrodens*, which are found in bites from humans or animals, may be associated with HIV-related osteomyelitis, as well as *Bartonella henselae*.

The management of osteomyelitis requires collaboration among various surgical and medical disciplines. Prolonged use of antibiotics and surgical infection control are the two main components of therapy. Since antibiotics do not easily penetrate infected fluid collections, such as abscesses and damaged or necrotic bone, surgical debridement of all affected bone is often necessary. Therefore, whenever possible, the removal of necrotic tissue and bone is recommended. The extent of the infection can be determined prior to surgery with the use of imaging modalities such as MRI. However, it can still be challenging for the surgeon to ascertain during surgery whether all necrotic bone and tissue have been successfully removed. The pathology report can aid in determining whether repeat debridement is required. In cases of osteomyelitis related to prosthetic joints, hardware removal is advised. However, in cases where the infection is caused by a highly susceptible organism, such as streptococci, and the infected prosthesis is in a stable joint, such as the hip, treatment with a prolonged antibiotic course for several months without removing the device has proven effective. Two-stage exchange arthroplasty is more frequently used when the prosthesis needs to be removed, as it has a lower risk of recurrent infection compared to one-stage arthroplasty, particularly when more virulent bacteria, such as *S. aureus*, are involved. In cases where the infection's location makes surgical debridement impractical, such as certain cases of pelvic osteomyelitis, months-long antibiotic treatment may be necessary. Surgical debridement is rarely necessary for nonverbal vowel osteogenesis unless there are neurological complications that require the relief of spinal cord compression, if medical treatment is ineffective, or if draining epidural or paravertebral abscesses is necessary. However, debridement is required in cases of osteomyelitis connected to spinal implants.

It is crucial to restore blood flow to the affected limb before proceeding with surgery if there is evidence of significant peripheral vascular disease. Additionally, managing diabetes mellitus and addressing other factors that may hinder wound healing, such as tobacco use, malnutrition, chronic hypoxia, weakened immune system, chronic lymphedema, and peripheral neuropathy, are essential. In the treatment of osteomyelitis, prolonged antibiotic therapy is key. Treatment should be guided by culture and sensitivity results whenever possible. In cases where this data is not available, starting empiric antibiotics is reasonable. A common empiric antibiotic regimen that covers both gram-positive and negative organisms, including MRSA, is vancomycin (15 mg/kg intravenously every 12 hours) in combination with either a third-generation cephalosporin (e.g., ceftriaxone 2 gm intravenously daily) or a beta-lactam/beta-lactamase inhibitor combination (e.g., piperacillin/tazobactam 3.375 intravenously every 8 hours). Once sensitivity data is obtained, the antibiotic therapy should be adjusted to specifically target the susceptible organisms.

- Pathogen-Specific Antibiotic Therapy for Osteomyelitis in Adults:
- ***Staphylococcus aureus* Penicillin-Sensitive: The** treatment of choice is penicillin G 4 million units every 6 hours.

Other regimens include, for example, a first-generation cephalosporin such as oxacillin or nafcillin 2 g IV every 4 hours, vancomycin 15 mg/kg IV every 12 hours, clindamycin 900 mg IV every 8 hours, and cefazolin 2 g IV every 8 hours.

- ***Staphylococcus aureus* Penicillin-Resistant:** Nafcillin 2 gm IV every 4 hours is the recommended course of treatment. Alternative therapies are cefazolin, clindamycin, or vancomycin (doses as above)
- ***Staphylococcus aureus* Methicillin-Resistant:** The treatment of choice is vancomycin IV
- A substitute dosage is 600 mg of linezolid intravenously every 12 hours.
- ***Streptococci* (Groups A, B, Beta Hemolytic, *Streptococcus pneumoniae*):** The preferred course of treatment is penicillin G, administered at a dosage of 4 million units every 6 hours. Alternative regimens include ceftriaxone, administered intravenously at a dosage of 2 grams daily, vancomycin administered intravenously, clindamycin administered intravenously, and cefazolin administered intravenously (dosages as mentioned above).
- ***Enterobacteriaceae* Quinolone Sensitive:** Levofloxacin 500–750 mg PO or IV daily, and ciprofloxacin 400 mg IV bid or 750 mg oral PO are the recommended courses of treatment.

Cefepime 2 gm IV every 12 hours, ceftriaxone 2 gm IV daily, and ceftazidime 2 gm IV every 8 hours are some alternative regimens.

- ***Enterobacteriaceae*, Quinolone-Resistant (*Escherichia coli*):** The treatment of choice is piperacillin/tazobactam 3.375 g IV every 8 hours, Ticarcillin/clavulanate 3.1 gm IV every 4 hours

An alternative regimen is ceftriaxone 2 g IV daily.

- ***Pseudomonas aeruginosa*:** Cefepime 2 gm IV every 12 hours and ceftazidime 2 gm IV every 8 hours are the recommended courses of treatment.

Meropenem 1 gm IV every 8 hours, Imipenem 500 mg IV every 6 hours, Ciprofloxacin 400 mg IV every 12 hours, or 750 mg PO daily are some alternative regimens.

- ***Enterococci:*** The treatment of preference is penicillin G, administered at a dosage of 4 million units every 6 hours. As an alternative, administer linezolid 600 mg IV or PO every 12 hours, daptomycin 6 mg/kg IV daily, and vancomycin 15 mg/kg every 12 hours.
- ***Anaerobes:*** Clindamycin 900 mg IV every 8 hours and ticarcillin/clavulanate 3.1 gm IV every 4 hours are the recommended courses of treatment. Alternatively, metronidazole 500 mg IV every 8 hours (for gram-negative anaerobes).

For adults with osteomyelitis, parenteral antibiotic therapy should be administered for 4 to 6 weeks to achieve acceptable cure rates and a reduced risk of recurrence. If the affected bone is completely removed or debrided with documented disease-free margins, a shorter course of antibiotic treatment is appropriate. After surgery, a 2-week course of antibiotics is adequate to treat any leftover tissue infection and promote wound healing at the surgical site. When used in the appropriate clinical context, vacuum-assisted wound closure devices are particularly useful in cases where deep or large wounds remain after extensive debridement. It has been demonstrated that these devices encourage wound healing through both direct and indirect effects. It is not usually advised to use hyperbaric oxygen therapy to treat osteomyelitis.

7.2.1.8. Differential Diagnosis

Osteomyelitis has a wide range of differential diagnoses, which should be considered when evaluating a patient who may have a bone infection. These differentials include:

- Charcot arthropathy especially in people with diabetes;
- SAPHO syndrome (synovitis, acne, pustulosis, hyperostosis, and osteitis);
- Arthritis including rheumatoid arthritis;
- Metastatic bone disease;
- Fracture, including pathological and stress fractures;
- Gout;
- Avascular necrosis of the bone;
- Bursitis;
- Sickle cell vaso-occlusive pain crises.

7.2.1.9. Prognosis

Acute osteomyelitis has a good prognosis with aggressive early treatment. However, if there is fresh trauma to the same area or if host immunity is weakened, there is a chance that the infection could recur years after successful treatment. After a year, the recurrence rate of chronic osteomyelitis in adults is approximately 30%. However, in cases where *P. aeruginosa* is involved, there could be a 50% chance of recurrence. Treating prosthetic device cases is more challenging, resulting in higher morbidity due to the need for more surgical procedures and longer antibiotic courses. Two strategies used to prevent postoperative infections are the use of surgical rooms with laminar airflow and practicing good preoperative preparation. Additionally, it is advised to use prophylactic preoperative antibiotic treatment with first-generation (cefazolin) or second-generation (cefuroxime) cephalosporins given parenterally 30 minutes before skin incision. It has been demonstrated that all of these actions improve patient outcomes by reducing the rate of postoperative infections from 0.5% to 2%.

7.2.1.10. Complications

It takes early intervention, including antibiotic therapy, to prevent complications from arising. The following are a few outcomes of untreated or insufficiently treated osteomyelitis:

- Septic arthritis;
- Pathological fractures;
- Squamous cell carcinoma;
- Sinus tract formation;
- Amyloidosis (rare);
- Abscess;
- Bone deformity;
- Systemic infection;
- Contiguous soft tissue infection.

7.2.1.11. Deterrence and Patient Education

Providing patients with education regarding the extended duration of therapy and the importance of adhering to treatment guidelines to promote sufficient wound healing and lower the likelihood of recurrence is a crucial aspect of their care.

7.2.1.12. Enhancing Healthcare Team Outcomes

Treating osteomyelitis is complex and typically requires a team of healthcare professionals, including primary care providers, radiologists, surgeons, podiatrists, infectious disease specialists, pharmacists, nurses, and sometimes plastic surgeons, pain specialists, or interventional radiologists. The primary care provider often plays a crucial role in diagnosing and coordinating care among these specialists. Treatment strategies are guided by the location of the infection and the presence of vascular issues. Minimally invasive procedures, such as aspiration of the affected area for testing, may be recommended for diagnosis. Antibiotic treatment is typically prescribed for six weeks, especially in cases with serious complications or when initial therapy is not successful.

Once again, effective management of osteomyelitis caused by vascular insufficiency requires good cooperation between the vascular and surgical teams, especially in cases where diabetes mellitus is present. Proper healing of the injured limb necessitates revascularization. Depending on the severity of vascular insufficiency, treatments to restore adequate blood flow may be employed prior to amputation, such as therapeutic angiograms performed by vascular surgery, interventional radiology, or femoral to popliteal bypass. Surgical revascularization techniques, such as local pedicle muscle flaps and myocutaneous flaps, are utilized to fill the space left by surgical debridement, prevent infection, and preserve vascular supply to the surgical site.

After surgical debridement, patients must receive meticulous wound care and long-term antibiotic follow up. Infectious disease specialists, who are involved in the patient's care, monitor the effectiveness of the therapy and make adjustments to the patient's antibiotic regimen when necessary. Many patients can complete their course of antibiotics by continuing their parental antibiotic regimen as an outpatient using peripherally inserted intravenous access. Depending on microbiological results, others can switch to highly bioavailable oral antibiotic therapy, such as quinolones. Patients who meet the eligibility requirements can receive multiple weekly home health wound nurse visits. Ambulatory patients are advised to use wound care clinics when they are open. In addition to being essential members of the care team, family members and caregivers also provide care and support between visits from medical professionals. This method is crucial for reducing osteomyelitis morbidity.

7.2.2. Hematogenous Osteomyelitis

Hematogenous osteomyelitis is an infection that primarily affects the highly vascularized areas of the developing skeleton in children. The disease's frequency, virulence, and extent of soft tissue involvement have all increased over time. Therefore, it is crucial to consider changes in clinical manifestations and management over the last 20 years when using imaging to treat the disease. Infection imaging should show one or more foci of involvement and the existence of drainable collections to determine the location accurately.

7.2.2.1. Microbial Etiology of Acute Hematogenous Osteomyelitis (AHO)

Most cases of acute hematogenous osteomyelitis (AHO) involve the femur, tibia, or humerus, and usually occur in the metaphysis of long tubular bones. Although multiple bacterial pathogens could be at play, *S. aureus* stands out as the primary pathogen, accounting for 70–90% of AHO infections in children. Other etiological agents include *Kingella kingae*, enteric Gram-negative bacilli (especially *Salmonella* spp.), coagulase-negative staphylococci (especially in implant-associated infections), *Streptococcus pyogenes, Streptococcus pneumoniae*, Group B streptococci (in infants), and so on. These are listed in no particular order. In sickle cell disease patients, anaerobic bacteria may also be involved. Childhood osteomyelitis was frequently caused by *Haemophilus influenzae* type b (Hib), but the Hib conjugate vaccine has reduced the incidence of Hib. Unusual causes of osteomyelitis include *Mycobacterium, Bartonella*, fungi (*Histoplasma, Cryptococcus,* and *Blastomyces*), *Candida*, and *Coxiella*. These patients typically have certain risk factors, such as immunosuppression or travel to/from areas where the offending pathogens are endemic. The etiology of AHO in children is still unknown in a large number of cases, despite the growing use of more sensitive diagnostic methods that are less dependent on the offending bacterium's culture, most notably PCR.

As an example, a recent report found that *K. kingae* was the most common cause of osteoarticular infections in French children younger than three years of age. However, approximately 70% of these cases were limited to septic arthritis, with only approximately 18% exhibiting clinical evidence of osteomyelitis. This is consistent with a review of pediatric cases in North America, which found that, other than Gram-positive cocci, *K. kingae* was a primary cause of osteoarticular infections in children younger than five years of age. This is also consistent with an experience at Arkansas Children's Hospital (AR, USA) where it was found that *K. kingae* is the most common cause of septic arthritis in children less than two years of age. *K. kingae* is a fastidious organism that is difficult to culture, and its apparently increasing prevalence as a causative agent of osteoarticular infections is unlikely to be due to a change in the overall epidemiology of the disease but rather to the increasing use of more sensitive diagnostic techniques, such as PCR, for the direct identification of pathogens present in joint fluid and bone specimens. These kinds of studies highlight the need for alternative methods of diagnosis that can direct the use of final antimicrobial therapy. They do not, however, change the conclusion that *Staphylococcus aureus* in particular and Gram-positive cocci in general are the most common causes of osteoarticular infections in children across all age groups.

The ongoing emergence of methicillin-resistant strains of *S. aureus* infection is a growing concern, as it is with all forms of the infection. The prevalence of osteomyelitis caused by methicillin-resistant *S. aureus* (MRSA) increased from 0.3 to 1.4 per 1,000 hospital admissions between 2002 and 2007, while the rate of osteomyelitis caused by methicillin-sensitive *S. aureus* (MSSA) remained stable, according to a survey of data from 33 different children's hospitals representing 17 of the 20 major metropolitan areas in the USA. In total, MRSA infections were present in 51% of the patients who were admitted with *S. aureus* infections. This is in line with what was observed at Arkansas Children's Hospital, where MRSA was responsible for about 65% of the *S. aureus* infections that occur in inpatients. Crucially, a study conducted on all children admitted between 1999 and 2003 with acute osteomyelitis to Children's Medical Center of Dallas (TX, USA) revealed that the complication rate of infection secondary to MRSA was significantly higher than that of patients with MSSA infections and patients with acute osteomyelitis caused by organisms other than *S. aureus*. Myositis, bone abscess, pathologic fracture, deep vein thrombosis, and disseminated illness were among the complications. It's important to note from that study that children with MRSA acute osteomyelitis who started appropriate antibiotic therapy within two days experienced a comparable rate of complications to those who delayed starting therapy for at least two days.

This suggests that treating MRSA-associated osteomyelitis may require more than just using the recommended antibiotics. This is especially true for infections brought on by CA-MRSA infections, as these patients frequently present with a more serious clinical picture, including increased inflammation, multifocal disease, and a higher frequency of bone abscesses that need to be surgically drained. This is why it's crucial to remember that the Dallas study's period corresponds to the beginning of the CA-MRSA infection epidemic, which hasn't yet reached its peak and may not even have done so yet.

7.2.2.2. Clinical Manifestations and Diagnosis of Acute Hematogenous Osteomyelitis (AHO)

The majority of children and teenagers affected by AHO report experiencing bone pain for a few days prior. AHO pain is characterized by its constant presence and gradual increase in intensity. It can be challenging to determine the exact location of pain in young children, but it tends to be more localized in older children. Generally, the affected limb is limited in its use due to the pain. Children often exhibit a limp, as the long bones in the lower limbs are commonly affected. If localized bone pain is accompanied by fever, it should raise suspicion of AHO. In cases where the joint is excessively immobile and there is no tenderness over the metaphysis, a diagnosis of septic arthritis may be considered in addition to or instead of osteomyelitis. Redness, warmth, and swelling are classic signs of inflammation, but they may not appear until the infection has spread from the metaphyseal cortex to the subperiosteal space. Infants and young children, with their thinner bone cortex, are more prone to this type of progression. AHO is frequently accompanied by elevated leukocytosis, erythrocyte sedimentation rate (ESR), and CRP, with elevated CRP being the most sensitive laboratory parameter. However, this also depends on the agent who committed the offense. For instance, a recent study discovered that only 58% of children with acute MSSA osteomyelitis had a significantly elevated CRP level (>4 mg/dl), compared to 86% of children with AHO caused by MRSA. Numerous imaging techniques have been employed to aid in the diagnosis of osteomyelitis because laboratory testing and physical examination are suggestive rather than conclusive. These include magnetic resonance imaging (MRI), computed tomography (CT), skeletal scintigraphy, and plain radiographs.

In order to rule out alternative diagnoses, such as a fracture, plain radiographs are crucial. While radiographic evidence of deep soft tissue swelling may be observed in the initial days following the onset of symptoms, osteopenia or osteolytic lesions resulting from bone deterioration typically take 2–3 weeks to manifest. Because of this, plain radiographs are only useful in diagnosing osteomyelitis in patients who have had their symptoms for a long time—a condition that typically does not apply to children. Consequently, the diagnosis of pediatric AHO is more frequently made using alternative imaging modalities. With a reported sensitivity of more than 90%, skeletal scintigraphy with technetium-99 m diphosphonate allows for a whole-body survey, which is helpful for patients with poorly localized symptoms or if multifocal osteomyelitis is a concern. However, skeletal scintigraphy is less helpful in this age group due to lower sensitivity and the need for neonates to be exposed to ionizing radiation. Distinguishing osteomyelitis from infarction linked to sickle cell disease and other non-infectious conditions, such as neoplasms and fractures, can be challenging. Furthermore, the diagnostic value of skeletal scintigraphy for community-acquired *S. aureus* osteomyelitis may be limited. According to a recent study, skeletal scintigraphy diagnosed osteomyelitis in only 53% of cases in children with community-acquired *S. aureus* osteomyelitis. The ability to obtain precise anatomical information regarding the state of infection is one advantage of CT scanning. When developing the overall therapeutic approach, CT is useful in defining subperiosteal abscesses, detecting intra-osseous gas, and detecting sequestra, which is indicative of chronic osteomyelitis. However, CT also necessitates radiation exposure. Studies have indicated that fluorodeoxyglucose positron emission tomography (FDG-PET) could be a good substitute for CT in adult diagnosis. However, this problem hasn't been sufficiently looked at in the particular setting of the young patient. By identifying intra-osseous, subperiosteal, and soft-tissue abscesses, magnetic resonance imaging (MRI) enables early abscess drainage without radiation exposure. An MRI can show edema and exudates in the medullary space, which are typical signs of acute osteomyelitis. These results, nevertheless, are also evident in other illnesses like infarct and fracture. An MRI can also be used to easily diagnose myositis. When surgery is necessary, MRI provides improved anatomic information and anatomic atlas for orthopedists. These factors have led to MRI's emergence as the preferred imaging technique for pediatric AHO. When diagnosing osteomyelitis, magnetic resonance imaging (MRI) has a sensitivity and specificity of 82–100% and 75–26%, respectively. Important restrictions on the use of MRI include cost, availability, and the requirement for sedation.

While laboratory testing, diagnostic imaging, and patient presentation are all significant, none of them can be used to definitively diagnose AHO. Moreover, none of them can reveal whether the offending organism is resistant to antibiotics. Due to this limitation, the only available method at present to establish a conclusive microbiologic diagnosis is the isolation of the causative organism, which remains the diagnostic gold standard. In a considerable number of cases, a definitive bacterial etiology cannot be determined due to the challenging cultivation of the offending organisms or compromised microbiologic analysis resulting from empirical antimicrobial therapy. Once the etiologic agent has been identified, empirical antimicrobial therapy should be modified in accordance with the particular susceptibility profile of the offending bacterial strain. It is advisable to include bone samples in cultured samples as they provide more diagnostic information compared to blood cultures. However, blood cultures should still be taken since approximately half of all AHO infections result in the recovery of an organism. For neonates and young children, relatively noninvasive techniques such as needle aspiration of the affected bone can be performed. However, older children and adolescents often require more invasive surgical techniques such as drilling or cutting into the bone. Direct inoculation of cultured material into a blood culture bottle increases the probability of recovering fastidious organisms such as *K. kingae*. The use of PCR to identify pathogens from bone specimens is also becoming increasingly common.

7.2.2.3. Treatment of Acute Hematogenous Osteomyelitis (AHO)

In all cases, the treatment of AHO necessitates the use of the proper antibiotics and may involve surgical incision and drainage. The continued emergence of CA-MRSA has made appropriate drainage especially important in recent years, for the reasons previously discussed. Anytime there is an abscess (intra-osseous, subperiosteal, or soft-tissue), incision and drainage should be carried out. It is necessary to remove devitalized bone surgically and debride the impacted soft tissues. Our experience has shown that, even with appropriate antibiotic therapy, multiple incision and drainage procedures are frequently required in children and adolescents with CA-MRSA osteomyelitis. If a child does not respond to empirical antibiotic therapy, surgical drainage should also be taken into consideration. In that instance, surgery might improve the course of care. Furthermore, tissue can be collected through surgical intervention and subsequently evaluated microbiologically for any uncommon etiologies of osteomyelitis, as well as histologically to confirm the diagnosis. Appropriate antibiotic therapy is necessary for the successful treatment of all forms of osteomyelitis, regardless of the need for surgical intervention. Antibiotics such as vancomycin, clindamycin, nafcillin, and first-generation cephalosporins have demonstrated effectiveness in treating *S. aureus* bone and joint infections. In our opinion, children (defined as those 3 months of age and older) should receive empirical therapy with either a first-generation cephalosporin (cefazolin) or an anti-staphylococcal penicillin (nafcillin and oxacillin) if MRSA is not a concern (communities with ≤10% CA-MRSA determined by local antibiogram). These agents are effective not only against MSSA but also against other causes of AHO, including *S. pyogenes* and *K. kingae.* Regretfully, the ongoing emergence of MRSA in isolates linked to the community has restricted available treatment choices, as all β-lactam antibiotics are ruled out.

Vancomycin or clindamycin (if local clindamycin resistance rates are ≤25%) should be used for empirical treatment of children in communities with 10% or more CA-MRSA. It should be mentioned, however, that neither clindamycin nor vancomycin is effective against *K. Kingae*. The D-test (an erythromycin-induction test that shows blunting of the clindamycin zone of inhibition on the side of a nearby erythromycin disk when the MLSB resistance phenotype is present) must be used to rule out the inducible macrolide, lincosamide, and streptogramin B (MLSB) resistance phenotype before considering clindamycin as a treatment option, as this phenotype has been linked to treatment failure. Vancomycin is, in our opinion, the drug of choice when treating patients with clindamycin-inducible resistance and in communities where the prevalence of clindamycin resistance exceeds 25%. If *K. kingae* is of particular concern in an area with significant MRSA, consideration should be given to therapy with cefazolin in addition to appropriate MRSA empiric therapy. It should be underlined once more that antimicrobial treatment should be promptly modified in accordance with the susceptibility profile of the offending organism if cultures produce a conclusive diagnosis. An example of the recommended first antibiotic therapy of AHO is shown in Figure 7.2.

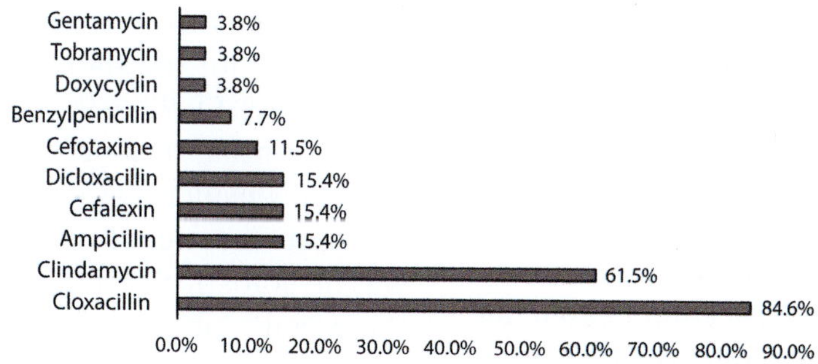

Figure 7.2. *Antibiotics used for the treatment of acute osteomyelitis.*

Source: *Thingsaker, E. E., Urbane, U. N., & Pavare, J., (2021). A comparison of the epidemiology, clinical features, and treatment of acute osteomyelitis in hospitalized children in Latvia and Norway. Medicina, 57(1), 36. https://doi.org/10.3390/medicina57010036.*

A successful treatment for CA-MRSA-caused skin and soft-tissue infections (SSTIs) is trimethoprim-sulfamethoxazole (TMP-SMX). However, there has been insufficient research conducted to determine the effectiveness of TMP-SMX in treating pediatric MRSA osteomyelitis. Similarly, doxycycline may be a useful treatment for susceptible MRSA SSTIs in children over the age of eight, but there is a lack of research on its efficacy in treating MRSA osteomyelitis in children. In recent years, new antimicrobial agents, such as the lipopeptide antibiotic daptomycin and the oxa-zolidinone antibiotic linezolid, have become available for the treatment of MRSA infections. Although there is limited clinical experience with these medications specifically in the context of pediatric bone infections, one study found that out of 13 children treated with linezolid as a step-down or alternative therapy for osteoarticular infections, 11 of them responded well. Two children experienced anemia during the course of the therapy, which lasted an average of twenty days. Prolonged therapy with linezolid has been associated with myelosuppression, peripheral neuropathies, and optic neuropathies. It is not recommended to exceed a treatment duration of 21 days due to these potential side effects. This limitation restricts the use of linezolid in the long-term antimicrobial therapy required to treat AHO in children. Research on the effectiveness of daptomycin in children is scarce. The use of daptomycin for AHO in children is restricted because lung surfactants inactivate daptomycin, making it ineffective for treating infections of this complexity. MRSA AHO complicated by pneumonia is a growing concern. It is also known that daptomycin elevates creatinine phosphokinase. When daptomycin is used, it is important to closely monitor creatinine phosphokinase levels because it can cause dangerous rhabdomyolysis. According to recent research, daptomycin is particularly useful in treating infections associated with biofilms, such as MRSA infections, especially in the context of a biofilm. This may be particularly significant when considering chronic osteomyelitis.

The typical course of treatment for AHO lasts between four and six weeks. There is a lack of evidence-based information regarding the best way to administer antibiotics to AHO, as well as unclear criteria for determining when to switch from parenteral to oral therapy. If there are remote foci of infection (i.e., endocarditis) or incomplete or delayed surgical evacuation, further antibiotic treatment may be required. The cost of catheter placement, home intravenous antibiotics, and home nursing care is significantly higher than that of oral therapy. However, interventional radiological placement of indwelling venous catheters in a peripheral vein is widely accessible. Relevant factors to take into account include complications related to the placement of a central venous catheter, such as bacteremia from the indwelling device and line malfunction. In an analysis comparing the outcome of a short (<7 days) versus a long (>7 days) course of intravenous treatment for AHO caused primarily by methicillin-susceptible Staphylococcus aureus (MSSA) in children aged 3 months to 16 years, 12 prospective studies revealed an overall cure rate of 95.2% (95%CI: 90.4–97.7) for the short course compared with 98.8% (95%CI: 93.6–99.8) for the longer course at 6 months. This difference is considered modest considering the potential complications and costs mentioned above. Furthermore, there was no statistically significant distinction in the therapeutic outcome between the two groups based on the length of oral therapy.

According to experience, if certain requirements are met, children can greatly benefit from sequential parenteral/oral therapy. Parenteral antibiotics should be administered until the child shows improvement as determined by laboratory testing and physical examination, and until they are no longer feverish. For bacteremic patients, we recommend parenteral therapy for 7–14 days; for nonbacteremic children, a shorter intravenous therapy course is acceptable. To assess the response to treatment at the beginning, CRP and ESR should be checked once a week. Typically, a week after starting effective therapy, the CRP returns to baseline, which many people use as an indicator to switch from parenteral to oral therapy. A complete blood count should be taken every week to evaluate treatment effectiveness and monitor for potential side effects of antibiotic therapy, including neutropenia. The duration of therapy should be determined based on symptom resolution and normalization of ESR, which usually takes 4–6 weeks. Reliable caregivers must be available, and regular outpatient follow-up appointments should be scheduled. The child must be able to take oral medications, the oral antibiotic must have good bone penetration, and it should provide the same antibacterial coverage as the parenteral drug. However, meeting these requirements may soon become challenging in the USA due to the increasing prevalence of CA-MRSA strains that are also resistant to clindamycin, as well as a lack of research on the use of other oral antibiotics in pediatric patients.

7.2.3. Chronic Osteomyelitis

A low-grade or recurrent infection that lasts for an extended period of time is known as chronic osteomyelitis. It is primarily characterized by bony sclerosis, periosteal new bone formation, and the presence of draining sinuses and/or sequestra. In children, it is not common. MRIs and CT scans are superior to traditional radiographs in defining the extent. The imaging findings are referred to as Garré sclerosing osteomyelitis if there is a significant amount of new bone formation. This condition is caused by multiple small foci of repeated infarction at the infection site, which leads to the formation of new bone.

7.2.3.1. Classification

There is disagreement over which classification system is best to use, despite the fact that many have been proposed. Osteomyelitis is generally classified as acute or chronic based more on the histopathological findings than the length of the infection. Usually manifesting two weeks following a bone infection, acute osteomyelitis is characterized by inflammatory changes in the bone. In contrast, sequestra formation and bone destruction are hallmarks of chronic osteomyelitis, which usually manifests six weeks or longer after bone infection. The Cierny–Mader classification is the most commonly utilized categorization scheme for adult chronic osteomyelitis (Table 7.1). It takes into account prognostic variables and defines the course of treatment for each clinical stage based on the host's anatomical type and physiological class.

Table 7.1. *Cierny–Mader Classification System*

Anatomical Type	
Type	**Characteristics**
I	Medullary osteomyelitis
II	Superficial osteomyelitis
III	Localized osteomyelitis

IV	Diffuse osteomyelitis
Physiological Class	
Type	Characteristics
A	Good immune system and delivery
B	Compromised locally (B^L) or systemically (B^S)
C	Requires suppressive or no treatment; minimal disability; treatment worse than disease; not a surgical candidate.
Factors Affecting Physiological Class	
Systemic Factors (^{S})	**Local Factors (^{L})**
Malnutrition	Chronic lymphedema
Renal or hepatic failure	Venous stasis
Diabetes mellitus	Major vessel compromise
Chronic hypoxia	Arteritis
Immune disease	Extensive scarring
Extremes of age	Radiation fibrosis
Immunosuppression	Small-vessel disease
Immune deficiency	Neuropathy
Tobacco abuse	
Alcohol abuse	
Malignancy	

Source: Michalis, P., & Peter, V. G., (2016). Chronic osteomyelitis: What the surgeon needs to know. EFORT Open Rev., 1(5), 128–135. doi: 10.1302/2058-5241.1.000017.

Additionally, osteomyelitis can be categorized as exogenous or hematogenous based on the pathogenesis or mechanism of infection. The most frequent cause of chronic osteomyelitis is a direct infection of the bone during trauma, which occurs as a consequence of surgical trauma (i.e., from persistent open wounds that are overlying or from contiguous soft tissue infections) after open reduction and internal fixation of fractures. Although hematogenous osteomyelitis primarily affects pediatric populations, the pathogens enter the bone through the systemic circulation. Adults usually experience it as a secondary consequence of a distal site of infection, which frequently involves the vertebral bodies of the lower spine and may also be linked to inflammation of the nearby intervertebral discs. Because vascular insufficiency is the secondary cause of osteomyelitis and exhibits many unique clinical and pathophysiological characteristics, some authors have proposed that this mechanism be distinguished from others. It usually results from a soft tissue infection of the foot that spreads to the bone, and it mostly affects patients with diabetes mellitus.

7.2.3.2. Epidemiology

Since the 1940s, when antibiotics were first developed, there has been a significant decline in the incidence and mortality of hemorrhagic osteomyelitis. However, it appears that the prevalence of chronic osteomyelitis after a contiguous focus of infection has increased, particularly in developed nations. The population's aging, the incidence of trauma rising, the incidence of diabetic foot infections increasing, and advancements in disease diagnosis are all potential etiological factors. The most frequent cause of osteomyelitis is still trauma. Infection rates in open long bone fractures range from 4% to 64%, while recurrence rates after bony infection have been reported to be as high as 20% to 30%. Conversely, infections in prosthetic joints are a relatively recent development in the field of chronic osteomyelitis. Though rates as high as 20% have been documented after revision surgery, their incidence is estimated to be as high as 1.5 to 2.5%.

7.2.3.3. Aetiopathogenesis

Bone is comparatively resistant to the spread of infection, unlike other tissue types. However, infection can occur following a significant inoculation of pathogens or even a smaller amount of highly virulent bacteria. Patient-related factors such as age, immunological status, trauma history, and geographic location significantly influence the type of pathogen that is isolated. Unlike contiguous-focus osteomyelitis, which is polymicrobial in nature, hematogenous osteomyelitis is typically caused by a single microorganism. *Staphylococcus aureus*, particularly methicillin-resistant *S. aureus* (MRSA), is the most commonly implicated pathogen in adult chronic osteomyelitis. Other pathogens that can cause harm include *Pseudomonas aeruginosa, Escherichia coli, Serratia marcescens*, and *Staphylococcus epidermidis*. Infections caused by fungi and bacteria are typically rare and are often associated with immunodeficiency.

Once bacteria like *S. aureus* enter the bone marrow cavity, they attach themselves to membrane proteins such as collagen receptors or fibronectin, leading to an infection. This process occurs regardless of the pathogen's mode of entry. Various microbial factors further hinder the penetration of surrounding tissues or access by the host defenses. To accomplish this, the extracellular matrix is degraded by attacking different types of host cells. Certain pathogens, like *S. aureus*, are also capable of surviving inside host cells. As a result, different pathogens form a multilayered, relatively impermeable polysaccharide/protein matrix known as a biofilm, which can be embedded in a slime layer or glycocalyx. Due to their biofilm-enclosed environment, these pathogens are shielded from the host's defense systems and the systemic effects of antibiotics. Consequently, they exhibit changes in their growth, gene expression, and protein synthesis. During the initial infectious phase, the bacteria remain in the planktonic phase, making them more susceptible to common antibiotics due to their high metabolic and generational rate. These pathogens can persist in this state for extended periods and trigger relapses years after the initial infection.

The primary mechanisms of tissue necrosis and bone destruction are the inflammatory factors generated by the pathogens and the host's leukocytes, as well as the compression and obliteration of the vascular network surrounding the affected area. The resulting avascular area is inaccessible to both inflammatory cells and antibiotic agents, making it a perfect harbor for bacteria. Reactive hyperemia and elevated osteoclastic activity are present in the vicinity of this avascular area, leading to localized bone loss and osteoporosis. The osteoblasts create new bone called periosteal bone at the same time.

7.2.3.4. Predisposing Factors

There have been several documented risk factors for the development of chronic osteomyelitis. The most frequent factors are a history of trauma, open fractures, and surgery. Peripheral vascular disease, diabetes, malnourishment, hypotension, chronic steroid use, cancer, alcoholism, smoking, systemic or local immunocompromised states, intravenous drug use, and the emergence of decubitus ulcers are additional factors. These days, one of the most significant risk factors is the existence of implants. They quickly acquire a coating of the host's proteins following implantation, which makes them a prime location for pathogen attachment. They are shielded from the host's defenses by the biofilm they produce, allowing them to reactivate months or even years later.

7.2.3.5. Clinical Features

It can be challenging to identify the clinical signs of chronic osteomyelitis because they are typically non-specific. Additionally, particularly in diabetic patients, it can be challenging to distinguish soft tissue infections from osteomyelitis symptoms. There have been reports of a wide range of symptoms, from open wounds over fractured bones to no skin lesions.

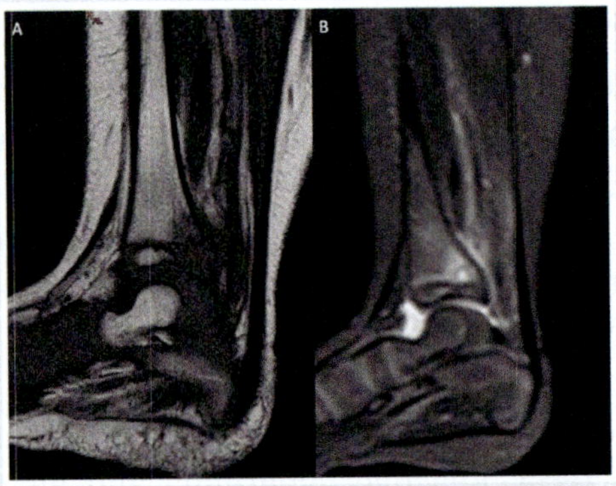

Figure 7.3. *Patient MRI of the left ankle showing primary metaphyseal acute hematogenous osteomyelitis with transphyseal extension to the distal tibia due to Kingella Kingae: (A) sagittal view of the left ankle with T1 sequence; and (B) sagittal view of the left ankle with T2 STIR sequence.*

Source: *Cochard, B., Habre, C., Pralong-Guanziroli, N., Gavira, N., Di Laura, F. G., Di Marco, G., Steiger, C. N., De Coulon, G., Dayer, R., & Ceroni, D., (2023). Transphyseal hematogenous osteomyelitis: An epidemiological, bacteriological, and radiological retrospective cohort analysis. Microorganisms, 11(4), 894. https://doi.org/10.3390/microorganisms11040894.*

Among the most frequently reported clinical symptoms are chronic pain, an erythematous area surrounding the affected bone, swelling and bone tenderness, decreased wound healing frequently linked to tissue necrosis, increased drainage or persistent sinus tracts, chills, low-grade fever, and general malaise (an example is shown in Figure 7.3). Patients who have their cases neglected usually describe a cyclical pain that flares up, goes away when pus escapes through the fistula and is accompanied by fever.

7.2.3.6. Imaging Features

Imaging is useful for both characterizing osteomyelitis and making a differential diagnosis. As a first-line imaging modality, plain radiography has extremely low sensitivity and specificity. However, it is helpful to distinguish osteomyelitis from other conditions like fractures and cancers, whether primary or metastatic. It may not be noticeable until there is a loss of 30 to 50% of the bone mineral content, but it can show soft tissue swelling, periosteal reaction, loss of definition, loss of bone density, and osteolysis as early as 10 to 21 days following the bone infection. Increased bone resorption, sequestra formation, and the creation of new bone in the periosteum or endosteum are examples of late symptoms.

The most detailed imaging of cortical bone is possible with CT, which is particularly helpful for identifying intra-osseous fistulae and sequestra. It also shows the early stage of the soft tissue condition and the involvement of the bone marrow, in addition to the periosteal reaction. Its quality diminishes in the presence of implants, but it is still commonly utilized for pre-operative planning and biopsy guidance. When evaluating the bone marrow and the soft tissues around it, MRI is advantageous because it can identify the edema and hyperemia that are present in the very early stages of the disease. It can be used as a supplement to estimate the margins needed for debridement or to gauge the effectiveness of therapy. It can also distinguish between infections of the soft tissues and those of the bone. However, in the case of implants, scar tissue, and recent surgeries, its usefulness is restricted.

Chronic osteomyelitis has also been diagnosed with routine bone scintigraphy. However, it is associated with low specificity and false-positive findings, especially in individuals with recent surgery, gout, diabetic arthropathy, and trauma. Therefore, it is not recommended to rely solely on this imaging modality. On the other hand, leucocyte scintigraphy is a reliable method for identifying chronic osteomyelitis in the peripheral skeleton, although its diagnostic accuracy in the axial skeleton is lower. False-positive results have also been reported in cases of peri-articular nonunions with accompanying post-traumatic arthropathy or mechanically unstable nonunions. The most sensitive and specific method for identifying lesions and their concurrent inflammatory activity in the early stages is Positron Emission Tomography (PET). However, its regular use is limited due to availability and associated costs. According to a meta-analysis examining the precision of diagnostic imaging for chronic osteomyelitis, Fluorodeoxyglucose PET, particularly in the axial skeleton, has the highest diagnostic accuracy for confirming or ruling out the diagnosis. In the early stages of the disease, ultrasonography (US) is primarily used to identify purulent collections within the soft tissues. Although reliable estimates of its specificity and sensitivity are not available, some authors argue that it may be diagnostic in certain circumstances.

7.2.3.7. Laboratory Evaluation

Although most laboratory tests are not very specific for chronic osteomyelitis, they can still aid in the diagnosis. Increased erythrocyte sedimentation rate (ESR) and CRP levels are examples of inflammatory markers that can be used in conjunction with other diagnostic tests to track a patient's clinical response to treatment. On the other hand, osteomyelitis is typically ruled out in cases where CRP and ESR levels are consistently normal, though this may not always be the case in the presence of a discharging sinus or a history of diabetes. Although they are not accurate markers, leukocytosis and increased alpha-1 acid glycoprotein levels may also be present. Conversely, the white cell count (WCC) may fall within normal ranges.

The most crucial factor in determining a final diagnosis of chronic osteomyelitis is the existence of positive microbial cultures from bone biopsies near areas of bone necrosis. These should not be taken from fistulae or superficial wounds as they have been linked to poor accuracy due to the presence of non-pathogenic microorganisms that colonize the wound. Due primarily to the uneven distribution of osteomyelitis lesions in the bone, false-negative results are also reported. Since multiple organisms are frequently involved—including anaerobic, mycobacterial, and fungal organisms—specific cultures and microbiological testing may be required. Samples from up to five sites surrounding the implant should be collected to increase the diagnostic yield, particularly in cases of implant-related osteomyelitis. Prolonged enrichment broth cultures are frequently required. Obtaining the cultures before initiating any antimicrobial treatment is crucial to prevent false-negative outcomes. Typically, hematogenous osteomyelitis is the only condition in which conventional blood cultures are helpful. Additional significant information can also be obtained from the histopathology of tissue specimens taken during biopsy or debridement. Positive special staining indicates the presence of pathogens earlier than the culture results, while a significant neutrophil presence is suggestive of infection.

7.2.3.8. Diagnostic Approach

Although diagnosing chronic osteomyelitis can be difficult, it is crucial to understand that an earlier diagnosis will result in a better prognosis. The diagnosis can be aided by a high index of clinical suspicion, recognition of the clinical symptoms, imaging, and laboratory investigations. Because the symptoms of chronic osteomyelitis are typically mild and lack systemic features, diagnosing the condition can be even more challenging, particularly in patients with impaired peripheral vasculature.

Finding a potential source of infection should be the main goal of the clinical examination. As previously indicated, the presence of positive bacterial cultures from bone biopsies taken from regions with bone necrosis is the most sensitive criterion.

7.2.3.9. Management

The management of chronic osteomyelitis is influenced by factors such as the length, intensity, and presence of coexisting medical conditions. It is crucial to consider that the affected area is often characterized by poor vascularization and compromised soft tissue envelope. The primary objectives of treatment are to eliminate the inflammatory process by removing all pathogens and devitalized tissue, and if necessary, to promote healing by optimizing the mechanical and biological environments.

This can be achieved through a combination of surgical debridement, antibiotic therapy, and dead space management. Special attention is required for patients with diabetes, as concurrent vascular compromise and peripheral neuropathy may complicate the diagnosis and treatment course, potentially masking the symptoms. In some cases, limb amputation may be necessary for a small but significant portion of these patients.

7.2.3.10. Antibiotic Treatment

It is best to initiate the initial empirical antibiotic treatment promptly upon acquisition of the culture samples. Subsequently, the antibiotic regimen should be tailored based on the sensitivities and outcomes of the cultures. The prevailing consensus among experts suggests a duration of four to six weeks for antibiotic treatment.

This recommendation is supported by the observation that bone revascularization typically takes three to four weeks, allowing sufficient time for the antimicrobial agents to penetrate the inflammatory area and target the pathogens that are susceptible to antibiotic treatment. However, there is limited evidence to substantiate this advice or demonstrate that prolonged antibiotic treatment reduces the recurrence rate. In fact, prolonged use of antibiotics increases the risk of side effects, expenses, and antibiotic resistance.

There is currently no conclusive data to support practice regarding the kind of antibiotics to use or the best way to administer them. The oral route of administration appears appealing because, if oral agents are as successful as parenteral antibiotics, they should carry comparable risks of side effects, be easier to administer, and result in shorter hospital stays and medical expenses. The antibiotic agent's ability to penetrate bone and whether or not it surpasses the minimal inhibitory concentrations for the pathogen that has been isolated are what matter most. The cultures' outcomes and the bone biopsies' sensitivities should inform the antibiotic regimen that is employed. A combination of antibiotic agents is advised in cases involving multiple microorganisms or when prosthetic infections are present, as this has been shown to lower the recurrence rate. Finally, it has been reported that pathogens like *S. aureus* develop resistance to several antibiotics, an aspect that further complicates treatment selection.

High dosages of local antibiotics can also be administered to the surrounding tissues by using polymethylmethacrylate (PMMA) beads. Their efficacy has been supported by numerous studies, and they also have the added benefit of controlling the dead space left over after debridement. The chosen antibiotic agent in the mixture should be effective against the specific bacterial pathogen. Calcium sulfate beads, which are biodegradable and do not require removal, offer a faster release of high concentrations of antibiotics compared to PMMA beads. Similarly, polylactide-polyglycolide co-polymer implants and hydroxyapatite-ceramic beads are biodegradable and effectively used in the management of chronic osteomyelitis.

It is recommended to customize the treatment for each patient based on the type and severity of osteomyelitis, any coexisting medical conditions, any isolated organisms, and whether this is the initial presentation or a recurrence when selecting antibiotics. In the case of methicillin-susceptible *S. aureus* (MSSA), we recommend treating the microorganism with IV Nafcillin or Cefazolin; for MRSA, we recommend treating it with IV Vancomycin. After a minimum of six weeks of antimicrobial therapy, it is usually advisable to reevaluate the patient and consult with microbiologists if necessary.

7.2.3.11. Surgical Treatment

Surgical management is the mainstay of treatment for chronic osteomyelitis. To eliminate all pathogens and their biofilms, as well as the sequestra (dead bone) that acts as a foreign substance and penetrates healthy and viable tissue, a sufficient surgical debridement should be performed. Additionally, the local soft tissue envelope needs to be debrided and, if necessary, rebuilt. When osteomyelitis has significantly spread into the medullary canal, debridement using the reamer-irrigator-aspirator (RIA) technique has been recommended, followed by the insertion of an intramedullary cement rod that has been impregnated with antibiotics. To reduce the chance of recurrence, a more aggressive strategy involving reaming the canal and, if it involves a joint, the two adjacent canals, is recommended. This is because macroscopic assessment of the degree of bone marrow infiltration is unreliable (Table 7.2 and Figure 7.4).

Table 7.2. *Different Randomized Controlled Trials: Oral Antibiotic Therapy or Short-Term Parenteral Therapy (<2 Weeks) Followed by Oral Antibiotic Therapy vs. Parenteral Antibiotic Therapy for Treating Chronic Osteomyelitis*

Article	Year	Osteomyelitis Type	Sample Size	Investigation	Exclusion Criteria	Results
Li et al. [12]	2019	Bone and joint infection, including infection of osteosynthetic material.	1,054	Standard oral vs. standard IV.	*S. aureus* bacteremia; endocarditis, concomitant infection requiring prolonged antibiotics; mild osteomyelitis; no suitable antibiotic choices to permit randomization; septic shock; unlikely to comply with trial; mycobacterial, fungal, parasitic, or viral infection.	Non-inferiority of oral therapy to parenteral therapy. Treatment failure at 1 year 13.2% vs. 14.6% respectively.
Azamgarhi et al. [1]	2021	Bone and joint infection	328	Standard oral vs. standard IV	Not available	OVIVA trial findings can be safely implemented into clinical practice.
Gentry et al. [7]	1991	Non-prosthesis osteomyelitis	33	Ofloxacin vs. cephalosporin	Multiple sites of infection, retained prosthetic material, bacteremia.	Ofloxacin statistically non-inferior to IV antibiotics.
Gentry et al. [6]	1990	Osteomyelitis after surgical debridement.	59	Ciprofloxacin vs. beta-lactam + aminoglycoside.	Septicemia, MRSA	Ciprofloxacin statistically non-inferior to IV antibiotics.
Gomis et al. [8]	1985	Osteomyelitis including prosthesis infection.	32	Ofloxacin vs. imipenem	Not available	Ofloxacin non-inferior to IV imipenem-cilastatin.

Euba et al. [5]	2009	Non-axial *Staphylococcus aureus* osteomyelitis.	50	TMP-SMX + rifampicin vs. cloxacillin	Prosthetic joint infection, polymicrobial.	Eight weeks of co-trimoxazole non-inferior to or 6 weeks of IV + 2 weeks of PO oxacillin.

Legend: IV: Intravenous; MRSA: methicillin resistant Staphylococcus aureus; and TMP-SMX: trimethoprim-sulfamethoxazole.

Source: *Besal, R., Adamič, P., Beović, B., & Papst, L., (2023). Systemic antimicrobial treatment of chronic osteomyelitis in adults: A narrative review. Antibiotics, 12(6), 944. https://doi.org/10.3390/antibiotics12060944.*

Since insufficient debridement has been linked to a high recurrence rate, concerns about the potential for osseous and/or soft-tissue defects should not be used as a reason to limit adequate debridement. To ensure the absence of malignant alterations, samples from the affected bone, sinus tract, and surrounding tissues should be sent for pathological examination after debridement. While there is no doubt that surgical debridement is necessary for chronic osteomyelitis, many people believe that it is not sufficient to maintain remission and that a combination of antibiotics and surgery produces better outcomes. It is important to consider, however, that not all cases of chronic osteomyelitis require surgery, as the patient's health and any coexisting conditions may make surgery contraindicated, particularly in the case of spinal involvement. In such situations, suppressive therapy with appropriate antibiotics may be considered.

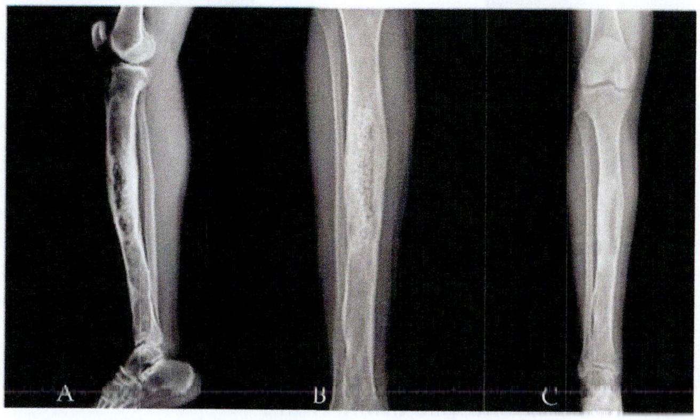

Figure 7.4. *X-rays of the leg in a patient treated with debridement and adjuvant PerOssal bead for chronic osteomyelitis of the tibia diaphysis. (A) Post-operative lateral view X-rays. Antero-posterior X-rays showing no filling at 6 months of follow-up (B); with complete filling at 12 months of follow-up (C).*

Source: Sambri, A., Cevolani, L., Passarino, V., Bortoli, M., Parisi, S. C., Fiore, M., Campanacci, L., Staals, E., Donati, D. M., & De Paolis, M., (2023). Mid-term results of single-stage surgery for patients with chronic osteomyelitis using antibiotic-loaded resorbable PerOssal® beads. Microorganisms, 11(7), 1623. https://doi.org/10.3390/microorganisms11071623.

7.2.3.12. Management of Dead Space

A sizable bone defect, or dead space, may develop after a forceful debridement that might be necessary to remove all devitalized tissue. In order to eradicate the infection and subsequently implant graft materials to facilitate bone regeneration, this area requires proper management. Broadly speaking, the features of the lesion after debridement and the host's physiological grade determine which reconstruction technique is best. The reason for the poor success rate of primary bone grafting procedures is usually the resorption of the bone graft as a result of persistent infection and/or inflammation. In two-stage procedures, antibiotic-impregnated cement spacers and antibiotic beads can be used to temporarily fill the dead space until reconstruction is completed. To manage critical size bone defects, other options include bone transport and circular external fixation devices. The induced membrane (Masquelet) technique has also been used with encouraging results. To optimize the compromised soft tissue envelope, local flaps such as muscle flaps, pedicled muscle flaps, myocutaneous flaps, and osseous flaps have been employed with positive outcomes. In cases where the local tissues are compromised, vascularized free flaps have also been used to cover large defects. Figure 7.5 shows a case report of a novel combination of arthroscopic techniques, namely "ossoscopy," bone grafting, and antibiotics for epiphyseal subacute osteomyelitis.

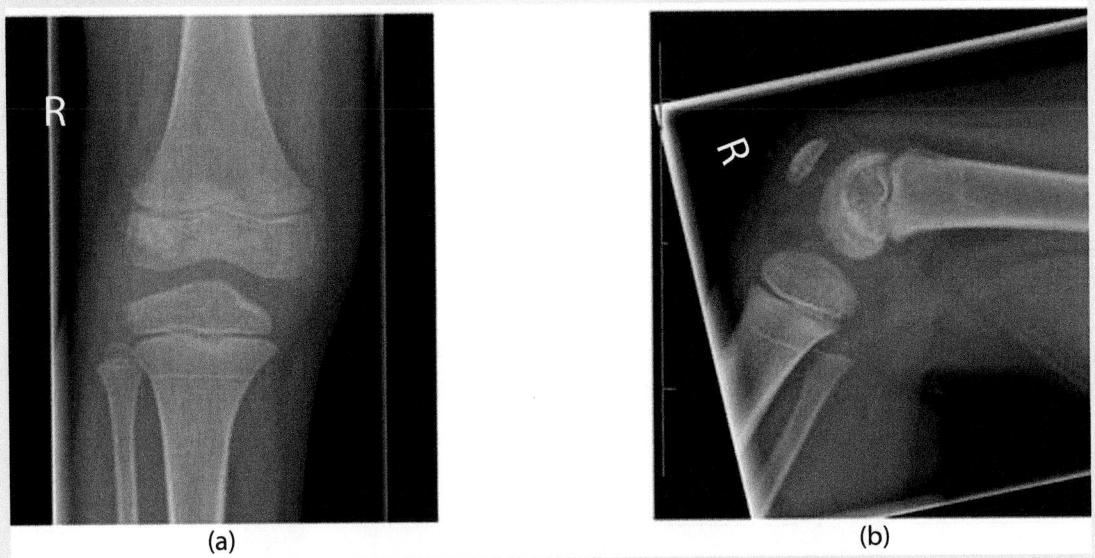

Figure 7.5. *Plain radiographs of the right knee in anterior-posterior (a); and lateral (b) views of the seven-year-old boy during a two-year follow-up. The bone defect of the epiphysis has healed. Please note the presence of the Harris line in the proximal tibia.*

Source: Weber, C. D., Migliorini, F., Delbrück, H., & Hildebrand, F., (2022). Surgical management of an osteomyelitis associated subchondral bone defect in the pediatric knee based on arthroscopy, "Ossoscopy" and bone grafting – A case report. Life, 12(11), 1754. https://doi.org/10.3390/life12111754.

7.2.3.13. Complications

The infective process and chronic inflammation can lead to many complications. Among the most frequent complications are sinus tracts, the development of abscesses, and extension to neighboring structures. However, the most significant—and frequently overlooked—complication is the malignant transformation of chronic osteomyelitis, or Marjolin's ulcer. While Marjolin's ulcer affects 1 in 6 to 23% of patients with chronic osteomyelitis, its occurrence is higher in developing nations with inadequate medical resources. Aggressive squamous cell carcinomas (SCC), which have a latent period of 27 to 30 years from the onset of osteomyelitis to malignant transformation, are the main cause of Marjolin's ulcers. The most significant predictor is the length of the chronic osteomyelitis.

7.2.4. Subacute Osteomyelitis

Although the organisms are present in the bone, they do not produce the symptoms of acute or chronic osteomyelitis, making it a unique type of bone infection. This can happen first when the organism's virulence is low or the host is resistant, or secondarily when acute osteomyelitis becomes subacute after treatment.

7.2.5. Brodie's Abscess

A Brodie abscess is a type of subacute osteomyelitis that can last for several years before developing into a chronic osteomyelitis. It typically manifests as a draining abscess that extends through the skin from the tibia. In rare cases, fibrous and granulation tissue may encapsulate an area affected by acute osteomyelitis. The most common causative organism is *Staphylococcus aureus*.

7.2.5.1. History

The term "Brodie abscess" is named after Sir Benjamin Collins Brodie, the 1st Baronet. In the 1830s, he first described a chronic inflammatory condition of the tibia without an apparent acute cause. Subsequently, it was discovered that infection was responsible for this condition.

7.2.5.2. Presentation

The presentation of a Brodie abscess includes localized pain, typically worse at night, which can be alleviated with aspirin. This pain is similar to the symptoms of osteoid osteoma, where the affected area is usually smaller than 1 cm.

7.2.5.3. Location

Brodie's abscess usually occurs at the metaphysis of long bones, such as the distal femur, proximal or distal fibula, distal radius, distal tibia, and proximal tibia.

7.2.5.4. Diagnosis

- **Radiographic Features:** Brodie's abscess appears as an oval, elliptical, or serpentine radiolucency, typically larger than 1 cm. It is surrounded by granulation tissue, highly reactive sclerosis, and a nidus that is often smaller than 1 cm. On radiographs, the margins often exhibit a scalloped appearance. The most effective imaging modality to visualize Brodie's abscess is a CT scan. Additionally, there may be corresponding soft tissue atrophy near the infection site and shortened bone in the affected area. Osteoblastoma can be a possible classic sign of Brodie's abscess (Figure 7.6).

- **Treatment:** The majority of the time, surgery is required. In the event that the cavity is small, curettage and surgical evacuation are carried out while administering antibiotics. After evacuation, the abscess space might need to be packed with cancellous bone chips if the cavity is large.

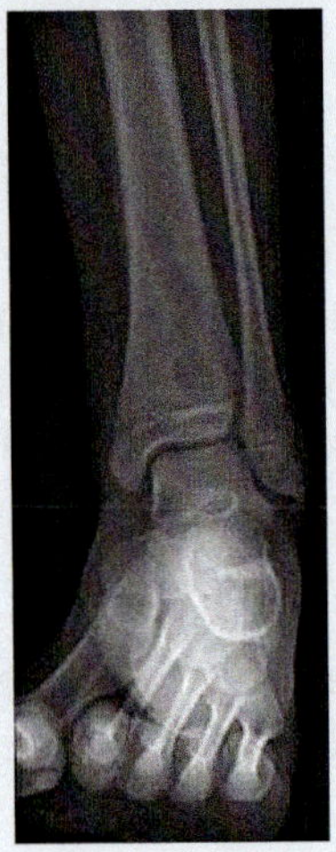

Figure 7.6. *Periostial reaction along the medial cortex indicates an aggressive lesion. Neoplasms such as Ewing sarcoma and osteomyelitis could both have this plain radiographic appearance. Staphylococcus was recovered during surgery.*

Source: By Jto410 – clinical work as a radiologist, CC BY-SA 3.0, https://commons.wikimedia.org/w/index.php?curid=25988436.

7.2.6. Sclerosing Osteomyelitis of Garre

Sclerosing osteomyelitis of Garré is an uncommon chronic inflammatory disease characterized by loss of the medullary canal and thickening of the corticosteal. It mainly affects the mandibular region in young children and adults, but can also rarely affect the metaphysis of long bones. Other names for this condition include ossifying periostitis, Garré's sclerosing osteomyelitis, nonsuppurative chronic sclerosing osteomyelitis, and chronic osteomyelitis with proliferative periostitis. This clinical feature is characterized by localized, episodic, nonprogressive pain with a subtle onset. It could last for several months or years, and it can also impact multifocal sites. The duration is highly unpredictable. The impacted bone usually retains its functionality. Cortical thickening and medullary canal loss are two of the radiographic features. Acute-phase inflammatory markers like erythrocyte sedimentation rate (ESR) and CRP may be elevated. In general, tissue and blood cultures come back negative, and the biopsy reveals chronic, nonspecific osteomyelitis. Focal dysplasia, syphilis, rectocolitis, pustulosis palmoplantaris, Crohn's disease, synovitis, acne, pustulosis, hyperostosis, and osteitis (SAPHO), osteosarcoma, Paget's disease, osteoid osteoma, Ewing's disease, chronic recurrent multifocal osteomyelitis, and eosinophilic granuloma are among the differential diagnoses.

The main objective of treatment is symptom relief. Although the precise mechanism is unknown, some patients respond to analgesics, and some respond to antibiotics. If the symptoms are unmanageable, surgical intervention may be necessary. This could involve anything from resection of the chronic osteomyelitis area to debridement of the affected bone, exposing the medullary canal.

7.2.7. Septic Arthritis

Joint inflammation caused by an infectious etiology, usually bacterial, but also occasionally fungal, mycobacterial, viral, or other uncommon pathogens, is known as septic arthritis. Typically, septic arthritis affects a single, large joint, such as the hip or knee. However, it can also occur in multiple, smaller joints, known as polyarticular septic arthritis. Septic arthritis is a rare orthopedic emergency that can result in severe joint damage and higher rates of morbidity and mortality. Early detection and intervention are crucial for maintaining joint function. According to a study on the healthcare burden of septic arthritis in the US, inpatient costs for septic arthritis increased by 24% and overall costs by 26% between 2009 and 2012. However, there were no time trends in the length of stay or admission outcomes. Older patients with septic arthritis are more likely to have comorbid predisposing conditions, which increases their long-term mortality.

7.2.7.1. Etiology

7.2.7.1.1. Etiology in Children

In children, arthritis, or inflammation of the joint, can have a variety of causes. The most prevalent type of bacterial pathogen worldwide is *Staphylococcus aureus.* Specific age groups and underlying medical conditions are linked to certain etiologic agents. The most frequent gram-negative bacterial cause of this in children under the age of three is *Kingella kingae.* Neonatals frequently contract gram-negative *Bacilli, Neisseria gonorrhea, Staphylococcus aureus,* and Group B streptococcus. In teenagers who are sexually active, *Neisseria gonorrhea* is a concern. Infection with *Salmonella* species is linked to sickle cell disease. Individuals receiving extended antibiotic therapy may develop fungal infections. *Pseudomonas aeruginosa*-related joint infections are linked to injection drug use and puncture wounds. In children, the hip joint is most frequently impacted.

7.2.7.1.2. Etiology in Adults

Adults are most commonly infected by *Staphylococcus aureus.* Although less frequent, Streptococcus pneumoniae is nevertheless a major cause of infection in adults. Additional unique situations include those previously mentioned (*Salmonella* in sickle cell patients and Pseudomonas in trauma/puncture wounds). *Neisseria gonorrhoeae* is the most common cause of nontraumatic acute monoarthritis in young, sexually active patients. *Neisseria gonorrhoeae* grows poorly from cultured synovial fluid; instead, it is best to culture the organism from other sites, such as the oropharynx, vagina, cervix, urethra, or anus, in high-risk patients. Mycobacterial and fungal organisms can be more difficult to diagnose because of their elusive presentation. While a synovial biopsy yields positive results in 95% of cases, an acid-fast smear of synovial fluid frequently yields negative results. Adults most frequently experience joint pain in the knee, then the hip. About 5% of patients develop polymicrobial joint infections as a result of abdominal infections or trauma. Patients who abuse IV drugs are susceptible to infections of the sternoclavicular and sacroiliac joints, which are typically caused by Serratia and Pseudomonas. Leukemia patients are particularly vulnerable to Aeromonas infections. Infection is very common in previously damaged joints, particularly in rheumatoid arthritis patients. The organisms cause damage to the articular cartilage on the lateral edges of the joint. Effusions are frequent and often associated with pain.

7.2.7.2. Epidemiology

Septic arthritis affects 2 to 6 persons out of every 1,00,000, though the exact number depends on risk factors. Compared to adults, children are more likely to develop septic arthritis. Septic arthritis is more common in men (2:1) and peaks between the ages of two- and three-years. However, children with hemarthroses who are hemophiliacs, immunocompromised children (e.g., human immunodeficiency virus infection, sickle cell anemia, and those undergoing chemotherapy), adults over 80 years old, diabetes mellitus, rheumatoid arthritis, recent joint surgery, joint prosthesis, prior intra-articular injection, cutaneous ulcers and skin infections, HIV, osteoarthritis, sexual activity (particularly in suspected gonococcal septic arthritis cases), and other causes of sepsis are risk factors.

7.2.7.3. Pathophysiology

Since the highly vascularized joint synovium lacks a limiting basement membrane, hematogenous seeding from systemic infection can cause infection. Perforation wounds, intra-articular injections, and direct injuries can also cause septic arthritis. It's possible for contiguous spread from nearby osteomyelitis. Contiguous spread poses a threat to the hip and shoulder. When bacteria invade the synovium and joint space, an inflammatory process ensues, leading to septic arthritis. Proteases and inflammatory cytokines are the mediators of joint degeneration. According to animal models, bacterial toxins and microbial surface elements like staphylococcal adhesins, which encourage the binding of the bacteria to intra-articular proteins, are additional factors that contribute to joint damage.

Prosthetic joint infections are classified into:

- Early within 3 months of implantation;
- Delayed within 3–24 months of surgery;
- Late: occurring after 24 months.

Staphylococcus is responsible for the majority of early prosthetic joint infections, while gram-negative and coagulase-negative staphylococcus are responsible for delayed cases. Late cases typically result from hematogenous spread from different foci.

7.2.7.4. History and Physical

Acute onset monoarticular joint pain, fever, swelling, and a reluctance or refusal to move the affected joint are the typical symptoms of septic arthritis. Fever is a nonspecific finding that may be present in 40–60% of cases. Most cases of septic arthritis affect the joints in the lower extremities, namely the hips, knees, and ankles, with the knee being the most commonly affected joint in adults. Around 20% of cases are oligoarticular, particularly when there are several comorbid conditions, such as rheumatoid arthritis, immune system compromise, or severe sepsis present. Injecting drug users may experience involvement of less common joints, such as the sternoclavicular or sacroiliac joint. Most adults who have gonococcal arthritis are sexually active, young, and in good health. They may exhibit dermatitis, tenosynovitis, non-erosive arthritis, and a migratory pattern of arthritis upon physical examination. Young patients with septic arthritis may present with systemic as well as local symptoms. Local symptoms include warmth, pain, edema in the affected joint, restricted range of motion, limping, and refusal to use or move the affected joint (pseudoparalysis). Symptoms affecting the entire body: Appearance of illness, fever, rapid heartbeat, irritability, loss of appetite.

7.2.7.4.1. Physical

The knee is the most frequently affected joint in septic arthritis, followed by the hip, ankle, and shoulder. Common effusions are examined to determine the causes. Restricted range of motion and pain upon palpation are observed. Staphylococcal infections often involve a single joint, while Neisseria commonly affects multiple joints simultaneously. Group B streptococci frequently affect the sacroiliac and sternoclavicular joints. Infections in prosthetic joints often result in a draining sinus.

7.2.7.5. Evaluation

Laboratory and imaging studies, along with arthrocentesis with synovial fluid analysis, are part of the evaluation process for suspected septic arthritis.

7.2.7.6. Laboratory Studies

A synovial fluid evaluation, including culture, Gram stain, crystallography, and white blood cell count with differential, is the most helpful diagnostic laboratory test for diagnosing septic arthritis. A synovial fluid with a white blood cell (WBC) count higher than 50,000 and a 90% neutrophil predominance suggests a bacterial source. The diagnosis is confirmed when a bacterial organism is identified in the synovial fluid. Additional helpful laboratory tests include a complete blood count, blood cultures, erythrocyte sedimentation rate (ESR), and CRP. An elevated peripheral blood WBC count is usually associated with a left shift. Although not conclusive, an elevated ESR and CRP can confirm the diagnosis. A low WBC count in synovial fluid can be observed in cases of disseminated gonococcal arthritis, early infection, peripheral leukopenia, and joint prosthesis.

In prosthetic joint infections, a synovial fluid WBC count of 1,100 and a neutrophil differential of 64% indicate septic arthritis. To rule out bacteremia, it is recommended to take two sets of blood cultures. If Neisseria is suspected, cultures from the throat, rectum, and cervix should be obtained.

7.2.7.7. Imaging Studies

Broadened joint spaces, soft tissue bulging, or subchondral bone changes (a late finding) can all be seen on plain radiographs. A standard plain radiograph does not rule out septic arthritis. In addition to assisting with needle aspiration of the joint, ultrasonography aids in locating and measuring the joint effusion. MRI can identify abnormalities in the surrounding soft tissue and bone, as well as the extent of cartilaginous involvement. It is highly sensitive for early detection of joint fluid.

Bone scans are non-specific and cannot differentiate between a sterile procedure and an infection. However, they are useful in evaluating isolated hip or sacroiliac joint infections.

7.2.7.8. Treatment/Management

Antimicrobial therapy and joint fluid drainage (arthrotomy, arthroscopy, or daily needle aspiration) are the two mainstays of treatment for septic arthritis. It is important to initiate empiric intravenous antibiotic therapy immediately after joint aspiration is completed and cultures are obtained. Empiric antibiotic coverage should include antistaphylococcal agents (nafcillin, oxacillin, or vancomycin) for all age groups and risk categories. Intravenous vancomycin, targeting gram-positive organisms, is typically used as an empirical antibiotic for nongonococcal septic arthritis, especially if MRSA is suspected based on community and institutional data. For additional gram-negative coverage, a third-generation cephalosporin such as ceftriaxone, ceftazidime, or cefotaxime should be added if the patient is immunocompromised, abuses intravenous drugs, or the gram stain is negative. Additional antibiotics should be guided by age, risk factors, and gram stain results (e.g., a third-generation cephalosporin for suspected *Salmonella* or *N. gonorrhea*). Prolonged antimicrobial treatment should be guided by cultures and sensitivities of blood and synovial fluid. An orthopedic surgeon should be involved as soon as possible. The method of draining joint fluid is chosen by the orthopedic surgeon based on several factors.

Treatment for nongonococcal septic arthritis typically consists of two weeks of intravenous antibiotics, followed by an additional one to two weeks of oral antibiotic therapy, for a total of three to four weeks. In cases of *Pseudomonas aeruginosa*, a longer antibiotic treatment period of four to six weeks may be appropriate. Intravenous ceftriaxone is a good treatment for gonococcal arthritis. After a 24–48-hour period of improvement in clinical symptoms, oral therapy is switched for the balance of the course of treatment. The joint should be re-aspirated and Lyme disease should be ruled out if no improvement is observed in five to six days. Reactive arthritis and the existence of fungi should also be taken into account. In these cases, imaging tests are required to rule out osteomyelitis. After two to three days, the joint does not require immobilization. To prevent muscle atrophy and restore joint function, aggressive physical therapy is required. A prosthesis must be removed or aggressively debrided in cases of prosthetic joint infection. After that, cement that has been treated with antibiotics is used to replace the new joint.

7.2.7.9. Differential Diagnosis

Differential diagnoses of acute monoarticular arthritis include:

- Infection: Bacterial, fungal, viral, spirochete, mycoplasma
- Crystal-induced arthropathies include hydroxyapatite crystals, acute and pseudogout, cholesterol, and calcium oxalate.
- Osteoarthritis
- Intra-articular injury: Meniscal tear, osteonecrosis, foreign body, fracture, and plant thorn synovitis.
- Inflammatory arthritis: Rheumatoid arthritis, systemic lupus erythematosus, sarcoidosis, and Still's disease are examples of seronegative spondyloarthropathies. These include ankylosing spondylitis, psoriatic arthritis, reactive arthritis, and arthritis associated with inflammatory bowel disease.
- Systemic infection: Bacterial endocarditis, human immunodeficiency virus, Lyme arthritis.
- Tumor: Metastasis, pigmented villonodular synovitis.
- Other: Avascular necrosis (AVN), neuropathic arthropathy, amyloidosis linked to dialysis, hemarthrosis, clotting disorders, or anticoagulant therapy.

7.2.7.10. Prognosis

In-hospital septic arthritis has a 7–15% mortality rate despite the use of antibiotics. In one-third of cases, patients with septic arthritis experience morbidity. Factors such as patient age, comorbid conditions like pre-existing joint disease, and previous use of synthetic intra-articular material all contribute to increased morbidity and mortality. This underscores the importance of maintaining a high index of suspicion, early diagnosis of septic arthritis, and prompt initiation of treatment, particularly in patients with comorbid conditions and known predisposing risk factors. Neisseria infections rarely result in death, whereas staphylococcus infections can have a mortality rate exceeding 50%.

7.2.7.11. Complications

Complications of septic arthritis include:

- Osteomyelitis;
- Chronic pain;
- Osteonecrosis;
- Leg length discrepancies;
- Sepsis;
- Death.

7.2.7.12. Consultations

Early in the course of the disease, it is advisable to seek a consultation with an orthopedic surgeon for synovial fluid drainage. In some cases, interventional radiology may be required to drain fluid from axial joints that are more difficult to access.

7.2.7.13. Deterrence and Patient Education

It is crucial to inform patients and caregivers about the severity of this illness and the potential for increased morbidity even after successful antibiotic treatment.

7.2.7.14. Pearls and Other Issues

When septic arthritis is suspected in an acutely inflamed joint, especially in a patient with risk factors, arthroscopy of the affected joint should be performed promptly. This aids in early diagnosis and the initiation of appropriate antibiotic therapy.

7.2.7.15. Enhancing Healthcare Team Outcomes

Septic arthritis is an uncommon orthopedic emergency that requires a high level of suspicion during diagnosis, particularly in patients with risk factors. Even with proper treatment, elderly individuals, those with a history of arthritis, or those with an intra-articular prosthesis have a higher rate of morbidity and mortality. Typically, septic arthritis presents as acute monoarticular joint inflammation, which has a broad differential diagnosis. Managing the infection with an interprofessional team is recommended due to its high morbidity and mortality rate. Arthrocentesis is a crucial part of the diagnostic process. Joint drainage is usually performed by orthopedic surgeons through daily needle aspiration, arthroscopy, or arthrotomy. However, for axial joint drainage, a consultation with interventional radiology may be necessary. Early in the treatment process, consulting with infectious disease specialists ensures appropriate antibiotic coverage and therapy duration based on culture results. It is important to ensure that the patient is receiving antibiotics that are effective against the specific organism, and to closely monitor culture results, as advised by the pharmacist.

An interdisciplinary team of healthcare professionals, including the primary care physician, nurses, wound care team, and physical and occupational therapists, is typically responsible for the initial management of patients with septic arthritis in an inpatient hospital setting. The primary care physician oversees the patient's care across disciplines and manages any co-existing conditions. These patients need to be monitored by a wound care nurse until full healing has taken place. Some patients can go home after being discharged, but others who require continued physical therapy at an acute or subacute rehabilitation facility may need more time away from their homes. The hospital's social workers assist in ensuring a smooth transition from inpatient to outpatient care. Patients must complete the prescribed antibiotic treatment and follow-up. Team members need to keep each other informed to provide the best possible care for the patient.

7.3. Specific Infections

The majority of bone and joint infections in small or premature infants are caused by repeated invasive procedures and prolonged nosocomial exposures. There is always a primary focus elsewhere in the body that takes precedence over the tuberculosis of the bones and joints. This primary focus is frequently invisible. Through the bloodstream, the bacilli penetrate the bone, dissemination occurs, and they lodge in various locations. Consequently, the lesion could be in the bone or the synovium. According to some reports, bone and joint tuberculosis does not appear for approximately 18 to 24 months following the onset of the primary lesion. The risk factors for the infection are inadequate resistance, poor nutrition, malnutrition, and poor sanitation. Bone and joint TB does not discriminate based on age. It may manifest at any age. However, the destruction of the growing bone causes severe deformities if it happens early in life. In the spine, this is especially true.

7.3.1. Tuberculosis of the Spine

Tuberculosis (TB) is a disease that affects approximately 25% of the world's population. Its symptoms include vulnerability, poverty, economic hardship, stigma, and discrimination. In 2021, there were 101.6 million cases of TB, which translates to 134 cases per 1,00,000 people. Around 16% of all TB cases were linked to HIV infection. The highest percentages of TB cases in 2021 were in Southeast Asia (45%), followed by Africa (23%) and the Western Pacific (18%). The regions with the lowest percentage of cases were Europe (2.2%), the Americas (2.9%), and the Eastern Mediterranean (8.1%).

Despite being a preventable and treatable disease, global control of TB remains inadequate. This is due to various factors such as rising HIV infection rates, drug abuse, population growth in developing countries, and migration to developed nations. Skeletal TB accounts for 1–2% of all TB cases and 10% of extrapulmonary TB cases. Spinal TB, which is expensive for families and countries, affects the productive age group and comprises more than half of all skeletal TB cases. Developing nations with high poverty rates, malnutrition, crowded living conditions, and poor hygiene are more likely to experience spinal TB. Gender does not influence a person's susceptibility to TB. The elderly are increasingly affected by spinal TB due to factors such as increased use of immunosuppressive medications, longer life expectancies, cancer treatment, diabetes, and HIV.

Spinal tuberculosis can have a mild clinical presentation. Symptoms may include anorexia, dysphagia, fever, and back pain that do not improve with physical therapy. In some cases, there may be no symptoms at all. Therefore, it is essential to obtain a complete medical history and perform a comprehensive examination of the spine and other joints. Factors such as a family history of tuberculosis, contact with an actively ill patient, lifestyle choices, and financial circumstances can all help in early diagnosis. After the clinical examination, the pathology and any new problems that might require additional testing and care should be identified.

7.3.1.1. Signs and Symptoms

Studies have found that the majority of patients with spinal tuberculosis suffer from issues with the lower thoracic and upper lumbar vertebrae. The cervical and lumbar regions are the most commonly affected areas, followed by the thoracolumbar junction. The transition from a rigid thoracic spine to a flexible lumbar spine can cause tiny injuries in the thoracolumbar region, which can facilitate the spread of tuberculosis bacteria. The bacteria typically move from a primary site, such as the lungs or genitourinary system, to the vertebral body through the blood. The vertebrae are easily infected because each one has a rich vascular plexus in the subchondral region. Moreover, since the same segmental artery supplies two nearby vertebrae, both are frequently affected simultaneously. The spine is connected to the intra-abdominal and intra-thoracic chambers via a valveless system known as Batson's venous plexus. When TB bacilli propagate through the anterior or posterior longitudinal ligaments, multiple contiguous vertebrae become involved, while core lesions in the vertebral body and involvement of non-contiguous vertebrae occur when TB spreads through Batson's plexus.

According to a published case series using FDG-PET SCAN, 63.6% of skeletal TB cases involved non-contiguous spinal involvement.

The clinical presentation of tuberculosis of the spine can be influenced by several factors, such as age, lesion location, and duration of the illness. The neurological symptoms can be further complicated by immunological conditions, co-morbidities, and the development of problems such as deformity, cold abscess, secondary infection, and neurological sequelae.

The most common symptom of spinal tuberculosis is chronic low back pain, which is usually dull and aching, and does not radiate. The pain starts mildly but worsens over time. Other symptoms such as weight loss, malaise and lack of appetite may also be present. Patients may have had contact with someone who had the illness, or may have had pulmonary tuberculosis that had healed in the past.

One of the defining symptoms of spinal tuberculosis is discomfort at night, which can awaken the patient. Sudden, intense pain is associated with the lack of a protective muscle spasm, a sign of the spine's instability. Severe pain during the night while lying flat is also associated with venous engorgement and swelling.

In cases of skeletal tuberculosis, back pain is especially resistant to conservative measures. Radicular pain may appear as a presenting symptom when a bone fragment or abscess develops and compresses a nerve root. Radicular pain in the abdomen may be misdiagnosed as other conditions, such as pancreatitis, appendicitis, cholecystitis, or renal disorders. This could lead to a delay in treatment and unnecessary tests and procedures.

Muscular spasms may also be present, which can manifest as sciatic pain from a unilateral spasm, or as prominent paraspinal muscles in the thoracolumbar spine. This can cause local sensitivity in the affected area, and patients may move very carefully to avoid exacerbating the pain. The "Tripod Sign" is a characteristic symptom of skeletal tuberculosis involving the thoracolumbar spine.

7.3.1.1.1. Neurological Deficit

Neurological involvement occurs in around 23 to 76% of spinal tuberculosis cases. Paraparesis is more common in the thoracic and cervical spines than below the L1 level, where the spinal cord ends and the canal is larger. Neurological symptoms can vary from mild gait issues to complete bladder and bowel incontinence. Patients in underdeveloped areas usually present after becoming weak, and initially walk slowly and awkwardly due to their discomfort and weakness. Cervical cord compression can cause weakness in all four limbs, while thoracic cord compression can lead to paralysis in both lower limbs, with or without bladder and bowel involvement. Lumbar spine involvement is characterized by symptoms of the lower motor neurons. Paresis may occur in cases of actively spreading disease or slowly healing bodies. The active state can result from intrinsic causes like inflammation, meningitis, infective thrombi, or vascular damage from endarteritis, or it can be directly caused by compression from an abscess, inflammatory tissue, sequestrum, or instability. Causes of paraplegia include scarring, disease recurrence in previously treated conditions, bony ridges, and the spinal cord growing over internal gibs.

Motor function usually deteriorates first after a spinal cord compression, followed by sensory and autonomic impairments. In an anterior lesion, compression usually begins anteriorly and moves posteriorly. The patient may not be aware of the onset of spasticity at first. It is distinguished during a clinical examination by an extensor plantar response and rapid deep tendon reflexes (DTR). Increased compression causes the anterior columns to become gradually implicated, leading to a loss of motor function. More compression causes the lateral spinothalamic pathways to become involved, which leads to a reduction in pain, warmth, and rough touch. When the posterior columns are affected, there is a complete loss of feeling, and irregularities in the bladder and bowel have already occurred. Long-term application of compression causes flexor spasms and flaccidity in place of spasticity. When bladder and bowel function are compromised early on, lesions at the conus medullaris or cauda equina may exhibit asymmetrical loss of feeling along with mixed symptoms of upper and lower motor neuron lesions. The Frankel and ASIA ratings, which were first created to identify neurological deficits in acute spinal injuries, can be used to classify neurological abnormalities in spinal tuberculosis. The modified Tuli classification is the most appropriate classification for Pott paraplegia involving the spinal cord. Five stages of Pott paraplegia were identified (Table 7.3). Neurological impairments in intraspinal granulomas, cauda equina syndromes, conus medullaris syndromes, or tuberculosis of other uncommon sites may not correlate to any of the phases described above, even though most neurologic abnormalities would fall into this category.

Table 7.3. *Classification of Paraplegia in Tuberculosis of the Spine*

Stage	Complaints	Motor	Sensory	Autonomic
I	Nil	Plantar extensor/ankle clonus; ASIA motor score – 100.	Nil	Nil
II	Able to walk with support	ASIA motor score; Tetra paresis (60–100); paraparesis (80–100).	Lateral column; involvement.	Nil
III	Confined to bed; can move limbs.	ASIA motor score; tetra paresis (0–30); paraparesis (50–80).	Lateral column; involvement.	May be present
IV	No limb movement	ASIA motor score; tetra paresis (0); paraparesis (50).	Both lateral and posterior column involvement.	May be present
V	Flexor spasms	Flaccid paralysis	Complete loss	Complete loss of bladder and bowel control.

Source: Wattana, L., Pathomthep, L., & Tawithep, L., (2023). Tuberculosis of the spine. World J. Orthop., 14(5), 275–293. doi: 10.5312/wjo.v14.i5.275.

7.3.1.1.2. Cold Abscess

Spinal tuberculosis is often accompanied by paravertebral abscesses, which can be present in at least half of the cases. A cold abscess is so named because it lacks typical inflammatory markers like redness, pain, and swelling. However, its presence suggests an ongoing infection. Most cold abscesses have well-defined borders that are smooth and uniform, and they can cause a fluctuation. When the abscess is large, the skin above it appears swollen and glossy. Stratified abscesses gradually erode subcutaneous and dermal tissue, resulting in a sinus that leaks. Pus from an abscess is usually white or pale yellow in color and contains caseous material with sequestered bone and detritus, but it does not have a foul odor that could indicate a fungal or pyogenic infection. If the underlying disease process is under control, tubercular sinuses heal over time, leaving a thin scar. A fibrotic scar that is anchored to the underlying tissue is a common symptom of inflammation caused by a secondary infection. The presence of pyogenic organisms in the pus does not rule out tuberculosis, as per culture. Paravertebral abscesses tend to migrate along the path of least resistance after damaging surrounding tissues such as the muscular, subpleural, sub-peritoneal, perivascular, perineural, and fascial planes. They can also appear as a superficial abscess distant from the original focus.

Enlargements in the axilla, subscapular area, or anterior or posterior neck triangles could be a sign of cervical spine retropharyngeal abscesses. Retropharyngeal abscesses don't have the typical pharyngo-vertebral crepitus, which is felt when the larynx is gently pressed against the vertebral column from side to side. This illness is life-threatening and can cause hoarseness, dysphagia, and stridor. If the infection travels through the brachial plexus, an abscess in the arm or forearm might develop. A fusiform paravertebral swelling in the thoracic area is recognized as a cold abscess. Rarely, it might stick to the diaphragm aperture or the arcuate ligament. It may also cause a protrusion in the chest wall by passing through the intercostal arteries. Usually, a lumbar spine cold abscess is found in the groin, or Petit's triangle. It might move down the psoas muscle and result in a deformity known as hip pseudo-flexion. It can follow the femoral or gluteal arteries and occasionally manifest as a tumor in the Scarpa's triangle or a gluteal abscess. The adductor region is where the abscess will appear if the obturator vessels are followed. If the sciatic nerve is suspected, the abscess may form in the popliteal fossa, the posterior thigh, or the gluteal area. It is essential to understand the pus distribution because it may divert the examiner's attention from the TB source. The focus on the cervical spine may manifest as an abscess in the mediastinum or elbow, even though the involvement of the thoracic spine may diffuse into the lumbar region through the diaphragmatic orifice. An abscess in the lumbar spine may manifest as swelling in the ankle, calf, or thigh.

7.3.1.1.3. Spine Deformity

During either the active or healed stages, patients may experience deformities. These deformities may appear immediately following a surgical debridement or may take years to manifest in older patients with compromised skeletal architecture due to osteoporosis. TB initially affects the anterior column, and as it progresses, kyphotic deformity and instability can occur. If treatment begins at this stage, the lesion usually heals with minimal deformity when the cancellous bones meet and the intervertebral disc is destroyed. However, delays in therapy can lead to further degradation and increased deformity. The clinical presentation is determined by the number of affected vertebrae, with additional collapse potentially causing the vertebral bodies to retropel and compress the spinal cord, impairing the nervous system. Regular follow-up is crucial for children's development until adulthood. If a child sustains facet damage during an active illness, they have an increased chance of developing severe deformities later in life. Severe abnormalities can lead to cerebral deficits, impede cardiac function, and lower the quality of life. Kyphosis is less problematic in the cervical and lumbar spines due to inherent lordosis, but it is more of an issue in the thoracic and thoracolumbar spines.

7.3.1.1.4. Pediatric Spinal TB

It is important to be cautious when a child reports back pain at the spine clinic, as children are more susceptible to spinal problems than adults. This is because their skeletons are still growing and developing, and they tend to be more active. Children have more cartilage in their vertebral bodies, which can be easily damaged by mechanical stress or active diseases. When the ring apophysis is loaded unevenly, it can cause new or existing spinal deformities to worsen, which can lead to neurological problems. Children who have been declared cured but still have residual deformities should undergo regular clinical and radiological examinations until they reach skeletal maturity, as physical activity and growth can exacerbate any pre-existing conditions. One-third of children with more than two of the four spine-at-risk indicators had an unfavorable outcome. Children with illnesses affecting more than three vertebral bodies, children under seven, and those with conditions affecting the thoracolumbar junction or lower thoracic region are more likely to experience spinal problems. The four signs that indicate a child's spine may be at risk are: (i) retropulsion of the damaged vertebra; (ii) facet subluxation; (iii) lateral translation of the vertebrae; and (iv) toppling of one vertebral column over another. Children who display two or more symptoms may have posterior facet dislocation and may require surgical intervention, according to Rajasekaran. He also proposed three categories for how the deformity develops in children: type 1 curves, where the curvature continues to increase until the child reaches skeletal maturity or stops growing, requiring surgery; type 2 curves which show a reduction in the deformity as the child grows; and type 3 curves, which show minimal change in the deformity during both the active and healed phases of the disease.

7.3.1.1.5. Spinal TB in Elderly

With the increase in life expectancy, more elderly patients are being diagnosed with spinal tuberculosis. As this population may have other health issues, such as co-morbidities and compromised health, medication interactions may occur. Elderly people are at a higher risk of dying, receiving the wrong diagnosis, or experiencing drug reactions. Factors that contribute to a higher incidence of spinal tuberculosis include malignancy, diabetes, poor nutrition, immunosuppression, prolonged hospitalization, and other conditions. It is important to be aware of symptoms of disseminated TB, TB meningitis, or other system involvement when evaluating an elderly patient. Low back pain is often disregarded when discussing degenerative conditions in the elderly.

7.3.1.1.6. Atypical Presentations

There are some rare clinical presentations that include pure intraspinal granulomas, isolated abscesses without skeletal involvement, and intervertebral disc prolapses. Additionally, there are some radiographic appearances that are considered atypical, such as concentric vertebral collapse, isolated posterior arch involvement, solitary or circumferential vertebral involvement, isolated meningeal, neural, or perineural involvement without any vertebral destruction, and multifocal osseous lesions.

7.3.1.1.7. Laboratory Diagnosis

Diagnosing spinal tuberculosis can be difficult, even when there is a strong suspicion of the disease. In addition to microbiological and histological markers, clinical and radiographic cues are used to aid diagnosis. However, clinical symptoms are not specific enough and tuberculosis infection test results may be inconsistent. Obtaining enough specimens from the infection sites for testing can also be challenging due to the low levels of bacteria in spinal TB. Despite these challenges, it is important to isolate Mycobacterium from clinical samples for drug susceptibility testing and diagnostic validation. Early diagnosis is important to minimize deformity and neurological damage and improve patient outcomes. Antitubercular drugs can effectively treat spinal TB if it is detected early to avoid surgery. Diagnosis is based on a strong clinical index of suspicion supported by biochemical and radiographic evidence, even with the advancements in technology.

7.3.1.1.8. Microscopy

Acid-fast bacilli (AFB) are a type of bacteria known as mycobacteria. Their cell walls contain high amounts of lipids, which cause them to attach to the fuchsin dye when it comes into contact with acid alcohol. This prevents the dye from leaving the cells, making the bacteria visible under a microscope. AFB microscopy, a history of constitutional TB symptoms, and evidence of pulmonary lesions on chest X-rays are all helpful in the early diagnosis of tuberculosis. Acid-fast smears can also be used to monitor therapeutic response in addition to supporting diagnosis. However, a drawback of smears is that they require at least 10,000 AFB per milliliter of material to be detected, which is usually not the case for paucibacillary illnesses like spinal TB.

Procedures for acid-fast staining consist of the following steps:

Carbol fuchsin stains are composed of phenol (carbolic acid) and fuchsin combined.

Ziehl-Neelsen (ZN, hot stain): The backgrounds in this smear appear bright blue, while the mycobacteria are stained red. The term "hot staining" refers to the use of heat to facilitate the penetration of carbol fuchsin into the bacilli. Subsequently, the smear is decolorized with 20% H_2SO_4 and counterstained with methylene blue. Due to their high lipid content in the cell wall, tubercular bacilli are resistant to the decolorizing ability of H_2SO_4, resulting in them being acid-fast. One advantage of Ziehl-Neelsen staining is that it is a cost-effective, reliable, and reproducible procedure that can also be utilized to evaluate the efficacy of antitubercular therapy. However, this technique has limitations in terms of its low sensitivity and inability to differentiate between different species of Mycobacteria.

Kinyoun staining, also known as "cold stain," requires less heat to penetrate carbol fuchsin due to the larger amount of phenol used in the process, in comparison to ZN staining. Mycobacteria look similar to ZN staining where they appear red against a light blue background. On the other hand, fluorochrome stains such as auramine O or rhodamine use a second fluorochrome and have the advantage of scanning a larger area of the smear than ZN staining. This leads to a shorter time required to scan the smear and increased sensitivity in detecting bacteria.

7.3.1.1.9. Culture

Compared to microscopy, culture techniques are less effective in detecting tubercle bacilli in specimens, with only 10–100/mL being detected. However, culture techniques do offer the advantage of being able to perform drug susceptibility testing and species identification using the isolated bacilli. Therefore, the gold standard for diagnosing tuberculosis is the presence of TB bacilli in culture. The drawback of conventional culture techniques is the time required to find appreciable growth, which can take anywhere from 4 to 8 weeks. The following categories apply to the various culture media that are used to cultivate Mycobacterium TB:

7.3.1.2. Solid Medias

There are different types of media used to grow mycobacteria:

- **Egg-based:** Egg-based media contain ingredients like potato flour, salts, glycerol, whole eggs, or egg yolks. They enable the growth of most mycobacteria and have a long shelf life. The most commonly used egg-based medium is the Lowenstein-Jensen (LJ) medium.
- **Agar-based:** On the other hand, agar-based media have a higher chemical definition than egg-based media. This allows colonies to emerge faster, usually in 10–12 days.
- **Selective Media:** These are designed to allow the growth of Mycobacteria alone by using antibacterial drugs to prevent contaminating germs. They are often used in conjunction with agar or non-selective egg media. Examples of selective media include the Gruft modification, which improves LJ media with penicillin and nalidixic acid, and the Mitchison selective medium, which enhances LJ media with carbenicillin, polymyxin B, trimethoprim, and amphotericin B.

7.3.1.3. Liquid Medias

The Mycobacteria Growth Indicator Tube (MGIT) is a method that uses fluorescence quenching to detect the growth of tubercle bacilli. It has an oxygen sensor that detects the growth of bacilli in a modified Middlebrook 7H9 culture that contains silicon rubber impregnated with ruthenium pentahydrate.

The BACTEC 460 TB system is a semi-automated process that uses 14C-labeled palmitic acid as the medium's carbon source. When bacteria break down the palmitic acid, $^{14}CO_2$ is produced, which the device detects. Bacilli in a smear-positive TB specimen can be found 9–14 days later. However, this approach has several drawbacks such as the inability to detect colony shape, difficulty in identifying mixed cultures, overgrowth of contamination, expensive cost, and hazardous radioactive waste disposal.

7.3.1.3.1. Automated Continuous Monitoring Systems

Automated continuous monitoring systems like the BACTEC 9000 MB system and the MB/BacT ALERT 3D system use different methods to detect the growth of microorganisms. The BACTEC 9000 MB system uses an oxygen sensor based on fluorescence quenching, just like the MGIT system. The MB/BacT ALERT 3D system, on the other hand, uses reflected light and a colorimetric CO_2 sensor in each bottle to monitor the amount and generation of CO_2 dissolved in growth media. As the bacilli grow, they produce CO_2, which dissolves in water and diffuses across the membrane to the sensor. This accumulation of hydrogen ions causes a drop in the pH of the sensor, which changes the color from dark to bright green or yellow.

7.3.1.3.2. Serological Tests

IgM levels, which are proteins produced by the immune system, tend to decrease three months after beginning treatment for tuberculosis (TB). This makes them a useful indicator of TB activity. On the other hand, IgG levels, another type of immune system protein, tend to increase during the same period. This suggests the presence of chronic or cured disorders, but it is not a definitive diagnosis.

To detect TB, doctors use a test called the Interferon Gamma Release Assay. This test measures the amount of interferon (IFN) gamma, a protein produced by the immune system in response to TB infection. One commonly used test is called QuantiFERON-TB Gold, which has an 84% accuracy rate in detecting IFN gamma in patients with spinal TB and vertebral body collapse. Although the Interferon Gamma Release Assay has made it easier to detect TB antibodies, it is still not able to distinguish between latent and active infections, or between extrapulmonary and pulmonary tuberculosis.

7.3.1.3.3. Molecular Testing Methods

Nucleic ACID probes: The method uses ribosomal RNA (rRNA) as the genetic target. This type of RNA is present in cells and culture. A single-stranded DNA probe, labeled with a radioactive (acridine ester), is used to hybridize with the rRNA and form stable DNA-RNA complexes. An instrument measures the amount of light produced by an unhybridized probe after it is deactivated, which is proportional to the amount of probe present. To determine if the sample is positive, a predetermined cutoff is used. The process takes two hours to complete. Another method, called *in situ* hybridization, uses a fluorescence-labeled oligonucleotide probe that is viewed directly through fluorescence microscopy for interpretation. This process is also known as fluorescence *in situ* hybridization (FISH) and is commonly used.

Nucleic acid amplification (NAA) techniques: The PCR (Polymerase Chain Reaction) method is widely used for both diagnostic and research purposes. In order to separate specific DNA sequences using gel electrophoresis, this technique multiplies certain DNA sequences into numerous copies. Synthetic oligonucleotide primers that complement a specific DNA sequence are used to achieve amplification. This technique results in a million-fold amplified target DNA. The IS 6110 repetitive element, which is present in many copies in the majority of *M. tuberculosis* strains, is the most commonly amplified target. The effectiveness of the PCR method for TB depends on the precision and expertise of the technician performing the assay. By using real-time PCR, the amount of *M. tuberculosis* in a clinical sample can be measured and the detection time can be accelerated. A single reaction vessel serves as the central hub for both amplification and detection processes in a closed system. This reduces the possibility of amplicon contamination in the laboratory. This procedure is fully automated, eliminating the need for electrophoresis or post-amplification processing.

The Xpert MTB/RIF Test, developed by Cepheid in Sunnyvale, California, is a fully automated polymerase chain reaction test that can detect tuberculosis (TB) and rifampicin resistance in less than two hours. The test involves mixing tissue samples obtained from a biopsy with lysis reagent and oscillating the mixture between the two. Then, two milliliters are removed and run through the GeneXpert machine, with results available in 90 minutes. The Xpert MTB/RIF test has several benefits, such as detecting rifampicin resistance simultaneously, identifying very small amounts of TB bacilli, and differentiating between typical and atypical mycobacteria. However, it only targets one gene, has no ability to detect mono drug resistance, and cannot identify non-viable pathogens.

Multiplex PCR: An alternative to amplifying a single *M. tuberculosis* gene is the multiplex PCR, which amplifies both the MPB 64 and IS 6110 genes found in mycobacterium. This method has higher sensitivity and specificity in detecting TB and rifampicin resistance. In addition, both genes can be amplified from a single tissue sample, which reduces the cost of the investigation.

7.3.1.3.4. Nanotechnology

Although there have been significant advancements in diagnosing tuberculosis (TB), accurate point-of-care tests for detecting *M. tuberculosis* in children, extrapulmonary TB, or HIV-associated TB are still lacking. The employment of nanotechnology, which uses particles ranging from 1–100 nm, can bridge this gap by providing a quick, efficient, and affordable point-of-care diagnosis. The potential of using various physiological fluids, such as blood, sputum, or urine samples, in nano-diagnostic methods to detect infectious diseases like tuberculosis is highly promising. This method can yield accurate and timely results using inexpensive and portable tools.

Among the nano-diagnostic techniques being explored for TB are:

- **Gold Nanoparticles (NPs):** These can be employed for the diagnosis of tuberculosis (TB). In this technique, DNA probes are combined with gold NPs. When complementary DNA is present in the samples, the nanoprobe solution remains pink at a wavelength of 526 nm. On the other hand, if complementary DNA is missing, the solution turns purple. This method is based on colorimetric detection of *M. tuberculosis* and is highly effective.
- **Dipstick with Gold NPs:** Alkanethiol derivatives were used to coat colloidal gold NPs with the *M. tuberculosis* antigen; this coating produced a pronounced red color when mixed with serum containing antibodies.
- **Indirect Immunofluorescence Microscopy:** It has been developed to detect *M. tuberculosis* using silica NPs linked with fluorescent dye.
- **A Detection System based on Quantum Dots:** It is used to identify the 23S rRNA gene of the mycobacterium. The process involves two probes. The first probe binds correctly to the 23S rRNA gene, while the second probe identifies the conserved sequence IS900 when the mycobacterium is exposed to sulfuric acid and chromium quantum dots. When mycobacterium DNA isolated from tuberculosis patients is hybridized with target gene sequences, a sandwich is formed. The conjugates of quantum dots and magnetic beads are then exposed to ultraviolet light, causing red fluorescence that can be seen with the naked eye.
- **Biosensor Detection:** It involves biosensors that detect short nucleotide sequences of *M. tuberculosis* DNA. There are four types of sensors: electrical, optical, biological, mass/piezoelectric.

7.3.1.3.5. Erythrocyte Sedimentation Rate and C-Reactive Protein (CRP)

The erythrocyte sedimentation rate (ESR), which falls with treatment response in spinal tuberculosis, is frequently more than 20 mm/hour (60–90% sensitivity). Still, it's not an especially sensitive test. ESR has a lower specificity (71% sensitivity) than CRP.

7.3.1.4. Imaging Modalities

7.3.1.4.1. Plain Radiographs

In the early stages of an illness, plain radiographs may not show any abnormalities. A loss of 30% mineral is necessary before the lesions become visible on radiography. Researchers have reported that the average degree of vertebral involvement ranges from 3.4 to 3.8.

Individuals with hemoglobinopathies, diabetes, and immunocompromised conditions may have significant spinal involvement. In 7% of patients, a skipped lesion occurs when two non-contiguous vertebrae are affected without involving neighboring vertebral bodies and intervertebral discs. This may happen due to infection transmission through Batson's plexus of veins (Figure 7.7). The lumbar area is the most frequently affected region, followed by the thoracic spine. The posterior arch is affected more frequently than the vertebral body. Para-discal, anterior, central, neural arch, or appendiceal (pedicles, laminae, spinous processes, or transverse processes) are the four radiographic forms of spinal involvement.

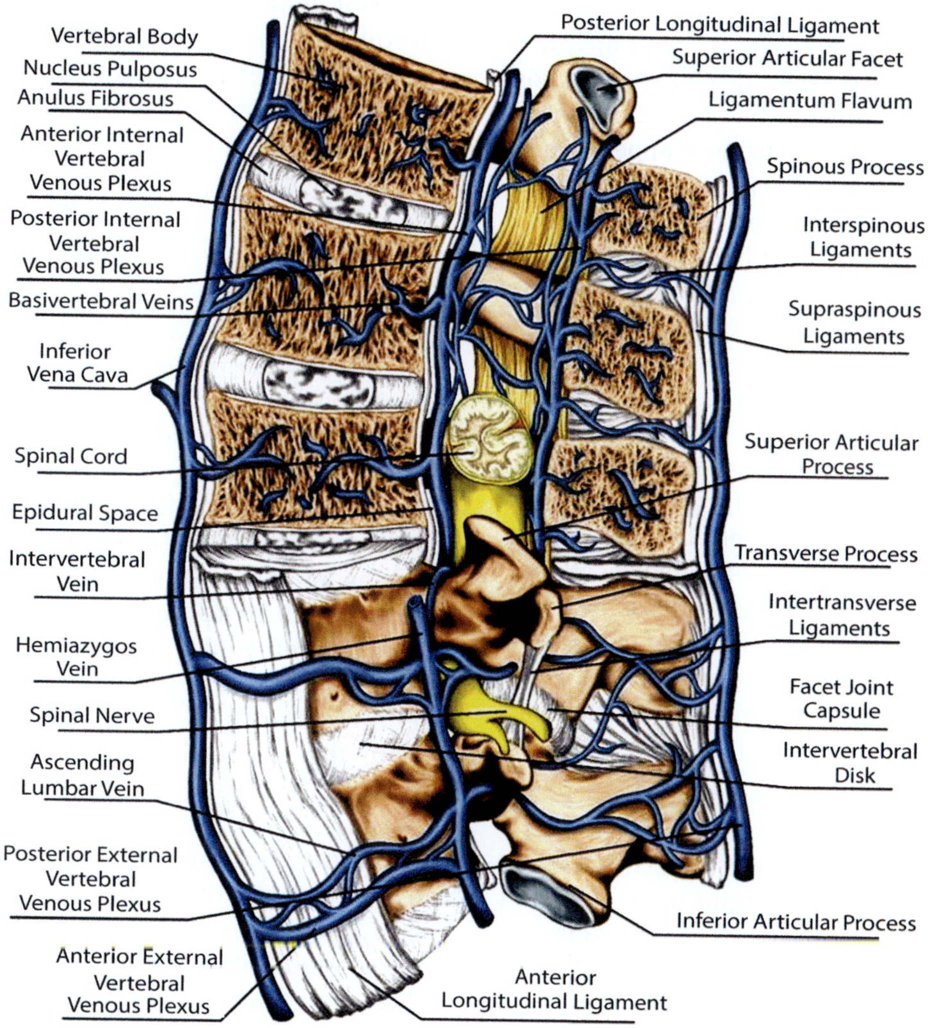

Figure 7.7. *The Batson venous plexus is a network of valveless veins that connect the deep pelvic veins and thoracic veins (which drain the inferior end of the urine bladder, breast, and prostate) to the internal vertebral venous plexuses in the human body.*

Source: Thibault, P. K., (2022). Cerebrospinal venous obstruction: Anatomy, clinical presentation, diagnosis, and treatment of chronic infective cerebrospinal venulitis. IntechOpen. doi: 10.5772/intechopen.102685.

7.3.1.4.2. Para-Discal Type

The most common type of vertebral involvement is when two adjacent vertebrae near the disc space are affected. This suggests that there is a common blood supply in that region. On radiographs, it appears as a reduction in the intervertebral disc space, which is linked to endplate irregularities in the nearby vertebrae. If there is an abscess or tuberculous granulation tissue in the paravertebral region, plain radiographs can reveal their development as soft tissue shadows adjacent to the spine. On a lateral radiograph of the cervical region, it appears as an enhanced prevertebral soft tissue shadow. Larger abscesses may have a broad posterior mediastinal shadow, but those below the T4 spinal level have a characteristic fusiform shape resembling a bird's nest. When an abscess is strained, a globular-shaped shadow may appear. When an abscess travels down the muscle, the psoas shadow enlarges in the lumbar area. In situations where the para-discal bodies have been destroyed over an extended period of time, the spine may angle, and one or both para-discal vertebral bodies may exhibit posterior convexity with wedge collapse. The most common spinal deformity is kyphotic deformity, as it affects the thoracic vertebrae. A significant kyphotic deformity may be the result of multiple involvement of neighboring vertebrae.

7.3.1.4.3. Central Type

The pattern of involvement described above occurs when an infection begins in the center of the vertebral body and spreads through Batson's venous plexus or the branches of the posterior vertebral artery. Eventually, the diseased vertebral body weakens and collapses due to trabecular bone loss caused by the infection. This collapse can occur under axial stress. It is sometimes mistaken for a neoplastic origin because the loss of disc space and paravertebral shadow is less than the para-discal type. However, a longer follow-up may result in a smaller surrounding disc area.

7.3.1.4.4. Anterior Type

This pattern is commonly observed when the disease process initiates directly beneath the periosteum and anterior longitudinal ligament. This results in erosion of the anterior aspect of the vertebral body, which can be seen as uneven cortical borders on lateral radiographs. If the infection spreads beneath the anterior or posterior longitudinal ligaments, it can affect several adjoining vertebrae. When adjacent disc space is lost, vertebral body collapse is usually mild and manifests later.

7.3.1.4.5. Appendiceal Type

The neural arch (pedicles and laminae), transverse processes, and spinous processes are either partially or fully involved in this. Radiographically, these lesions may be suspected when there are indirect signs of involvement, such as paravertebral shadows or erosive alterations with an undamaged disc. It is challenging to observe posterior spinal joint involvement with routine radiography. Additionally, there may be damage to the posterior spinal articulations, which can lead to lateral translation and an unusual deformity. Radiography's primary flaw is that it is insensitive when a disease is first developing. It can be challenging to locate the cervicodorsal and craniovertebral junctions on X-rays, two different locations in the spine. Assessing spinal cord alterations, soft tissue involvement, and the precise location and extent of abscesses is challenging with plain X-rays. Therefore, the emergence of any radiographic indicator could indicate a moderate advancement of the disease process.

7.3.1.4.6. Computed Tomography (CT)

Computed tomography (CT) is a medical imaging technique that provides greater detail on bone irregularities, disruptions, sclerosis, and disc collapse. This technique can reveal findings much earlier than normal radiography. There is documented evidence of fragmentary, osteolytic, sclerotic, and subperiosteal bone disintegration patterns. CT is very helpful in identifying bone fragments in epidural lesions or calcification inside an abscess. It is also critical for assessing paraspinal abscesses more accurately than normal radiography. CT is very useful in giving instructions for percutaneous diagnostic sampling, especially in hard-to-reach places. However, when assessing the impact of the disease on brain structures, magnetic resonance imaging (MRI) performs better than CT.

Radiological evidence of healing in spinal tuberculosis (TB) trails clinical and laboratory findings. Many patients may not show any improvement on X-rays or CT scans even several months after starting combination therapy. This should not be interpreted as a sign that the treatment is not working. However, if images are repeated more than six months after the treatment started and show no improvement, the possibility of an additional lesion or a condition that is resistant to treatment should be considered.

7.3.1.5. Magnetic Resonance Imaging

MRI is considered a superior imaging modality due to its ability to provide enhanced soft tissue contrast and identify abnormalities in the spinal cord, bone marrow, and intervertebral disc. It is the preferred method for a full examination of the tuberculous spine and is particularly useful in diagnosing disorders in challenging areas such as the sacrum, coccyx, neural arch components, sacroiliac joint region, cervicodorsal junction, craniovertebral junction, and vertebral appendages. Standard MRI procedures involve contrast-enhanced T1W sequences following gadolinium contrast injection, as well as fat-suppressed T1W, T2W, and short tau inversion recovery sequences in the axial, sagittal, and coronal planes.

Abnormal marrow signal intensity that appears hypointense on T1W sequences and hyperintense on T2W sequences, exhibiting heterogeneous enhancement and a lack of cortical definition indicates the involvement of the vertebral body. Disc degeneration is common in contiguous vertebral body disease, and a lost normal internuclear cleft, post-contrast enhancement, and increased signal on T2W images are signs of disc involvement. In contrast to pyogenic spondylitis, disc involvement happens later in mycobacterium because it lacks proteolytic enzymes. Severe spinal damage with disc sparing may occasionally result in the "floating disc sign." The disc is more susceptible to infection and is highly hydrated in children.

As the paraspinal collection narrowly breaches the anterior longitudinal ligament in the thoracic region, it may surround the intercostal space, mediastinum, pleural cavity, or even the intercostal arteries themselves. In the lumbar region, the psoas muscle shows uniform signal intensity, increased muscular size, and a loss of typical muscle shape when it is involved. On T2W imaging, the psoas abscess appears as a dense peripheral post-contrast enhancement and high-signal fluid. Although posterior element involvement is more common in TB infections, it is less common than in pyogenic infections. The affected area shows up as a homogeneous amplification and an aberrant signal. While posterior elements are usually found in conjunction with anterior element abnormalities, they can also be affected independently. When a lesion affects both the anterior and posterior components, it is referred to as a composite or panvertebral lesion. Granulomatous lesions within the spinal canal may involve the spinal cord, the epidural/subdural space, or both. An MRI may reveal epidural extension in approximately 61% of affected vertebrae. Pressure applied to the spinal cord from either the front or the back may result in compression myelopathy.

7.3.1.6. Medical Management

7.3.1.6.1. Multidrug Antitubercular Therapy

There are four types of mycobacteria present in the human body. These are – (i) extracellular fast dividing; (ii) extracellular slow dividing; (iii) intracellular intermittently dividing; and (iv) dormant bacilli. Treating tuberculosis (TB) is different from treating other infections as it requires the use of multiple drugs. This is because TB is caused by different types of bacteria that require different types of drugs to be treated effectively. For instance, ethambutol (EMB) is used to kill bacteria inside macrophages, streptomycin kills bacteria that multiply quickly, and rifampicin kills bacteria that grow slowly. Drugs like streptomycin, EMB, and isoniazid are used to kill rapidly multiplying bacteria.

The slow growth rate of mycobacteria is both a blessing and a curse. While it allows for longer treatment duration, it also limits the effectiveness of medication options that act as quick multipliers. Additionally, the limited permeability of intra-macrophage bacilli and mycobacterial cell walls results in low drug permeability. Treating TB, therefore, requires specific drugs that can penetrate bacterial cell walls and macrophages.

It is common knowledge that mycobacteria quickly develop resistance to antibiotics when treated alone. The frequency of isoniazid resistance mutations is 1 in 10^6, while the frequency of rifampicin resistance mutations is 1 in 10^8. Resistance to both drugs is present in 1 in 10^{14} individuals. To prevent the emergence of resistance, a minimum of two drugs are given together during treatment.

The majority of antitubercular drugs, apart from thioacetazone, exhibit a prolonged duration of action referred to as the lag-effect. This characteristic allowed for the intermittent administration of medication, which was crucial for the effectiveness of directly observed therapy.

7.3.1.7. First-Line Drugs

After years of intensive research, only a few drugs have been found to be effective against tuberculosis. The five primary medications used in current anti-tubercular treatments are isoniazid (INH), RIF, EMB, pyrazinamide (PZA), and streptomycin. These medications are the most effective and least toxic, so it is advisable to use them with caution and ensure compliance to prevent the emergence of resistance. Long-term use of multiple medications may increase the risk of various side effects and complications. Therefore, a thorough understanding of drug interactions, side effect profiles, and pharmacokinetics is necessary to ensure safe and effective therapy. It is also important to monitor patients monthly to ensure the treatment is working effectively.

7.3.1.7.1. INH

Isoniazid is a key medication used for the prevention and treatment of tuberculosis. When activated by the catalase-peroxidase KatG, the prodrug INH produces different types of radicals. These radicals bind to nicotinamide adenine dinucleotide (NAD) and form the INH-NAD adduct which inhibits the enoyl-ACP reductase InhA of the fatty acid synthase type II (FASII) pathway. As a result, cell death occurs. INH is particularly effective against mycobacteria that grow quickly and can act on both intracellular and extracellular bacteria. It is also able to cross the blood-brain barrier. However, INH is not effective against stationary-phase mycobacteria, as it can only destroy dividing bacteria.

INH becomes bactericidal after the first one to four days of being bacteriostatic and is not acid-fast. Several genes can cause INH resistance, with mutations in the *katG* gene being the most common reason, followed by mutations in other genes such as *ndh, ahpC, inhA,* and *kasA.* The recommended dosage of INH is 5 mg/kg for adults and 10 mg/kg for children.

There are some side effects of INH, including peripheral neuropathy, lethargy, hepatitis, convulsions, insanity, and a lupus-like condition. However, the risk of peripheral neuropathy can be reduced by taking pyridoxine (10–25 mg/d). INH can also increase the plasma levels of drugs like acetaminophen, benzodiazepines, anticonvulsants, and oral anticoagulants by inhibiting cytochrome P450.

7.3.1.7.2. RIF

Rifampicin is a derivative of rifamycin that binds to the β-subunit of RNA polymerase to prevent messenger RNA elongation. It has a sterilizing effect on bacteria that have irregular metabolisms, and works both intracellularly and extracellularly to suppress bacteria that multiply swiftly but metabolize slowly.

It is recommended that adults take 10 mg/kg and children take 15–20 mg/kg. However, due to the potential for liver damage associated with high dosages, the daily maximum dose should not exceed 600 mg.

Some of the side effects associated with rifampicin include hemolytic anemia, gastrointestinal distress, purpura, and orange-red urine stains. Rifampicin induces cytochrome P450, which means that dose adjustments are necessary for other drugs that are metabolized in the liver, including non-nucleoside reverse transcriptase inhibitors, oral hypoglycemics, anticonvulsants, antifungals, protease inhibitors, and cardiac therapies.

The most common cause of rifampicin resistance is a mutation in the 81-bp *rpo*B gene (codons 507–533), which codes for RNA polymerase's β-subunit.

7.3.1.7.3. PZA

PZA is a prodrug that needs to be converted into its active form, pyrazinoic acid, by an enzyme called amidase. This enzyme is produced by the pncA gene. PZA is believed to inhibit the production of coenzyme A, membrane transport, and trans-translation, which are all necessary for bacterial growth. PZA is particularly effective in combating non-replicating persisters in an acidic and inflammatory environment. It is most effective in the first two months of treatment when acute inflammatory changes are still noticeable. PZA is crucial in reducing the duration of chemotherapy and has a strong sterilizing effect. The dosage for children is 35 mg/kg, and for adults, it is 25 mg/kg. However, PZA has some known adverse effects, including pruritis, exanthema, hyperuricemic arthralgia, and hepatotoxicity. Patients with gout on cyclosporine require dosage modifications. In *M. tuberculosis*, resistance to PZA is mainly caused by mutations in the *Pnc*A gene's 561 bp open reading frame or an 82 bp putative promoter region.

7.3.1.7.4. EMB

Ethambutol (EMB) is a medication that works by inhibiting the production of arabinogalactan in mycobacteria. It does this by blocking the activity of the enzyme arabinosyltransferases. However, it is only effective against bacteria that are actively growing and reproducing. It is considered a bacteriostatic medication. In addition to its effects on arabinogalactan biosynthesis, EMB also disrupts RNA synthesis and can affect glycerol metabolism. The recommended dosage for adults is 15 mg/kg, while children should take 15–25 mg/kg.

EMB can have some significant side effects, including retrobulbar neuritis, which is dose-dependent. This condition affects the nerves that supply the eye, resulting in a loss of visual acuity, scotomas (blind spots), and difficulty distinguishing between red and green colors. However, if the medication is stopped early, these effects can be reversed. Other side effects of EMB include myocarditis, eosinophilia, peripheral neuritis, abdominal discomfort, and hypersensitivity. Children should not take this medication because it can be challenging to measure visual acuity accurately in young children. Patients with low creatinine clearance (30 mL/min) may require dosage adjustments.

Finally, it's worth noting that one of the most common causes of resistance to EMB is a specific mutation in the *emb*B gene, which codes for arabinosyltransferases. This mutation is found in codon 306.

7.3.1.7.5. Streptomycin

Streptomycin is an aminocyclitol glycoside produced by *Streptomyces griseus.* It is highly effective against actively proliferating bacilli in cavities when injected intramuscularly. It inhibits the translation of ribosomal proteins S12 and 16S rRNA, encoded by the genes *rps*L and *rrs*, respectively, and acts best at an alkaline pH. For adults, the recommended dosage is 15 mg/kg, while children should take 15–25 mg/kg. Possible side effects include rashes, eosinophilia, fever, ototoxicity, vestibulotoxicity, and nephrotoxicity. Streptomycin resistance is commonly caused by a lysine to arginine substitution in codon 43 of *rps*L. Streptomycin should not be used during pregnancy because it can cross the placenta and damage the developing fetus's kidneys and ears. Other first-line drugs are safe to use while pregnant. Children have different pharmacokinetics than adults, requiring larger dosages based on body weight due to their faster metabolism and significantly lower blood concentrations.

Table 7.4 summarizes the dose, pharmacological activities, and side effects of the first-line anti-tubercular medications.

Table 7.4. *The First-Line Anti-Tubercular Medications' Dose, Pharmacological Activities, and Side Effects*

Anti-Tuberculosis Drugs	Dose (mg/kg)	Pharmacological Activities	Side Effects
Isoniazid	5	☐ Inhibits the enoyl-ACP reductase *Inh*A of the fatty acid synthase type II (FASII) pathway.	☐ Peripheral neuropathy, lethargy, hepatitis, insanity, convulsions, and a lupus-like condition.
Rifampicin	10	☐ Inhibits messenger RNA elongation by binding to the β-subunit of the RNA polymerase.	☐ Hemolytic anemia, gastrointestinal distress, purpura, and orange-red urine stains.

Ethambutol	15	Inhibits enzyme arabinosyltransferases, glycerol metabolism, and RNA synthesis.	Abdominal discomfort, eosinophilia, peripheral neuritis, myocarditis, and hypersensitivity.
Pyrazinamide	25	Disrupts membrane energetics and inhibits membrane transport function.	Hepatotoxicity, pruritis, hyperuricemic arthralgia, and exanthema.
Streptomycin	15	Binds to the small 16S rRNA of the 30S ribosomal subunit irreversibly, interfering with the binding of formylmethionyl-tRNA to the 30S subunit.	Ototoxicity, rashes, fever, nephrotoxicity, eosinophilia, and vestibulotoxicity.

Source: Wattana, L., Pathomthep, L., & Tawithep, L., (2023). The article "Tuberculosis of the spine" was published in World J. Orthop. You can find it at: doi: 10.5312/wjo.v14.i5.275.

7.3.1.8. Second-Line Drugs

Antibiotic resistance has become a concern, and as a result, second-line treatments are frequently used. However, these treatments are more expensive, more toxic, and less effective compared to first-line treatments. The most commonly used second-line drugs are fluoroquinolones, injectable aminoglycosides, ethionamide, and cycloserine.

7.3.1.8.1. Fluoroquinolones

Antibiotics known as fluoroquinolones (FQs) have a broad spectrum of action against TB bacteria *in vivo* and *in vitro*. They have a bactericidal effect and work by inhibiting DNA synthesis. Commonly used fluoroquinolones include moxifloxacin, levofloxacin, ofloxacin, and ciprofloxacin. A 400–600 mg daily dose is advised. It is rare to experience side effects like headaches, nausea, rashes, and lightheadedness. The most common pathway for drug resistance is a mutation in DNA gyrase, the biological target of FQs.

7.3.1.8.2. Aminoglycosides

Injectable aminoglycosides, such as Amikacin (AMK), Kanamycin (KAN), and Capreomycin (CAP), are important for treating multidrug-resistant tuberculosis. These medications are made of streptomyces and have bactericidal properties. While CAP attaches to the 70S ribosome to inhibit mRNA-tRNA translocation, AMK and KAN work by blocking protein translation. All three medications are taken once daily at a dose of 15 mg/kg. However, it is important to monitor renal function and hearing regularly due to their side effects, including ototoxicity, renal toxicity, and electrolyte abnormalities. Resistance to AMK and KAN is often linked to changes in the 16S rRNA, and cross-resistance between the two medications is common. CAP resistance is associated with *Tly*A mutations, which can increase the risk of treatment failure and death.

7.3.1.8.3. Cycloserine

Cyclorine is a type of bacteriostatic medication that is made from *Streptomyces orchidaceus*. This medication works by inhibiting the formation of mycobacterial cell walls. Due to its ability to penetrate bone and reach comparable levels to plasma, it is commonly used in the treatment of osteoarticular tuberculosis. The recommended dosage is one gram administered once per day. However, it's important to note that this medication may cause seizures, headaches, and psychosis, so it's not recommended for use by individuals with mental illnesses or renal insufficiency. Nonetheless, Cyclorine is effective in treating both MDR and extremely drug-resistant (XDR) tuberculosis, as it has high stomach tolerance and low drug interactions.

7.3.1.8.4. Ethionamide/Prothionamide

Protionamide and ethionamide are bacteriostatics that are made with iso-nicotinic acid. The way it works is comparable to that of INH in that it prevents the synthesis of mycolic acid by inhibiting InhA. The drug is taken once daily in a dosage of one gram. Among the side effects are depression, hepatitis, peripheral neuropathy, hypothyroidism, and severe gastrointestinal intolerance. The two drugs have a great deal of cross-resistance.

7.3.1.8.5. Para-Aminosalicylic Acid

Para-aminosalicylic acid (PAS) was one of the first drugs developed for the treatment of tuberculosis. However, it was discontinued due to rapid development of resistance and gastrointestinal intolerance. Some of the known side effects of using this drug include hypersensitivity, hepatic dysfunction, and hypothyroidism. The recommended dosage for PAS is 12 grams, which can be taken all at once or divided into two doses.

7.3.1.9. Novel Drugs

In light of the increasing rate of treatment failure in *M. tuberculosis*, there is an urgent need for innovative drugs that target new receptors, have higher efficacy, fewer drug interactions, and a lower toxicity profile.

7.3.1.9.1. Delamanid

The prodrug delamanid is a dihydro-nitroimidazo-oxazole derivative that, when activated by the enzyme deazaflavin-dependent nitroreductase (Rv3547), inhibits the formation of components of mycobacterial cell walls. QT prolongation, headache, nausea, and dizziness are all adverse effects. With the least amount of toxicity and no significant drug interactions with other anti-TB medications, the safety profile is good. WHO advises against using the medication except in longer-term MDR regimens when no other effective treatment can be found due to the inconsistent results of effectiveness trials.

7.3.1.9.2. Bedaquiline

In 2012, a new medication called bedaquiline was introduced to treat tuberculosis. It works by binding to a component of the mycobacterial ATP synthase to prevent it from functioning. It is recommended for patients with MDR and XDR-TB, just like other second-line treatments. Compared to other anti-TB drugs, bedaquiline is less likely to cause cross-resistance due to its unique mode of action. Some of the side effects that have been reported include hepatic transaminase elevation, nausea, arthralgia, headaches, hemoptysis, chest pain, anorexia, and rashes. It should not be used with other medications that prolong the QT interval due to the main side effect, which is QT prolongation. Mutations affecting the *rv0678* gene, which encodes the MmpL5 efflux pump repressor, have been associated with cross-resistance to clofazimine and low-level bedaquiline resistance.

7.3.1.10. Surgical Management

When it comes to treating spinal tuberculosis, chemotherapy is the primary form of treatment. Long-term antitubercular chemotherapy is an essential aspect of treating spinal tuberculosis. The decision to have surgery for spinal tuberculosis is controversial, as there is no clear agreement on when it is necessary. However, in some cases, surgery may be necessary to prevent and treat complications from spinal tuberculosis, such as cold abscess, deformity, and neurological issues. Recent studies have demonstrated that antitubercular therapy and excisional treatment are equally effective. However, excisional treatment alone may result in anterior column deficiency, deformity, and delayed neurological damage.

The following circumstances warrant surgical intervention:

- **Progressive Neurological Deficit:** Early surgical decompression is crucial in reducing morbidity and improving quality of life for patients with a progressive neurological deficit.
- **Progressive Spinal Deformity:** When it comes to progressive spinal deformity, it is important to note that if the lumbar spine is compensating, then more kyphosis in the thoracic spine may be tolerated. However, if there is an excessive loss of lordosis in the lumbar spine, it is not acceptable. In cases where there is a 60° kyphosis, it should be surgically corrected because it can impair circulation and result in paraplegia.
- **Failure of Conservative Treatment:** Any increase in discomfort or neurological deficit after 3–4 weeks of chemotherapy, whether or not a brace or bed rest is required, should be treated surgically as a therapeutic failure.
- **Uncertain Diagnosis:** In cases where there is no abscess on the surface or percutaneous biopsy samples are insufficient or unavailable, it can be challenging to diagnose or determine medication sensitivity. In such situations, surgery may be required to obtain adequate tissue samples.

7.3.1.11. End Point of Pharmalogical Treatment

One of the major issues with spinal tuberculosis is the absence of clear criteria for determining the status of healing. This makes it difficult to determine when to stop taking anti-tubercular drugs. Unlike pulmonary tuberculosis, where repeated biopsies and culture conversion are the gold standard, these methods are not practical for spinal tuberculosis due to their invasive and time-consuming nature, and low yield because of the paucibacillary nature of the TB spine. Additionally, there is no universally accepted technique for predicting clinical outcomes or calculating the entire body burden of *M. tuberculosis*. Therefore, a combination of radiographic evaluation, laboratory markers, and clinical improvement are still considered valid measures for determining the healing status of spinal tuberculosis.

7.3.1.11.1. Clinical Improvement

Pain: While the majority of spinal tuberculosis patients who are making a full recovery report that their pain has decreased, this is not an absolute indicator because back pain can have multiple etiologies.

More importantly, healing can occur in the absence of a strong bony fusion, which can lead to ongoing pain from spinal instability even after the disease has recovered. Furthermore, there is not yet a reliable metric to gauge pain intensity.

- **Deformity:** Spinal deformity typically worsens or persists as the disease progresses.
- **Neurology:** In some cases, chronic bone compression may cause persistent neurologic dysfunction, even though the patient's neurology may improve when the soft tissue that is compressing the neural components is reduced.

7.3.1.11.2. Laboratory Improvement

- **ESR:** It is commonly elevated and is used to monitor patients' response to treatment. If normalcy does not return after therapy, concerns about primary medication resistance or alternative causation should be raised.
- **CRP:** Patients with spinal tuberculosis (TB) have been found to have up to 75% higher levels of CRP. This protein primarily targets inflammatory and viral lesions. Unlike erythrocyte sedimentation rate (ESR) which takes around 4 weeks to detect a change, CRP takes only about 2 weeks to detect a change. Therefore, CRP is more relevant for tracking therapy response.

7.3.1.11.3. Imaging Improvement

MRI – to assess whether spinal TB has healed, several established standards are used. Magnetic resonance imaging (MRI) is one of them. However, even after the infection has been fully cleared, soft tissues and sterile abscesses may still be visible on an MRI. MRI often lags behind clinical recovery by up to 3 mo.

When MRI is relied upon as the sole diagnostic tool to determine the severity of an active disease, it may be overly sensitive. The emergence of new lesions during treatment, worsening of pre-existing lesions, marrow swelling, and fresh bone damage or abscesses are indications of poor disease management, particularly when accompanied by a decline in clinical status.

7.3.1.12. Prognosis

Positive prognostic factors have been reported to include younger age and earlier diagnosis. The clinical outcome is influenced by the degree of spinal degeneration (instability, deformity, abnormalities) and the severity of the disease (number of damaged vertebrae). When paraplegic symptoms are present at the time of diagnosis, the prognosis is poor. Other risk factors include poverty, malnutrition, and immunodeficiency (HIV, drug addiction, and alcoholism).

Prompt diagnosis and treatment improve the prognosis for tuberculosis of the spine. A high level of clinical suspicion should be applied to people who seem to have persistent back pain, even in the absence of neurological symptoms and indicators. Treatment with medicine is usually successful. Molecular techniques for diagnosing spinal TB and drug resistance should be used to detect MDR/XDR TB, which is on the rise. Surgical intervention is necessary in advanced cases involving significant bone involvement, the development of an abscess, or paraplegia. Since spinal TB can affect young people, effective prevention measures need to be implemented. Stopping the disease's spread is the only way to prevent spinal TB.

7.3.2. Tuberculosis of the Hip

Hip joint tuberculosis accounts for 15% of all cases of skeletal tuberculosis, making it the second most common site after the spine. Hip tuberculosis is the term used to describe tuberculosis that has spread from the lungs to the hips in an individual.

The initial infection may start in the:

- Acetabular roof (most common);
- Epiphysis;
- Metaphysis;
- Greater trochanter (least common).

7.3.2.1. Causes of Hip Tuberculosis

When tuberculosis infection spreads from the lungs to the hip area, it results in hip tuberculosis. The spread of tuberculosis to other organs is facilitated by blood vessels, where it usually affects the lungs first. While lung tuberculosis can be transmitted through the exchange of bodily fluids, such as blood, hip tuberculosis cannot be transmitted from person to person. Malnutrition, unsanitary living conditions, slum housing, and environmental factors are some of the factors that contribute to the development of tuberculosis.

7.3.2.2. Symptoms of Hip Tuberculosis

- Most affected children are between 5 and 15 years of age.
- A painful limb is the most common and earliest symptom.
- The patient starts to walk with a limp. The patient puts a little pressure over the affected side of the hip and walks with an antalgic gait.
- The patients start to feel excessive pain in their hips, especially during nighttime.
- Additionally, deformity, stiffness, shortening, and fullness around the hips can also be experienced by the patients.
- Other symptoms like fever, weight loss, and loss of appetite can be seen.
- On examination, tenderness may be present and the joints may be elicited down from their original position.

7.3.2.3. Stages of Hip Tuberculosis

- **Stage 1 (Stage of Tubercular Synovitis):** It is possible that the effusion in the hip joint may cause pain and swelling. The hip needs to be positioned in its maximum configuration, which involves maximum external rotation, flexion, and abduction.
- **Stage 2 (Stage of Early Arthritis):** As hip tuberculosis worsens; the articular cartilage deteriorates and eventually disappears. This can lead to deformities in flexion, adduction, and internal rotation due to abrupt movement of the flexors. It is highly recommended to shorten the distance between the joints after diagnosis since the damaged cartilage results in less than 1 centimeter of space.
- **Stage 3 (Stage of Late Arthritis):** As damage to the joint increases, the affected limbs may begin to shorten or shrink. This can lead to limitations in movement. In addition, the cartilage, acetabulum, and head of the joint may become damaged or destroyed. An X-ray can reveal if there is complete loss of joint space,

as well as damage to the head or acetabulum. If the shortening of the limb is more than 1 cm, it is considered to be a significant and genuine shortening.

- **Stage 4 (Late Arthritis with Dislocation):** The upper portion of the thigh bone may move upward and backward, causing the lower portion of the hip socket to be left empty. This happens when the hip socket, the ball of the thigh bone, and the connecting ligaments are destroyed. This can also lead to the ball of the thigh bone breaking off and getting dislocated.

7.3.2.4. Diagnosis of Hip Tuberculosis

To determine the type and stage of hip tuberculosis, the doctor may recommend certain diagnostic tests that are designed differently for adults and children.

7.3.2.4.1. In Children

Perthes disease is most commonly found in children between the ages of 4 and 8. The children may display typical signs such as a painful limp and restricted range of motion. During clinical examination, they may exhibit restricted abduction and internal rotation, with their entire range of motion being painful. The femoral head and acetabulum are found to have been destroyed on the children's MRI. In cases of low-grade septic arthritis, pus may be observed along with other symptoms in hip tuberculosis.

7.3.2.4.2. In Adults

Osteoarthritis: The X-ray may reveal sclerosis and consistent constriction of the hip joint space may indicate rheumatoid arthritis, a rare form of arthritis that affects a single joint.

7.3.2.5. Treatment of Hip Tuberculosis

In cases where an individual is experiencing severe hip pain accompanied by symptoms such as fever, weight loss, and reduced appetite, hip tuberculosis is considered to be active. Upon examination, the hip may appear tender, the range of motion could be painful, and the local temperature may have increased. Patients in such cases are typically given the following therapies:

- **Nonoperative Treatment:** Upon admission, patients will receive antitubercular therapy (ATT). Skeletal or skin traction is used to rest the injured hip, which helps prevent or correct the deformity, eases pain and spasms, and keeps the hip from dislocating. Once the patient begins to feel less pain, certain exercises may be recommended.
- **Operative Treatment:** The damaged bone or tissue is removed if conservative therapy is unsuccessful. This involves opening the joint, removing pus, injured tissue, swollen synovium, and other decomposing tissues.

7.3.2.6. Prognosis

The outlook for hip TB can be good if treatment is received promptly and appropriately. Delays in diagnosis and treatment, however, can result in permanent complications, severe joint destruction, and disability.

7.3.2.7. Prevention

General TB prevention strategies, including the BCG vaccination, infection control, and the early detection and treatment of active TB cases in the community, can prevent TB. The difficult ailment known as TB-x can significantly lower a person's quality of life. To avoid long-term joint damage and complications, prompt diagnosis and treatment are crucial.

7.3.3. Tuberculosis of the Knee

After the hip and spine, the knee is the third most common location for skeletal tuberculosis. Best knee tuberculosis is a term for tuberculosis that originates in the lungs and spreads to the knee through blood vessels. Patients who are commonly impacted are typically older children and young adults.

The origin of TB in the knee can be:

- Synovial;
- On the bone articular surface of the patella, femur, and tibia;
- On the bone non-articular parts of the tibia and femur.

The majority of TB knee cases begin as synovial and often stay that way for a considerable amount of time. The joint space was subsequently reduced as the infection moved to the cartilage.

7.3.3.1. Causes of Knee Tuberculosis

When tuberculosis infection spreads from the lungs to the knee area, it results in knee tuberculosis. Tuberculosis can spread from the lungs to other organs through blood vessels, and it first affects the lungs. While lung tuberculosis can be transmitted through the exchange of bodily fluids such as blood, knee tuberculosis cannot spread from one person to another because it affects different organs. Malnourishment, unsanitary living conditions, slum housing, and environmental factors are some of the factors that contribute to tuberculosis.

7.3.3.2. Symptoms of Knee Tuberculosis

- The majority of patients typically arrive with chronic knee pain, stiffness, and swelling.
- Sinuses can manifest as healing little folds of skin or as discharging.
- Pain in flexion and extension may be experienced by patients.
- Examining the area around the patella may reveal a doughy thickening.
- An MRI may reveal soft tissue swelling in the knee area three to four weeks after the infection.

7.3.3.3. Diagnosis of Knee Tuberculosis

- **X-Ray:** These initially reveal articular erosions and a decrease in joint space. In late cases, the knee deformity is complete.
- **MRI:** It is essential when X-ray results are inconclusive, as it can show pus collection, synovial thickening, and bone deformities.
- **Biopsy:** Generally speaking, an arthroscopic biopsy is recommended. The rice bodies within the joints are readily visible thanks to an arthroscopic biopsy.

7.3.3.4. Treatment of Knee Tuberculosis

The same treatment is used for tuberculosis in the hip and knee. When there is severe hip pain accompanied by fever, weight loss, and loss of appetite, it is considered an active case of tuberculosis in the knee. Upon examination, the knee will be tender, range of motion will be painful, and the local temperature will have increased. The procedure used to treat tuberculosis in the knee is as follows:

- Anti-tubercular therapy (ATT) is started in all patients. Double traction can be used to reduce knee deformity.
- Once the deformity decreases and the injury begins to heal, traction is stopped and a plaster cast is applied to allow gradual return of range of motion as the injury continues to heal.
- After 18 to 24 months, patients can begin walking without assistance, though they may still use walkers or crutches during this time.

7.3.4. Tuberculosis of the Ankle and the Foot

Rarely, the infection can present in synovial or bony structures such as the lower tibia and talus calcaneum. Other commonly affected bones include the talus and calcaneum. The infection can spread to the ankle joint from calcaneal tuberculosis after involving the subtalar joint. Diagnosis and treatment methods align with previously discussed general principles.

7.3.5. Tuberculosis of the Shoulder and Elbow

Shoulder tuberculosis of the synovial type is an extremely rare condition that can cause the development of a draining sinus and a cold abscess. The dry form of tuberculosis that affects the shoulder is known as "caries sicca." This condition is believed to be an atrophic form of tuberculosis and is often seen in adults. Symptoms include pain, restricted mobility, and noticeable muscle atrophy, as well as visible radiological degradation of the cavities and articular surfaces. Treatment follows the broad guidelines previously covered. When it comes to elbow tuberculosis, the infection primarily affects the bone, occasionally the synovium. This condition typically affects adults and older children, presenting similar symptoms to other cases of bone and joint tuberculosis. Diagnosis and treatment follow general principles.

7.3.6. Tuberculosis of the Wrist

Tuberculosis of the bone and joint is a condition that frequently occurs in adults but is not very common. It usually begins as a focus in the bone or synovial tissue, with the lower end of the radius and the capitate being the most commonly affected sites. It spreads rapidly to surrounding structures, including the extensor and flexor tendon sheaths. The signs and symptoms of bone and joint tuberculosis are similar to other cases of tuberculosis. Therefore, the general principles are followed for diagnosis and treatment of the condition.

7.3.6.1. Spina Ventosa

Spina, which means short bones, and ventosa, which means air, combine to create the meaning of a short bone filled with air, also known as tuberculous dactylitis. This condition is commonly seen in children and affects short tubular bones such as the metacarpals, metatarsals, and phalanges. The blood supply to these bones is rich, with the nutrient artery entering at the center, where the focus of infection occurs. Initial central destruction gives the appearance of a bone filled with air, followed by layers of new bone formation around the lesion, resulting in a spindle-shaped expansile lesion. Sinus formation can lead to secondary infection, but appropriate treatment with antibiotics and anti-tuberculosis therapy can lead to complete resolution.

7.3.7. Mycotic Infections of the Bone

Fungal bone infections are categorized as either superficial or deep.

- **Superficial Mycoses:** Begin with infection of the skin and mucous membrane as the initial site, then proceed to infect nearby soft tissue and bone. Examples include *Maduramycosis*, *Candida*, and others.

- **Deep Mycoses:** Bone infections typically do not affect healthy individuals but can impact those with weakened immune systems, such as those from *Aspergillus*, *Cryptococcus*, and *Blastomyces*.

7.3.8. Maduramycosis

Maduromycosis was first identified in Madura, India, between 1842 and 1846. It is mostly found in the tropics and affects the feet due to a penetrating trauma infection caused by soil and thorns. People who work outdoors, come into contact with dirt, or participate in outdoor activities regularly are more vulnerable to getting infected. Human-to-human transmission instances have also been reported. Various types of organisms, such as actinomycetes, which are false fungi, and eumycetes, or true fungi, can produce mycetoma. *Petriellidum boydii* is the organism that typically causes maduromycosis in North America, *Madurella mycetomi* in Africa and India, *Nocardia brasiliensis* in Mexico, and *Nocardia asteroides* in Japan. In the US, maduromycosis is rare (Figure 7.8).

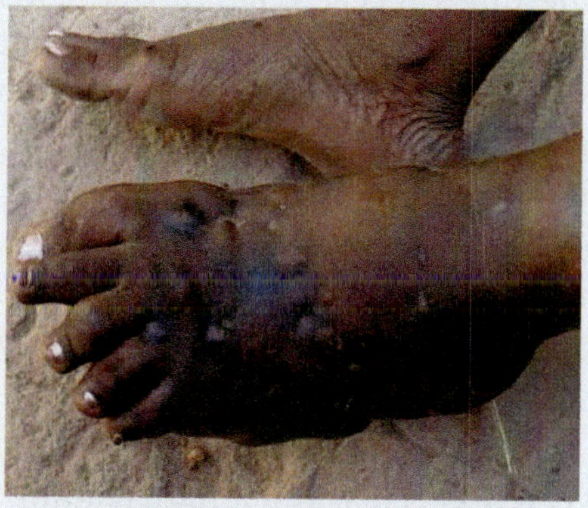

Figure 7.8. *Madura foot.*

Source: By Mohammad (2018) – Own work, CC BY-SA 4.0, https://commons.wikimedia.org/w/index.php?curid=65398084.

7.3.8.1. Pathogenesis

Mycetoma is a condition that is more commonly found in adult men than women, especially those who work in agriculture. However, it can occur in individuals from other professions as well. The condition is caused by organisms that are transmitted through penetrating injuries such as thorn punctures. These organisms can be found in plants, plant residues, and soil. While fungi are responsible for most cases of mycetoma, *Nocardia* species have been found in soil. The organisms have developed various strategies to survive in the human body, such as producing melanin, thickening the cell wall, and immunomodulation, which allow them to evade the immune system.

7.3.8.2. Clinical Features

The early sign of mycetoma is small swelling on the skin, which gradually grows larger over time. Sinuses may also appear on the surface of the nodule. Pain may be felt on the skin before the sinus ruptures. In the early stages, the sinuses may heal. In well-established lesions, there are persistently discharging sinuses, significant woody swelling, and deformity. The hands, lower legs, and feet are the primary areas affected, although some infections can become widespread and spread over a limb. Dissemination is uncommon, except in cases where it involves the skull, which can be life-threatening.

Radiological findings may show cortical thinning or hypertrophy, periosteal proliferation, and lytic lesions. Magnetic resonance imaging (MRI) is the most precise method for determining the size and scope of these lesions.

7.3.8.3. Differential Diagnosis

- Osteomyelitis caused by bacteria or actinomycosis;
- Botryomycosis;

- Chromoblastomycosis;
- Sporotrichosis.

7.3.8.4. Laboratory Diagnosis

The grains are typically obtained by using a sterile needle to open a sinus where a small amount of pus is present beneath the skin's surface. The grains are typically visible to the unaided eye in the pus and blood emerging from the sinus tract. Microscopy can be done directly. Grains are immersed in a solution of 5–10% potassium hydroxide (KOH) and they get a light squeeze. If the filaments are visible through an ×40 objective, a fungus is the cause. Nevertheless, if these are not apparent, an actinomycete is probably the cause. Actinomycetes under a microscope have long chains of spores, a profusion of aerial mycelium, and branching filaments as typical characteristics. After formalin fixation, grains can be extracted straight from the sinuses for histology and embedded. Haematoxylin and eosin-stained sections typically show a variety of grains, so using specific fungal stains like periodic acid Schiff or methenamine silver is not strictly necessary.

The ZN staining technique is superior in discriminating between actinomycotic agents. *Nocardia* spp. are ZN positive, whereas *A. madurae* and *S. somaliensis* are ZN negative. Actinomycetes or fungi can be grown on a range of media and have typical appearances when cultivated; however, their identification requires a specialized laboratory. The commonly recommended media are blood agar, brain-heart infusion agar, Löwenstein agar, and Sabouraud agar supplemented with 0.5% yeast extract.

If this method is not successful in obtaining grains, a wide and deep biopsy is required, and the specimen is sent for histology and culture. Separating fungal and actinomycete causes is a primary goal of laboratory diagnosis since each cause requires a different course of treatment.

7.3.8.5. Management

The treatment of mycetoma depends on the identification of the causative agent, whether caused by an actinomycete or a fungus. Antibiotics like sulfonamides, sulfones, or co-trimoxazole are used to treat actinomycetes. Additional drugs such as rifampicin or streptomycin may be used in combination for better results, with alternatives like AMK, ciprofloxacin, and imipenem used for more challenging cases. The treatment may last for several weeks. However, eumycetomas are more challenging to treat, with only around 40%–50% of *Madurella mycetomatis* infections responding to antifungal medications like ketoconazole, itraconazole, or voriconazole. Therapy may need to continue for over a year. In severe and debilitating cases, surgery, particularly amputation, may be necessary.

7.3.9. Parasitic Infestation of Bone

7.3.9.1. Hydatid Cysts in the Bone

The dog tapeworm, *Echinococcus granulosus*, is responsible for the formation of hydatid cysts in the bones. It measures 5 mm in length and has 3 segments. Dogs are the definitive hosts for this tapeworm, as it resides in their intestines. The tapeworm's segments, called scolices, are passed out in the dog's feces. When a dog consumes infected meat, the tapeworm life cycle continues and new generations of tapeworms develop. Man, sheep, and cattle are intermediate hosts and can become infested by ingesting food that has been contaminated with dog feces. When the scolices are ingested, they hatch into larvae and enter the bloodstream through the portal system. These larvae may then become lodged in the bones, particularly affecting the pelvis, vertebrae, ribs, and femur, leading to the formation of hydatid cysts.

The cysts gradually destroy the affected bones, with the growth plate unable to prevent the destruction. The destruction may even reach the epiphysis. Cystic lesions can appear either as solitary or multiloculated and can cause extensive damage to the cortex and medulla. If the spine is affected, the patient may experience neurological symptoms. Paraskeletal cysts can be diagnosed through CT and MRI scans. Confirmatory tests include needle biopsy and Casoni's complement fixation test. Treatment with albendazole is recommended, to be administered every four weeks for a minimum of 6–8 weeks. Precautions may be necessary to prevent fractures. Surgical removal and bone grafting may be required for persistent cysts. Hypertonic saline can be used to irrigate the cavity to help prevent recurrences.

A Closer Look

Chemical Composition and Physical Properties of Bones

In most higher animals, bone cells make up only 5% of the volume of mature bone. The nonliving intercellular material of bone is composed of inorganic mineral components in the form of rod-shaped crystals, and small amounts of protein polysaccharides, glycoaminoglycans that are chemically bound to protein and distributed within and around the collagen fiber bundles. Collagen is an organic component of bone that is arranged in long strands or bundles. Many of these crystals lie in voids within the collagen bundles themselves, and they are arranged parallel to the long axes of the bundles. The intercellular composite is composed of 50% organic material and 30% dry weight, with minerals making up the remaining portion. The two main minerals found in the intercellular composite are phosphate and calcium. When first deposited, the mineral is amorphous in crystal structure, but matures and takes on characteristics of other apatite minerals, with hydroxyapatite as the main constituent. Carbonate exists in two different phases, calcium carbonate and a carbonate apatite, and ranges from 4% of bone ash in fish to 8% in most mammals and over 13% in turtles. There is little free water (about 8% of total volume) in adult mammalian bone, and diffusion from surfaces into the intercellular substance occurs at sluggish rates typical of diffusion from solid surfaces rather than within liquids.

The hardness, rigidity, and compressive strength of bone is contributed by mineral crystals, but they are weak in tension due to defects that can lead to breakage. In contrast, collagen fibrils in bone are highly elastic and possess significant tensile strength, but have low compressive strength. The combination of minerals and collagen fibrils gives bone overall tensile strength, allowing it to exhibit properties found in two-phase materials like fiberglass and bamboo. By dispersing a rigid, brittle material within a flexible matrix, stress failure is prevented in the brittle material, enabling bone to approach the maximum strength of single crystals.

Determining the true strength of the mineral-matrix composite at the "unit" structural level has been difficult due to the fine structure of bone. However, cortical bone specimens have been found to have a tensile strength in the range of 700–1,400 kg per square cm (10,000–20,000 pounds per square inch) and compressive strengths in the range of 1,400–2,100 kg per square cm (20,000–30,000 pounds per square inch). These values are similar to those of aluminum or mild steel, but bone has an advantage over such materials in that it is considerably lighter. The strength of bone is greatest along its long axis and is roughly parallel to both the collagen fiber axis and to the long axis of the mineral crystals.

It has been difficult to determine the actual strength of bone at the individual structural level due to its complex structure. However, it has been found that compact (cortical) bone is extremely strong. It has a compressive strength of 1,400–2,100 kg per square centimeter (20,000–30,000 pounds per square inch) and a tensile strength of 700–1,400 kg per square centimeter (10,000–20,000 pounds per square inch). These strengths are similar to those of mild steel or aluminum, but bone is much lighter. The long axis of the bone, which runs parallel to the mineral crystals and collagen fibers, is primarily responsible for its strength. Bones are also elastic and can withstand impact due to the significant degree of elasticity present in them, despite their apparent stiffness. Bone has an estimated modulus of elasticity of between 420 and 700 kg per square centimeter (6,000 to 10,000 pounds per square inch), which is significantly less than steel. This indicates that bone is much more elastic than steel. Bones exhibit perfect elasticity up to 30% to 40% of their breaking strength, beyond which they exhibit gradual deformation or "creep" which is likely to occur along inherent flaws in the bone structure. The rate at which loads are applied to bones has a significant impact on their modulus of elasticity. During rapid deformation, bones become stiffer than during slow deformation, suggesting the presence of viscous flow during deformation.

Since bone is made up of two phases, it is not surprising that the ratio of minerals to collagen affects the physical characteristics of the bone. Less mineral content makes the bone more flexible while more mineral content makes it more brittle. The weight-bearing bones of mammals have an ash content of about 66%, which corresponds to optimal ratios for maximal tensile strength.

Summary

- Osteomyelitis is the term for bone infection. It's an inflammatory process, either acute or chronic, that affects the bone and its supporting structures due to pyogenic organism infection, caused by bacteria, fungi, or mycobacteria.
- The infection known as hematogenous osteomyelitis mainly affects the most vascularized areas of the developing skeleton in children. The frequency, virulence, and extent of soft-tissue involvement in the disease have all increased.
- Hematogenous osteomyelitis is an infection that affects the highly vascularized areas of the developing skeleton in children.
- Chronic osteomyelitis, on the other hand, is a low-grade or recurrent infection that persists for an extended period. It is characterized by bony sclerosis, periosteal new bone formation, and the presence of draining sinuses and/or sequestra.
- Subacute osteomyelitis, which is also known as a Brodie abscess, can last for several years before progressing to chronic osteomyelitis.
- Sclerosing osteomyelitis of Garré is an infrequent chronic inflammatory ailment characterized by loss of the medullary canal and thickening of the corticosteal layer. Primarily impacting the mandibular region in young children and adults, it can also occasionally affect the metaphysis of long bones (e.g., femur, tibia).
- Joint inflammation resulting from an infectious etiology, commonly bacterial but occasionally fungal, mycobacterial, viral, or other infrequent pathogens, is referred to as septic arthritis. Typically, septic arthritis affects a solitary, sizable joint, such as the hip or knee.
- The majority of skeletal and articular infections in diminutive or premature infants are attributable to recurrent invasive procedures and protracted nosocomial exposures. There has consistently been a principal emphasis elsewhere in the anatomy that has taken precedence over the tuberculosis of the bones and joints. This principal emphasis is frequently imperceptible (i.e., not easily detected).
- It's important to note that fungal infections of the bone are typically categorized into two types: superficial, which are more common, and deep, which are much rarer.

References

1. Azamgarhi T., Shah A., Warren S. Clinical Experience of Implementing Oral Versus Intravenous Antibiotics (OVIVA) in a Specialist Orthopedic Hospital. *Clin. Infect. Dis.* 2021;73:2582–2588. doi: 10.1093/cid/ciaa985.
2. Bader, M. S., (2008). Diabetic foot infection. *Am. Fam. Physician, 78*(1), 71–79.
3. Calhoun, J. H., & Manring, M. M., (2005). Adult osteomyelitis. *Infect. Dis. Clin. North Am., 19*(4), 765–786.
4. Concia, E., Napoleon, P., Massari, L., et al., (2006). Osteomyelitis: Clinical update for practical guidelines. *Nucl. Med. Commun., 27*(8), 645–660.
5. Euba G., Murillo O., Sabé N., Mascaró J., Cabo J., Pérez A., Tubau F., Verdaguer R., Gudiol

F., Ariza J. Long-term follow-up trial of oral rifampin-cotrimoxazole combination versus intravenous cloxacillin in treatment of chronic Staphylococcal osteomyelitis. *Antimicrob. Agents Chemother.* 2009;53:2672–2676. doi: 10.1128/AAC.01504-08.

6. Gentry L.O., Rodriguez G.G. Oral Ciprofloxacin Compared with Parenteral Antibiotics in the Treatment of Osteomyelitis. *Antimicrob. Agents Chemother.* 1990;34:40–43. doi: 10.1128/AAC.34.1.40.
7. Gentry L.O., Rodriguez-Gomez G. Ofloxacin versus Parenteral Therapy for Chronic Osteomyelitis. *Antimicrob. Agents Chemother.* 1991;35:538–541. doi: 10.1128/AAC.35.3.538.
8. Gomis M., Barberán J., Sánchez B., Khorrami S., Borja J., García-Barbal J. Imipenem/Cilastatin in the Treatment of Osteomyelitis. *Rev. Esp. Quimioter.* 1999;12:244–249.
9. Hatzenbuehler, J., & Pulling, T. J., (2011). Diagnosis and management of osteomyelitis. *Am. Fam. Physician, 84*(9), 1027–1033.
10. Kaplan, S. L., (2005). Osteomyelitis in children. *Infect. Dis. Clin. North Am., 19*(4), 787–797.
11. Lazzarini, L., Mader, J. T., & Calhoun, J. H., (2004). Osteomyelitis in long bones. *J. Bone Joint Surg. Am.,* (10), 2305–2318.
12. Li H.-K., Rombach I., Zambellas R., Walker A.S., McNally M.A., Atkins B.L., Lipsky B.A., Hughes H.C., Bose D., Kümin M., et al. Oral versus Intravenous Antibiotics for Bone and Joint Infection. *N. Engl. J. Med.* 2019;380:425–436. doi: 10.1056/NEJMoa1710926.
13. Matteson, E. L., & Osmon, D. R., (2020). Infections of bursae, joints, and bones; Chap 256. In: Goldman, L., & Schafer, A. I., (eds.), *Goldman-Cecil Medicine* (26th edn.) Philadelphia, PA: Elsevier.
14. Paluska, S. A., (2004). Osteomyelitis. *Clin. Fam. Pract., 6*(1), 127–156.
15. Pineda, C., Vargas, A., & Rodriguez, A. V., (2006). Imaging of osteomyelitis: Current concepts. *Infect. Dis. Clin. North Am., 20*(4), 789–825.
16. Raukar, N. P., & Zink, B. J., (2018). Bone and joint infections; Chap 128. In: Walls, R. M., Hockberger, R. S., & Gausche-Hill, M., (eds.), *Rosen's Emergency Medicine: Concepts and Clinical Practice* (9th edn.) Philadelphia, PA: Elsevier.
17. Stengel, D., Bauwens, K., Sehouli, J., et al., (2001). Systematic review and meta-analysis of antibiotic therapy for bone and joint infections. *Lancet Infect Dis., 1*(3), 175–188.
18. Tande, A. J., Steckelberg, J. M., Osmon, D. R., & Berbari, E. F., (2020). Osteomyelitis; Chap 104. In: Bennett, J. E., Dolin, R., & Blaser, M. J., (eds.), *Mandell, Douglas, and Bennett's Principles and Practice of Infectious Diseases* (9th edn.). Philadelphia, PA: Elsevier.

Chapter

BONE TUMORS

8

Contents

8.1. Introduction

When cells inside a bone divide uncontrollably, an abnormal mass of tissue known as a bone tumor results. The majority of bone tumors are not malignant. Benign tumors typically do not pose a threat to life and do not usually spread to other body parts. Treatment options vary widely depending on the type of tumor and can range from straightforward observation to surgical removal of the tumor. There are some malignant (cancerous) bone tumors. Malignant bone tumors have the potential to metastasize or spread cancer cells throughout the body. Chemotherapy, radiation therapy, and surgery are almost always used in conjunction with the treatment of malignant tumors.

Orientation and Directional Terms

Term	Definition	Illustration
Multiple myeloma	Multiple myeloma is the most common primary bone cancer. It is a malignant tumor of the bone marrow, which is the soft tissue in the center of many bones responsible for producing blood cells. This cancer can affect any bone.	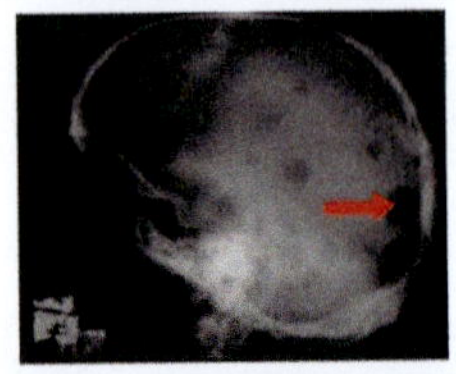
Osteosarcoma	Osteosarcoma is the second most common primary bone cancer. It occurs in two to five people per million each year, with most cases in teenagers and children. Most tumors develop around the knee in either the femur or tibia. Other common locations include the hip and shoulder. Osteosarcoma is typically treated with chemotherapy and surgery.	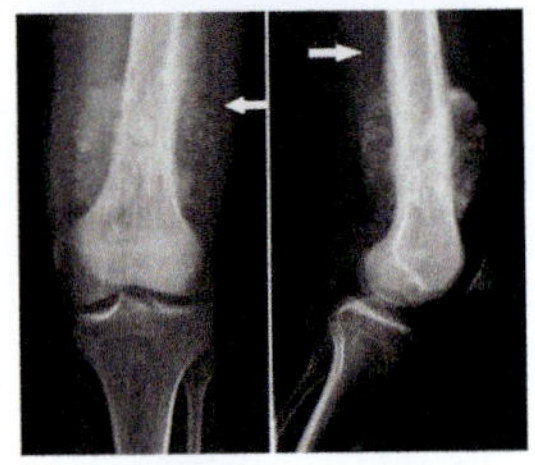
Ewing's sarcoma	Ewing's sarcoma typically occurs in patients between the ages of 5 and 20. The most common locations affected are the upper and lower leg, pelvis, upper arm, and ribs. Treatment for Ewing's sarcoma usually involves chemotherapy and either surgery or radiation therapy.	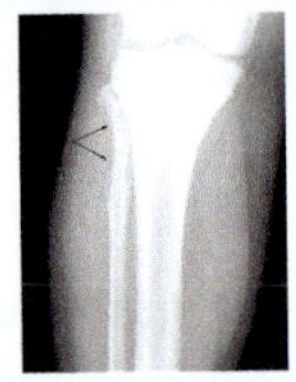
Chondrosarcoma	Chondrosarcoma is a malignant tumor composed of cartilage-producing cells. It is most often seen in patients between the ages of 40 and 70. Most cases occur around the hip, pelvis, or shoulder area. In most cases, surgery is the only treatment used for chondrosarcoma.	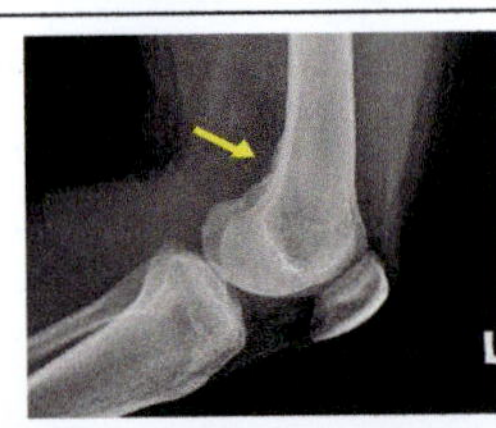
Osteoblastoma	Osteoblastoma is a rare tumor that grows in the spine and long bones, primarily affecting young adults.	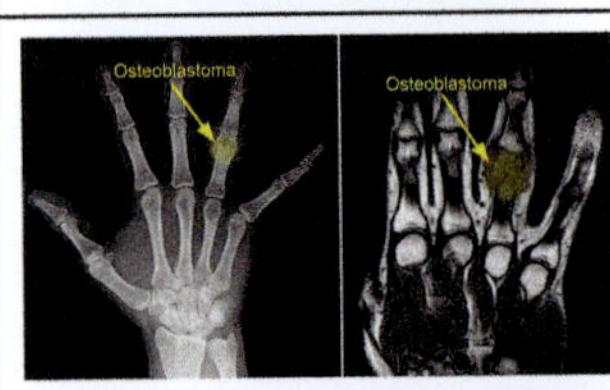
Enchondroma	Enchondroma typically manifests in the bones of the hands and feet, often without any accompanying symptoms. It is the most prevalent form of hand tumor.	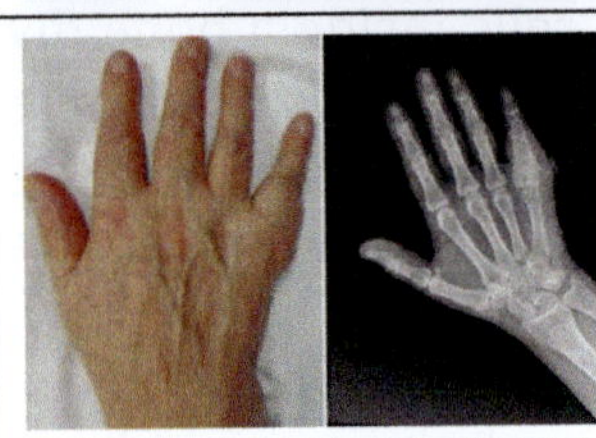

8.2. Common Benign Bone Tumors (BBTs)

The majority of bone tumors are benign (not cancerous). This implies that benign tumors do not metastasize to other areas. Any part of a bone, or any bone in the skeletal system, has the potential to develop a tumor. The femur, tibia, humerus, pelvis, spine, and ribs are among the largest bones that are typically affected. Certain tumor types are more commonly found in specific locations, such as the spine or near the growth plates in the shoulder, hip, or knee. Osteochondroma, osteoma, osteoid osteoma, osteoblastoma, giant cell tumor, aneurysmal bone cyst, fibrous dysplasia, and enchondroma are the most common types of benign bone tumors (BBTs). These tumors are further classified based on the type of cells they contain, including vascular, connective tissue, bone-forming, and cartilage-forming tumors. Due to their often asymptomatic nature and challenges in detection, determining the incidence of BBTs is difficult. Certain rare types of BBTs will not be covered due to their low frequency. Generally, these tumors occur in individuals under 30 years of age and are often associated with hormones that promote growth (such as osteochondroma).

8.2.1. Bone-Forming Tumors

8.2.1.1. Osteoid Osteoma

Bone-forming tumors, which make up 12% of BBTs, are benign osteoblastic tumors. Although they can appear before the age of three, they usually do so in the second decade of life, and they affect boys more than girls—by a factor of two to four. There have been reports of infrequent metachronous presentations, which are typically solitary. They are made up of a nidus that is encircled by sclerotic tissue, which is usually less than 1.5 cm in diameter. Given their similar morphology and genetic makeup, an osteoblastoma may be diagnosed if the lesion has a greater diameter. The scientific community is still divided over whether these two distinct entities should be distinguished from one another.

- **Sites of Development:** Although the spine, particularly the lumbar region, is a common site of presentation, bone-forming tumors primarily affect the long bones of the lower limbs.
- **Micro-Macroscopic Features:** The histopathological examination reveals a central nidus lined by osteoblasts and composed of small osteoid islands. The nidus contains unmyelinated nerve fibers that are responsible for pain. Osteoclastic resorption makes the area around the nidus appear more distinct, and the nidus is surrounded by dense sclerotic tissue. Some research indicates that the nidus may also produce osteocalcin in addition to prostaglandins. Its genetic features are similar to those of osteoblastoma; in fact, osteoidosteoma expresses Runx2 and Osterix, transcription factors involved in osteoblastic differentiation.
- **Clinical Features:** Bone-forming tumors can cause excruciating pain, which might worsen at night. One of their primary features is that the pain is usually relieved in less than 30 minutes with NSAIDs (prostaglandin inhibitors); if this does not occur, the condition is most likely not an osteoid osteoma, and other treatment options need to be explored. Bone-forming tumors can also cause muscular atrophy, erythema,

swelling, and tenderness. The site of presentation may influence the clinical symptomatology. Differential diagnosis is essential because patients with spine osteoid osteomas may exhibit a scoliotic posture. The affected bone may lengthen or develop an angular deformity as a result of this lesion affecting open physis. Moreover, a precise assessment of the femoroacetabular impingement is required if it affects the hip joint and results in hip impingement. When a lesion appears intra- or juxta-articular, synovitis may be the result.

- **Imaging:** A bone-forming tumor appears as a nidus surrounded by sclerotic tissue on an X-ray examination. When something is intra-articular, it might be difficult to diagnose, necessitating further investigation. A CT scan, which is the second level examination, reveals a small, well-defined nidus encircled by a sclerotic reaction that may contain calcifications. Bone scintigraphy detects arterial phase uptake in the nidus, with lower concentration in the reactive surrounding bone compared to the high vascular concentration found in the nidus. The double-density sign is a common and diagnostic indicator. It is important to consider growth plates, as they may mask the signal if an osteoid osteoma is located close to them. Therefore, evaluating the contralateral side may be beneficial. Additional imaging modalities may assist in the diagnostic process, but each situation needs to be evaluated individually (Figure 8.1).

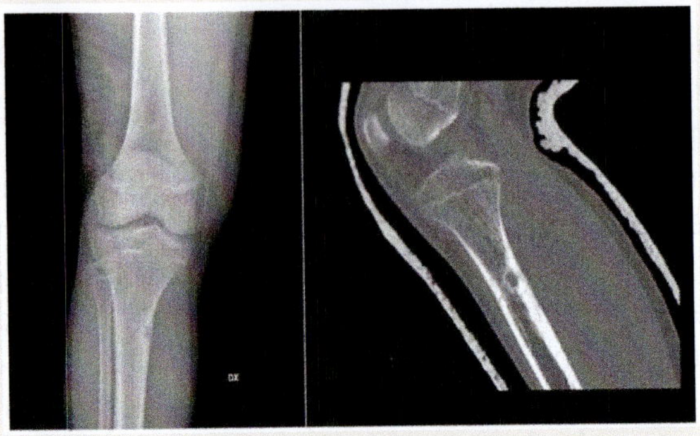

Figure 8.1. *X-rays and CT scan of a tibial fracture that occurred in the development site of an Osteoid osteoma.*

Source: De Salvo, S., Pavone, V., Coco, S., Dell'Agli, E., Blatti, C., & Testa, G., (2022). Benign bone tumors: An overview of what we know today. J. Clin. Med., 11(3), 699. doi: 10.3390/jcm11030699.

- **Differential Diagnosis:** In order to accurately diagnose a patient, it is important to rule out osteoblastoma, which may have no pain or mild pain, does not respond well to NSAIDs, and typically has a more widespread and intricate appearance compared to osteoid osteoma. The presentation of osteoid osteoma may mimic that of subacute or chronic osteomyelitis, but it usually originates from growth plates.
- **Treatment and Prognosis:** The tumor's natural course calls for spontaneous resolution in 6 to 15 years; if symptoms do not appear, cautious waiting is advised. However, NSAIDs are the recommended medication if symptoms are present. According to studies, taking aspirin or NSAIDs for treatment could shorten the

healing process by two or three years. Lesions that cause scoliosis, length discrepancy, and other morpho-functional disorders can be surgically removed, and treated with radiofrequency, cryotherapy, and MRI-guided high-intensity focused ultrasound, among other approaches. The nidus must be removed as the primary goal of the resection; the sclerotic margins do not need to be removed. Recurrences may occur if the nidus is not completely removed following resection.

8.2.1.2. Osteoblastoma

Osteoblastoma is a bone-forming neoplasm that primarily affects young adults (mean age of 20 years), with a higher incidence rate in males (two to three times more common than females) and accounts for about 14% of BBTs. As the age at presentation increases, the tumor becomes more aggressive. They consist of a central nidus encircled by sclerotic tissue, similar to osteoid osteomas. It does not produce prostaglandins and has fewer nerve fibers, despite the nidus being more vascularized and the lesions being less organized. Its diameter can reach up to 15 cm, although its average size is only about 3 cm.

- **Sites of Development:** Osteoblastoma most commonly originates from the sacrum and posterior elements of the spine. Cementoblastoma is the term used for the long tubular bones of the lower limb, which is another common site of presentation along with the mandible.
- **Micro-Macroscopic Features:** An osteoblastoma is a reddish-brown, richly vascularized lesion. It typically has a border that separates it from the bone marrow, and the cortical surface's margins press up against it. Usually, a layer of fibrous tissue divides it from other bone structures. As the tumor grows more aggressively, the borders penetrate deeper. The formation of immature and osteoid bone trabeculae is a crucial characteristic of the osteoblastoma lesion. Osteoblastoma and osteosarcoma can be distinguished from each other using immunohistochemistry because the former has nuclear beta-catenin staining, whereas the latter has cytoplasmic or membranous staining. As mentioned for osteoid osteoma, osteoblastoma is characterized by genetic mutations of FOS and FOSB.
- **Clinical Features:** Osteoblastoma grows slowly and most patients do not experience any symptoms, similar to most benign tumors. This clinical characteristic can aid in distinguishing osteoblastoma from osteoid osteoma. When symptoms are present, they may include soft tissue swelling and dull, localized pain. As with other cases, the location of the tumor can impact the symptoms. Involvement of the spine can lead to postural scoliosis, muscle weakness, and compression of the nerve roots. Individuals with lower extremity involvement may exhibit a limp. A rare variant of this tumor, known as toxic osteoblastoma, presents with systemic symptoms such as fever, anorexia, and diffuse periostitis.
- **Imaging:** MRI, CT scans, and plain radiographs are utilized in the evaluation of osteoblastoma. Plain radiographs may reveal various

patterns. While it may resemble an osteoid osteoma, it is larger (>2 cm) and exhibits less reactive sclerosis around it. A typical characteristic is benign periosteal reaction. Lesions growing in the axial skeleton can mimic aneurysmal bone cysts. Additionally, when the tumor is larger in size (>4 cm), aggressive osteoblastomas can mimic malignant lesions, resulting in disruption and thinning of the cortical layer.

- **Differential Diagnosis:** Several potential conditions could be causing the symptoms, including osteoid osteoma, osteomyelitis, stress fracture, osteosarcoma, giant cell tumor of bone, and aneurysmal bone cyst. To accurately diagnose the specific condition, more advanced radiographic imaging may be required.
- **Treatment and Prognosis:** In contrast to osteoid osteoma, osteoblastoma has the potential to develop aggressively; therefore, surgical treatment is the preferred course of action. Depending on the lesion's aggressiveness grade, different procedures are preferred. Curettage and resection en-bloc are the most common options, depending on how aggressive the tumor is. Although intralesional curettage is less invasive, its recurrence rate makes it a less common procedure, only used when there is minimal suspicion of cancerous growth. However, en-bloc resection is used on more aggressive lesions because it has a lower recurrence rate than other techniques. Chemotherapy and radiation therapy, among other therapeutic approaches, have not shown promise in treating this tumor. To rule out potential recurrences, it is essential to keep the patient under follow-up care following surgery, including imaging exams. A growing osteoblastoma has the potential to harm nearby bone or nerve structures if left untreated.

8.2.1.3. Giant Cell Tumor

Giant cell tumors represent 15–20% of benign bone neoplasms in the United States, with even higher incidence rates in other countries such as China. Unlike other benign tumors, they exhibit local aggressiveness, resulting in osteolysis, and have the potential to metastasize, typically to the lungs. The main demographic affected by this condition is young adults in their third decade of life.

- **Sites of Development:** Development of giant cell tumors often occurs in the meta-epiphyses of long bones, particularly the proximal tibia and distal femur, which make up the knee joint.
- **Micro-Macroscopic Features:** Microscopically, giant cell tumor of bone (GCTB) is characterized by its friable and red/brown appearance. The multinucleated giant cells are surrounded by a stromal background consisting of monocytes and spindle cells. Various patterns may be observed, including hemosiderin, necrosis, and hemorrhage. The neoplastic cells primarily consist of mononuclear spindle cells. Genetic studies have shown that 20% of GCTBs exhibit p53 overexpression, which is associated with tumor recurrence and metastases. Increased telomerase activity and prevention of telomere shortening have also been observed. Additionally, a study found that 54% of GCTB

had a 20q11 amplification. RANKL overexpression is the most common molecular feature in GCTB, particularly in osteoblast-like mononuclear stromal cells, which recruit osteoclast cells. The presence of osteoclast cells leads to osteolysis. Histone modification, found in over 90% of these tumors, may be one of the initial steps in neoplastic formation.

- **Clinical Features:** Most patients arrive in pain. During a physical examination, palpable tenderness, swelling, and joint effusion in cases where the joints are close together may be discovered. Antalgic gait is another common observation. Pathologic fractures, which frequently affect the joints, can be an oblique indicator of the lesion's existence.
- **Imaging:** The imaging study includes MRIs, CT scans, and standard X-rays. Basic radiography can reveal several patterns, most commonly a radiolucent meta-epiphyseal lesion. Campanacci developed one of the most popular classifications in 1987 (Table 8.1).

Table 8.1. *Campanacci Grading*

Grade	Radiological Finding
I	Lesions confined in the bone cortex, which is intact (cystic lesions).
II	Lesions confined in the bone cortex, which appears thinned but not perforated.
III	Lesions extended over the bone, that invade the cortex and expand to the soft tissues.

Source: Paul, C. J., (2022). "Benign Bone Tumors: An Overview of What We Know Today," JCM, 11(3), 699. doi: 10.3390/jcm11030699.

The purpose of this classification is to impact the level of surgery. To clarify the aggressiveness of the tumor, other histopathological and genetic factors need to be assessed, even if doing so makes the diagnostic study simpler. CT can be used to further define the lesion's boundaries. MRI findings are often nonspecific, with the T1-weighted sequence showing a decrease in signal intensity and an increase in the T2-weighted signal: these sequences can also have a low signal intensity. Another nonspecific but frequent feature of GCTB in scintigraphy is the "donut sign" due to the intense uptake of radionuclide in the periphery and the necrosis in the center of the lesion. Chest CT imaging is suggested in recurrent GCTB to spot eventual pulmonary metastases.

- **Differential Diagnosis:** Brown tumors linked to hyperparathyroidism and metastases of other body tumors are examples of benign and malignant tumors rich in giant cells and osteoclasts that are included in the differential diagnosis.
- **Treatment:** Surgery is the gold standard for treating GCTB. Intralesional curettage combined with PMMA (polymethylmethacrylate) cavity filling is a common method. If the tumor is situated in a disposable bone, like the fibula or distal ulna, extensive bone resection is usually necessary. Numerous strategies, including denosumab, radiotherapy, bisphosphonates, and chemotherapy, can be considered in the event of extraosseous extension and metastases. There is disagreement regarding the follow-up, but imaging exams must be performed on these patients on a regular basis.

Metastases primarily originate from the lungs and affect 2–3% of GCTB cases (especially if the primary tumor originates from the spine). However, because these metastases preserve the morphological and histological characteristics of the original tumor, they are frequently referred to as "benign" pulmonary implants. These are most frequently found in recurrent lesions.

8.2.2. Cartilage-Forming Tumors

8.2.2.1. Osteochondroma

As the most common benign tumor of the bone, osteochondroma accounts for 20–50% of benign tumors and 10–15% of all tumors. Usually, it forms in developing bones. Some studies suggest that they most likely originate from the epiphyseal growth plate. Males are more frequently affected than females. It is visible as a bony protrusion on the outside of the bone that is covered in cartilage. In multiple hereditary osteochondromas, there may be one or more lesions. The single osteochondroma (85%) typically manifests at the age of 20. A growth plate fragment that has herniated through the periosteum and formed a sessile or pedunculated lesion is thought to be the source of this tumor. This herniation may develop spontaneously, following trauma or radiation exposure, or both. Recent research has discovered a mutation in the tumor suppressor exostin-1 (EXT1). This lesion was discovered incidentally while conducting other tests. Multiple osteochondromas usually present with an earlier age of onset and more pronounced symptoms. With an incidence of 1/50,000–1,00,000, autosomal dominant inheritance with incomplete penetrance is the primary cause of the majority of these lesions. Exostin-1 and exostin-2, two tumor suppressor genes, frequently undergo mutations. Lesions may enlarge in both situations as they mature; when skeletal maturity is reached and the lesion grows, a malignant lesion should be suspected (Figure 8.2).

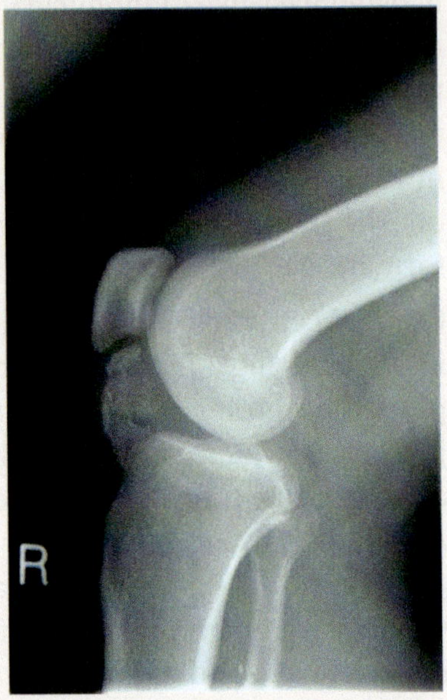

Figure 8.2. *Lateral radiograph of the knee demonstrating ossification in the peritendinous tissues in a patient with osteochondroma.*

Source: Michael, R. C., Sian, D., Daniel, Ge. V. P., & Robin, R. Accelerated para-articular osteochondroma formation within the knee: A case report. Cases Journal. https://commons.wikimedia.org/w/index.php?curid=4280855 (accessed on 23 March 2024).

- **Sites of Development:** The metaphysis is the primary bone segment that is affected. The most frequent site is the distal femur, followed by the proximal tibia and humerus. Osteochondromas may cause spinal involvement.
- **Micro-Macroscopic Characteristics:** The bluish cartilage covering the bone usually measures 1–3 cm in children and a few millimeters in adults (if the thickness of the cartilage in an adult is greater

than 1 cm, malignancy needs to be suspected). Lesion continuity from the cortex to the medulla is a pathognomonic feature of osteochondroma.

- **Clinical Features:** While multiple osteochondromas can result in multiple bone deformities, short limbs, short stature, leg length discrepancy, coxa valga, or valgus knee, a single osteochondroma only manifests as a painless mass.
- **Imaging:** When X-rayed, osteochondroma is typically found in the metaphysis, with its cortex continuing into the original bone cortex through a marrow cavity. Further MRI, CT, or US investigations might be required for symptomatic patients. When assessing the thickness of the adult bone and cartilage cap, as well as potential side effects like bursae, neurological, and vascular involvement, MRI is a useful tool. Scintigraphy is not a useful test for diagnosis because it exhibits enhancement in both benign and malignant lesions (Figure 8.3).

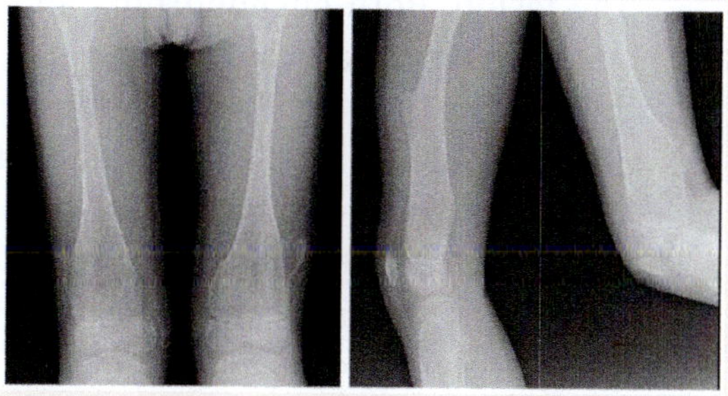

Figure 8.3. *X-rays of multiple osteochondromas.*

Source: Paul, C. J., (2022). The article Benign Bone Tumors: An Overview of What We Know Today, 11(3), 699. Published in JCM. doi: 10.3390/jcm11030699.

- **Differential Diagnosis:** This disease must be differentiated from hemimelic dysplasia of the epiphysis (Trevo disease), which is characterized by the presence of multiple osteochondromas in the lower limbs, parosteal osteosarcoma, a subtype of osteosarcoma originating from the surface of long bones, and subungual exostosis (Dupuytren's exostosis), where lesions develop on the back of the phalanx near the nail and can cause pain and ulcers. Radiographs reveal large, lobulated, dense bone masses; in advanced stages, the lesion may invade the medullary space. None of these conditions show continuity of the lesion from the cortex to the medulla.
- **Treatment and Prognosis:** Individual osteochondromas typically develop asymptomatically over time. Excision is recommended if a single osteochondroma is symptomatic or if there is a risk of malignant transformation. After partial excision of the cartilage cap, the recurrence rate is 2%, and this can only occur during the developmental stages. The prognosis for osteochondroma is generally good, with only 1% of cases progressing to malignancy; hereditary osteochondroma carries a 2.5–5% risk of malignant transformation.

8.2.2.2. Enchondroma

Enchondroma is a benign tumor that forms inside the medullary cavity of the bone, originating from hyaline cartilage. It is the second most common noncancerous primary bone tumor, accounting for 3–10% of all bone tumors and 13% of noncancerous bone tumors. Typically diagnosed between the ages of 15 and 35, it affects both males and females equally. In 40% of cases, enchondroma occurs due to a sporadic mutation in the IDH1 and IDH2 genes, resulting in increased levels of D-2-hydroxyglutarate. This mutation hinders cell differentiation during bone development and promotes the formation of chondroid tumors. Rare mutations in PTHR1 and genetic abnormalities in certain chromosomes are also associated with enchondromas. While generally noncancerous, these tumors have the potential to become malignant, such as chondrosarcoma.

- **Sites of Development:** Around 90% of enchondromas originate from solitary lesions in the medullary cavity, which are the result of an ectopic cartilage nest. Enchondroma is believed to arise from growth plate fragments that became trapped in the bone metaphysis during development. Instead of undergoing ossification, the trapped chondrocytes retain their chondroid characteristics. Chondroma develops in the metaphyseal segment of tubular bones such as those in the hand, foot, femur, and humerus. The usual site of development is the proximal metaphysis of the proximal phalanx on the ulnar side. The most commonly affected phalanges are the proximal phalanges, followed by the middle, metacarpal, and distal phalanges.
- **Micro-Macroscopic Characteristics:** Enchondroma is a nodular lesion that appears translucent, hypocellular, bluish-gray in color, and consists of a significant amount of hyaline cartilage without vascular components. The nuclei are regular and well-defined, with low mitotic activity. Chondroid calcified matrix and chondrocyte necrosis suggest adult enchondroma. Hypercellularity and cytologic abnormalities are characteristics shared by both chondrosarcoma and enchondroma of the hand.
- **Clinical Features:** Encephalomas are typically asymptomatic, and their discovery often occurs incidentally during other examinations. Pain may occur as a result of a pathologic fracture or malignant transformation.
- **Imaging:** One of the radiographic characteristics of enchondroma is a single, oval, radiolucent lesion located in the metaphysis of the bone. In adults, calcifications with a higher signal radiodensity may be visible in the center of this lesion. CT can detect the classic "arcs and rings" pattern of chondroid mineralization. MRI provides detailed information about the erosive and aggressive nature of the lesion. Both enchondroma and chondrosarcoma exhibit a low-intensity signal on T1 and a high-intensity signal on T2. Distinguishing between the two is facilitated by the absence of perilesional edema around chondrosarcoma and its presence around enchondroma. Unless the lesion is atypical or in cases of doubt, a biopsy is not recommended.
- **Differential Diagnosis:** Bone infarction, low-grade chondrosarcoma (progressive

destruction of the chondroid matrix, an expanding lesion that may invade soft tissue, with pain as the main symptom), and tuberculous dactylitis (spina ventosa) all require differential diagnosis. Distinguishing enchondroma from chondrosarcoma is still difficult. In middle-aged adults (40–50 years old), chondrosarcoma typically manifests in the axial skeleton and is frequently accompanied by subtle, progressive, nocturnal pain. From a radiographic perspective, the lesion appears as a lobular lytic lesion with a poorly defined margin and a mineralized matrix. Enchondroma typically manifests in young adults (30–40 years old) in the appendicular skeleton. It is frequently an asymptomatic lesion that is discovered by accident. From a radiographic perspective, the lesion appears to be well-defined in the center and has the characteristic "arcs and rings calcification" pattern. Mutations such as IDH1 and IDH2 and similar histological features are shared by chondrosarcoma and enchondroma. A potential chondrosarcoma diagnosis can be made based on the presence of periostin, alpha-methyl-acyl-CoA racemase (AMACR) in the stroma during the immunohistochemistry exam, and perilesional edema in MR imaging.

- **Treatment and Prognosis:** Treatment is not necessary for asymptomatic and small enchondroma; observation is sufficient. The outcomes of early or delayed surgical treatment are comparable in these situations. Symptomatic enchondroma requires bone grafting and basic curettage. Synthetic bone substitutes, autogenic bone, or allogeneic bone can all be used for bone grafting. When a lesion represents more than 50% of the cortex's diameter or has a diameter of more than 25 mm, there is an increased risk of fracture. In these cases, early surgical intervention is debatable. Surgery is advised in cases of fractures. Since enchondroma is a benign and self-limiting lesion, it has a favorable prognosis. Recurrence following curettage and bone grafting surgery is uncommon.
- **Enchondromatosis:** It is defined as the presence of multiple enchondromas with a unilateral predominance. The most common mutations are those in IDH1 and IDH2. Ollier disease and Maffucci syndrome are two diseases that are similar to this condition. Ollier disease is a rare, sporadic illness that affects 1 in 1,00,000 people. Enchondromas typically appear at age 10 and develop prior to solitary enchondroma. Several enchondromas develop in the epiphyses or in the space between the metaphysis and the diaphysis. The development site may obstruct appropriate bone formation, metaphysis enlargement, and bone bending.

Multiple enchondromas, soft tissue hemangiomas, and vascular anomalies are the hallmarks of Maffucci syndrome. Maffucci syndrome patients frequently experience the development of malignant non-skeletal lesions, such as ovarian or pancreatic carcinomas, or gliomas. Chondrosarcoma carries a 40% risk of malignant transformation in both conditions; specifically, the risk is 50% higher in Maffucci syndrome and 35% higher in Ollier disease. Both conditions exhibit cellular atypia and hypercellularity as histological features (Figure 8.4).

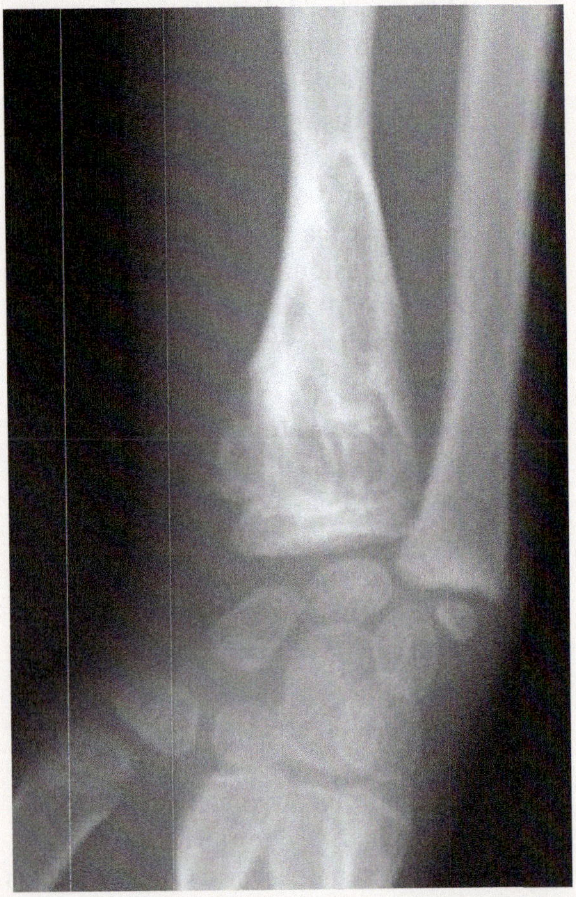

Figure 8.4. *X-ray image showing enchondromas localized in the lower part of the radius of a seven-year-old girl with Ollier disease.*

Source: Silve, C., & Jüppner, H., (2006). Ollier disease. Orphanet Journal of Rare Diseases, 1, 37. PMID 16995932 doi: 10.1186/1750-1172-1-37. CC BY 2.0. https://commons.wikimedia.org/w/index.php?curid=2576382 (accessed on 23 March 2024).

8.2.2.3. Chondroblastoma

The most immature cartilage cells, called chondroblasts, are the source of chondroblastoma, a benign tumor. It accounts for less than 1% of all bone tumors and nearly 5% of BBTs. It usually manifests in adolescence and affects boys 2:1 more frequently than girls. Its exact cause is unknown, but a combination of environmental and predisposing factors is thought to be responsible. Chromosomes 5 and 8 frequently reorganize. Specific mutations (K36M) of gene H3F3B or H3F3A have been discovered, both associated with the H3.3 histone.

- **Site of Development:** Teens with skeletal immaturity are more likely to develop chondroblastoma, which usually appears as a single lesion on the apophysis or epiphyses of long bones. Most often, the proximal humerus is affected first, followed by the proximal tibia and distal femur.
- **Micro-Macroscopic Characteristics:** Chondroblastomas typically display pinkish-brown lesions with occasional bleeding and cystic formations. Histologically, these tumors are characterized by polygonal cells with distinct cytoplasm and round nuclei. Giant cells, known as osteoclasts, are always present. A unique feature of chondroblastomas is the presence of a pericellular calcification net, resembling 'chicken wire.' Immunohistochemistry testing shows positive results for vimentin, neuron-specific enolase, protein S-100, SOX9, DOG1, as well as keratins 8, 18, and 19 (Figure 8.5).

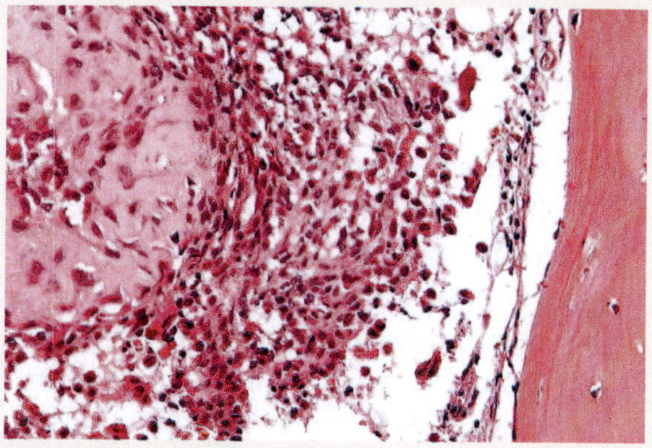

Figure 8.5. *Very high magnification micrograph of a chondroblastoma. H&E stain.*

Source: By Nephron – Own work, CC BY-SA 3.0, https://commons.wikimedia.org/w/index.php?curid=12522989.

- **Clinical Features:** Symptoms of chondroblastoma include limping, edema, joint stiffness, and persistent low-grade joint pain. Physical examinations often reveal muscle atrophy, reduced range of motion, and joint effusion.
- **Imaging:** On radiography, chondroblastoma typically appears as a small, well-defined lesion with sclerotic borders in the epiphyses. The lesion usually measures 3–6 cm in diameter. CT scans can show cortical erosion, calcifications in the matrix, and extension into soft tissues. MRI can detect perilesional edema, and post-contrast imaging can reveal gadolinium localization in the center of the lesion.
- **Differential Diagnosis:** It is crucial to differentiate chondroblastoma from other conditions such as giant cell tumor, chondromyxoid fibroma, aneurysmal bone cyst, and osteomyelitis.
- **Treatment and Prognosis:** Reduction of pain, prevention of lesion spread in the joint and surrounding soft tissues, and reduction of recurrence are the objectives of treatment. Surgery is performed to achieve these goals. The type of surgery will vary depending on the location, degree of involvement in the bone or joint, and stage of the lesion (latent, active, or aggressive). Surgical options include en-bloc bone resection, complete curettage with or without bone graft, and occasionally amputation. To minimize the risk of recurrence, chemical cauterization with phenol or cryotherapy is preferred in addition to surgical therapy. Following surgery, it is crucial to have regular follow-up. The preferred option in the event of a recurrence is en-bloc bone resection. If surgery is not feasible, radiofrequency can be used as an alternative. Adjuvant chemotherapy and radiation therapy have not been established as effective in the management of chondroblastomas. Following surgical treatment, the prognosis for chondroblastoma is favorable. The recurrence rate ranges from 8.3% to 21%, and it increases if the lesion is localized in the hip or pelvis or if the surgery is inadequate.

8.2.3. Fibrous Lesions

8.2.3.1. Fibrous Dysplasia

Fibrous tissue that proliferates and replaces the normal bone matrix is the hallmark of FD, a benign bone lesion. It makes up about

5–7% of BBTs. In both sexes, it is equally prevalent. FD comes in two flavors: polyostotic fibrous dysplasia (PFD) and monostotic fibrous dysplasia (MFD). Around 70% comes from MFD. Lesions in polyostotic patients may be bilateral or unilateral. Endocrine disorders (MAS) are only 2–3% of cases involving FD.

- **Sites of Development:** Lesions are most frequently found in the craniofacial bones as well as the long bones of the arms, legs, ribs, and pelvis. The spine is involved in 1.4–5.5% of FD lesions. MFDs typically reach adulthood, reach full skeletal maturity, and then stop growing. In contrast, PFDs continue to grow even after reaching adulthood, creating weak spots that could lead to pathological fractures. In 2–3% of cases, PFD could be linked to endocrine disorders such as Mazabraud syndrome (a rare benign condition characterized by the association of multiple or single intramuscular myxomas with polyostic fibrous dysplasia) or McCune-Albright syndrome (MAS). Due to FD's impact on the hormone that regulates phosphate metabolism, it can also lead to the development of hypophosphatemic osteomalacia, with the calcaneus and distal femur being the next most common sites. FD is a non-inherited illness; a potential etiological factor could be a mutation in the GNAS1 gene on chromosome 20q13.2–13.3 that occurred in somatic cells during embryonic development. The occurrence of fewer mutant cells with age accounts for the incidence rates up to the 20s. After amplifying the genomic DNA of patients using polymerase chain reaction analysis, mutations were discovered in the gene's coding region 8.
- **Clinical Features:** Fibrous dysplasia is typically seen in teenagers or young adults in their 20s and can affect any bone, but is most commonly found in the proximal femur, tibia, ribs, and skull. While it usually does not cause symptoms, swelling, and pain can occur in some cases. Severe cases may lead to repeated fractures. A common deformity associated with fibrous dysplasia is the "shepherd's crook" varus deformity of the proximal femur, which can cause pain and eventual limping.
- **Microscopic Features:** Histologically, bone trabeculae with irregular shapes and no osteoblastic rimming are surrounded by a low to moderate cellular fibrous stroma in fibrous dysplasia.
- **Imaging:** Fibrous dysplasia presents on X-rays as a radiolucent, ground-glass expansive lesion, sometimes bowing, with no discernible trabecular pattern. The inner cortex may exhibit endosteal scalloping in the absence of periosteal reaction. Abnormal curvature of the proximal shaft (coxa vara) and femur neck characterize Shepherd's crook deformity, which can lead to pathologic fracture. In most cases, periosteal reaction is nonexistent unless a pathologic fracture occurs.
- **Differential Diagnosis:** Simple bone cysts, non-ossifying fibromas, osteofibrous dysplasia, adamantinoma, low-grade

intramedullary osteosarcoma, and Paget disease are among the lesions that may mimic fibrous dysplasia. Simple bone cysts are less dense than fibrous dysplasia and have a thinner layer of lamellar bone surrounding them. As the skeleton develops, simple cysts move away from the metaphysis and appear more radiolucent on X-rays. Aspirating fluid from the straw-colored cyst is a possibility. Non-ossifying fibromas typically occur in the growing metaphysis of weight-bearing long bones, intracortically and eccentrically. NOFs typically appear painlessly and spontaneously recede with age. The intracortical location, smaller size, absence of intralesional ossification, and spontaneous regression following skeletal maturity set non-ossifying fibromas apart from fibrous dysplasia. The distal third of the tibia or fibula is typically the only location where osteofibrous dysplasia or ossifying fibroma is found. Usually, children under the age of 10 experience it. One important radiographic distinction between osteofibrous dysplasia and fibrous dysplasia, despite their striking similarity, is that the former typically occurs intracortically, whereas the latter is more centrally distributed.

- **Treatment and Prognosis:** Bisphosphonates are considered the standard of care. Surgical treatment is considered in cases of vertebral collapse instability, spinal cord compression injury, possible pathological fracture, or persistent pain. A biopsy is not recommended when radiographic findings are characteristic. It is advised to take a series of radiographs every six months to assess for any progression. In cases of polyostotic disease, the patient should undergo endocrine and metabolic testing due to the common association with endocrine disorders. Surgical treatment options for correcting or preventing bony deformities in extensive lesions include curettage and bone grafting, as well as osteotomy with internal fixation. FD growth ceases once skeletal development slows down, and the occurrence of cancer is extremely rare. Malignant transformation is not typical, with a prevalence ranging from 0.4 to 6.7%. However, the risk of malignant transformation increases in patients with PFD. Malignant transformation can cause unexplained pain, and X-rays will show visible mineralization and osteolysis of the lesion.
- **Non-Ossifying Fibroma:** As the most common benign lesion of the skeletal system, a non-ossifying fibroma (NOF) is one of the five most common bone lesions. The World Health Organization (WHO) classifies this bone lesion as a tumor-like lesion based on its histologic classification. Various synonyms have been used, such as fibrous xanthoma, histiocytic xanthogranuloma, fibrous cortical defect, and metaphyseal fibrous defect. Non-ossifying fibromas may or may not be associated with other

extra-skeletal abnormalities (non-syndromic).

- **Clinical Features:** Non-ossifying fibromas (NOFs) affect children and adolescents, with an estimated prevalence of 30%–40% among all children, predominantly females. These fibromas are commonly found in the fibula and upper extremities, but they are most frequently observed in long bones, particularly in the distal femoral and distal tibial metaphyses. NOFs are typically asymptomatic and are incidentally discovered through radiographs.
- **Macroscopic and Microscopic Features:** Macroscopically, NOFs appear as fibrous, fleshy, yellow, or tan-brown lesions with areas of bleeding. Microscopically, NOFs are characterized by swirls of fibrous tissue containing hemosiderin, foamy histiocytes, and multinucleated giant cells.
- **Sites of Development:** NOF lesions arise from tendons inserting into the perichondrium of the epiphyseal plate, causing a tug lesion. In the case of NOF in the distal femoral metaphysis, there is a clear correlation between the pull on the bone and the origin of tendinous/fibrous structures. This theory explains why the primary sites of onset for NOFs are the origin of the medial or lateral gastrocnemius or the insertion of the adductor magnus.
- **Imaging:** NOFs appear as solitary, eccentric, lytic lesions in the metaphysis of long bones on radiographs. They often have a polycyclic shape. The lesion is typically lucent, and the cortex may show thinning or thickening. The margins may appear densely sclerotic or indistinct. When multiple lesions are present, the longest dimension of the lesion aligns with the long axis of the bone. The spread of NOF can lead to thinning of the cortical bone in the diaphysis, with interspersed sclerosis and anterior or anterolateral bowing (Figure 8.6).

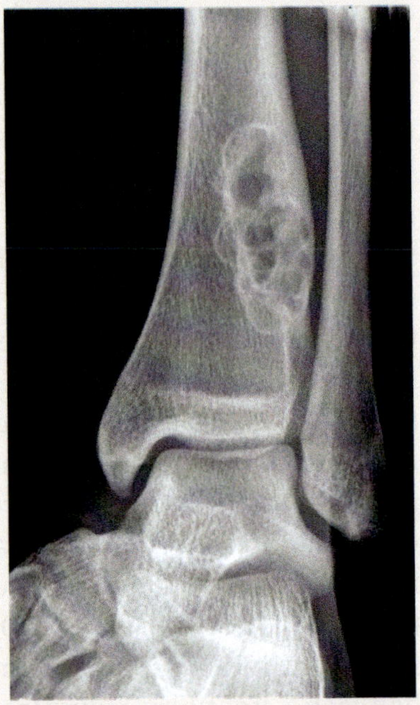

Figure 8.6. *X-ray of nonossifying fibroma of the distal tibia.*

Source: By Hellerhoff – Own work, CC BY-SA 3.0, https://commons.wikimedia.org/w/index.php?curid=9815560.

- **Differential Diagnosis:** Focal cortical dysplasia (FCD) is the primary entity frequently included in the histologic differential diagnosis of NOF; both disorders refer to the same histopathological process, but NOF can be identified by its larger size (>3 cm). The FCD is a small, lytic intracortical lesion that is usually located eccentrically and has a distinct outline. It is an osteolytic defect covered in a thin layer of reactive bone. NOF is always ovoid and eccentric, and it frequently causes the cortex above to enlarge and thin. Both periosteal response and overt cortex violation are typically absent. Desmoids, which normally form inside the cortex, can be radiographically distinguished from NOFs, which are enlarged cortical defects that have spread into the medullary cavity. Proliferative cortical irregularities are known as cortical desmoids. Desmoids and NOF are histologically identical; their radiographic appearance is the only difference between them.

- **Treatment:** Lesions with no symptoms do not require care. A surgical procedure is required if a NOF encompasses more than 33 mm of length or more than 50% of the bone width in two straightforward X-ray views, as these conditions can lead to fracture. Local intralesional curettage or resection combined with bone graft filling is the course of treatment.

8.2.4. Cystic Tumors

8.2.4.1. Unicameral Bone Cyst

Unicameral bone cysts, also known as solitary bone cysts, are lesions filled with fluid and lined with fibrous tissue. UBC is a common nonmalignant condition, with a higher prevalence in males with a ratio of 2:1. Around 80% of cases involving teenagers or patients in their 20s are associated with UBC lesions. It is believed that the development of UBCs is linked to venous circulation disorders, specifically a blockage in the venous flow that leads to bone resorption due to increased pressure. There is also a correlation between UBCs and elevated levels of inflammatory proteins in the intracystic fluid.

- **Sites of Development:** Unicameral bone cysts primarily affect long bones, such as the femur and humerus, in the metaphyseal region.
- **Clinical Features:** UBCs tend to exhibit more aggressive clinical behavior during the first decade of life. Approximately 80% of UBCs present with no symptoms, while in other cases, symptoms may include localized tenderness, swelling, mild pain, or even a pathologic fracture. Due to their usually mild or asymptomatic nature, UBCs are often discovered incidentally.
- **Micro-Macroscopic Features:** Histologically, these lesions have a cementum-like material lining the inner surface of the cyst, along with a membrane that exhibits several ridges. The fluid within the cyst is serous or serous-bloody and may occasionally contain giant cells, reactive new bone, or hemosiderin.
- **Imaging:** The gold standard for diagnosis is an X-ray. The cyst develops towards the diaphysis with the long axis running parallel to the length of the bone, emerging from the medullary cavity in the metaphyses of long bones. The lesion has a "rising bubble" appearance, which is a

pathognomonic indication of UBCs (Figure 8.7).

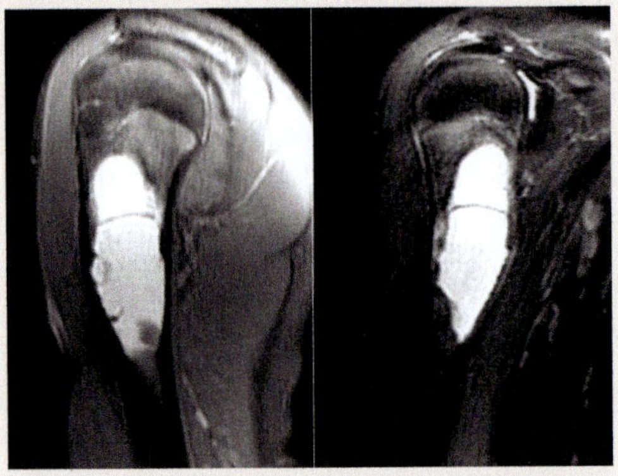

Figure 8.7. *T2-weighted sagittal MRI depicting the lesion of the bone cyst of the proximal humeral in a 13-year-old boy.*

Source: Suat, Ç., et al., (2016). Unicameral (simple) and aneurysmal bone cysts: The effect of insufficient curettage on recurrence. Pan African Medical Journal, 24, 311. doi: 10.11604/pamj.2016.24.311.9624.

- **Treatment and Prognosis:** Corticosteroids are directly injected, once or more, into the cyst as part of the treatment. Two more invasive procedures that are only used for larger bone cysts or those that jeopardize the integrity of the bone are curettage and bone grafting. The patient's age, the cyst's size, and the strength of their entire bone are taken into consideration when selecting the best course of action. Only 15% of childhood simple bone cysts resolve on their own without medical intervention; the majority, however, continue or worsen.

8.2.4.2. Aneurysmal Bone Cyst

Aneurysmal bone cysts are uncommon, benign, blood-filled cyst neoplasms made of vascular channels that have a propensity to enlarge and can cause harm to bone tissue. Though it usually occurs alone, it can also develop on its own or alongside other benign tumors. It typically manifests in young adults and children, mostly in girls.

- **Sites of Development:** ABCs can originate from any bone, but they are most commonly found in the proximal femur, tibia, humerus, and posterior spine bones. When it affects the long bones, the metaphyseal district is where it ideally develops.
- **Micro-Macroscopic Features:** The Capanna system (Table 8.2) allows ABCs to be categorized based on their morphology.

Table 8.2. *Capanna Classification System*

Type 1	Central well contained metaphyseal lesion.
Type 2	Lesion involving an entire segment of bone with cortical expansion and thinning.
Type 3	An eccentric metaphyseal lesion with no or minimal cortical expansion.
Type 4	Subperiosteal reaction with no or minimal cortical erosion.
Type 5	Periosteum displaced with the erosion of cortex and extension into cancellous bone.

Source: Paul, C. J., (2022). Benign bone tumors: An overview of what we know today. J. Clin. Med., 11(3), 699. doi: 10.3390/jcm11030699.

Most of these lesions (70%), when primary, are associated with recurrent chromosomal translocations causing gene fusions with ubiquitin-specific peptidase 6 (USP6). The other 30% arise with other benign bone tumors (BBTs).

- **Clinical Features:** ABCs are typically asymptomatic but can produce mild discomfort, soreness, and edema. Their rapid growth may resemble a cancerous tumor, which needs to be ruled out. Additional symptoms may manifest depending on the origin of the problem; if it originates from the spine, torticollis, scoliosis, or neurologic deficits may result. Additionally, when it arises near growth plates, it may lead to pathologic fractures or growth disorders.

- **Imaging:** ABCs are clearly defined by a sclerotic rim on plain X-rays. Pathologic fractures or periosteal reactions may result from them. The "soap bubble" appearance caused by the remaining trabeculae is a common finding. Usually, the cortical bone contains them. CT is a reliable tool for further investigation, particularly in sensitive areas such as the spine and pelvis. Multiple blood-filled cavities can be observed on an MRI. Conversely, septations within the lesion may become more apparent. In any case, a biopsy is necessary for confirmation due to similar malignant behavior (Figure 8.8).

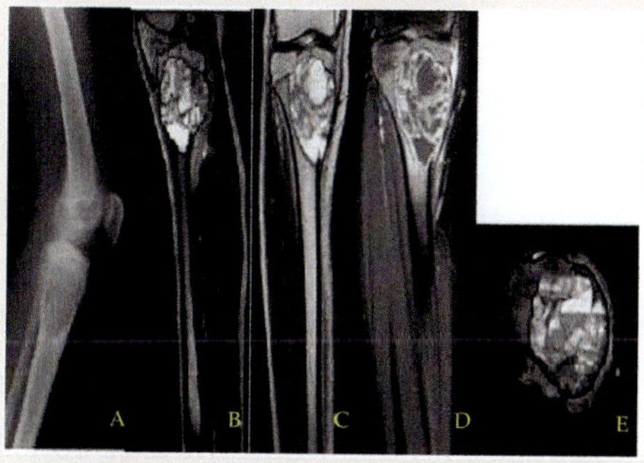

Figure 8.8. *Radiography (A) shows a very limited oval metaphyseal tibial osteolytic lesion. MRI cuts include sagittal T1-weighted (B), coronal T2 (C); T1 post-contrast (D); and axial T2 FATSAT (E); revealing partitions with a typical intralesional contrast-enhanced liquid level, indicative of an aneurysmal cyst.*

Source: Meryem, B., et al., (2013). Aneurysmal bone cyst primary. About eight pediatric cases: Radiological aspects and review of the literature. Pan African Medical Journal, 15, 111. doi: 10.11604/pamj.2013.15.111.2117.

- **Differential Diagnosis:** Unicameral bone cysts, giant cell tumors, telangiectatic osteosarcomas (malignant, exhibiting tissue enhancement during MRI examination), osteoblastomas, and chondroblastomas all require treatment.
- **Treatment:** The recommended course of care is surgery combined with curettage, resection, or bone grafting. Selective arterial embolization is a viable option when other treatments are ineffective for reaching central locations. Cryotherapy, chemical cauterization, sclerotherapy with polidocanol, and radionuclide ablation are additional options. Embolization is often performed before surgery to prevent excessive blood loss. In cases where surgical excision is not feasible, denosumab nonsurgical treatment may be considered. Although low doses of radiation can cause the lesion to ossify, they are not used due to the risk of malignant transformation. Certain injections, such as those containing zein (corn protein), absolute alcohol, and calcitonin and steroids administered under CT guidance, have shown success in certain trials. Despite being benign, this tumor tends to grow and can be locally aggressive and destructive, making excision treatment the preferred approach.

In routine clinical practice, BBTs are commonly encountered, especially in pediatric patients. It is crucial for clinicians to be able to identify them based on radiographic findings, clinical presentation, and symptoms, and take appropriate action to prevent misdiagnosis, as it can significantly impact the treatment course for patients.

8.3. Common Malignant Bone Tumors

Malignant (cancerous) tumors are more dangerous and rare than benign ones. Malignant tumors have a moderate to high chance of spreading from their original site of development. The lymphatic or blood vessels serve as routes for the spread of cancer cells. The most common sites for malignant bone tumors to metastasize are other bones or the lungs. Malignant bone tumors can occur at any age. Osteosarcoma and Ewing's sarcoma, two of the most common malignant bone tumors, typically affect individuals who are 30 years of age or younger. On the other hand, chondrosarcomas are malignant tumors that develop as cartilage-like tissue and usually manifest after the age of thirty. Primary malignant bone tumors, especially in adults, are far less common compared to metastatic bone tumors. Examples of primary malignant bone tumors include bone lymphoma, malignant giant cell tumor, fibrosarcoma, osteosarcoma, adamantinoma, chondrosarcoma, chordoma, Ewing sarcoma of bone, and fibrosarcoma and undifferentiated pleomorphic sarcoma.

8.3.1. Multiple Myeloma

One type of cancer that develops in white blood cells, known as plasma cells, is multiple myeloma. Healthy plasma cells aid in the fight against infections by producing antibodies. Antibodies are responsible for seeking out and combating pathogens. In multiple myeloma, the bone marrow becomes overpopulated with cancerous plasma cells. Blood cells are formed in the soft tissue called bone marrow, which is found inside bones. The cancer cells push out healthy blood cells from the bone marrow. Instead of producing beneficial antibodies, the cancer cells produce malfunctioning proteins. This leads to complications associated with multiple myeloma. Not every case of multiple myeloma requires immediate attention. If the multiple myeloma is not causing symptoms and is growing slowly, close observation may be the initial course of action. For those who require treatment for multiple myeloma, there are several ways to help control the disease.

8.3.1.1. Symptoms

In the early stages of multiple myeloma, there may be no symptoms or indicators.

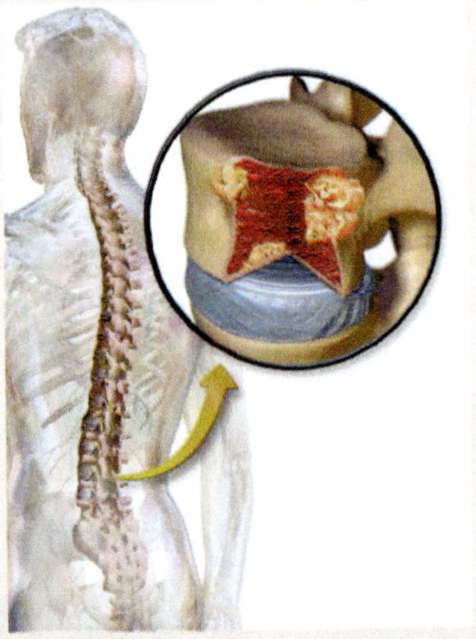

Figure 8.9. *Illustration showing the most common site of bone lesions in vertebrae.*

Source: Blausen Medical Communications, Inc., CC BY 3.0, https://commons.wikimedia.org/w/index.php?curid=27639943.

However, when they do appear, they may include:

- Bone pain, especially in the spine, chest, or hips;

- Nausea;
- Constipation;
- Loss of appetite;
- Mental fogginess or confusion;
- Tiredness;
- Infections;
- Weight loss;
- Weakness;
- Thirst;
- Needing to urinate often.

If concerned about any symptoms, please schedule a visit with a physician or other health care provider (Figure 8.9).

8.3.1.2. Causes

The cause of myeloma is unknown. The initial indication of multiple myeloma is the presence of a single plasma cell in the bone marrow. The bone marrow, which is the soft substance inside bones, is responsible for the production of blood cells. Due to an unknown factor, the plasma cell transforms into a malignant myeloma cell. This myeloma cell then rapidly divides, giving rise to numerous additional myeloma cells. Unlike healthy cells, which have a regulated growth rate and lifespan, cancer cells disrupt these regulations and produce an excessive number of cells. While healthy cells die as part of their natural cycle, cancer cells continue to survive. In individuals with myeloma, these cancer cells accumulate in the bone marrow, displacing healthy blood cells. This leads to fatigue and a weakened ability to fight infections. Myeloma cells persist in their production of antibodies, similar to healthy plasma cells. However, these antibodies, known as monoclonal proteins or M proteins, are not utilized by the body. Instead, the body experiences an accumulation of M proteins, which can result in various issues such as kidney damage. Additionally, myeloma cells have the ability to weaken bones and increase the risk of fractures.

8.3.1.2.1. A Connection with MGUS

MGUS, or monoclonal gammopathy of unknown significance, is the earliest diagnosis of multiple myeloma. M protein levels in the blood are low in MGUS. The body is not harmed by the M proteins.

8.3.1.3. Risk Factors

Factors that may increase the risk of multiple myeloma include:

- Getting older. Most people are diagnosed in their late 60s.
- Being male. The disease is more common in men than in women.
- Being Black. Multiple myeloma is more common in Black people than in other racial groups.
- Having multiple myeloma in one's family increases the likelihood of developing the illness if one's parent or sibling has it.
- Possessing MGUS, or monoclonal gammopathy of unknown significance, raises the risk of developing multiple myeloma as MGUS is its precursor.

It is impossible to avoid multiple myeloma.

8.3.1.4. Diagnosis

Multiple myeloma can occasionally be discovered by a medical professional during a blood test conducted for another illness. In some cases, the symptoms may prompt the medical provider to perform a multiple myeloma test.

Tests and procedures used to diagnose multiple myeloma include:

- **Blood Tests:** A blood sample can reveal the presence of M proteins produced by myeloma cells. Blood tests may also detect the production of beta-2-microglobulin, another protein produced by myeloma cells.

Additional blood tests, such as those for blood cell counts, calcium levels, uric acid levels, and kidney function, can provide further insights for the healthcare team.

- **Urine Tests:** Urine samples may contain M proteins, which are known as Bence Jones proteins.
- **Bone Marrow Tests:** Samples of bone marrow are obtained through bone marrow aspiration and bone marrow biopsy. Bone marrow consists of a solid and a liquid component. During a bone marrow biopsy, a small sample of solid tissue is taken using a needle. A bone marrow aspiration involves taking a sample of fluid with a needle. The hip bone is typically used to obtain these samples.

The samples are then tested in a laboratory to search for myeloma cells. Additional specialized testing, such as the fluorescence *in situ* hybridization test, can provide further details about the genetic material (DNA) of the cells.

- **Imaging Tests:** These tests can reveal bone abnormalities associated with multiple myeloma. Examples of imaging tests include MRI, CT scan, X-ray, and PET (positron emission tomography) scan.

8.3.1.4.1. Stages

The stage of the myeloma is determined by patient's healthcare team based on the results of their tests. There are three stages of multiple myeloma. The stage indicates to medical team the rate of growth of the myeloma. A multiple myeloma in stage 1 is expanding slowly. The myeloma gets more aggressive as the stages rise. A multiple myeloma in stage 3 is rapidly worsening. A risk level can also be assigned to multiple myeloma. This is another method of expressing the disease's level of aggression. The medical team plans the treatment based on the prognosis and the multiple myeloma stage and risk level.

8.3.1.5. Treatment

Treatment for multiple myeloma is not always required immediately. If the myeloma does not exhibit any symptoms, testing may be conducted to monitor its progression. The initial approach to managing multiple myeloma symptoms typically involves medication. Therapy can help alleviate discomfort, manage side effects, and inhibit the growth of myeloma cells. There are cases when multiple myeloma is asymptomatic, referred to as smoldering multiple myeloma by doctors. Immediate treatment may not be necessary for this type of multiple myeloma. If the myeloma is small and growing slowly, regular examinations may be recommended to monitor the cancer. A medical professional may conduct blood and urine tests to detect any signs of worsening myeloma. If multiple myeloma symptoms arise, treatment may be initiated in consultation with the healthcare team.

Treatment options may include:

- **Targeted Therapy:** This treatment utilizes drugs that specifically target certain chemicals present in cancer cells. By inhibiting the function of these substances, targeted therapies can effectively kill cancer cells.
- **Immunotherapy:** It is a medical treatment that stimulates the immune system to eliminate cancer cells from the body. While the immune system naturally targets

foreign cells and bacteria to prevent illness, cancer cells can evade detection. Immunotherapy enhances the immune system's ability to recognize and eliminate cancerous cells.

- **CAR-T Cell Therapy:** Also known as chimeric antigen receptor T cell therapy, this treatment modifies immune system cells to combat multiple myeloma. Blood is first treated by removing some white blood cells, including T cells. The cells are then sent to the laboratory where they are altered to produce unique receptors. These receptors enable the cells to identify a surface marker on myeloma cells.
- The modified cells are reintroduced into the body, where they can locate and eliminate the numerous myeloma cells.
- **Chemotherapy:** It involves administering potent medications to kill cancer cells. These medications target rapidly proliferating cells, including myeloma cells.
- **Corticosteroids:** These medications help regulate inflammation, swelling, and irritability in the body. They also combat myeloma cells.
- **Bone Marrow Transplant:** Also known as a stem cell transplant, involves replacing diseased bone marrow with healthy bone marrow.

Blood-forming stem cells are extracted from the body prior to a bone marrow transplant. The diseased bone marrow is then eradicated using high doses of chemotherapy. The stem cells are subsequently infused into the body, where they migrate to the bones and initiate the regeneration of bone marrow. Autologous bone marrow transplants involve the use of the individual's own cells in the transplantation process.

Occasionally, the donor of the stem cells may be a healthy individual. This type of transplant is referred to as an allogenic bone marrow transplant.

- **Radiation Therapy:** Strong energy beams are employed in radiation therapy to eliminate cancer cells. Protons, X-rays, and other energy sources can be utilized. Radiation can effectively halt the growth of myeloma cells. If myeloma cells form a mass called plasmacytoma, radiation therapy may be employed. It can also be used to manage a bone-destroying or painful plasmacytoma.

8.3.1.5.1. How Treatments Are Used?

The course of the treatment will be determined by the likelihood of a bone marrow transplant. The healthcare team takes a number of factors into account when determining whether a bone marrow transplant is the best option for you. These include patient's age, general health, and the likelihood that their multiple myeloma will worsen.

- When a transplant of bone marrow is a possibility, the treatment plan will likely start with a combination of medications if the medical team determines that a bone marrow transplant is a good option for you. Corticosteroids, immunotherapy, targeted therapy, and occasionally chemotherapy may be included in the combination.

Blood stem cells are extracted from the blood following several months of therapy. The transplant of bone marrow may occur shortly after the cell collection. If there is a relapse, the patient could also wait until after it has occurred. For patients with multiple myeloma, doctors may recommend two bone marrow transplants.

Immunotherapy or targeted therapy will probably follow the bone marrow transplant. By doing so, the myeloma may be prevented from returning.

- When a bone marrow transplant is not a viable alternative, treatment options may include a combination of medications. This combination may consist of corticosteroids, immunotherapy, targeted therapy, and occasionally chemotherapy.
- In cases where the cancer returns or does not improve with treatment, repeating the same treatment could be considered as part of the treatment plan. Additionally, trying one or more of the available multiple myeloma treatments is another option.

8.3.1.5.2. Treating Complications

Treating complications associated with multiple myeloma is also an important part of the overall regimen. For example:

- Bone pain can be managed using radiation therapy, painkillers, and surgery.
- Severe kidney damage may require dialysis.
- Vaccines can help prevent infections such as pneumonia and the flu.
- Medications that promote bone growth can help prevent bone loss.
- Persistent anemia can be alleviated by medications that boost red blood cell production in the bloodstream.

8.3.2. Osteosarcoma (Osteogenic Sarcoma)

Osteosarcoma is the most prevalent primary bone cancer in children and is caused by primitive mesenchymal cells that form osteoid tissue. It accounts for approximately 20% of all primary bone tumors and occurs in two forms: primary (without underlying bone pathology) and secondary (underlying pathology that has undergone malignant degeneration/conversion). The manifestation of osteosarcoma is highly heterogeneous, allowing for subtyping based on the degree of differentiation, location within the bone, and histological variation. The biological behavior, demographics, and imaging appearance of these subtypes differ.

8.3.2.1. Signs and Symptoms

Many patients initially experience pain that may worsen at night, be sporadic, and range in severity, often persisting for an extended period of time. Active teenagers engaged in sports frequently report pain in the lower part of the thigh or just below the knee. A large tumor may cause noticeable localized swelling. In some cases, a sudden fracture could be the first sign due to the weakened state of the affected bone. Deep-seated tumors, like those originating in the pelvis, may not result in visible swelling on the skin's surface.

8.3.2.2. Causes

Numerous research teams are investigating the possibility of cancer stem cells causing tumors, as well as the genes and proteins responsible for various phenotypes. Rarely, radiation therapy for unrelated illnesses could be a contributing factor.

- The tumor cells of low-grade osteosarcoma (OS), such as low-grade central OS and paraosteal OS, contain a small supernumerary marker chromosome or a giant rod chromosome that carries multiple potentially cancer-causing genes and is assumed to play a role in the development of these OS.

- A higher risk of developing osteosarcoma is linked to familial cases where the retinoblastoma gene is rendered inactive due to chromosome 13q14 loss.
- Osteosarcoma is more common in people with bone dysplasias, such as Paget's disease of the bone, fibrous dysplasia, enchondromatosis, and hereditary multiple exostoses.
- Li-Fraumeni syndrome, caused by a germline TP53 mutation, increases the risk of developing osteosarcoma.
- Rothmund-Thomson syndrome (i.e., This disease is more common in people with an autosomal recessive association of congenital bone defects, hypogonadism, hair and skin dysplasias, and cataracts.
- High levels of Sr-90, known as the "bone seeker," elevate the likelihood of bone cancer and leukemia in animals, and it is believed to have similar effects on humans.

Water fluoridation has no conclusive link to cancer or cancer-related deaths, either for osteosarcoma or bone cancer in particular or for cancer in general. Numerous studies have concluded that there is no correlation between fluoride concentration in water and osteosarcoma. The US National Toxicology Program study from 1990, which revealed equivocal evidence of a connection between fluoride and osteosarcoma in male rats, is the source of the beliefs surrounding the relationship between fluoride exposure and osteosarcoma. However, there is still no conclusive proof that fluoride causes cancer in mice. Worldwide, water fluoridation has been implemented to enhance the oral health of the public. It is also considered a significant health achievement. Water supplies are subject to regulations regarding fluoride concentration levels. For example, the United States Environmental Protection Agency limits fluoride levels to 4 milligrams per liter. Although fluoride is naturally present in water supplies, many communities have chosen to supplement with fluoride to the extent that it can prevent tooth decay. It is also well known that fluoride can promote the growth of new bone. Further investigation, however, reveals no human risk of osteosarcoma from fluoridated water. The majority of the research involved tallying the number of cases of osteosarcoma patients in specific regions with varying fluoride concentrations in drinking water. There is no discernible difference in the incidence of osteosarcoma cases across fluoridated regions, according to the statistical analysis of the data. Another significant study was conducted to compare the fluoride concentration of bone samples from patients with osteosarcoma to that of newly diagnosed malignant bone tumors. As a result, there is no discernible difference between the median fluoride concentrations in bone samples from patients with osteosarcoma and tumor controls. The fluoride exposures and concentrations in the bones of osteosarcoma patients are similar to those of healthy individuals.

8.3.2.3. Mechanism

Osteosarcomas typically develop at locations where bone is growing, most likely due to the proliferation of osteoblastic cells in this area and their increased likelihood of acquiring mutations that could cause cellular transformation (p53 and the RB genes are frequently implicated in this process). The tumor is usually located at the end of a long bone, specifically in the metaphysis. The distal end of the femur or the proximal end of the tibia or humerus are the most frequently affected sites. Osteosarcoma typically affects the knee in 60% of cases, followed by the hip in 15%, the shoulder in 10%, and the jaw in 8% of cases. On X-ray examination, the tumor appears solid, hard, and irregular due to tumor spicules of calcified bone radiating at right angles (resembling a fir-tree, moth-eaten appearance, or sunburst pattern). The Codman triangle, formed by these right angles, is a characteristic feature of osteosarcoma, although not diagnostic. Surrounding tissues may become infected (Figure 8.10).

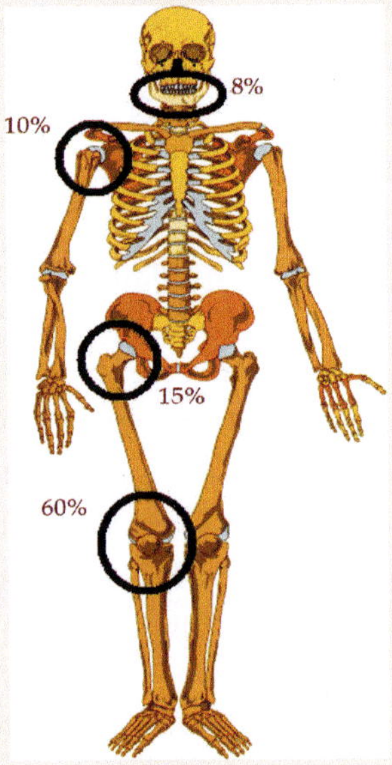

Figure 8.10. *Predilections of osteosarcoma.*

Source: By Human_skeleton_front_-_no_labels.svg: Mikael Häggströmderivative work: Madhero88 – Human_skeleton_front_-_no_labels.svg, CC BY-SA 3.0, https://commons.wikimedia.org/w/index.php?curid=5805909.

Microscopically, the presence of osteoid, or bone formation, within the tumor is a characteristic feature of osteosarcoma. Anaplastic tumor cells exhibit pleomorphism, with some displaying giant size and multiple atypical mitoses. Osteoid, which describes irregular trabeculae (amorphous, eosinophilic/pink) with or without central calcification (hematoxylinophilic/blue, granular), is produced by these cells and refers to tumor bone. Tumor cells are found within the osteoid matrix. Tumors can be classified into different groups based on the characteristics of the tumor cells, such as whether they resemble bone, cartilage, or fibroblast cells. Multinucleated osteoclast-like giant cells have been observed in osteosarcomas.

8.3.2.4. Diagnosis

X-rays are the primary imaging method for diagnosing osteosarcoma. On X-rays, osteosarcoma can be identified by features such as a sunburst appearance and the Codman triangle, which is the result of the tumor elevating the bony cortex and creating new bone. A CT scan can be used to define the bony anatomy, evaluate ossification (the laying down of new bone materials) and cartilage calcification, as well as to detect pathologic fractures. However, an MRI scan provides a better image of the medullary cavity and soft tissue (Figure 8.11).

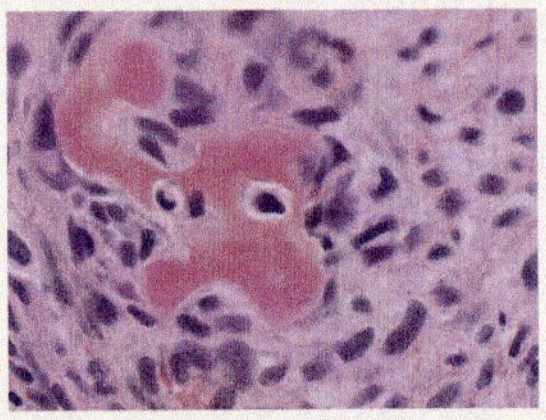

Figure 8.11. *Histopathology of osteosarcoma, showing tumor cells with high nuclear pleomorphism, but relatively less so in cells entrapped in neoplastic bone matrix (appearing pink on this H&E stained slide).*

Source: By Mikael Häggström, M.D. Author info – Reusing images – Conflicts of interest:NoneMikael Häggström, M.D. Consent note: Consent from the patient or patient's relatives is regarded as redundant, because of absence of identifiable features (List of HIPAA identifiers) in the media and case information. – Own work, CC0, https://commons.wikimedia.org/w/index.php?curid=105063019.

Early symptoms of osteosarcoma are typically detected on X-rays obtained during routine dental examinations. Dentists, who are trained to recognize potential warning signs of the disease, can often identify a symmetrical widening of the periodontal ligament space. If a dentist suspects osteosarcoma or another underlying condition, they would refer the patient to an oral and maxillofacial surgeon for a biopsy. If osteosarcoma is suspected outside of the face, an orthopedic oncologist with the necessary training should perform the biopsy. According to the American Cancer Society, it is particularly important to carry out this treatment correctly in the case of osteosarcoma. Incorrect biopsy procedures could result in the affected limb needing to be amputated. Osteosarcoma can also spread to the lungs, where it typically appears as one or more spherical nodules on a chest X-ray, usually in the lower regions.

Variants include:

- Conventional: osteoblastic, chondroblastic, fibroblastic OS;
- Telangiectatic OS;
- Small cell OS;
- Low-grade central OS;
- Periosteal OS;
- Paraosteal OS;
- Secondary OS;
- High-grade surface OS;
- Extraskeletal OS.

8.3.2.5. Treatment

The preferred course of treatment for osteosarcoma is a total radical surgical en-bloc resection of the cancer. While most patients can undergo limb-salvage surgery, complications can necessitate additional surgery or amputation, especially in cases of infection, prosthetic loosening, and non-union, or local tumor recurrence. In order to lower the risk of cancer recurrence, mifamurtide is administered to patients following surgery to remove the tumor and in conjunction with chemotherapy to eradicate any remaining cancer cells. Additionally, after the tumor is removed, rotationplasty is an option.

The best doctors to treat patients with osteosarcoma are medical oncologists and orthopedic oncologists who have dealt with sarcomas before. Neoadjuvant chemotherapy, or chemotherapy administered before surgery, is the current standard of care, which is followed by surgical resection. An indication of the prognosis and information on whether to modify the chemotherapy regimen following surgery can be obtained from the percentage of tumor cell necrosis (cell death) observed in the tumor following surgery. Conventional treatment involves limb-salvage orthopedic surgery (or amputation in certain cases) and a combination of intra-arterial cisplatin, adriamycin, ifosfamide with mesna, BCD (bleomycin, cyclophosphamide, and dactinomycin), etoposide, and muramyl tripeptide in addition to high-dose methotrexate with leucovorin rescue. Rotationplasty is an option. If the rate of necrosis is low, ifosfamide may be used as an adjuvant treatment.

Even though osteosarcoma responds well to chemotherapy, it has one of the lowest rates of survival for pediatric cancers. With an aggressive intra-arterial regimen that individualizes therapy based on arteriographic response, the best reported 10-year survival rate is 92%. In certain studies, the five-year survival rate varies from 60% to 85+%, while the three-year event-free survival (EFS) rate falls between 50% and 75%. Approximately 65–70% of patients who received treatment five years ago will still be alive today. The overall averages of these survival rates differ significantly based on the rate of necrosis in each individual case. Pegfilgrastim and filgrastim aid in neutrophil and white blood cell counts. Epoetin alfa and blood transfusions are helpful for anemia. While phenotypes have demonstrated an increased role for tumor microenvironments, computational analysis on a panel of osteosarcoma cell lines has revealed new shared and specific therapeutic targets (proteomic and genetic) in osteosarcoma.

8.3.2.6. Prognosis

Prognosis is separated into three groups.

- Rarely, stage I osteosarcoma can be low-grade central osteosarcoma or parosteal osteosarcoma. With wide resection, it has an excellent prognosis (>90%).
- The prognosis of stage II depends on various aspects such as the site and size of the tumor, among others. Other pathological factors, including the degree of p-glycoprotein, whether the tumor is cxcr4-positive or Her2-positive, are also important. Metastasis to the lung is another aspect where fewer metastases are associated with better survival.
- The degree of necrosis in the primary tumor, the number of metastases, and the resectability of the lung nodules are the determining factors in the initial presentation of stage III osteosarcoma with lung metastases. The overall probability of survival is approximately 30%.

The number of children's cancer deaths attributed to malignant neoplasms of the bones and joints is unknown. The annual decline in osteosarcoma-related mortality has been approximately 1.3%. Osteosarcoma long-term survival rates increased significantly in the latter half of the 20th century, reaching approximately 68% in 2009.

8.3.2.7. Epidemiology

Osteosarcoma represents 2.4% of all pediatric cancer cases and approximately 20% of all primary bone cancers, making it the eighth most common type of childhood cancer. The prevalence of osteosarcoma in the U.S. Incidence rates for osteosarcoma in U.S. patients under 20 years of age are estimated at 5.0 per million per year in the general population, with a slight variation between individuals of black, Hispanic, and white ethnicities (6.8, 6.5, and 4.6 per million per year, respectively). It is slightly more common in males (5.4 per million per year) than in females (4.0 per million per year). The femur accounts for 42% of its genesis, the tibia for 19%, and the humerus for 10% of the cause. It is more commonly found in the metaphyseal region of tubular long bones. Around 8% of cases involve the skull and jaw, and 8% involve the pelvis.

Each year, about 300 out of the 900 Americans who receive a diagnosis will pass away. An underlying bone pathology, such as Paget's disease of the bone, is typically linked to a second peak in incidence that occurs in the elderly.

8.3.3. Adamantinoma

Adamantinomas are uncommon bone tumors that are typically found in the tibia and are considered to be low-grade malignant. The origin of these tumors is uncertain, but they share histological similarities with ameloblastoma, a tumor commonly found in the jaw. Adamantinoma is characterized by a mixture of epithelial cells and osteofibrous components. There are two types of adamantinomas – classical and differentiated, with the latter resembling osteofibrous dysplasia. While imaging techniques have improved, a definitive diagnosis of adamantinoma still requires histopathological examination.

8.3.3.1. Etiology

The cause of adamantinoma is still unknown at this time. According to a widely recognized pathogenesis theory, the skin's basal epithelial cells migrate early in the embryonic process. The anterior tibia, where the enchondral bone formation is closest to the skin's surface, is the most frequently occurring site of adamantinoma, which lends credence to this theory.

Certain findings from ultrastructural and immunohistochemical studies indicate that adamantinoma may have an epithelial genesis. It is still up for debate, though, whether osteofibrous dysplasia and adamantinoma are related. The diagnosis, prognosis, and course of treatment for patients with adamantinoma are all impacted by the potential correlation between these two conditions.

8.3.3.2. Epidemiology

Adamantinoma represents 0.4% of primary malignant bone tumors, making it a rare tumor. With a male-to-female ratio of 5:4, this tumor shows a slight male predominance. Adamantinomas primarily affect people in their 20s to 40s; they are uncommon in younger and elderly populations. Even though they most frequently affect the tibia's anterior metaphysis or diaphysis, adamantinomas can also affect the fibula, ulna, femur, humerus, and radius.

8.3.3.3. Pathophysiology

Both classic and osteofibrous dysplasia-like adamantinomas exhibit a consistent pattern of numerical abnormalities, with extra copies of chromosomes 7, 8, 12, 19, and 21.

8.3.3.4. Histopathology

8.3.3.4.1. Macroscopic Findings

Typically, well-defined, yellowish-gray cortical tumors are the outward manifestation of classical adamantinomas. These tumors are lobulated and have a firm-to-bony consistency. Peripheral sclerosis is frequently present in conjunction with these tumors. Sometimes the tumors present as multiple lesions, but other times they present as a single lesion. Macroscopically, the tumor's visible cystic spaces are often filled with a blood-like or straw-colored fluid.

8.3.3.4.2. Histological Findings

Differentiable epithelial and osteofibrous components, which can be combined in different ratios and with different patterns of differentiation, define classical adamantinomas. In classic adamantinoma, four main patterns of differentiation are seen: spindle cell, squamous, tubular, and basaloid. The tubular and basaloid patterns of classic adamantinoma are the most commonly observed, though all four patterns may coexist. Spindle cells are frequently found lining cystic spaces, in recurrences, and in metastases. The osteofibrous component consists of storiformly arranged spindle cells, usually associated with woven bone trabeculae in or close to the lesion center. At the margin of the tumor, osteoblasts prominently surround these trabeculae and show differing degrees of transformation to lamellar bone.

Mast cells or multinucleated giant cells are infrequently found, and foam cells or myxoid changes may be present. Typically, there is little mitotic activity within the tumor. The predominance of osteofibrous tissue characterizes the osteofibrous dysplasia-like variant, which is the fifth histological pattern. Small clusters of epithelial cells in this variation can only be found by immunohistochemistry or close inspection. It is important to sample adamantinoma extensively, particularly when it is differentiated and the epithelial component is only present in specific areas.

8.3.3.4.3. Immunohistochemical Study

Adamantinoma is characterized by the coexpression of keratin, vimentin, p63, epithelial membrane antigen (EMA), and podoplanin in the epithelial cells, while the fibrous tissue component tests positive for vimentin. In contrast to osteofibrous dysplasia-like adamantinoma, classic adamantinoma exhibits the presence of estrogen, progesterone, and N-cadherin. The epithelial component of classic adamantinomas is encircled by a continuous basement membrane made of collagen IV, laminin, and galectin 3. In less distinct epithelial islands, however, there might be several breaks or no basement membrane at all. Only the epithelial component expresses both the epidermal growth factor (EGF) and the epidermal growth factor receptor (EGFR). Conversely, both components contain fibroblast growth factor 2 (FGF2) and fibroblast growth factor receptor 1 (FGFR1). Adamantinoma cells also express receptor activator of nuclear factor kappa-B ligand (RANKL) and macrophage colony-stimulating factor (M-CSF) in culture, which may be involved in the osteolysis seen.

8.3.3.5. History and Physical

The clinical course of adamantinomas is usually prolonged and characterized by slow, progressive growth. The main issue raised by patients is the gradual enlargement, which may or may not be accompanied by pain. Patients may also need to seek medical attention due to bone deformities and the possibility of pathological fractures. Furthermore, when the spine is impacted, some patients may show neurological deficits. It is noteworthy that pathological fractures may occur in up to 23% of patients with adamantinoma. Because of the disease's mild symptoms and slow course in the beginning, it may go unnoticed. Delays in diagnosis and treatment occur because patients frequently endure symptoms for years before seeking medical attention.

8.3.3.6. Evaluation

8.3.3.6.1. Plain Radiograph

Adamantinoma typically presents on X-ray as a well-circumscribed, multilobulated, osteolytic tumor of the cortical structure. Peripheral sclerosis, septation, and intralesional opacities may also be observed. Multiple foci within the same bone are commonly seen.

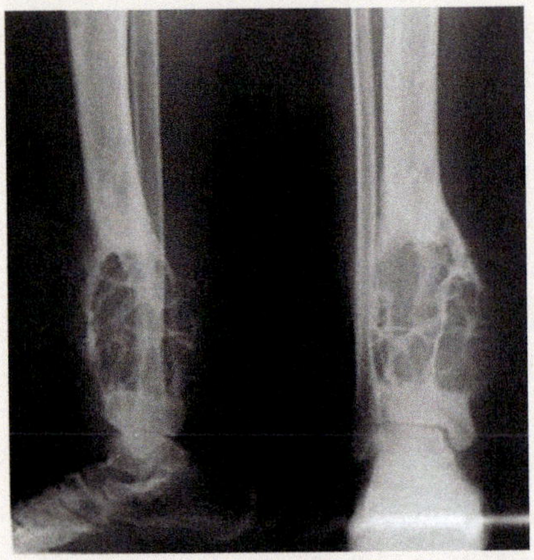

Figure 8.12. *Radiograph showing an adamantinoma in the distal tibia with lytic expansive changes.*

Source: By T-rex89 (Original) and Hellerhoff (cutting part of image and retouching) – File: Adamantinoma.jpg, CC BY-SA 4.0, https://commons.wikimedia.org/w/index.php?curid=98360985.

This characteristic "soap-bubble" appearance is created by ring-shaped densities encircling the multifocal radiolucencies. Generally, the lesion is confined to the intracortical area and extends along the length of the bone. However, in some cases, it can cause cortical destruction and infiltrate the surrounding soft tissues, periosteum, or medullary cavity. In such situations, the lesion is usually accompanied by a lamellar or solid periosteal reaction (Figure 8.12).

8.3.3.6.2. Computed Tomography (CT) Scan

An efficient way to visualize the soft tissue extension and cortical involvement of adamantinomas is through a computed tomography (CT) scan. However, CT scans may not provide detailed imaging of the intraosseous extension of these tumors. CT scans are useful in detecting pulmonary metastases and are an essential part of the standard diagnostic evaluation of adamantinomas.

8.3.3.6.3. Magnetic Resonance Imaging

The use of magnetic resonance imaging (MRI) is crucial for the locoregional staging of adamantinomas as it allows for precise visualization of soft tissue extension, intramedullary involvement, and distant cortical foci. Establishing tumor-free margins is a critical aspect of surgical planning to ensure complete tumor removal, and MRI serves as a valuable tool in this process. When reconstructive surgery is required, MRI helps determine the most appropriate course of action by assessing the extent of the disease.

MRI reveals two morphological patterns of adamantinoma:

- Multiple small nodules in one or more foci; and
- A solitary lobulated focus.

On T1-weighted images, adamantinomas typically exhibit low signal intensity, while on T2-weighted images, they show high signal intensity. However, it is important to note that these results are nonspecific and can be applicable to various other conditions.

8.3.3.7. Treatment/Management

Treatment for Adamantinoma: The initial step is crucial and necessitates a meticulous biopsy without curettage. Curettage is associated with recurrence, and after intralesional curettage, the recurrence rate in typical adamantinoma can reach up to 90%. Following marginal excision, the local recurrence rate of these adamantinoma tumors can reach 32%. In one study, the local recurrence rate for patients who underwent resection was 29%, while the local recurrence rate for patients who underwent curettage was 100%.

8.3.3.7.1. Resection

The primary approach in treating adamantinoma is to surgically remove the bone tumor through wide-margin excision and en-bloc removal. Reconstruction of the resulting bony defect is performed after tumor removal. Various methods can be employed to fill the bone defect, including distraction osteogenesis, endoprosthesis or tailored prostheses, vascularized autografts, and intercalary allografts.

8.3.3.7.2. Recurrence of Adamantinoma

It is widely acknowledged that the behavior of adamantinoma can be highly unpredictable. Therefore, individuals diagnosed with adamantinoma should undergo long-term monitoring, often exceeding 15 years. Routine monitoring should include physical examinations to check for lymphadenopathy and lung imaging, typically conducted annually or in the event of local recurrence. Surgical resection is recommended for the treatment of metastatic lesions and recurrences detected during routine monitoring.

8.3.3.7.3. Metastasectomy of Pulmonary Recurrences

Metastasectomy is the standard of care for pulmonary recurrences. A Dutch study found no discernible effects on tumor volume or survival from chemotherapy or radiation therapy. The effectiveness of radiation therapy and chemotherapy in treating adamantinoma has been shown to be limited.

8.3.3.7.4. Radiation Therapy

Radiation therapy can help alleviate back pain and potentially reduce the need for opioid analgesics, although it is generally ineffective in directly treating adamantinoma. Additionally, targeted treatment with tyrosine kinase inhibitors has shown long-lasting results in some patients.

8.3.3.7.5. Amputation

In cases where local recurrence occurs and limb salvage or en-bloc resection are not feasible options, amputation may be necessary for adamantinoma. Importantly, there is no significant difference in survival rates between limb salvage and amputation. Curestigation is not recommended due to the high rate of recurrence.

8.3.3.8. Differential Diagnosis

Several authors have reported a strong correlation between osteofibrous dysplasia and differentiated adamantinoma, also known as osteofibrous dysplasia-like adamantinoma. This connection can pose challenges in the differential diagnosis due to their common location in the tibia, similar histological and radiological features, and other factors. Adamantinoma can mimic various bone tumors clinically, radiologically, and histologically. These include bone cysts, giant cell tumors, and malignant tumors such as chondrosarcoma, angiosarcoma, and metastases.

8.3.3.9. Prognosis

Adamantinoma is a neoplasm that is highly aggressive locally and has the potential to metastasize. Without proper surgical treatment, the tumor frequently recurs.

The following are risk factors for recurring or spreading diseases:

- Symptoms lasting for less than five years;
- Male gender;
- Patients younger than 20;
- Pain upon presentation;
- Initial treatment involving curettage or resection;
- Absence of squamous differentiation within the tumor;
- An increase in the epithelium-to-stroma ratio.

About 15% to 30% of cases of adamantinomas have the potential to spread, usually through hematogenous or lymphatic routes. The lungs, lymph nodes, bones, and viscera of the abdomen are common sites for metastasis.

8.3.3.10. Complications

The recurrence rate of adamantinoma ranges from 30% to 35%. Adamantinoma-related deaths occur at a rate of 6% to 18%. In 12% to 29% of cases, there is a possibility of metastasis to the lung or lymph nodes.

8.3.3.11. Consultations

Evaluation of adamantinoma should be conducted by orthopedic and oncology specialists, as mentioned below.

- **Orthopedics:** Surgeons specializing in orthopedics play a crucial role in identifying, treating, and reconstructing bone tumors, including adamantinoma.
- **Oncology:** Medical or radiation oncologists provide their expertise in adjuvant therapies and systemic treatment for adamantinoma.

- **Surgical Oncology:** It involves comprehensive surgical care and coordination of treatment plans for patients diagnosed with adamantinoma.

8.3.3.12. Deterrence and Patient Education

The management of adamantinoma must include patient education. Healthcare professionals should discuss the following important points with patients when providing education:

- **Explanation of the Condition:** Healthcare professionals' main duty is to give patients a succinct and straightforward explanation of adamantinoma, emphasizing its uncommonness and aggressive characteristics as a bone tumor. They should also emphasize to the patients the locally invasive nature of adamantinoma and its primary location in the bones, such as the anterior tibia.
- **Symptoms and Metastasis:** A slow-growing swelling with or without pain is one of the common symptoms that healthcare professionals should talk about with patients when educating them. Additionally, it should be disclosed to patients that 15%–30% of cases of adamantinoma have the potential to metastasize to the lungs or lymph nodes.
- **Recurrence:** It is important to draw attention to the high recurrence rate of adamantinoma, which remains at roughly 33% even following excision. To detect recurrences early, healthcare professionals should stress the value of patient monitoring and long-term follow-up care.
- **Patience and Timeliness:** Medical practitioners should inform patients that adamantinoma recovery is a gradual process to set reasonable expectations. Potential options for reconstructive procedures following tumor excision should be discussed with patients to restore both function and esthetics.
- **Mental Health:** Key elements of an effective treatment plan include stressing the importance of mental health, providing counseling to patients and their families, and pointing out resources that can be used to address patients' emotional needs. Healthcare professionals ought to advise patients that experiencing anxiety or depression is a typical psychological reaction to receiving an adamantinoma diagnosis.

8.3.3.13. Enhancing Healthcare Team Outcomes

Patients with adamantinoma require the best possible care, which necessitates a multidisciplinary team of specialists from various medical fields, including orthopedics, pathology, medical and surgical oncology, and imaging. The combined expertise of these specialists is crucial to ensure accurate diagnosis, prognosis, and comprehensive patient care. To reach a definitive diagnosis and determine the most effective treatment plan, the involvement of musculoskeletal radiologists and pathologists in the interpretation of imaging data and tissue samples is essential. Additionally, the inclusion of a pain management expert is important to alleviate discomfort and improve the quality of life for adamantinoma patients, as effective pain management is vital to their overall care. Given that adamantinoma patients often experience anxiety and depression, it is advisable for patients and their families to seek counseling from a mental health nurse.

In the oncology unit, nurses play a vital role in patient education, follow-up, and care coordination. It is their responsibility to inform patients and their families about the available treatment options, pain management techniques, and support services. For patients with advanced adamantinoma, a palliative care team is crucial. This specialized team focuses on alleviating symptoms and improving the overall well-being of patients. Orthopedic oncologists are essential in developing and implementing a comprehensive treatment plan for patients, which includes tumor extraction and reconstructive surgery when necessary. Their expertise is crucial in accurately diagnosing the condition and selecting the most appropriate treatment approach based on microscopic, radiographic, and gross findings. After therapy, patients need to be closely monitored for an extended period to detect any extraosseous metastases or tumor recurrence. To enhance patient outcomes and quality of life, a collaborative interprofessional team approach is necessary.

8.3.4. Chondrosarcoma

Malignant cartilaginous neoplasms, or chondrosarcomas, can exhibit a variety of morphological characteristics and clinical manifestations. Approximately 20% of all primary malignant bone tumors belong to this category. Typically, they originate in the pelvis or long bones. Unlike the less common secondary tumors that develop within an existing enchondroma or osteochondroma, primary or conventional chondrosarcoma arises from preexisting normal bone. The three subgroups of conventional chondrosarcoma—the central, periosteal, and peripheral subgroups—account for 85–90% of all chondrosarcomas. Variants of non-conventional chondrosarcoma include dedifferentiated chondrosarcoma, mesenchymal chondrosarcoma, and clear cell chondrosarcoma. A definitive diagnosis of chondrosarcoma can often be made solely through imaging examination, as the radiographic features of the disease are frequently highly distinctive (Figure 8.13).

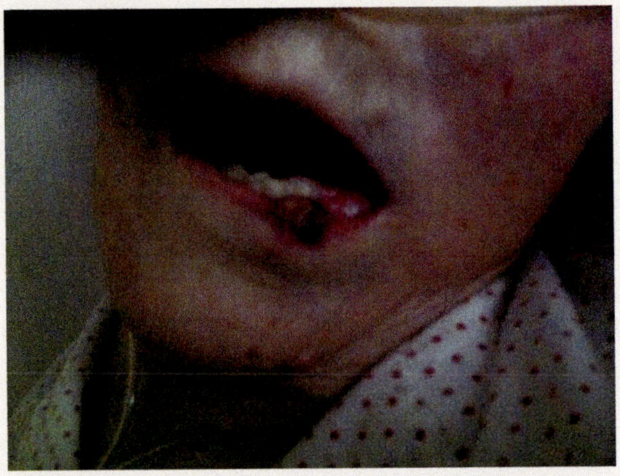

Figure 8.13. *Metastatic chondrosarcoma at the lower lip.*

8.3.4.1. Etiology

The malignant transformation of osteochondromas and enchondromas can lead to chondrosarcomas, although most of these cases are sporadic. Out of all osteochondromas, 5% develop multiple or solitary forms of malignant transformation.

8.3.4.2. Epidemiology

Primary central chondrosarcoma ranks third among primary bone cancers, following osteosarcoma and myeloma. Chondrosarcoma is a tumor that typically occurs in individuals of maturity and advanced age. When diagnosed, the majority of patients are older than 50, with a slight male predominance. The axial skeleton (pelvis, scapula, sternum, and ribs) and the proximal femur and proximal humerus are the most frequently involved locations of chondrosarcoma. Involvement of the hands and feet is uncommon.

8.3.4.3. Pathophysiology

Certain types of chondrosarcoma have been linked to chromosomal abnormalities such as 9p21, 10, 13q14, and 17p13. Genetic instability and chromosomal structural abnormalities have been documented in well-differentiated chondrosarcomas examined by cytogenetics. Furthermore, amplification of AP-1 and MYC transcription factors is essential to the pathophysiology of chondrosarcoma.

8.3.4.4. Histopathology

8.3.4.4.1. Macroscopic Findings

Chondrosarcomas are large tumors that typically measure more than 4 cm. The presence of hyaline cartilage is indicated by their translucent lobular, blue-gray, or white-cut surface. There might be areas with cystic changes and myxoid or mucoid material. Mineralization commonly occurs, characterized by yellow-white chalky areas of calcium deposit. Visible erosion and destruction of soft tissue may be observed.

8.3.4.4.2. Microscopic Findings

Chondrosarcomas exhibit abundant production of the blue-gray cartilage matrix. Irregularly shaped cartilage lobules of varying sizes and forms are present. Fibrous bands penetrate the bone trabeculae or divide these lobules. Calcified regions indicating the existence of a preexisting enchondroma are often found. The chondrocytes in chondrosarcomas differ from other chondrocytes; they have enlarged hyperchromatic nuclei and vary in size and shape. Binucleation is commonly observed. Chondroid matrix liquefaction or myxoid changes are typical characteristics of chondrosarcomas. Mitoses and necrosis are visible. Bony trabeculae are frequently trapped due to penetration into the marrow space and cortical bone.

Chondrosarcoma grading is crucial and helpful in predicting histological behavior. Three grades of chondrosarcomas are distinguished based on their histopathology:

- **Grade I:** Sometimes referred to as an atypical cartilaginous tumor, it is thought to be low-grade (locally aggressive). Lesions of grade I frequently resemble benign enchondroma or normal cartilage. The ability to distinguish between a benign and malignant tumor in this case typically rests on the ability to show a "chondrosarcoma permeation pattern," in which the tumor penetrates the marrow cavity rather than being contained by the natural architecture. Moderately cellular grade I chondrosarcomas have plump, hyperchromatic nuclei that are all the same size.
- **Grade II:** Tumors exhibit increased nuclear atypia, hyperchromasia, nuclear size, and cellularity. One can find mitoses.
- **Grade III:** Comparing tumors to grade II chondrosarcomas, they are more atypical and pleomorphic. Mitoses are easier to find. The cells surrounding the lobules become spindled and less differentiated.

Mesenchymal and clear cell chondrosarcomas are two other, less frequent forms of chondrosarcomas.

8.3.4.4.3. Immunophenotype

An IDH1 R132H antibody specific to a given mutation can identify only 20% of all IDH1 mutations.

8.3.4.5. History and Physical

Pain and swelling locally are the most common initial symptoms. Typically, the symptoms last for months or even years. Brain tumors can produce symptoms related to the nervous system.

8.3.4.6. Evaluation

8.3.4.6.1. Plain Radiography

Initially, plain radiography is used for assessment. Simple X-rays make it possible to determine whether a lesion is aggressive or cartilaginous. Simple X-rays could show the following results (Figure 8.14):

- Lytic lesions in 50% of the cases;

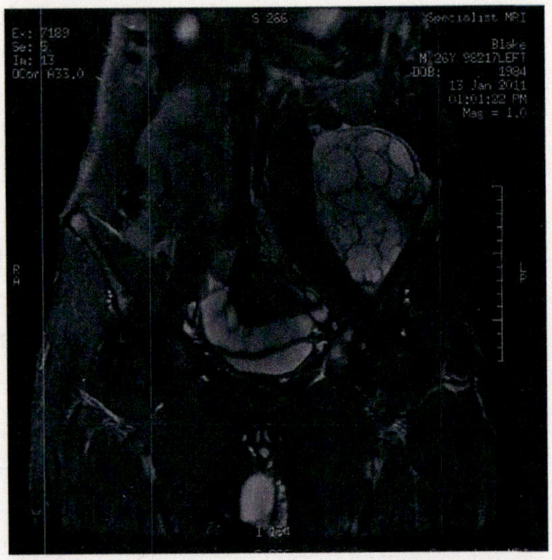

Figure 8.14. *MRI of a left-pelvis chondrosarcoma in a 26-year-old male.*

Source: By An MRI Machine – Magnetic Resonance Image, CC0, https://commons.wikimedia.org/w/index.php?curid=14710757.

- About 70% of cases have intralesional calcifications (also known as rings and arcs calcification or popcorn calcification);
- Endosteal scalloping;
- In high-grade chondrosarcomas, a permeative or moth-eaten appearance is observed;
- Thickening, remodeling, and periosteal response of the cortex.

8.3.4.6.2. Computed Tomography (CT) Scan

A computed tomography (CT) scan can reveal the following findings:

- Calcification of the matrix in 94% of the cases;
- Endosteal scalloping;
- About 90% of long bone chondrosarcomas have a cortical breach;
- Heterogenous contrast enhancement.

8.3.4.6.3. Magnetic Resonance Imaging

MRI typically shows a lobulated lesion with low or intermediate signal on T1-weighted images and high signal intensity on T2 images.

8.3.4.6.4. Tissue Biopsy

Tissue biopsy is necessary for the diagnosis and differentiation of chondrosarcoma from other benign or malignant bone tumors. The biopsy should be performed at the most aggressive area of the cancer, as identified by imaging.

8.3.4.7. Treatment/Management

Treatment/management of chondrosarcoma will be determined by the healthcare provider based on:

- Patient's medical history, age, and general state of health;
- Cancer type, stage (extent), and location;
- Patient's tolerance for specific medicines, procedures, and therapies;
- Expectation for the course of the disease;
- Patient's opinion or preference.

In order to treat chondrosarcoma, the mass must be removed and the chance of its recurrence must be decreased. It might be essential to closely monitor the health care provider. Treatment may include:

8.3.4.7.1. Surgery

The location and histologic grade of chondrosarcoma dictate the treatment strategies. Surgical excision is the principal treatment modality for chondrosarcoma. Intralesional curettage, burring, and surgical adjuvant application, such as hydrogen peroxide, are treatment options for low-grade central chondrosarcoma. Larger tumors, axial or pelvic tumors, intraarticular or soft tissue involved tumors, and these tumors need to be treated with wide excision. The preferred surgical method for intermediate or high-grade chondrosarcoma is wide en-bloc excision.

8.3.4.7.2. Chemotherapy

In cases of conventional chondrosarcoma, chemot herapy is typically ineffective. Nevertheless, in dedifferentiated chondrosarcomas with a high-grade spindle cell component, it might play a part.

8.3.4.7.3. Radiation Therapy

In order to mitigate the high local failure rates following incomplete resection of high-risk chondrosarcomas, radiation therapy is recommended. These include tumors in locations where surgical resection is difficult or impossible, as well as locally recurrent, intermediate- to high-grade tumors. Unresectable tumors may also benefit from definitive radiation therapy.

8.3.4.7.4. Differential Diagnosis

- Chondromyxoid fibroma;
- Enchondroma;
- Chondroblastic osteosarcoma;
- Fracture callus.

8.3.4.8. Prognosis

Predicting metastasis and local recurrence is primarily determined by histological grade. The prognosis is favorable for low-grade chondrosarcomas because they grow slowly and rarely spread. The five-year survival of grade I chondrosarcoma is 83%. In contrast, high-grade chondrosarcoma and dedifferentiated chondrosarcoma have a worse prognosis due to their propensity for early metastasis and rapid tumor growth. Three- and grade II chondrosarcomas have a five-year survival rate of 53%.

8.3.4.9. Complications

- Recurrence of the tumor.
- Distant metastases: The lung is the main location of metastases. The grade of chondrosarcoma affects the rate of metastasis.
    - Low-grade: less than 10%;
    - Intermediate-grade: 10%–50%;
    - High-grade: 50%–70%.

8.3.4.10. Deterrence and Patient Education

It is important to educate patients and their families on how to identify early symptoms of bone tumors. Individuals who experience bone pain, joint or bone swelling, or detect any palpable mass on their bones should seek immediate assistance. The primary treatment for chondrosarcoma is surgery. After surgery, it is important to closely monitor these patients for the possibility of local recurrence over the long term.

8.3.4.11. Enhancing Healthcare Team Outcomes

To achieve optimal outcomes in managing chondrosarcoma, a multidisciplinary team consisting of orthopedists, radiologists, surgical oncologists, oncologists, pathologists, and specialty care nurses is ideal. A conclusive diagnosis of chondrosarcoma requires correlation between the gross, radiographic, and microscopic features of the lesion. Long-term follow-up is necessary for patients after surgery due to the potential for distant metastases and tumor recurrence. The prognosis for those with low-grade disease is generally very good.

In addition to reviewing prescriptions, pharmacists also play a role in identifying drug interactions and educating patients. Specialty care nurses in the fields of orthopedics, oncology, perianesthesia, and operating rooms are responsible for monitoring patients, providing patient education, and keeping the team updated on the patient's condition. By working together, the team can improve patient outcomes.

8.3.5. Chordoma

Tumors known as chordomas can develop anywhere in the base of the skull or the spine. Chordomas most frequently occur in the base of the skull (approximately one-third of cases) and the lower back (sacral area), accounting for one-third to one-half of cases. The remaining embryonic tissue known as the notochord, which eventually becomes the core of spinal discs, gives rise to chordomas. Although they usually grow slowly, these tumors are thought to be malignant and have the potential to spread. Even chordomas with a slow growth rate have the potential to become aggressive and grow quite large locally, pressing against or invading vital areas of the spine or brain. This can result in pain, nerve problems, or even be fatal.

8.3.5.1. Etiology

The notochord is the source of chordomas. The mesodermal structure in the embryo known as the notochord aids in signaling tissues for differentiation and organization. In humans, the notochord eventually regresses to become the nucleus pulposus.

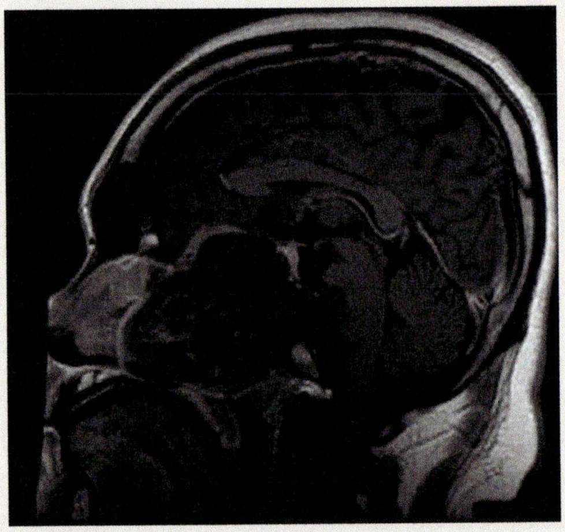

Figure 8.15. *MRI of an extensive clival chordoma in a 17-year-old male patient, sagittal view. A tumor in the nasopharynx extending from the nasal cavity to the brainstem posteriorly is clearly visible.*

Source: Hassan, S., Abdullah, J. M., Wan, D. S. J., & Idris, Z., (2008). Combined use of maxillomandibular swing approach and neurosurgical ultrasonic aspirator in the management of extensive clival chordoma: A case report. J. Med. Case Rep., 2, 49. doi: 10.1186/1752-1947-2-49.

The brachyury gene, the mechanistic target of rapamycin (mTOR) signaling pathway, phosphatase, and tensin homolog (PTEN) gene deficiency, INI-1, and platelet-derived growth factor receptor beta (PDGFR-beta) are among the genes linked to chordoma formation, though no conclusive genetic marker has been found as of yet. Currently, a few familial clusters of chordomas have been reported (Figure 8.15).

8.3.5.2. Epidemiology

Although they usually affect people in their 40s to 60s, choreomas have also been documented in young children and the elderly. It is commonly believed that there is a male-to-female ratio of approximately 2:1 among affected individuals, with a new diagnosis incidence rate of 1:1,000,000 per year. Chordomas account for about 20% of primary spinal tumors and only 3% of all bone tumors. The majority of chordomas (50%) are found in the sacrum/coccygeal region, with another 35% found in the spheno-occipital region, and the remaining 10 to 15% found in the mobile spine.

8.3.5.3. Pathophysiology

Chordomas initially present as slowly expanding, locally invasive tumors that only occasionally and towards the end of the disease develop distant metastases. Despite being considered indolent tumors, there is a significant risk of multiple local recurrences.

8.3.5.4. History and Physical

The precise location of the chordoma determines the patient's history and physical examination findings. Although the lower cranial nerves can also be impacted, headaches and/or dysfunctions of cranial nerves, most commonly cranial nerve VI (abducens nerve), are the most common presentations of skull base and clival chordomas. Seldom will a clival chordoma exhibit rhinorrhea as a result of a CSF leak. Usually, neck, shoulder, or arm pain without any specific cause is the first symptom of cervical chordomas. Occasionally, the mass effect causes dysphagia. Cervical chordomas can also invade the brain, compressing the spinal cord or nerves that exit the brain, resulting in myelopathy or radiculopathy, respectively, as well as lower cranial nerve dysfunction. In addition to causing non-specific localized pain, thoracic and lumbar chordomas can also result in pathologic fractures, radiculopathies, or myelopathies. When a tumor affects the lumbosacral plexus, sacral chordomas present similarly to thoracic and lumbar chordomas, causing localized pain, potential radiculopathy, and possibly even malfunctioning of the bladder, bowel, or autonomic nervous system (ANS).

8.3.5.5. Evaluation

The two primary methods utilized for the evaluation of chordomas are imaging and biopsy. A lytic lesion that exhibits local destructiveness can be visualized on a plain X-ray. It is preferable to employ CT imaging to depict the destructive lytic chordoma. Sclerosis may occasionally be observed at the chordoma's margin. On CT, chordomas appear hypodense in comparison to bones and may exhibit irregular dystrophic calcification. Contrast-enhanced CT imaging reveals moderate to significant enhancement of chordomas. Magnetic resonance imaging (MRI) is the most accurate technique for determining the extent of a chordoma. Chordomas demonstrate decreased signal intensity on T1-weighted imaging and may exhibit areas of hyperintensity, indicative of intratumoral hemorrhage. T1-weighted imaging with gadolinium contrast reveals a heterogeneous contrast enhancement resembling a honeycomb pattern. Chordomas typically appear hyperintense on T2-weighted imaging. Gradient-echo MRI imaging can confirm the presence of intratumoral hemorrhage. Bone scans are occasionally performed as part of the diagnostic process, with chordomas typically displaying normal to decreased uptake. A needle or open biopsy is frequently employed to confirm the diagnosis of chordoma. Due to the potential spread of chordoma along the biopsy tract, caution must be exercised during the organization and execution of the biopsy. Therefore, to minimize the risk of local recurrence, the biopsy tract should be included in any subsequent chordoma resection.

8.3.5.6. Treatment/Management

Chordomas can become life-threatening if they grow large and start to press on important parts of the brain, or if they metastasize, or spread to other parts of the body. Chordomas can grow extremely large and harm brain and spinal nerves, potentially resulting in permanent disability even in cases where they have not spread. Chordomas must be treated as soon as possible while they are still controllable. Preoperative planning, surgery (known as an en-bloc resection, which entails removing the entire tumor along with any surrounding tissue that may have been invaded by cancerous cells), and postoperative therapy are all part of the treatment. Because chordomas can spread, the initial surgery must be successful. Surgical intervention offers the greatest opportunity for tumor control and cure. The surgical team may include more than one surgeon, depending on the location, size, and appearance of the chordoma. Experts in neurosurgery, surgical oncology, orthopedic oncology, urology, vascular surgery, plastic surgery, and anesthesiology may work together during a chordoma procedure. Preoperative planning with medical specialists may also be part of surgery to guarantee the best possible result.

After the surgery, the patient will be admitted to the neurosurgical intensive care unit (NCCU) for postoperative care, which is critical to the outcome of the procedure. The patient will be continuously observed in the NCCU to ensure that the recovery from the procedure is going well. When the time is right, the team will work to develop a plan for physical medicine, rehabilitation, and occupational therapy. To maximize the functional recovery, therapists and rehabilitation physicians may recommend that the patient to remain in an inpatient rehabilitation center after their release from the hospital. If radiation therapy is not able to shrink the tumor further or prevent it from spreading, the doctor might determine that it is. A radiation oncologist, who can assess patient's situation and develop a treatment plan, is one of the healthcare professionals that will work with during radiation treatment.

8.3.5.7. Differential Diagnosis

Clival/Spheno-occipital lesions:

- Benign notochordal cell tumor;
- Chondrosarcoma;
- Ecchordosis physaliphora;
- Meningioma;
- Pituitary macroadenoma;
- Plasmacytoma.

Vertebral lesions:

- Chondrosarcoma;
- Giant cell tumor;
- Plasmacytoma;
- Spinal metastases;
- Spinal lymphoma.

8.3.5.8. Pearls and Other Issues

It is important to emphasize that, in order to reduce the risk of local recurrence, the biopsy tract must be included in the final resection of chordoma if chordoma is being considered in the differential diagnosis. Chordomas have a significant mortality rate and a high recurrence rate despite their low-grade status. The overall five-year survival rate is approximately 50%, but it increases to 65% with complete resection and negative margins. Approximately 50% of patients who undergo surgical resection with positive margins will survive for five years, while 40% of patients with inoperable chordoma will survive for five years.

Chordomas are soft, gelatinous tumors that may exhibit bleeding when viewed under a microscope. Microscopically, they consist of rare mitotic figures and lobules of physaliferous (bubbly) cells separated by fibrous septa with a large myxoid stroma. There are four subtypes of chordomas: chondroid, dedifferentiated, poorly differentiated, and conventional. The most common type, known as conventional or classic chordomas, may show areas of dedifferentiation. Skull base chordomas and poorly differentiated chordomas are more frequently seen in young adult and pediatric patients. Chordomas with poor differentiation typically exhibit loss of the INI-1 gene. Dedifferentiated chordomas are the most aggressive and rapidly growing type, more commonly seen in pediatric patients, and may also show loss of INI-1. Chordomas that are difficult to differentiate from chondrosarcoma on histology are referred to as chondroid chordomas. Chordomas typically express the brachyury gene, which is not expressed by chondrosarcomas. There have been reports of chordomas dedifferentiating into high-grade spindle cell tumors, indicating a worse prognosis.

8.3.6. Ewing Sarcoma of Bone

Ewing sarcoma is a type of cancer that primarily develops in the bone or soft tissue. It is commonly found in the hip bones, ribs, or long bones such as the femur, tibia, or humerus. It can also affect the surrounding soft tissues and muscles. Ewing sarcoma cells have the ability to metastasize, or spread, to other parts of the body including the kidneys, heart, bone marrow, adrenal glands, and other soft tissues. Under a microscope, Ewing sarcoma cells appear small, spherical, and blue. The tumor is named after Dr. James Ewing, who first described it in the 1920s.

8.3.6.1. Epidemiology

In terms of epidemiology, Ewing sarcoma is the second most common primary bone cancer in teenagers and young adults, typically affecting individuals around 15 years old. It accounts for less than 5% of all soft tissue sarcomas and there are over 200 reported cases per year in the United States. From 1973 to 2004, the incidence of Ewing sarcoma in the US was 2.93 per million. The peak occurrence is between the ages of 10 and 15, with 30% of cases occurring in children under 10 and another 30% in adults over 20. Males have a higher prevalence compared to females, with a ratio of 3 to 1. Whites are more commonly affected by this cancer compared to other racial groups, although there is limited research on this racial disparity. The prevalence of Ewing sarcoma in older populations is currently unknown.

8.3.6.2. Pathophysiology

The origin of Ewing sarcoma from a specific cell type remains unclear. Ewing sarcoma is characterized by nonrandom gene rearrangements involving the EWS and ETS (E26 transformation-specific or E-twenty-six) gene families. The most common gene rearrangement is t(11;22)(q24;q12). In over 80% of reported cases, a hybrid gene called EWS–FLI1 is formed through the fusion of the FLI1 gene on 11q24 and the EWS gene on 22q12. The resulting aberrant transcription factor, the EWS-FLI1 fusion protein, may contribute to the pathophysiology of Ewing sarcoma. The underlying cause of the translocation remains unknown. The second most frequent rearrangement of the EWS–ETS gene family is the t(21;22)(q22;q12) translocation, which leads to the fusion of EWS with the ERG gene on 21q22 and is observed in approximately 15% of cases.

8.3.6.3. Histopathology

Ewing sarcoma is characterized by small round cells with an elevated nuclear-cytoplasmic ratio. It belongs to the family of childhood small round blue cell tumors, which also includes retinoblastoma, neuroblastoma, rhabdomyosarcoma, and nephroblastoma. Ewing cells rarely exhibit eosinophilic cytoplasm, which is rich in glycogen and can be detected by staining with periodic acid-Schiff. Strong CD99 expression is observed in over 80% of cases. This highly sensitive immunohistochemical biomarker lacks specificity because it can also be found in other sarcomas and lymphomas, but it probably plays a major role in promoting leukocytes' continued migration to endothelium. Ewing cells frequently express CD45, synaptophysin, chromogranin, vimentin, keratin, desmin, neuron-specific enolase, and S-100 in addition to the MIC2 gene product CD99. However, the requirement for greater specificity has also placed limitations on this immunohistochemistry panel. To establish a definitive distinction, molecular genetic studies utilizing reverse transcription-polymerase chain reaction and fluorescence *in situ* hybridization are needed.

8.3.6.4. History and Physical

Ewing sarcoma patients frequently experience localized symptoms for a few weeks or months, such as pain, stiffness, or swelling. More than half of Ewing sarcoma patients experience sporadic pain that worsens at night. Although it can present differently and occur in various locations, Ewing sarcoma is typically found in the diaphysis of long bones. Pathological fractures in the long bone may result from bone or metastatic lesions. Back pain may manifest as a symptom of Ewing sarcoma located in the pelvis. Metastatic disease is often indicated by the presence of systemic symptoms, such as fever and weight loss. Approximately 20% of patients have metastatic disease at the time of initial diagnosis, and of those cases, over 20% involve the lungs or pleura. In patients with central nervous system (CNS) involvement, a thorough physical examination and neurologic assessment are crucial. Individuals may exhibit dysphonic breathing, pleural effusions, or rales in cases of lung and pleura metastases. Patients with bone marrow metastases may experience purpura or petechiae due to thrombocytopenia. When a patient's CNS is involved, a neurologic examination is crucial. An X-ray of the affected area taken during the initial study may reveal a periosteal reaction with an onion skin appearance. Initial staging requires a CT scan, magnetic resonance imaging, and bone scan.

8.3.6.5. Evaluation

Imaging studies should assess both the primary site and any potential metastatic locations. Destructive confluent "moth-eaten" lesions, the "Codman triangle" of the elevated periosteum, or a multilayered onion-skin periosteal reaction can all be observed on plain radiographs of the affected area. Primary site imaging, which may involve MRI or CT with contrast, is essential as it allows for evaluation of disease severity, operability, level of edema, and involvement of adjacent organs. Additional imaging techniques such as CT thorax, positron emission tomography (PET)/CT, bone scan, and MRI of the spine and pelvis can be utilized to identify potential lymph node involvement or metastatic sites.

If a biopsy is necessary, patients with symptoms should be referred to an orthopedic surgeon. While a diagnosis can be made with a core needle biopsy guided by CT, an open biopsy provides adequate sampling. Molecular cytogenetic analysis of biopsy specimens to assess the t(11;22) translocation should be included in the diagnostic study. Considering bone marrow aspiration with smear and bone marrow biopsy is advisable. Initial measurement of serum lactate dehydrogenase is recommended as it holds prognostic value. Prior to initiating treatment, patients should be offered fertility counseling (Figure 8.16).

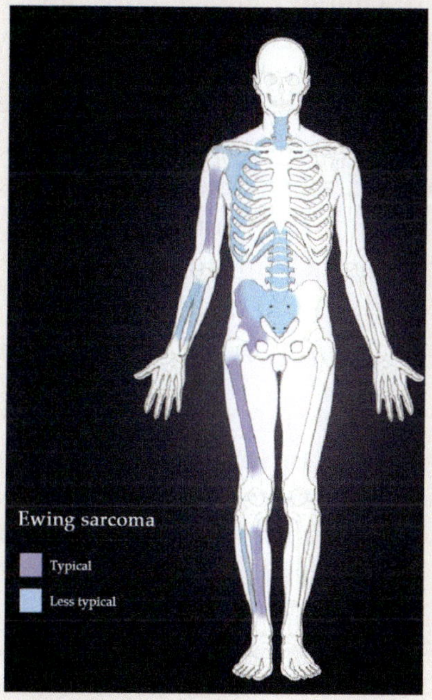

Figure 8.16. *Distribution of Ewing sarcoma: The most frequent locations are the large long bones and the pelvis.*

Source: By Frank Gaillard, CC BY-SA 3.0, https://commons.wikimedia.org/w/index.php?curid=17938132.

8.3.6.6. Treatment/Management

Patients receiving chemotherapy and local therapy, such as radiation and surgery, are routinely treated by multidisciplinary teams, regardless of the presence of metastases. The mainstay of care for all patients with Ewing sarcoma is systemic therapy in general. In the US, this is administered as alternating IE (ifosfamide/etoposide) and VDC (vincristine/doxorubicin/cyclophosphamide). Usually, doctors advise local therapy involving radiation, surgery, or a combination of the two following induction chemotherapy. While the five-year survival rate for metastatic disease is approximately 30%, it is 75% to 80% for nonmetastatic disease.

8.3.6.7. Differential Diagnosis

The differential diagnosis of Ewing sarcoma can be narrowed down by combining immunohistochemical and morphological findings with pertinent clinical history. This includes other small round cell tumors such as neuroblastoma, rhabdomyosarcoma, lymphoma, neuroectodermal tumors, desmoplastic small round cell tumor, and synovial sarcoma. In the differential diagnosis of Ewing sarcoma, take into account osteomyelitis, osteogenic sarcoma, and eosinophilic granuloma.

8.3.6.8. Surgical Oncology

One of the mainstays of local therapy for Ewing sarcoma is surgical resection, which serves as a diagnostic tool and gauges tumor response. Furthermore, compared to radiation therapy (RT), this treatment modality is thought to have fewer long-term side effects, especially in terms of growth restriction and the emergence of secondary cancers. Amputation has become much less common in this context, and function-preserving surgery using custom endoprostheses has become more common, especially since the introduction of 3D printing technologies. The preferred approach for local control is surgery, particularly for tumors originating from bones that are replaceable, such as the scapula, iliac wings, ribs, fibula, and distal four-fifths of the clavicle. There haven't been any prospective randomized trials comparing radiotherapy and surgery, but a meta-analysis of multiple prospective trials indicates that, in circumstances involving intralesional resections, wide resections of the tumor, or poor histologic response, only local control may be preferable to surgery when combined with postoperative radiotherapy.

8.3.6.8.1. Biopsy

Depending on the treatment plan, either a core needle biopsy or an open incisional biopsy is advised. Even though a core needle biopsy may be sufficient for diagnosis, more tissue may be required due to the increasing reliance on biologic studies, which may not be possible to obtain through multiple needle biopsies. Consensus guidelines, however, still permit either strategy. During surgery, biopsy tracts are frequently removed, just like in other types of sarcoma. Biopsies should also be performed on regions where metastasis is suspected, such as lymph nodes or bone lesions.

8.3.6.8.2. Limb Sparing Surgery

Preoperative imaging is crucial for evaluating the surgical feasibility of these tumors. An MRI can provide information on tumor size and peri-tumoral edema. PET/CT can detect metastatic disease and involvement of lymph nodes. Anatomical considerations are essential to ensure complete disease eradication and minimize postoperative morbidity. Tumors that require the removal of a visceral organ or cross the midline, such as sacral tumors, are typically incurable. Patients with incurable diseases are not recommended candidates for debulking surgeries. In the case of spinal tumors, excision may be considered for carefully selected individuals who respond well to chemotherapy. Immediate surgical decompression therapy is necessary for individuals with cord compression and neurological compromise. Alternatively, chemotherapy or radiotherapy may be viable options. For tumors involving the chest wall, resection of the affected chest wall, pleura, and usually adjacent ribs is necessary, especially when the ribs are involved. Ewing sarcoma of the scapular body can be removed without compromising function if it does not involve the chest wall. Resection of the sternum and the lateral four-fifths of the clavicle can be performed without reconstruction. Resection of the proximal humerus and diaphyseal region is possible, but reconstruction with metallic implants or allografts is often required. Intercalary resection, preserving the native joint, may be performed on the ulna and radius, but allografting or autografting may be necessary. Tumors in the mandibular and base of the skull regions are complex and require the expertise of multiple subspecialists.

It is recommended to consider wide excision of the primary tumor and peritumoral edema once a patient meets the criteria for surgical candidacy. A sufficient surgical margin consists of a normal tissue rim surrounding the tumor.

8.3.6.8.3. Amputation

Amputations are infrequent procedures, but they may be taken into account in situations where less aggressive methods fail to achieve a negative margin, in limbs with low baseline function, or in cases of locally recurrent disease.

8.3.6.8.4. Metastatic Disease

In the context of widespread metastatic disease, it may be difficult to justify surgical removal of the primary tumor. However, in cases of limited metastatic burden or for palliative purposes, this option may be considered. Despite the poor prognosis associated with metastatic disease, individuals with isolated metastasis in the lungs may benefit from surgical resection. In select patients, metastasectomy has demonstrated a three-year overall survival rate of 60% and an EFS rate of 45%. The decision to proceed with surgery should be made on an individual basis.

8.3.6.8.5. Recurrent Disease

Within the first two years following diagnosis, approximately 70% of relapses occur. A single metastatic site or an isolated local recurrence may arise in 10 to 15% of patients, despite distant spread being the most common site of relapse. It can be hypothesized that these patients would benefit from more localized therapy. A retrospective review of earlier Ewing sarcoma trials revealed that patients with local relapse who were able to undergo repeat resection had a five-year probability of survival of 30% compared to 9% in those who could not undergo resection. However, the small number of patients and selection biases must be acknowledged when considering treatment options for relapsed patients.

8.3.6.8.6. Complications

About 25% of patients experience problems directly related to surgery or resulting from treatment using multiple modalities. These problems include the development of an abscess, fibrosis, thrombosis, delayed wound healing, and hardware failure or loosening. It seems that the location of the tumor (e.g., pelvis vs. extremity) influences the risk of postoperative complications.

8.3.6.9. Radiation Oncology

In the field of Radiation Oncology, patients with Ewing sarcoma who have metastatic or inoperable disease, or who are unable to achieve negative margins, undergo radiation treatment. Retrospective data suggests that local failure rates are lower with surgery (4% vs. 15%), and local failure appears to be higher in older patients with pelvic tumors. However, no direct prospective trials have been conducted to compare radiotherapy to surgical resection. The local failure rate among patients who required both radiotherapy and surgery was 6.6%. There is no noticeable difference in survival between local therapy plus surgery, radiotherapy alone, or a combination of both. In the context of metastatic disease, radiotherapy has also been used to control the disease and may improve EFS.

8.3.6.9.1. Preoperative Radiotherapy

For adults with sarcomas, preoperative radiation therapy is usually recommended. This therapy offers smaller margins, a clear target, and lower radiation doses compared to postoperative radiotherapy. However, radiation therapy is generally not advised for pediatric patients with Ewing sarcoma due to limited evidence supporting its use, despite these potential benefits. A retrospective analysis of non-selective preoperative radiation therapy for pelvic Ewing sarcoma showed higher rates of adequate surgical margins (81% vs 59.1%), five-year local recurrence-free survival (88% vs 66.5%), and better responses to chemotherapy (96.3% vs 63.6%) compared to a more conservative approach. However, overall survival and metastasis-free survival did not differ significantly. The widespread use of preoperative radiation therapy raises concerns about potential overtreatment, interference with pathological assessment of chemotherapy response, and long-term toxicity. According to consensus guidelines, patients who have not responded well to chemotherapy, have large tumor volumes, tumors close to critical structures, and are expected to have close or positive surgical margins may benefit from preoperative radiotherapy. Current AEWS protocols allow for the use of preoperative radiotherapy.

8.3.6.9.2. Definitive Radiotherapy

Patients with Ewing sarcoma who have an incurable disease or where resection would be extremely morbid are advised to receive definitive radiotherapy. Radiotherapy is still an option, particularly for patients with large pelvic tumors, even though it has never been prospectively compared to surgical resection. Compared to other sarcoma subtypes, Ewing sarcoma is thought to be more radiosensitive. Several retrospective reviews have shown that local control rates range from 70% to 80%.

There have been indications that local control rates for smaller lesions (less than 8 cm) treated with radiation therapy alone may be extraordinarily high (90% vs 52%).

8.3.6.9.3. Adjuvant Radiotherapy

Patients who have intraoperative tumor spill, microscopic or gross residual disease after surgical resection, or who do not respond well to chemotherapy are typically considered as candidates for adjuvant radiotherapy. However, after a total resection, patients should not receive adjuvant radiation therapy. Similar to preoperative radiation therapy, the available data are contradictory and the evidence of benefit is not well established. Retrospective reviews have shown that patients receiving adjuvant radiation therapy following insufficient resection experienced relapse rates comparable to those of inadequate resection alone (12% vs. 14%).

8.3.6.9.4. Intraoperative Radiotherapy

Intraoperative radiotherapy is allowed on current protocols and delivered as a single fraction. This treatment modality offers the advantages of shorter treatment durations and lower treatment volumes. To reduce the number of external beam radiation therapy (EBRT) treatments required, a boost dose of intraoperative radiotherapy may be administered. This therapy is indicated for the treatment of recurrent or residual disease in the surgical tumor bed. The local control rates over a five-year period ranged from 70% to 77%. The toxicities associated with this treatment include soft tissue necrosis and peripheral neuropathy, which have a dose limit.

8.3.6.9.5. Proton Therapy

Theoretically, proton therapy's Bragg peak has fewer radiation doses to normal tissue, no exit dose, and lower overall toxicity than photons. Dosage escalation may also be possible with proton therapy if necessary. Proton therapy evaluation is more challenging than photon therapy due to the absence of prospective randomized data. The evidence is still biased and retrospective in nature. Proton therapy is thought to be most beneficial for tumors in the pelvis, base of the skull, chest wall, and axial skeleton that are near the spinal cord. When compared to photon therapy, ovarian doses for women with pelvic sarcomas were significantly lower when using proton therapy. Due to the smaller amounts of normal tissue exposed to radiation when compared to photons, there would also be a decreased chance of developing secondary cancer.

In terms of oncologic results, the local control after three years using proton therapy was 92% when radiotherapy was used alone and 100% when combined with surgery. These results were similar to those of other series with treatments based on photons. Proton therapy patients with non-metastatic skull base Ewing sarcoma had a 96% local control rate after four years. However, there were some late toxicities associated with this, including bilateral vasculopathy and hearing loss. Proton therapy has some theoretical advantages over photons when administered to children; however, in many cases, normal tissues and protons can also be spared with highly conformal treatments such as stereotactic body radiotherapy or brachytherapy.

8.3.6.9.6. Metastatic Disease

Upon reflection, it has been determined that local treatment using surgery, radiation, or a combination of both can significantly increase EFS in patients with disseminated disease. Research has shown that radiotherapy results in a three-year EFS of 23%, while patients who do not receive local treatment only have an EFS of 13%. This is especially evident in the treatment of lung metastasis, where whole lung irradiation is recommended for patients with any number of lung metastases regardless of their response to chemotherapy. Efforts to replace whole lung irradiation with high-dose therapy have not been successful. In patients with limited metastasis, stereotactic body radiotherapy (SBRT) has been explored as a treatment option. SBRT has shown promising results in patients with pulmonary metastasis, with 88% experiencing a partial response without any severe toxicity. SBRT has also been studied in the treatment of extrapulmonary metastasis. While SBRT for bony metastasis is generally well tolerated, the risk of significant toxicity depends on factors such as location, radiation dosage, and the use of chemotherapy.

8.3.6.9.7. Acute Toxicity

Radiation can cause dermatitis, cystitis, mucositis, nausea, vomiting, or diarrhea, among other acute side effects that vary greatly depending on the area that was exposed to radiation. Although these side effects can cause patients some inconvenience, they usually pass quickly and resolve in the days to weeks following radiation therapy.

8.3.6.9.8. Late Toxicity

For long-term survivors, the late toxicities—which can manifest months or even years after treatment—usually present greater challenges than the acute side effects. Similar to acute side effects, they are mostly specific to the location.

8.3.6.9.9. Secondary Malignancies

Chemotherapy or radiation therapy can lead to the development of secondary cancers. Radiotherapy has been associated with osteosarcomas, but there have also been reports of various other solid tumors. According to a recent systematic review of Ewing sarcoma patients, the cumulative incidence of solid tumors (63%) at 30 years was 20.5% for secondary malignancies. A retrospective analysis reveals a dose-dependent cumulative risk of second malignancies, with 130 cases reported at doses greater than 60 Gy and no cases at doses less than 48 Gy.

8.3.6.9.10. Pathological Fracture

Pathological fractures are more common in weight-bearing bones. The femur is the most frequent location as a result. There is a 20%–33% variation in the fracture rate. If possible, it is advisable to avoid the 50 Gy isodose line crossing the entire circumference of the bone, and no more than half of the bone volume should receive 50 Gy.

8.3.6.9.11. Edema

Patients with limb-encompassing irradiation for Ewing sarcoma may develop edema. This is caused by fibrotic changes that lead to lymphatic blockage, resulting in edema in the distal extremities. Once edema has started, it cannot be reversed. During radiation planning, a strip of skin is usually spared to allow lymphatic drainage and reduce the risk of edema. Approximately 20% of patients exhibit this condition.

8.3.6.9.12. Fibrosis/Loss of Mobility

Compared to preoperative treatment, fibrosis can occur in up to 90% of cases and is more common following surgery-related radiotherapy. Roughly 20–40% of patients experience limb mobility issues. Meticulous radiation planning and strict dose limitations are effective ways to reduce this toxicity.

8.3.6.9.13. Wound Healing

Research has shown that patients who receive preoperative radiotherapy have higher rates of delayed wound healing after surgery (35% vs. 17%).

8.3.6.9.14. Growth Deficiency

The growth plates have moderate radiation sensitivity. Growth stunting may occur with doses of 10 Gy to the epiphyseal plate, and complete arrest may result from doses exceeding 20 Gy. This can lead to noticeable differences in length between the irradiated and unirradiated limbs. Patients under the age of 15 typically experience limb shortening, while those over the age of 15 do not seem to be at risk, possibly due to growth plate closure. Limb atrophy is present in as many as 80% of cases.

8.3.6.9.15. Timing

The clinical situation determines when to initiate radiation and chemotherapy. Radiation therapy and chemotherapy are often administered concurrently. However, anthracyclines are typically withheld during radiation therapy. In cases of emergency, such as cord compression, blindness, or severely compromised organ function, the full course of radiation therapy may be administered immediately on day 1. From a clinical perspective, this is an uncommon scenario. In the adjuvant setting, local therapy (i.e., surgery, radiotherapy, or both) is usually administered concurrently with consolidation chemotherapy during weeks 12 to 14. During the first week of consolidation therapy, patients receive treatment if pre-operative radiotherapy is scheduled. If a postoperative boost is necessary, it should commence two weeks after surgery or as soon as the patient feels sufficiently recovered. Delays in local therapy lasting longer than 16 weeks were associated with poorer 10-year overall survival outcomes (70.3% vs 57.1%).

8.3.6.9.16. Target Delineation

Prior to any surgical resection or chemotherapy, the initial gross tumor volume (GTV1) —which would include any clinically involved lymph nodes—is determined by radiographic and palpable disease. A variety of imaging modalities, such as MRI, PET, and CT scans that can be fused to the simulation CT, can be utilized to help outline gross disease. In addition to covering occult disease surrounding the gross disease by adding a 1 to 2 cm margin and the draining lymph node chain surrounding any involved nodes, the initial clinical target volume (CTV1) will include the initial GTV1. It is important to respect the CTV's natural barriers to spread and to exclude it. Depending on the availability and sophistication of the institution's image guidance, the initial PTV1 consists of the CTV1 with a 0.5 to 1.0 cm margin. Motion control and the creation of an internal target volume may be necessary, depending on the location of the tumor. The boost volumes might be necessary. Gross target volume (GTV2) will include soft tissue in patients who have not had their cancer removed, but it will also include the disease that existed in bone before chemotherapy. Gross residual tumor, tumor bed, and pretreatment disease in the bone are included in the GTV2 of patients who have undergone partial resection and have macroscopic disease. The GTV2 comprises disease from post-induction chemotherapy imaging for microscopic residual disease. A margin of 0.5 to 1.5 cm around the GTV2 is the clinical target volume for the boost. With a margin of 0.5–1.0 cm, the PTV2 is built around the CTV2. Changes to these volumes might be necessary, depending on where the tumor is located.

8.3.6.10. Medical Oncology

8.3.6.10.1. Localized Disease

In the past, adjuvant chemotherapy using VACA (vincristine, dactinomycin, cyclophosphamide, and doxorubicin) rather than VAC (vincristine, dactinomycin, and cyclophosphamide) produced better outcomes with RT plus IESS-II and IESS-II trials. Subsequent trials showed that the omission of dactinomycin had no discernible effect on clinical outcomes because of the dose limitation of doxorubicin in dactinomycin regimens. A number of studies assessed the addition of etoposide and ifosfamide to conventional chemotherapy. The VACD-IE group had significantly higher survival rates than the VACD group, according to the Pediatric Oncology Group-Children's Cancer Group study INT0091. Additionally, there was a lower incidence of local failure in the VACD-IE group.

In the European Intergroup Cooperative Ewing Sarcoma Study (EICESS-92), VACA (vincristine, dactinomycin, cyclophosphamide, and doxorubicin) and VAIA (vincristine, dactinomycin, ifosfamide, and doxorubicin) were compared to reveal similar effects for cyclophosphamide and ifosfamide; the former had higher toxicity.

The three-year EFS rates were 73% and 74% for VACA and VAIA, respectively. Patients on the standard arm of a phase III trial (AEWS0031) from the Children's Oncology Group (COG) received VDC alternating with IE every three weeks, while patients on the same chemotherapy arm received the same treatment every two weeks. Without increasing toxicity, the study showed that 2-week intervals were more effective than 3-week intervals. Because of this study, VDC/IE is now considered the gold standard of care in the US. Chemotherapy is initiated before local therapy and may be continued after surgery in the event that no progression is observed. Six cycles of alternating VDC/IE induction are given over a period of 12 weeks in the non-metastatic setting. Local therapy is started during the 13–14 week period after induction. Chemotherapy is started as soon as possible, usually one to two weeks after surgery, if one is scheduled. Chemotherapy is usually administered concurrently with radiotherapy, except for anthracyclines, which are administered at a different time. Depending on the protocol, systemic treatment is usually finished at weeks 42 to 48.

8.3.6.10.2. Metastatic Disease

About 25% of all patients with Ewing sarcoma present with de novo metastatic disease, which is typically associated with a poor prognosis. This group has an overall five-year survival rate of about 30%. On the other hand, some patient subgroups might have a better prognosis.

There have been proposed risk stratification schemes based on the overall disease burden and the location. In contrast to patients with diffuse involvement of multiple organs, where the expected overall survival is 5–10% over the same time frame, patients with isolated pulmonary metastasis, for instance, have an overall survival of 30–40% for five years.

8.3.6.10.3. Recurrent Disease

Relapses following definitive treatment have a dismal five-year survival rate of only 13% of patients. Recurrence time is thought to be a predictor of post-recurrence survival; patients who have had their disease for more than two years have a five-year survival rate of 30%, compared to 7% for those who have had it for less than two years. Long-term relapses are possible, though the majority happen during the first two years of treatment. At 20 years, the cumulative risk of recurrence is 13%. A number of agents, such as topotecan and cyclophosphamide, irinotecan and temozolomide, gemcitabine, and docetaxel, or high-dose ifosfamide, were studied in the multiarm Phase II/III rEECur trial. With a median survival of sixteen months, this trial proved the superiority of high-dose ifosfamide in extending survival. Additional systemic agents are being developed, including eribulin plus irinotecan and nab-paclitaxel plus gemcitabine. Additionally intriguing have been targeted chemical agents. Tyrosine kinase inhibitors like cabotezantinib have shown antitumor activity in patients who have received extensive pretreatment.

The combination of the CDK4 inhibitor palbociclib with the anti-IGFR antibody ganitumab resulted in unsatisfactory outcomes. Additional agents, like TK216, that target the EWS-FL11 fusion protein are being studied. Pembrolizumab or nivolumab, two immunotherapy agents that target PDL-1, have not shown any tumor responses.

Low PDL expression (19% of all tumor cell samples), a low tumor mutational burden, and a limited number of lymphocytes infiltrating the tumor could be the cause of the lack of response. Autologous stem cell transplantation combined with high-dose chemotherapy (HDT-ASCT) is being studied, but no prospective clinical trials are currently underway. Only a small percentage of relapsed candidates may be qualified for this rigorous systemic regimen. An HDT-ASCT single-institution experience showed a 46% overall survival rate at 10 years, including relapsed and metastatic Ewing sarcoma. An especially low OS is seen in patients with early relapses, less than two years.

8.3.6.10.4. Toxicity

Adverse health outcomes are associated with an increased risk of Ewing sarcoma. Despite the administration of granulocyte colony-stimulating factor, patients undergoing current therapies are prone to developing severe neutropenia, which can be complicated by recurrent fever, opportunistic infections, and mucositis. The elevated risk of developing a second malignant neoplasm is one of the potential side effects of radiation and chemotherapy. In large series, less than 2% of cancer survivors have experienced the cumulative incidence of a second neoplasm, typically occurring three years after the initial diagnosis. Acute myeloid leukemia, myelodysplastic syndrome, and sarcomas are the most common cancers observed in the radiation field. Medications such as alkylating agents (e.g., cyclophosphamide), topoisomerase II inhibitors (e.g., etoposide, teniposide), and anthracycline agents (e.g., doxorubicin) can lead to secondary leukemias. However, the IESS trial, which compared VAC and VAC-IE, demonstrated that the addition of etoposide did not increase the risk of developing a second cancer. The C-arm of the INT-0091 study revealed that very high cumulative doses of ifosfamide and cyclophosphamide were associated with a 10% incidence of therapy-related leukemia. Ifosfamide and cyclophosphamide are also known to be linked to infertility. Additionally, ifosfamide may cause renal tubule cell dysfunction, renal failure, or progressive chronic renal failure.

Cardiotoxicity related to cumulative dose is a well-known side effect of anthracyclines, such as doxorubicin. Cardiomyopathy is a side effect of doxorubicin treatment that can develop many years after initiation and is dependent on the dose administered. If doxorubicin is administered prior to dexrazoxane or through prolonged infusion, the risk of cardiotoxicity can be mitigated.

8.3.6.11. Staging

The Musculoskeletal Tumor Society has established a widely utilized staging system for Ewing sarcoma, which categorizes the disease into three grades: low grade (Stage I), high grade (Stage II), and distant metastasis (stage

III). Additionally, the staging system assesses the disease's compartmental status (whether it is confined to the bone cortex or extends beyond it). The American Joint Committee on Cancer employs the TNM classification scheme, which considers factors such as tumor size, distant metastasis, lymph node metastasis, and tumor grade (cellular differentiation, mitotic rate, and extent of necrosis).

8.3.6.12. Prognosis

Patients with Ewing sarcoma who have involvement in their distal extremities are expected to have a better prognosis than those who have lesions in their proximal extremities. The presence of metastatic disease significantly affects prognosis evaluation. Unilateral lung involvement is associated with a better prognosis than bilateral lung involvement, and patients with solitary pulmonary metastases are more likely to have a better prognosis than patients with extrapulmonary metastatic sites. Extensive tumors and the development of lung and bone metastases are linked to a poor prognosis. In studies, the size of the tumor is a significant prognostic factor. According to the data, another important clinical prognostic factor is being younger than 15 years old. According to clinical research, patients who had little to no viable tumor remaining at the time of surgery after receiving neoadjuvant chemotherapy appeared to fare better than those who had larger than usual amounts of viable tumors. Furthermore, there is a higher chance of recurrence when neoadjuvant chemotherapy is not responded to adequately. The translocation of EWSR1-ETS is no longer regarded as a poor prognostic factor.

8.3.6.13. Complications

Metastases, local recurrence, secondary malignancies, pathological fractures, surgery, and morbidities related to chemotherapy and radiation therapy can complicate Ewing sarcoma. For information on complications unique to each treatment modality, please refer to each subsection.

8.3.6.14. Deterrence and Patient Education

There are no safeguards against Ewing sarcoma. To improve results, it is important to educate parents and patients about the significance of adhering to all treatment modalities.

8.3.6.15. Enhancing Healthcare Team Outcomes

Ten to 15% of bone sarcomas are Ewing sarcomas, an aggressive tumor primarily affecting adolescents and young adults. Ewing sarcoma can develop in various locations and its appearance can also vary. The pelvis, axial skeleton, and femur are the most common anatomical sites for Ewing sarcoma, but it can develop in any soft tissue or bone. Patients with Ewing sarcoma often experience local symptoms such as pain, stiffness, or swelling for a few weeks or months. More than 50% of Ewing sarcoma patients have sporadic pain that worsens at night. Lesions in the bone or metastases can cause pathological fractures in the long bone. Back pain may be a symptom of Ewing sarcoma located in the pelvis. Systemic symptoms like fever and weight loss often indicate metastatic disease. Approximately 20% of patients are diagnosed with metastatic disease initially, and over 20% of these cases involve the lungs or pleura.

The management of localized disease has significantly advanced over the past 40 years, thanks to both local therapy and multiagent adjuvant chemotherapy. As a result, the five-year survival rate has increased from less than 20% to more than 70%. However, the recurrence rate remains high, with approximately 25% of patients experiencing a relapse after initially having a localized disease. For patients with relapsed and refractory Ewing sarcoma, there is currently no standard treatment. The survival rate is less than 30% for patients with isolated lung metastases and less than 20% for those with bone and bone marrow involvement.

If the patient experience joint pain, palpable mass, or bone pain, it is important to undergo evaluation. A thorough physical examination is essential, as these presenting symptoms may be connected to an osseous neoplasm. The best management strategy for Ewing sarcoma involves an interprofessional team approach. Primary clinicians should maintain a high degree of suspicion and make early referrals to pediatric oncologists for the best possible treatment of childhood cancer. The team should include skilled radiologists, orthopedic surgeons, radiation oncologists, pathologists, nurses, and pharmacists. Early diagnosis and intervention can help reduce morbidity and complications associated with the disease.

8.3.7. Fibrosarcoma and Undifferentiated Pleomorphic Sarcoma

Soft tissue cancer, or sarcoma, is one kind of undifferentiated pleomorphic sarcoma (UPS). Soft tissues help to support and connect the body. They include:

- Blood vessels;
- Fat;
- Fibrous tissues, including tendons, ligaments, and cartilage;
- Muscles;
- Nerves;
- Skin.

This type of sarcoma typically affects soft tissues, but it can also occur in the bones, behaving similarly to osteosarcoma, which is one of the more common types of sarcomas originating in the bones. UPS predominantly affects the arms and legs, although it occurs less frequently in the retroperitoneum, which is the posterior abdominal area. It is usually a malignant and aggressive cancer, with a roughly 40% chance of spreading to other parts of the body. The lungs are the most common site of metastasis, while lymph nodes are less frequently involved. Due to its aggressive nature, this cancer may recur locally, meaning it can return to the original site from which it was surgically removed.

8.3.7.1. Etiology

The precise pathogenic mechanisms underlying UPS are still unknown. Generally, stem cell syndromes (STSs) consist of diverse cell populations with mesenchymal characteristics that may arise from simple genetic modifications or complex genomics. UPS belongs to the latter group, exhibiting a variety of possible cellular origins, mutational signatures, and altered signaling pathways. Reports suggest that a subset of cells known as side population (SP) cells, detectable by the Hoechst dye efflux assay, are responsible for the tumorigenesis of UPS. An elegant xenograft experimental model indicates that these cells have a higher capacity for proliferation, growth, self-renewal, and tumor formation. Hedgehog and Notch signaling pathways, along with their downstream transcriptional targets, are known to be significantly upregulated at the subcellular and tissue levels, as demonstrated by UPS-derived SP cells and *in situ* analyzes of UPS.

Vestigial-like family member 3 (VGLL3) and yes1-associated transcriptional regulator (YAP1) cofactors were found to be highly amplified in a genome sequencing study, suggesting that the Hippo pathway may also be involved in the biology of UPS tumors. Well-established loss or deletion mutations of phosphatase and tensin homolog (PTEN) and overexpression of phosphorylated protein kinase B (pAKT) in UPS, implicated in the PIK3/PTEN/AKT/mTOR pathway, have been reported in several other studies. Similarly, UPS had a different level of overexpression of Dickkopf-related protein 1 (DKK1), an inhibitor of the Wnt/B-catenin signaling pathway, than other STSs. The UPS genetic signature and human mesenchymal stem cells (hMSC) exhibited a strong correlation, as demonstrated by hierarchical cluster analysis of stem cell genes in the same publication. Dkk1's requirement for hMSC differentiation was also confirmed.

Tumor protein 53 (TP53), retinoblastoma-associated protein (RB1), cyclin-dependent kinase inhibitor 2A (CDKN2A), transcriptional regulator ATRX (ATRX), PR domain zinc finger protein 10 (PRDM10), and triple functional domain protein (TRIO) gene fusions have all been linked to mutations in UPS. A known risk factor for the development of STS, aside from genetic abnormalities, is radiation therapy (RT). In fact, 1–3% of patients with a sarcoma diagnosis also have radiation-associated STS. In particular, 51.1% of patients in a set of 1068 UPS cases had radiation exposure in the past.

8.3.7.2. Epidemiology

UPS is included in the 2020 WHO classification of STSs under the heading of malignant tumors of uncertain differentiation. UPS was the second most common STS after leiomyosarcoma, regardless of the primary tumor site, accounting for 17.1% of 26,758 cases, according to the Surveillance, Epidemiology, and End Results (SEER) program. Males exhibited noticeably higher incidence rates than females, with white males being impacted more frequently than black males. Additionally, the incidence increased linearly with age, peaking after the sixth decade of life.

8.3.7.3. Histopathology

A histopathology examination is necessary in order to diagnose UPS. When conducting an initial evaluation, the core needle technique is recommended over open incisional biopsy. With the future resection incision in mind, a skilled surgeon should carry out the latter to reduce the risk of dissection and bleeding. Because of inadequate sampling, fine-needle aspiration is not advised. In the event that the diagnosis cannot be made using the initial biopsy specimen, an image-guided core needle biopsy is recommended. For deep thoracic, abdominal, or pelvic tumors, endoscopic needle biopsy should be taken into consideration. Under light microscopy, UPS exhibits pleomorphic, atypical spindle cells with a high number of mitotic figures. The deep dermis, hypodermis, fascia, and striated muscle can all be infiltrated to varying degrees. The tumor within the fibrous stroma may present a storiform, fascicular, or sheet-like pattern. Deep tumors are defined by the superficial fascia and beyond, as per the guidelines of the National Comprehensive Cancer Network (NCCN). Only a prognostic indicator can accurately distinguish between superficial and deep UPS. However, visualization of deep-tissue invasion and absence of solar elastosis in UPS is helpful in ruling out atypical fibroxanthoma.

To confirm the diagnosis of UPS and rule out other cancers, a panel of immunohistochemical markers is utilized. These markers include keratins, S100 protein and/or SOX10, smooth muscle actin (SMA), and desmin, which are expressed in melanoma, pleomorphic myogenic sarcomas, and metastatic sarcomatoid carcinomas, respectively. MDM2 and CDK4 help exclude dedifferentiated liposarcoma in cases of internal, intrathoracic, or intraabdominal tumors. Contrary to previous reports suggesting high sensitivity of LN2 for UPS, a recent study demonstrated similar expression of LN2, CD10, and ezrin markers in UPS and atypical fibroxanthoma. Vimentin, p53, and Ki67, three other IHC markers reported to be expressed in UPS, do not show a disease-specific relationship.

A comprehensive post-operative histopathology report should include tumor, node, and metastasis (TNM) staging, vascular involvement, mitotic rate, depth of invasion, size, histologic grade, presence or absence of necrosis, and excision margin status.

8.3.7.4. History and Physical

UPS typically presents as a rapidly growing, asymptomatic, subcutaneous or cutaneous nodule without any visible skin abnormalities. Symptoms of internal, intrathoracic, and intraabdominal UPS may be constitutional or result from mass effect. In a recent retrospective analysis of 100 UPS cases, the extremities were the most commonly affected site (55%). The trunk (35%), retroperitoneum (9%), and left atrium (1%) were the next most frequently involved locations. Another series of 266 cases reported an average tumor size of 8.8+/−6.6 cm. In cases of radiation-associated UPS, the median latency time between radiation exposure and tumor development was 9.33+/−1.31 years.

8.3.7.5. Evaluation

Imaging of the primary tumor, lymph nodes, and distant metastases is an integral part of the evaluation and study conducted after histopathology and immunohistochemistry confirm the diagnosis. The location of the tumor determines the specific TNM staging criteria.

When internal viscera or retroperitoneal involvement is suspected, non-contrast CT of the chest, abdomen, and pelvis should be considered. In certain cases, a head, neck, and total spine MRI or CT scan may be requested. Sentinel lymph node biopsy (SLNB) and positron emission tomography (PET) are not recommended for UPS due to insufficient evidence. However, it is important to note that a recent meta-analysis and systematic review concluded that the (18)F-fluorodeoxyglucose PET scan is a valuable predictive tool for patients with bone sarcomas and STSs. Further research efforts should focus on this matter for better characterization, prognosis, and treatment purposes, as molecular diagnosis has not yet been formally established for UPS.

8.3.7.6. Treatment/Management

The standard of care for head, neck, trunk, and extremities UPS is en-bloc surgical excision with microscopically negative margins, particularly for stage I tumors. This can be accomplished by performing a broad local excision with 2 cm margins of unaffected tissue; however, in certain cases, the involvement of significant neurovascular structures may make the procedure more challenging. When margins are small (<1 cm), microscopically positive, involve bone, major blood vessels, or nerves, postoperative radiotherapy (RT) is recommended. A 5 cm margin should be covered by effective radiation therapy (RT), which can be given by high-dose equivalent (HDR), low-dose brachytherapy (LDR) (45 Gy), intraoperative radiation therapy (IORT) (10–16 Gy), or external beam radiation therapy (EBRT) (50 Gy). Subjects treated with insufficient margins (marginal or intralesional) had a 1.82 higher death rate than those who received wide margin excision in a retrospective analysis involving 266 patients. Additionally, adjuvant RT decreased metastatic disease and mortality in 68% and 66% of UPS patients, respectively. When attempting to preserve healthy tissue, Mohs micrographic surgery (MMS) has also been used in the past. Since limb-sparing surgery did not result in better overall survival rates, extremity amputation is the last option.

Chemotherapy, utilizing distinct antineoplastic agents, is commonly employed for advanced, extensive, or incurable stages of various sexually transmitted infections. To determine the appropriateness of pre- or postoperative chemotherapy and radiation, a multidisciplinary approach should be taken during stages II and III. Incurable cases may benefit from chemoradiation, regional limb therapy, or chemotherapy. However, there is insufficient data available to support a specific treatment plan for patients in stage IV, and consultation with STS-trained oncologists is recommended. A comparative study involving 286 patients with high-risk STSs found that histotype-tailored neoadjuvant chemotherapy did not outperform standard chemotherapy (epirubicin plus ifosfamide). In fact, patients with UPS who received standard chemotherapy had a higher disease-free survival rate (HR 2.17, 95% CI, 0.98–4.80) compared to those who received the histotype-specific regimen (gemcitabine plus docetaxel). An expanded, open-label, randomized, controlled trial involving 435 STS patients from four nations also supported this, indicating that the recommended course of treatment should continue to be anthracycline plus ifosfamide. Presently, immuno-checkpoint inhibition using pembrolizumab (anti-PD1), nivolumab (anti-PD1), and ipilimumab (anti-CTLA4) is being studied as an alternative to conventional chemotherapy for UPS.

The management of internal, retroperitoneal, or intraabdominal undifferentiated pleomorphic sarcomas (UPSs) follows similar guidelines. The preferred course of treatment for resectable disease is excision with negative margins, either with or without intraoperative radiation therapy (IORT). For cases that cannot be surgically removed, high-dose rate (HDR) brachytherapy, chemotherapy, or chemoradiation are recommended.

8.3.7.7. Differential Diagnosis

The most frequent differential diagnoses for UPS are different types of soft tissue sarcomas (STSs), which need to be differentiated using immunohistochemistry markers, the clinical history, and physical examination. The conditions that fall under this category include malignant peripheral nerve sheath tumor, dermatofibrosarcoma protuberans, osteosarcoma, liposarcoma, leiomyosarcoma, angiosarcoma, fibrosarcoma, and myxofibrosarcoma. Histopathological or clinical features of UPS may also be observed in metastases, spindle-cell squamous cell carcinoma, and desmoplastic melanoma.

8.3.7.8. Prognosis

The most crucial interventions to enhance overall prognosis are early disease recognition and a suitable treatment plan. Recurrences and metastases occurred in 14.1% and 7.8%, respectively, of the 319 patients in a recent retrospective study from three tertiary care centers. Advanced American Joint Committee on Cancer (AJCC) staging, invasion beyond the subcutaneous fat, and preoperative tumors larger than 5 cm all significantly increased the risk of recurrence. In addition, the risk of metastasis was markedly elevated for tumors ranging from 2 to 5 cm as well as those exhibiting lymphatic or vascular invasion. Post-treatment local recurrence (15%) was statistically correlated with advanced age and insufficient surgical margins, according to a UPS-specific report, while post-treatment metastatic disease (37.6%) was significantly relevant in tumors ≥ 5 cm.

In terms of overall survival, the 5- and 10-year rates were 60% and 48%, respectively. Contrary to popular belief, radiation-associated UPS has considerably lower five-year disease-specific survival and recurrence rates than sporadic UPS. This suggests that the two types of UPS may have different mutational profiles. Visits for follow-up are crucial in order to identify metastases or local recurrences. For the first two years, a physical examination of stage I tumors should be done every three to six months, and after that, once a year. Unless clinical signs and symptoms are present, imaging studies are generally not indicated. Stage II to IV disease requires annual follow-up after the first two years of every two to six months, then every two years for the next two years. Primary tumor site assessment is advised using either contrast CT or post-operative MRI with or without contrast. Depending on each patient's unique risk of recurrence, more imaging of the affected and surrounding regions might be necessary.

8.3.7.9. Complications

The most frequent side effects, similar to those of many other high-grade STSs, include metastasis, local recurrences, and death. These adverse events may also be treatment-related and present as limb amputation disability, organ damage sequelae, wound complications, or neurovascular compromise, depending on the affected area.

8.3.7.10. Deterrence and Patient Education

To ensure proper follow-up, treatment adherence, and reassurance, patient education regarding UPS is of utmost importance. According to a study, up to 45% of individuals diagnosed with sarcoma experience symptoms of psychological distress. Among the primary concerns expressed by these patients are the impact on daily activities and finances, the lack of information resources, the need for group support, and the complexities of the healthcare system.

8.3.7.11. Enhancing Healthcare Team Outcomes

Treatment decisions should involve an interprofessional healthcare team, as recommended by current guidelines. This typically includes medical specialists (radiation oncology) and surgical specialists (general, plastic, reconstructive, vascular, orthopedic) with extensive experience in dealing with STSs. It is important to note that most patients will initially be seen by general practitioners, and some may receive specialized treatment before proceeding to occupational therapy and physical therapy. Therefore, training programs for non-specialists and primary care providers can also improve overall patient care. Pharmacy and nursing professionals will contribute from their respective areas of expertise. Community-level education is crucial to raise awareness of the disease and promote the establishment and growth of sarcoma organizations and support groups. This interprofessional approach to care will yield the best patient outcomes.

8.3.8. Lymphoma of Bone

White blood cells called lymphocytes are the source of lymphoma, a type of cancer. Even though the lymph nodes are where most lymphomas start, the illness can originate anywhere in the body. Bone marrow, the spongy tissue found inside most bones, is where primary lymphoma of bone (PLB) begins. PLB makes up only 3% of all malignant (cancerous) bone tumors, making it an extremely uncommon occurrence. Chemotherapy and radiation are typically used in conjunction for PLB treatment.

8.3.8.1. The Role of Lymphocytes

One kind of cancer that starts in lymphocytes, which are white blood cells, is called lymphoma. The immune system in the body is made up of lymphocytes. The two primary lymphocyte subtypes are:

- T lymphocytes (T cells); and
- B lymphocytes (B cells).

Both T cells and B cells have specialized roles in helping the body fight infection.

8.3.8.2. Types of Lymphoma

Lymphoma is categorized into two main types depending on the presence of specific cells known as Reed-Sternberg cells when examined under a microscope.

The two main types of lymphoma are:

- Hodgkin's Lymphoma; and
- Non-Hodgkin's Lymphoma.

Doctors differentiate between the two types of lymphomas based on whether the tumors start in the body's B or T cells. Diffuse large B cell lymphoma (DLBCL), a non-Hodgkin's lymphoma of B cell origin, accounts for the majority of primary bone lymphoma cases. Numerous different types of lymphomas cause the remaining cases.

8.3.8.3. Primary Lymphoma of Bone

Bone primary lymphoma is extremely uncommon. Compared to tumors that originate in bone, cancers that begin elsewhere in the body and then metastasize—or spread—to bone are far more common. One or more destructive bone lesions—those that break down healthy bone—may be present in PLB patients. Though they can develop in any bone, these lesions most frequently affect those with red bone marrow. This comprises:

- Flat bones — such as the pelvis, spine, and ribs;
- Long bones — such as the femur (thighbone) and humerus (upper arm bone).

Although PLB can strike anyone at any age, individuals over the age of 30 are more frequently diagnosed with it. Men are more affected than women.

8.3.8.4. Cause

Physicians are uncertain about the exact cause of PLB, but individuals who have undergone organ transplants and are infected with certain viruses (such as Epstein-Barr and HIV) are more susceptible to the illness.

8.3.8.5. Symptoms

The most typical symptom of PLB is persistent pain, even at rest. Some patients may also experience swelling or notice a lump near the tumor. Additionally, PLB can lead to bone fractures as it destroys healthy tissue and weakens the bones. These fractures, known as pathologic fractures, can sometimes be the reason for the discovery of the cancer. When patients seek treatment for the fracture, the tumor may be detected through physical examination or imaging tests. The femur (thighbone), pelvis, and spine are the most commonly affected weight-bearing bones in pathologic fractures.

Other symptoms of PLB may include:

- Fatigue;
- Feeling ill;
- Fever;
- Night sweats;
- Weight loss.

In rare instances, if a tumor compresses the spinal cord, neurological symptoms may appear. Neurological symptoms could include any of the following:

- Shooting pain;
- Numbness or tingling in the legs;
- Bowel or bladder incontinence.

8.3.8.6. Doctor Examination

8.3.8.6.1. Physical Examination

The doctor will:

- Talk with the patient about the general health and medical history;
- Ask about the symptoms;

Examine the painful area, looking for:

- Tenderness over the bone;
- Swelling or a mass;

- Enlarged or hard lymph nodes.

The physician will diagnose primary lymphoma of the bone with the aid of imaging and other tests

8.3.8.6.2. Laboratory Tests

Laboratory tests will probably be ordered by the doctors to look for abnormalities (levels outside of normal ranges) in the blood.

- Blood count;
- Electrolytes;
- Inflammation;
- Hormone levels;
- Cancer markers.

Blood tests may also be prescribed by the doctors to look for variations in the kinds and quantities of various blood cell types. Potential discoveries consist of:

- Anemia (low red blood cell count);
- Thrombocytopenia (low platelet count).

8.3.8.6.3. Imaging Tests

Radiology images: X-rays can produce images of dense materials such as bone. The inner portion of the bone in PLB will appear mottled, or "moth-eaten," on an X-ray.

- Erosion (small craters or holes) of the bone;
- A soft tissue mass or swelling;
- Change in the normal shape of the bone due to tumor expansion.

The doctor will use the results of the X-rays to determine whether further imaging tests are necessary.

Additional imaging tests: The doctor may request further imaging to help assess the tumor if more detailed information is required.

Other imaging tests may include:

- Computerized tomography (CT) scan;
- Magnetic resonance imaging (MRI) scan;
- Positron emission tomography (PET) scan;

These tests can assist the physician in determining whether the cancer has grown into adjacent soft tissues or migrated to other areas of the body.

Biopsy: A bone biopsy is a procedure used to make a final (and definitive) diagnosis of primary lymphoma of the bone. A tiny sample of the tumor is taken out during a bone biopsy and examined under a microscope.

The procedure can be carried out as a minor incision or as a needle procedure under local anesthesia. An interventional radiologist or an orthopedic surgeon may carry out this procedure. Under a microscope, lymphomas typically show up as a large number of tiny, round, blue cells. The diagnosis of primary lymphoma of the bone can be difficult. To confirm the diagnosis, numerous specialized studies are required, and multiple biopsies are required for certain patients.

8.3.8.7. Staging

To stage the tumor, The doctor will perform additional tests after determining that the tumor is PLB.

Tumor stage is determined by several factors, including:

- The size and location of the primary tumor;
- Lymph node involvement;
- Whether the cancer has metastasized (spread to other parts of the body).

The doctor will be able to choose the best course of action for treatment based on the tumor's stage.

8.3.8.8. Treatment

8.3.8.8.1. Chemotherapy

PLB is typically managed with a combination of radiation therapy and multi-agent chemotherapy (CHOP, vincristine, doxorubicin, and prednisone), either alone or in combination. The specific combination of drugs used will depend on the tumor's stage and the results of imaging tests. In some cases, an additional medication such as rituximab, which specifically targets tumor cells, may be necessary.

8.3.8.8.2. Radiation Therapy

Radiation therapy is commonly employed to destroy tumor cells in primary bone lymphomas. By utilizing high doses of X-rays, radiation therapy kills cancer cells in the bone and promotes bone healing. A radiation oncology expert oversees meticulous strategies to selectively eliminate lymphoma cells while safeguarding healthy, normal cells.

8.3.8.8.3. Surgical Treatment

Surgical intervention is generally not required to remove the tumor in most cases of primary bone lymphoma. However, in situations where there is a pathologic fracture or an imminent pathologic fracture (i.e., one that is expected to occur soon), some patients may need surgery to stabilize the affected bone and enhance its security. By inserting metal rods, plates, and screws during the procedure, the surgeon can address existing fractures or prevent future bone breakage. This surgical intervention often helps alleviate pain and improve mobility, as PLB can cause significant pain and immobility.

The surgeon fixes an existing fracture or stops bone breakage before it happens by inserting metal rods, plates, and screws during the procedure.

8.3.8.9. Outcome

The outcome after treatment will depend on several factors, including:

- Age;
- The size, location, and stage of the tumor;
- The method of treatment.

The patient's doctor will see them following treatment to evaluate their response and ensure that the tumor has not returned or developed complications. Routine follow-up appointments are necessary to monitor the patient's progress.

8.3.9. Malignant Giant Cell Tumor

An uncommon and aggressive non-cancerous tumor is the giant cell tumor of the bone. Adults typically experience it between the ages of 20 and 40, when skeletal bone growth is finished. It typically appears at the end of a bone, close to a joint. Giant cell tumors typically affect the knee, but they can also affect the bones of the arms and legs. Additionally, flat bones such as the pelvis and breastbone may be affected.

8.3.9.1. Causes

Although the precise etiology of giant cell tumors is still unknown, they have occasionally been connected to a bone disease called Paget's disease. This is a long-term bone disease that causes enlarged and malformed bones.

8.3.9.2. Symptoms

These are the most typical signs of a tumor with giant cells. However, every individual may have a unique set of symptoms. Among the symptoms are:

- A visible mass;
- Bone fracture;
- Fluid buildup in the joint nearest the affected bone;
- Limited movement in the nearest joint;
- Pain at the nearest joint.

Giant cell tumor symptoms can mimic those of other illnesses. For a diagnosis, always consult the healthcare provider.

8.3.9.3. Diagnosis

In addition to a complete medical history and physical exam, other tests may include:

- **Biopsy:** A biopsy is a diagnostic procedure in which tissue samples are taken from the patient and analyzed under a microscope to look for the presence of cancer or other abnormal cells.
- **Radionuclide Bone Scans:** A nuclear imaging test used to identify tumors and diseases of the bones as well as the source of inflammation or pain in the bones.
- **X-Rays:** A diagnostic procedure that creates pictures of internal organs, bones, and tissues on film by using invisible electromagnetic energy beams.

8.3.9.4. Treatment

The specific treatment for giant cell tumors will be determined by the healthcare provider based on:

- Patient's age, overall health, and medical history;
- Extent of the disease;
- Patient's tolerance for specific medications, procedures, or therapies;
- Expectations for the course of the disease;
- Patient's opinion or preference.

The aim of treating a giant cell tumor is to eradicate the tumor while averting any harm to the bones. The course of treatment could involve:

- Amputation, in severe cases;
- Bone grafting;
- Bone reconstruction;
- Physical therapy to regain strength and mobility;
- Surgery to remove the tumor and any damaged bone.

Radiation therapy is frequently used to control and occasionally even eradicate tumors that cannot be surgically removed. Tumors with giant cells may recur. One may need to consult their healthcare provider for several years following that.

A Closer Look

Paget Disease of Bone

Paget's disease is a chronic bone disease that primarily affects middle-aged individuals. It is characterized by excessive formation and breakdown of bone tissue. This condition can be localized, affecting multiple bones or even the entire skeleton. In some cases, it may only affect a single bone. Paget's disease is classified as one of the metabolic bone diseases. It is named after Sir James Paget, an English surgeon and pathologist who first described the condition. Individuals of northern European descent are more susceptible to developing Paget's disease of the bone, while those of Asian and African descent are less affected. The disease is characterized by both excessive bone formation, mediated by osteoblasts (cells that synthesize bone), and excessive bone resorption, mediated by osteoclasts (cells that dissolve and absorb bone). When osteoclasts isolated from patients with Paget's disease of the bone are examined under an electron microscope, structures resembling viruses can be observed. These osteoclasts are highly active, rapidly resorbing bone and stimulating the activation of a "coupling factor" that leads to increased bone production by local osteoblasts. This uncontrolled and disorganized increase in bone formation can result in regions of excessive bone formation and resorption, leading to bone deformities and weakening.

Men are more likely than women to have advanced Paget's disease of the bone, but both sexes are affected in roughly equal amounts. The bony abnormalities are detected through radionuclide bone scans or X-rays, which are performed for other purposes, as many patients are asymptomatic. The bone-forming enzyme alkaline phosphatase (ALP) is found in high concentrations in the serum of certain patients. Bone overgrowth may be associated with pain or may solely affect the affected bone. A significant amount of pain, for example, may be caused by an overgrowth of a vertebrae or skull bone impinging on the spinal cord or nerves. Bones also become softer and experience increased blood supply during the bone-destructive stages, which can lead to heart or circulatory issues. Bones that are still developing are brittle, dense, and prone to fractures. The disease most commonly affects the femur, pelvis, skull, and spine, although it can affect almost any bone. Pathological fractures and arthritis are common in patients with classic, advanced Paget's disease of bone. These patients also exhibit macrocephaly, a shortened spine, and bowed thighs and legs. Bone cancer rarely exacerbates the condition.

There is currently no known cure for Paget's disease of the bone. Treatment typically involves medication that inhibits bone cell activity, such as calcitonin or bisphosphonates. Additionally, individuals with Paget's disease of the bone should engage in regular exercise and ensure adequate daily intake of calcium and vitamin D.

8.4. Summary

- The majority of bone tumors are non-malignant (not cancerous). This signifies that non-malignant tumors do not relocate from their original site to another area.
- Bone-forming tumors, constituting 12% of non-malignant bone tumors, are non-malignant osteoblastic tumors.
- Being the most prevalent non-malignant tumor of the bone, osteochondroma accounts for 20–50% of non-malignant tumors and 10–15% of all tumors. Typically, it develops in growing bones. Due to this, some studies have suggested that they most likely originate from the epiphyseal growth plate.
- Fibrous tissue that proliferates and replaces the normal bone matrix is the characteristic feature of Fibrous Dysplasia (FD), a benign bone lesion. It constitutes approximately 5–7% of benign bone tumors (BBTs).
- Unicameral bone cysts, also known as solitary bone cysts, are lesions lined with fibrous tissue and filled with fluid.
- Malignant (cancerous) tumors are more perilous and uncommon compared to benign ones. Malignant denotes a tumor that had a moderate to high likelihood of spreading from its original site of development. The lymphatic or blood vessels serve as the conduits through which the cancer cells disseminate.
- Multiple myeloma is a form of cancer that arises in leukocytes referred to as plasma cells. Through the production of antibodies, these plasma cells, when healthy, contribute to the defense against infections. Antibodies actively search for and engage in the battle against pathogens.
- Osteosarcoma is the most prevalent primary bone cancer in children and is caused by primitive mesenchymal cells that form osteoid tissue.
- Adamantinomas are uncommon bone tumors that are typically found in the tibia and are considered to be low-grade malignant.
- Malignant cartilaginous neoplasms, or chondrosarcomas, can have a variety of morphological characteristics and clinical manifestations. Approximately 20% of all primary malignant bone tumors are of this type.
- Tumors known as chordomas can develop anywhere in the base of the skull or the spine. Chordomas most frequently occur in the base of the skull (approximately one-third of cases) and the lower back (sacral area), accounting for one-third to one-half of cases.
- Ewing sarcoma is a cancer that primarily occurs in the bone or soft tissue. Although it can develop in any bone, it is most commonly found in the hip bones, ribs, or long bones such as the femur, tibia, or humerus.
- Soft tissue malignancy, or sarcoma, is one type of undifferentiated pleomorphic sarcoma (UPS). Soft tissues aid in the support and connection of the human body.
- Lymphocytes, a type of white blood cells, serve as the origin of lymphoma, a form of malignancy. Although lymph nodes are the primary site of lymphoma development, the

disease can originate from any part of the body. Primary lymphoma of bone (PLB) begins in the bone marrow, the spongy tissue located within most bones.

- An atypical and assertive benign neoplasm is the giant cell tumor of the bone. Adults generally encounter this condition between the ages of 20 and 40, once skeletal bone growth has concluded.

References

1. Davies, A. M., Murali, S., & Steven, L. J. J., (2009). *Imaging of Bone Tumors and Tumor-Like Lesions*. Berlin, Heidelberg: Springer Berlin Heidelberg. http://dx.doi.org/10.1007/978-3-540-77984-1.
2. Kang, H. S., Joong, M. A., & Yusuhn, K., (2017). *Oncologic Imaging: Bone Tumors*. Singapore: Springer Singapore. http://dx.doi.org/10.1007/978-981-287-703-1.
3. Paulos, J., & Dominique, G. P., (2021). *Bone Tumors*. London: Springer London. http://dx.doi.org/10.1007/978-1-4471-7501-8.
4. Santini-Araujo, E., Ricardo, K. K., Franco, B., & Yong-Koo, P., (2020). *Tumors and Tumor-Like Lesions of Bone*. Cham: Springer International Publishing. http://dx.doi.org/10.1007/978-3-030-28315-5.
5. Santini-Araujo, E., Ricardo, K. K., Franco, B., & Yong-Koo, P., (2015). *Tumors and Tumor-Like Lesions of Bone*. London: Springer London. http://dx.doi.org/10.1007/978-1-4471-6578-1.
6. Wu, J. S., & Mary, G. H., (2012). *Bone Tumors*. New York, NY: Springer New York. http://dx.doi.org/10.1007/978-1-4419-0808-7.

Chapter 9

SCFE, PERTHES' DISEASE AND OTHER OSTEOCHONDRITIS

Contents

9.1. Introduction

A common hip pathology in pre-adolescents and adolescents is slipped capital femoral epiphysis, also known as slipped upper femoral epiphysis. It occurs when there is an abnormal displacement of the femoral epiphysis inferiorly and posteriorly in relation to the femoral head and neck. Young adults who complain of atraumatic hip, thigh, or knee pain—which may be accompanied by a limp or an inability to bear weight—often present with this condition. The majority of SCFE cases are idiopathic. Frequently, no past trauma or injury exists prior to the onset of symptoms. Osteochondrosis is a group of diseases characterized by disruptions in endochondral ossification that arise during periods of rapid growth. Legg-Calvé-Perthes disease is one instance where a systemic etiology has frequently been proposed. It is characterized by disruption of the blood supply to the femoral head epiphysis. About 3% of adults who had Legg-Calvé-Perthes disease as children develop osteochondritis dissecans after skeletal maturity is reached.

Orientation and Directional Terms

Term	Definition	Illustration
Osteoarthritis	Osteoarthritis is the most common type of arthritis. It occurs when the cartilage that lines the joints is worn down or damaged, causing the bones to rub together when you use that joint. A healthcare provider will assist you in finding a combination of treatments to manage the symptoms.	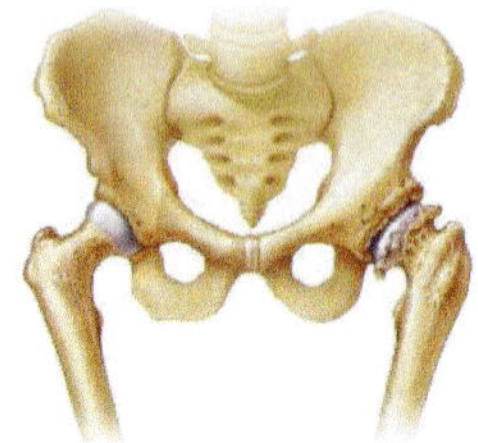
Osteochondroplasty	Osteochondroplasty is a surgical procedure utilized to repair and reshape damaged cartilage and protruding bony surfaces of the femur or acetabulum in the hip joint.	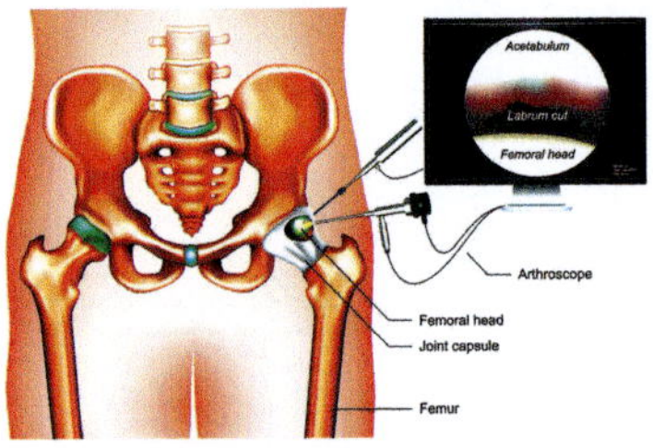
Osgood-Schlatter disease	The bony bump where the patellar tendon attaches to the tibia.	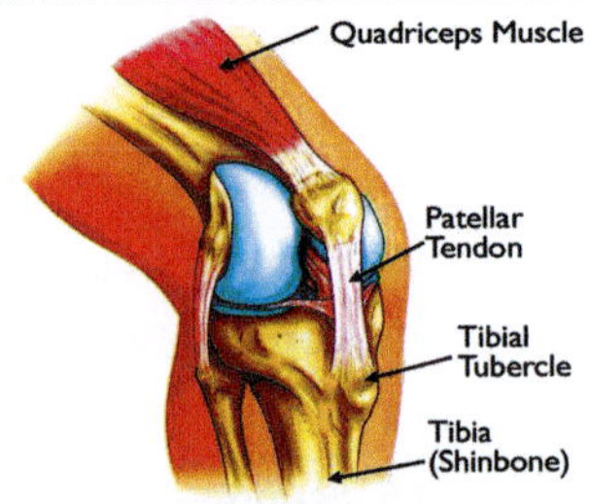
Chondrolysis	Chondrolysis of the hip is characterized by the rapid and progressive destruction of the articular cartilage of the femoral head and acetabulum, resulting in joint space narrowing and restricted movement.	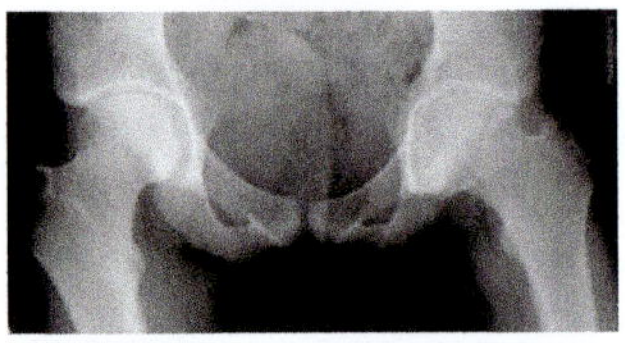
Epiphyseal dysplasia	Multiple epiphyseal dysplasia is a type of skeletal dysplasia. Skeletal dysplasias are conditions that cause problems with cartilage.	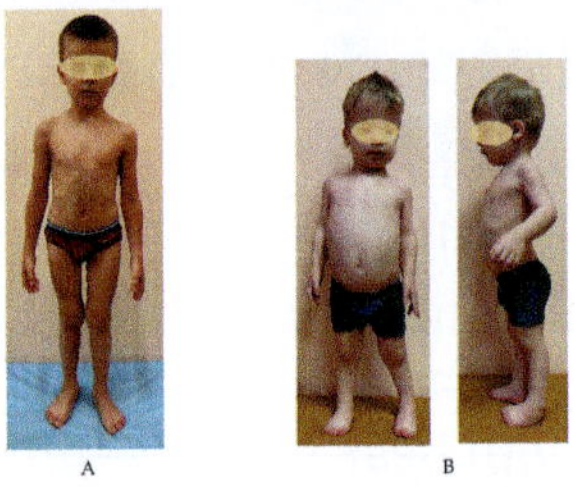

9.2. Slipped Capital Femoral Epiphysis (SCFE)

The most prevalent hip pathology in pre-adolescents and adolescents is slipped capital femoral epiphysis (SCFE), also known as slipped upper femoral epiphysis (SUFE). However, due to the chronic nature of the presentation or its unusual presentation, such as thigh or knee pain, this diagnosis is often overlooked or delayed. When a preteen or adolescent presents with leg pain, there are numerous potential diagnoses to consider. Therefore, it is essential for medical professionals to always rule out SCFE. There is a correlation between increased rates of complications, such as femoral head osteonecrosis, and a delay in the diagnosis of SCFE.

9.2.1. Etiology

The majority of slipped capital femoral epiphysis (SCFE) cases are of an idiopathic nature. Frequently, there is an absence of previous trauma or injury prior to the onset of symptoms. Furthermore, a correlation has been documented between the onset of SCFE and individuals who suffer from Down syndrome, renal problems, and endocrine disorders such as hypothyroidism, hyperthyroidism, panhypopituitarism, and growth hormone deficiency. The most frequent cause of nonidiopathic SCFE has been found to be hypothyroidism. Therefore, an endocrine test is indicated when a child under the age of 10 or weighing less than the 50th percentile exhibits symptoms of SCFE.

9.2.2. Epidemiology

Regarding pre-adolescent and adolescent patients, SCFE is one of the most prevalent hip pathologies, occurring in roughly 10.8/1,00,000 (Range: 0.33/1,00,000 to 24.8/1,00,000). Obesity is the single biggest risk factor for SCFE. Male sex, phases of rapid growth, radiation therapy to the hip in the past, and retroversion of the acetabulum or femoral head—both of which increase mechanical shear forces across the physis—are additional risk factors. The average age of onset is 11.2 years in females and 12.0 years in males. The left hip is more commonly affected, but approximately 25% (Range: 8 to 50%) of cases are bilateral.

9.2.3. Pathophysiology

The precise mechanism is still unknown. Displacement is thought to result from a high physiologic axial load passing through a comparatively weak physis. Obesity and other conditions increase the mechanical weight and force transmitted, while certain renal or endocrine disorders can weaken the physis. The metaphysis externally rotates with anterior translation, while the epiphysis remains in the acetabulum. This slippage takes place at the physis's hypertrophic zone. A number of factors increase the risk of slippage of the physis during adolescence. This results in the physis being in a vertical position where it is more vulnerable to shear forces, weakening, and thinning the perichondrial ring of la Croix, and further destabilizing it by unlocking the physis's mamillary processes. SCFE is a Salter-Harris type I fracture that can be differentiated with preceding epiphysiolysis, more steady displacement, and intact periosteum in chronic cases or partially torn in acute cases.

9.2.4. History and Physical Details

A pre-adolescent, adolescent, or young adult patient complaining of atraumatic hip, thigh, or knee pain should always be evaluated for SCFE by the clinician, especially if it is accompanied by limping or an inability to bear weight. Although the hip is where SCFE-related pain is most frequently reported (52%), other common locations for reports of pain include the groin (13.9%), thigh (35%), and knee (26%). Medial obturator nerve pain is typically the cause of knee pain. The average time for a patient to experience symptoms before being diagnosed with SCFE is four to five months; however, a patient may present with symptoms in as little as three weeks. Even though the majority of patients do not disclose any past trauma or injury prior to the onset of symptoms, a history of trauma or injury does not rule out SCFE. The patient might favor crossing one leg over the other while sitting. Examining the affected extremity may reveal a limited internal rotation, and passive internal rotation may cause pain. Internal rotation, abduction, and hip flexion would all be lost. The patient may demonstrate the Drehmann sign, which is obligatory external rotation with passive hip flexion to 90°. The patient may also walk with a Trendelenburg, antalgic, or shuffling gait, or they may not be able to bear any weight at all. There may or may not be thigh atrophy.

9.2.5. Evaluation

Anteroposterior (AP) and frog-leg lateral views on bilateral hip radiographs should be the initial step in evaluating patients with suspected SCFE. Bilateral radiographs are necessary for comparison purposes. Klien's line, a radiographic finding, is used to identify SCFE on plain radiographs. A line is drawn along the superior border of the femoral neck on the AP view. In a healthy hip, the line intersects the lateral aspect of the superior femoral epiphysis. The absence of this intersection, known as the Trethowan sign, indicates the presence of SCFE. However, the diagnostic sensitivity of this method for SCFE is relatively low.

Additional techniques for identifying SCFE in plain radiography include the Southwick slip angle and the "S" sign. The Southwick slip angle measures the degree of epiphyseal displacement in relation to the diaphysis and is considered a more sensitive technique for identifying SCFE. The "S" sign involves drawing a line from the proximal femoral head-neck junction to the proximal femoral physis along the inferior cortical outline of the femur in the frog-leg lateral view. In a normal hip, the cortical outlines are symmetrical, without sharp turns or broken continuity. Asymmetrical cortical outlines, sharp turns, or broken continuity suggest the presence of SCFE. Combining the "S" sign with Klein's line has been found to improve the sensitivity and specificity of SCFE detection.

The expansion or lucency of the growth plate, or epiphysiolysis, may be an early radiographic sign. Another indication that can be observed on AP radiographs is the metaphyseal blanch sign of steel, which refers to the blurring of the proximal femoral metaphysis due to overlapping with the displaced epiphysis.

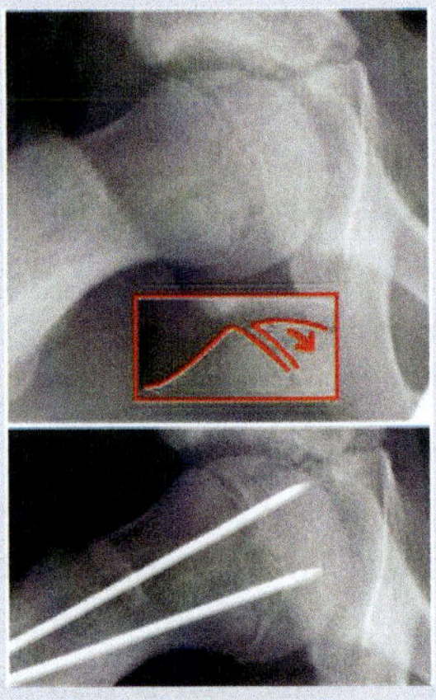

Figure 9.1. *X-ray showing a slipped capital femoral epiphysis, before and after surgical fixation.*

Source: By Dr. Jochen Lengerke – Praxis Dr. Jochen Lengerke, Public Domain, https://commons.wikimedia.org/w/index.php?curid=6637014.

In cases where there is a high clinical suspicion but radiographs do not show findings consistent with SCFE, obtaining an MRI for further assessment may be considered by the clinician. In diagnosing pre-slip cases, magnetic resonance imaging (MRI) can be valuable in identifying metaphyseal edema and growth plate widening. Although more research on the use of ultrasound is needed, several recent small studies suggest that it may be a more sensitive modality than radiographs for diagnosing SCFE (Figure 9.1).

If the patient is under 10 years old or prepubescent, has short stature (more than two standard deviations below the mean for age), or weighs less than the 50th percentile for age, the clinician should consider laboratory testing to assess potential underlying medical conditions such as endocrine or renal disorders. Thyroid-stimulating hormone (TSH), thyroxine (free T4), blood urea nitrogen (BUN), and serum creatinine levels are among the initial laboratory tests that may be performed. In consultation with relevant pediatric specialists, such as pediatric endocrinologists, additional testing can be conducted.

9.2.6. Treatment/Management

The primary function of management is to oversee both stable and unstable SCFE. This comprises:

9.2.6.1. In Situ Fixation with Percutaneous Screws

The objective is to prevent further slippage of the epiphysis. *In situ*, the epiphysis is immobilized. If a reduction is required to minimize the risk of osteonecrosis, a gentle reduction is performed rather than a forceful one. The use of one or two screws is a subject of controversy. While biomechanical stability can be achieved with a single screw, using two screws carries a higher risk of complications, such as violation of the articular surface. In both the AP and lateral views, the screw should be centrally positioned in the head and perpendicular to the physis. To achieve this, the entry point in the proximal femur should be anterior. However, caution must be taken not to be medial to the intertrochanteric line to prevent impingement between the screw head and the acetabulum during flexion. To halt the progression of slippage, screws should be advanced until they are 5 mm away from the subchondral bone in all views. At least five threads should engage the epiphysis.

The process is carried out with the assistance of fluoroscopy. In any view, the screw tip should not penetrate the articular surface. The approach-withdraw method has been utilized to verify the correct positioning of the screw. Under live fluoroscopy, this is achieved by rotating the hip internally and externally to the maximum extent. It is believed that the screw tip approaches the subchondral bone before retracting from it. The accurate positioning of the screw is the main focus of this procedure. After surgery, patients with stable slips are allowed to bear weight following fixation, while those with unstable slips are allowed to partially bear weight for six weeks. It has been demonstrated that capsulotomy reduces intracapsular pressure in unstable SCFE. However, it does not appear to decrease the incidence of avascular necrosis (AVN). Another controversial technique is the prophylactic fixation of the contralateral hip, which is recommended when there are significant risk factors for a contralateral slip, such as endocrine disorders, obesity, male gender, and the first slip occurring at a younger age than ten.

9.2.6.2. Open Reduction and Internal Fixation of the Slipped Epiphysis (Modified Dunn Procedure)

The objective is to stabilize the epiphysis and correct the deformity of the proximal femur while ensuring the preservation of blood supply to the femoral head. The Gibson approach is employed, wherein the hip is surgically dislocated during the procedure. The patient assumes a decubitus position on the side. A straight lateral incision is made over the greater trochanter to access the space between the Medius and gluteus maximus. To expose the metaphysis, a trochanteric flip osteotomy, specifically a Z-shaped anterior capsulotomy, is performed. Prior to hip dislocation, the slipped epiphysis is primarily stabilized using K-wires, followed by the application of a traction hook around the femoral neck. After hip dislocation, the periosteum is incised along the anterior neck, proximal femur, and lesser trochanter. Anterior and posterior periosteal flaps are created bluntly. The epiphysis is fully separated from the metaphysis using a chisel, and the metaphysis is subsequently debrided. Two or three K-wires, inserted in both antegrade and retrograde fashion, are utilized to reduce and fix the epiphysis to the metaphysis. Patients are advised to bear partial weight for a period of six weeks post-surgery.

This contentious management technique is also recommended for severe and unstable slips. Capital realignment, a modified Dunn procedure, is used to carry it out. Following the initial course of treatment, patients may experience symptomatic consequences that can also be addressed surgically, such as femoroacetabular impingement due to a cam lesion from a metaphyseal bump or cases of SCFE deformity with a slip angle of less than 30°. Osteochondroplasty is a treatment option for both. Proximal femoral osteotomy, however, is a treatment option for severe SCFE deformity with a slip of greater than 30° to 45°, which is painful or limits function in the absence of hip osteoarthritis or osteonecrosis. There have been several descriptions of proximal femoral osteotomies; the intertrochanteric (Imhauser) osteotomy is the most widely performed. Femoral neck cuneiform osteotomy is the procedure that can correct deformities the most. There have also been descriptions of subtrochanteric (Southwick) osteotomies.

In cases of mild to moderate chronic SCFE deformity, where a prominent metaphyseal bump causes pain and limited range of motion, osteochondroplasty is recommended. Osteochondroplasty can be performed through a modified Smith-Peterson approach via a limited anterior arthrotomy, or arthroscopically using a burr. Additionally, a curved osteotome can be utilized to remove the bump, and a burr can be employed to reshape the head-neck junction after the hip is surgically dislocated.

9.2.7. Differential Diagnosis

Infectious etiologies such as septic arthritis and osteomyelitis should be considered in the differential diagnosis of SCFE, particularly if the patient presents with symptoms of fever or malnutrition. Etiologies such as avulsion fracture of the anterior iliac spine(s), adductor muscle strain, ligamentous knee injury, and femur or pelvic fractures should be taken into consideration if the onset of pain is reported in the context of a sports injury or other traumatic event. In the appropriate clinical setting, inflammatory processes like Osgood-Schlatter disease, Legg-Calve-Perthes disease, and transient synovitis can also be considered. Even if other clinical features are atypical, the clinician should seriously consider obtaining plain radiographs of the hips if the patient's clinical examination is consistent with a possible SCFE.

9.2.8. Staging

The Southwick Slip Angle Classification, Temporal Classification, and Loder Classification are the three classification schemes used in SCFE. Introduced in 1993, the Loder Classification aids in the prediction of osteonecrosis and is based on weight-bearing capacity. If the patient is able to bear weight, with or without crutches, the case can be considered stable, with a lower than 10% chance of osteonecrosis. If the patient is unable to support their own weight, they may be deemed unstable, with a higher risk of osteonecrosis (24–47%). The Southwick Slip

Angle Classification assesses the severity of SCFE by measuring the difference in the epiphyseal diaphyseal angle between the affected hip and the unaffected/contralateral hip, both in AP and lateral hip radiographs. Mild cases are classified as <30°, moderate cases as 30–50°, and severe cases as more than 50°.

Temporal classification is based on the duration of symptoms. However, it is rarely used as it does not affect prognosis. When a patient experiences worsening symptoms for longer than three weeks, SCFE is classified as acute on chronic. If symptoms persist for longer than three weeks, it is classified as chronic. Another grading system for SCFE is based on the percentage of slippage. Grade I is assigned to cases with up to 33% slippage, Grade II to cases with 34 to 50% slippage, and Grade III to cases with more than 50% slippage.

9.2.9. Prognosis

The prognosis heavily depends on the Loder classification. When SCFE was initially studied in 1993, it was found that 47% of patients with SCFE who were considered unstable eventually developed osteonecrosis, whereas no patient classified as stable experienced this condition.

9.2.10. Complications

The development of femoral head osteonecrosis, chondrolysis, femoroacetabular impingement, labral tears, infection, chronic pain, and femoral growth arrest due to premature closure of the physis are among the complications associated with SCFE. Early-onset hip osteoarthritis is one of the later consequences of SCFE.

- The first injury may cause femoral head osteonecrosis, which is more likely in cases of unstable SCFE. Furthermore, metalwork positioned in the posterosuperior aspect of the femoral neck may cause it to develop as a postoperative complication, as there is a chance of it impairing the femoral neck's blood supply.
- Articular surface penetration may result in chondrolysis. Usually, patients will appear with a limited range of motion and pain. A CT scan would be the most effective modality to evaluate metalwork penetration, as radiographs will reveal less joint space.
- Failure of proximal femoral remodeling results in femoroacetabular impingement (pistol grip deformity). As previously mentioned, proximal femoral osteotomy is one way to address this.

Slip progression: This has been reported in 1 to 2% of cases with single screw fixation.

9.2.11. Deterrence and Patient Education

Strict non-weight-bearing status instructions are needed for patients and their families. They will also need counseling regarding appropriate pain management. Anticipatory guidance regarding SCFE and the need for urgent orthopedic follow-up should be provided to patients and their families if, following pediatric orthopedic consultation, urgent operative management is not carried out. Admission with pediatric orthopedic consultation should be seriously considered if there is any reason to believe that the family might not be able or willing to follow up with an orthopedic surgeon.

9.2.12. Enhancing Healthcare Team Outcomes

The most prevalent hip pathology in pre-adolescent and adolescent patients is slipped capital femoral epiphysis (SCFE), also known as slipped upper femoral epiphysis (SUFE). Nevertheless, the diagnosis may go unnoticed or be delayed. When making a differential diagnosis for pre-adolescent and adolescent patients experiencing leg pain, primary care (family medicine, internal medicine, or pediatrics) and emergency medicine clinicians—including clinicians and advanced practice providers—should always take SCFE into account. To ensure the best possible care, it is imperative that clinicians—including specialists in radiology and orthopedics—work together effectively with nurses, pharmacists, physical therapists, and patient care technicians. Patients who have been diagnosed with SCFE must be put on strict non-weight bearing precautions right away and given enough analgesia. Prioritizing urgent pediatric orthopedic consultation to provide definitive management is necessary. In addition, clinicians ought to take into account any clinical indicators of potential underlying renal or endocrine disorders and further assess patients as needed in collaboration with the relevant subspecialists. For the best possible patient outcomes, interprofessional collaboration and honest communication are essential.

9.3. Legg-Calve-Perthes' Disease

The childhood hip disorder Legg-Calvé-Perthes disease (LCPD) is caused by a disruption in blood flow to the femoral head. The bone stops growing and dies (osteonecrosis or avascular necrosis) due to reduced blood supply. The femoral head weakens and loses bone mass as new blood vessels penetrate the dead bone and eliminate the necrotic bone over time. Although it can affect children as young as two years old, children between 4 and 8 are most likely to have the condition. It may result in a permanent femoral head deformity, increasing the risk of osteoarthritis in adults. One type of hip osteochondritis is called Perthes. It's important to consider bilateral Perthes, which affects both hips, to rule out multiple epiphyseal dysplasia.

9.3.1. Epidemiology

Perthes' disease is a common hip disorder in young children, with a prevalence of 5.5 per 1,00,000 children annually. The lifetime risk of developing the disease is approximately one in 1,200 individuals, with boys being affected three to five times more often than girls. New cases of Perthes' disease rarely occur after age 14, with cases diagnosed after this age typically being from early childhood or a different cause of AVN.

White northern Europeans tend to have a higher incidence of Perthes' disease compared to other ethnicities, although data is limited in the Southern Hemisphere. Children of individuals with the disease may have a slightly increased risk, possibly due to genetics or shared environmental factors. The disease is most commonly seen in children aged three to twelve, with a median age of six. Incidence rates in the UK show a pattern of lower rates in London and higher rates in more northern areas like Scotland. Some evidence suggests that socioeconomically deprived communities may have a higher risk of developing the disease, possibly due to factors like tobacco smoke exposure. However, this association is complicated by the common socioeconomic gradient seen in both smoking and Perthes' disease.

9.3.2. Signs and Symptoms

The majority of children with the condition are between the ages of 4 and 10. Hip pathology can cause pain to be felt in a normal knee or ankle, so common symptoms include pain in the knee, ankle, or hip. This pain is worsened by movement of the hips or legs, particularly internal hip rotation, which twists the lower leg away from the center of the body when the knee is flexed 90°. The patient has a limp when they first arrive, and their range of motion is limited, especially in abduction and internal rotation. Usually, the pain is not too severe. Elasticity in the thigh muscles can result from both imbalanced leg length and inactivity. There are situations when certain activities, such as standing, walking, running, kneeling, or bending over time, can seriously irritate or inflame the injured area. When femoral osteonecrosis is severe, the pain is typically a persistent, throbbing sensation that worsens with movement.

The child's complaints of pain, which are frequently dismissed as growing pains, and limping or other joint guarding, especially when fatigued, are the initial symptoms. While it typically originates in the hip, referred pain can also be experienced in the knee. When a child favors their injured side and puts most of their weight on their 'good' leg, it can result in pain in the unaffected hip and leg. Males are primarily affected (4:1 ratio). Although it has been identified as early as 18 months, Perthes is typically diagnosed between the ages of 5 and 12. Approximately 10% of children with the condition have bilateral Perthes, although the condition usually only affects one hip.

9.3.3. Cause

Childhood hip disorders, such as Perthes disease, are caused by a disturbance in blood flow to the head of the femur. This leads to the cessation of bone growth and subsequent osteonecrosis or AVN due to reduced blood supply. Legg proposed that LCP disease is caused by a disruption in the blood supply to the femoral epiphysis, Calvé suggested rickets, and Perthes hypothesized that an infection leading to degenerative arthritis is the cause. Currently, various factors have been associated with this condition, including altered circulatory hemodynamics, inflammation, trauma, endocrine dysfunction, and heredity. Some examples of risk factors include low birth weight, delayed skeletal maturity, short stature, systemic hormonal changes, low economic index, and impaired and disproportionate growth. Although the exact cause is unknown, Perthes disease is believed to be a result of decreased blood flow to the joint.

The condition is thought to be caused by the constriction or blockage of the ligamentum teres femoris artery, which hinders the takeover of the medial circumflex femoral artery. The medial circumflex femoral artery is the primary blood supply to the femoral head. This idiopathic vascular restrictive condition is known as LCP disease. Common symptoms include femoral head deformity, flattening, and collapse, primarily affecting male children of Caucasian descent between the ages of four and ten. Children with LCP disease often experience an uneven gait, limited range of motion, and varying degrees of groin pain. For example, a child may exhibit bone maturity equivalent to a four-year-old, despite being six years old chronologically. Consequently, the child may engage in activities appropriate for a six-year-old, but due to the lack of bone strength, they are at risk of hip joint fractures or flattening. While a deficiency in blood factors with anticoagulant properties may cause vessel blockages supplying the joint, genetics does not appear to be a determining factor in this case. There may be a deficiency in proteins C and S, which also function as blood anticoagulants. However, no evidence has been found to support this theory. Over the years, numerous theories have been proposed, but none have withstood rigorous scientific scrutiny.

9.3.4. Pathology

The femoral head weakens and experiences bone mass depletion due to the infiltration of new blood vessels into the necrotic bone, resulting in its elimination over time. The loss of bone leads to a certain degree of collapse and deformity of the femoral head, as well as occasional secondary alterations to the shape of the hip socket. The disruption of blood supply to the femoral head in the hip joint, for which no known cause exists, is commonly referred to as idiopathic avascular osteonecrosis of the capital femoral epiphysis. Adults with osteoarthritis are more prone to developing a permanent deformity of the femoral head as a consequence of Perthes. While other forms of osteochondritis can affect the elbows, knees, ankles, and feet, Perthes exclusively affects the hip. To exclude the possibility of multiple epiphyseal dysplasia, bilateral Perthes, which affects both hips, should always be thoroughly investigated.

9.3.5. Diagnosis

Hip X-rays can confirm or suggest the diagnosis. X-rays typically show a flattened and eventually fractured femoral head. In cases where X-rays are not conclusive, an MRI or bone scan may help make the diagnosis. In order to make an early diagnosis, bone scintigraphy and MRI are typically performed because plain radiographic changes take six weeks or longer to manifest clinically. MRI results are more accurate, i.e., 97–99% against 88–93% in plain radiography. A positive diagnosis for capital femoral epiphysis, or the growing femoral head, depends on patchy areas of vascularity, should an MRI or bone scan be required.

9.3.6. Treatment

Reducing pain, minimizing hip deformity, and preventing or lessening permanent femoral head deformity are the objectives of treatment to lower the chance of adult-onset severe degenerative arthritis. To assess risks and treatment options, a consultation with a pediatric orthopedic surgeon is recommended. The prognosis is more favorable for younger children compared to older children. Until the illness has progressed, the primary focus of treatment has always been to alleviate mechanical pressure from the joint. Remedial measures include the use of braces (typically for several months, with an average duration of eighteen months) to restore range of motion, traction (to separate the femur from the pelvis and reduce wear), physical therapy, and surgery (if permanent joint damage necessitates it). Custom orthotics can be utilized to maintain everyday activities. Overnight traction can be used in addition to or instead of walking aids. These devices abduct the leg(s) at a 45° angle and internally rotate the femoral head. A lumbar spine orthosis can begin proximally and extend all the way to the limbs. Waist belts and thigh cuffs, inspired by the Scottish-Rite orthosis, are the most common forms of functional bracing. Typically, an orthotist prescribes these devices after consultation with a doctor. Some research has indicated poor clinical outcomes with the Scottish Rite orthosis, leading to its decreased usage. The only recommendation for many children, particularly those whose disease first manifests before age six, is to avoid contact sports and other activities that put stress on the hips. Uncertainty surrounds the optimal course of treatment for older children (onset of Perthes after age 6). A femoral, pelvic, or shelf osteotomy, as well as the hip distraction method—which involves using an external fixator to relieve the hip of the weight bearing on it—are the current treatment options for older children beyond the age of eight. The top of the femur can grow again because of this. Children can stay active during treatment for Perthes disease by participating in a variety of other activities that reduce mechanical stress on the hip joint, even though running and high-impact sports are not advised. Swimming is highly recommended because it minimizes stress and provides a full range of motion exercise for the hip muscles. Another excellent option that reduces stress is cycling. Daily exercises are typically part of physical therapy, and progress is tracked with weekly meetings with a physiotherapist. The goal of these exercises is to enhance and preserve the femur's full range of motion inside the hip socket. In order to guarantee a flawlessly smooth interface between the femur and hip socket, these exercises must be performed throughout the healing process. This will lessen the disease's long-term effects. Investigations into the use of bisphosphonates, such as zoledronate or ibandronate, are ongoing, but firm guidelines are not yet accessible.

Perthes disease resolves on its own, but long-term issues may arise if the femur head remains malformed. The goal of treatment is not to "cure" the disease, but to minimize damage while the illness progresses. Alcohol and steroids are advised to be avoided as they lower blood oxygen levels, which are essential for healthy joints. As the affected person ages, aberrant posture and gait adopted to protect the injured joint can lead to issues with the knee and back. Hip arthritis is also associated with the condition, though this does not seem to be a definite outcome. Although this varies from person to person, hip replacements are generally necessary anytime after the age of 50 due to the regular wear and tear already placed on the already damaged hip.

9.3.7. Prognosis

The prognosis is best for children under six years old because they have more time for the dead bone to remodel and revascularize, increasing the likelihood that the disease will eventually resolve and the femoral head will heal and remain spherical. After the age of ten, children diagnosed with Perthes' disease are highly susceptible to developing osteoarthritis and coxa magna. When a diagnosis of LCP disease is made after the age of eight, surgical intervention yields better results than nonoperative measures. The most significant predictor of risk for degenerative arthritis is the shape of the femoral head at the time that Legg-Calvé Perthes disease heals; for this reason, hip congruence and femoral head shape are the most useful outcome measures (Figure 9.2).

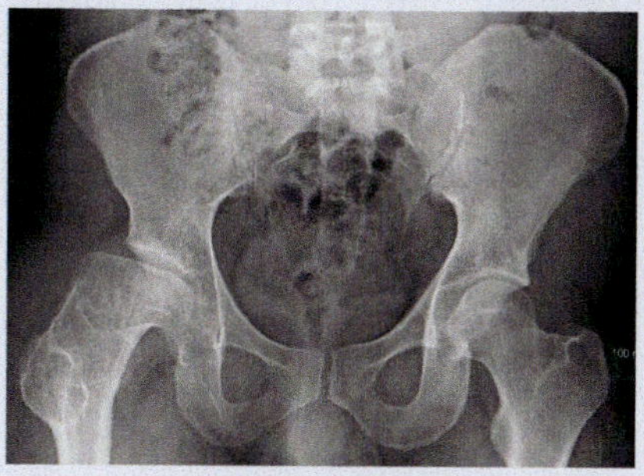

Figure 9.2. *An X-ray showing the deformity by Legg–Calvé–Perthes disease of the right hip (left side of the X-ray).*

Source: By James Heilman, MD – Own work, CC BY-SA 4.0, https://commons.wikimedia.org/w/index.php?curid=45600367.

9.4. Idiopathic Avascular Necrosis (AVN)/Osteochondritis

A degenerative bone disease called osteonecrosis is defined by the death of the bone's cellular constituents as a result of a disruption in the subchondral blood supply. It is also referred to as ischemic bone necrosis, aseptic necrosis, and AVN. At weight-bearing joints, it usually affects the epiphysis of long bones. In severe cases, a joint may collapse completely or the subchondral bone may be destroyed. AVN most commonly affects the femoral head, knee, talus, and humeral head. In general, the hip is the most frequent site. Less frequently, AVN affects other body bones like the jaw and carpus. Osteonecrosis must thus be diagnosed and treated as soon as possible. The etiology and pathogenesis of the disease are covered in this activity. It also covers the symptoms and available treatments for the most prevalent types of osteonecrosis.

9.4.1. Etiology

Osteonecrosis is caused by a decrease in the blood supply to the subchondral region. There are, however, a lot of risk factors and theories regarding how this vascular impairment develops. These can be easily divided into six groups. These are:

- Direct cellular toxicity
  - Chemotherapy
  - Radiotherapy
  - Thermal injury
  - Smoking
- Extraosseous arterial fracture
  - Hip dislocation
  - Femoral neck fracture
  - Iatrogenic post-surgery
  - Congenital arterial abnormalities
- Extraosseous venous
  - Venous abnormalities
  - Venous stasis
- Intraosseous extravascular compression
  - Hemorrhage
  - Elevated bone marrow pressure
  - Fatty infiltration of bone marrow due to prolonged high-dose corticosteroid use
  - Cellular hypertrophy and marrow infiltration (Gaucher disease)
  - Bone marrow edema
  - Displaced fractures
- Intraosseous intravascular occlusion
  - Coagulation disorders such as thrombophilias and hypofibrinolysis
  - Sickle cell crises
- Multifactorial

Mutations in the COL2A1 gene, which codes for the production of type 2 collagen, have occasionally shown evidence of autosomal dominant inheritance patterns. However, frequently a cause cannot be found, and these patients are diagnosed with idiopathic osteonecrosis. Over time, repetitive trauma—such as working on an assembly line—can result in AVN. Nontraumatic risks for AVN include any factor that might affect the blood supply to the bone. Changes in the bone marrow brought on by radiation can result in AVN. Significant small blood vessel blockage brought on by hyperlipidemia lowers the amount of blood that nourishes the bone. Diseases such as sickle cell anemia can also reduce the blood flow to the bone (Figure 9.3).

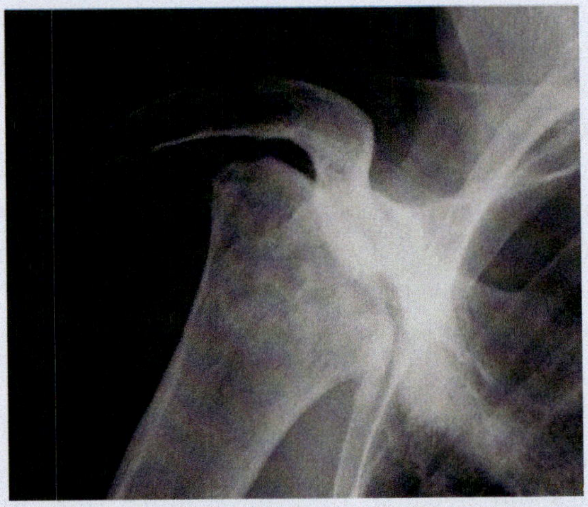

Figure 9.3. *Radiography of total avascular necrosis of the right humeral head. The patient is an 81-year-old woman with long-standing diabetes.*

Source: By Jmarchn – Own work, CC BY-SA 3.0, https://commons.wikimedia.org/w/index.php?curid=16749539.

Necrosis is more likely in anatomy with low collateral capabilities or retrograde vasculature, such as the carpus. The unique anatomy of the talus is also responsible for its limited blood flow, as articular cartilage comprises a significant portion of its surface area.

High doses and prolonged use of glucocorticoids can cause osteonecrosis through osteocyte apoptosis. Apoptosis delays the lacunar-canicular system. Additional risk factors for AVN include misuse of alcohol, blood dyscrasias, autoimmune illnesses like lupus, etc. For 25% of patients with AVN, the reason for the disruption in blood flow is unknown. For instance, the precise cause of AVN in Kienböck and Preiser disease is typically unknown.

9.4.2. Epidemiology

Osteonecrosis most frequently affects the hip, but it can also affect the talus, knee, and humerus. Less frequently, it affects the smaller wrist bones, such as the lunate. AVN causes 10% of all hip arthroplasties performed in the US, typically affecting patients between the ages of 30 and 65. In general, men are more likely to be affected by ON, but autoimmune diseases like lupus that affect women are also significant. Less common variations, such as Preiser disease (osteonecrosis of the scaphoid), typically affect middle-aged men more on their dominant hand. Conversely, middle-aged men who engage in physical labor are more prone to developing Kienböck disease (osteonecrosis of the lunate); there have even been case reports involving children.

9.4.3. Pathophysiology

A decrease in blood supply to the subchondrium causes hypoxia, resulting in the destruction of cell membrane integrity and necrosis of the cells. The majority of the necrosis will exhibit pathological appearances of neutrophils and macrophages. Macroscopically, this leads to subchondral collapse and subsequent joint degeneration. An MRI will reveal osteosclerotic alterations due to impaired osteoclast function, which reduces bone resorption. Specifically, fat cell edema/ischemia of the bone marrow will cause the T2 signal to increase and the T1 signal to decrease.

9.4.4. Histopathology

Osteocytes cannot be phagocytosed; instead, they undergo apoptosis. As a consequence, the osteocytes are not replenished. Osteosclerosis and poor bone remodeling are the outcomes of this process.

9.4.5. History and Physical Details

Non-traumatic cases typically present as mechanical pain with variable onset and severity, often difficult to localize. Physical examinations in the early stages of the disease are usually unremarkable, leading to delayed diagnosis. A comprehensive medical history should include recent trauma, steroid use, autoimmune disease, sickle cell disease, alcoholism, tobacco use, manual labor, altered gait, connective tissue disorders, pain with subtle onset, and decreased range of motion. In the early stages, hip osteonecrosis is often asymptomatic. The most common presenting symptoms are hip and groin pain, which typically indicate advanced disease. Referred pain in the thigh and buttock may also be present. Resting pain is experienced by most patients, along with gait abnormalities and stiffness.

In cases of knee osteonecrosis, the most typical symptom is sudden knee pain that worsens with weight-bearing, particularly at night. A history of osteoporosis or osteopenia and the absence of recent trauma are often reported. Physical examination findings may include reduced range of motion and palpable pain over the medial femoral condyle. Osteonecrosis of the shoulder affects the proximal humerus and is frequently associated with trauma and osteonecrosis in other areas of the body. Key features include reduced active range of motion and pulsating pain radiating to the elbow. Talar osteonecrosis is linked to trauma and polyarticular disease. Patients often report pain and difficulty walking well beyond the expected recovery period following a traumatic event.

The majority of the time, osteonecrosis of the scaphoid and lunate presents without a history of trauma. Patients typically report unilateral dorsal and radial wrist pain; they are skilled laborers. Reduced wrist edema, weakened grip strength, and reduced range of motion are other frequent observations.

9.4.6. Evaluation

Although they frequently appear normal in the early stages of the disease, the initial diagnostic standard is an evaluation using plain radiographic films that show two orthogonal views. Because magnetic resonance imaging has a high sensitivity for identifying bone edema, it is advised for identifying the disease at an earlier stage.

9.4.7. Classification

- **Osteonecrosis of the Hip:** There are two types of femoral head osteonecrosis: traumatic and atraumatic. Up to 70% of the atraumatic cases might be bilateral. The Ficat, Arlet, and Steinberg classifications are frequently used to map the stages of hip osteonecrosis. Ficat and Arlet delineate the four phases of the disease's progression, taking into account both radiographic and clinical findings. The first stage of the disease is when there are no radiological signs. The femoral head collapse, flattening, and narrowing of the joint space characterize stage IV, which is the terminal stage. The Steinberg classification takes into account the use of MRI for both lesion size assessment and pre-clinical lesion detection.
- **Osteonecrosis of the Knee:** The most prevalent type is known as spontaneous osteonecrosis of the knee (SONK). As previously mentioned, secondary osteonecrosis is more common in younger individuals and is often associated with various risk factors that are shared among all forms of osteonecrosis. Post-arthroscopic osteonecrosis, which occurs in 4% of patients who have undergone arthroscopic meniscectomy, is the third and rarest type. SONK is more frequently observed in women and typically presents in the sixth decade of life. The classical pattern involves the medial femoral condyle in up to 94% of cases, as demonstrated by subsequent cadaveric studies revealing a watershed area in this region. The primary symptom is mid-knee pain, often resembling a torn meniscus. The Koshino classification outlines the four stages of disease progression. Stage 1 refers to clinical illness that is not detectable on radiological examination. Stage 4, the degenerative phase, is characterized by osteosclerosis and the development of osteophytes around the condyles (Figure 9.4).

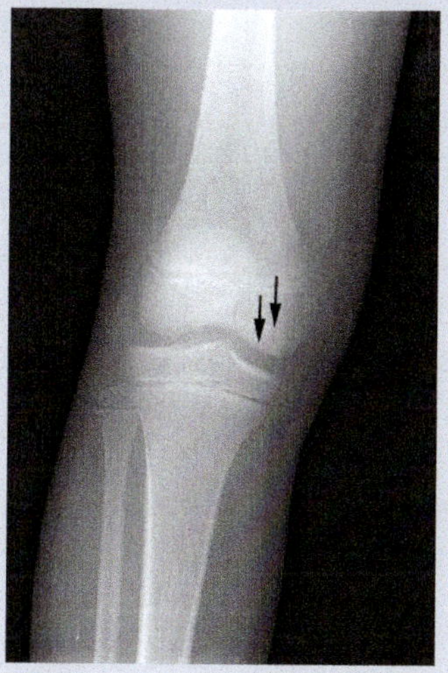

Figure 9.4. *Front X-ray of the right knee of an adolescent (epiphyseal plates are open): arrows point to avascular necrosis and developing osteochondritis dissecans in the outer medial condyle of the femur.*

Source: By Pil Kang, Affiliation: Uniformed Services University – Walter Reed Army Medical Center. Obtained from MedPix Database: http://rad.usuhs.edu/medpix/medpix_image.html?imageid=14465, Public Domain, https://commons.wikimedia.org/w/index.php?curid=4967854.

- **Osteonecrosis of the Shoulder:** Although trauma is the most common cause of osteonecrosis of the shoulder, other factors such as long-term high-dose corticosteroid use can also contribute to the condition. The length of the posteromedial metaphyseal head extension and the integrity of the medial hinge are found to be important factors in the development of osteonecrosis, and certain combinations of fracture planes are linked to reduced head perfusion. A neck component is present in the majority of fracture patterns associated with an elevated risk of AVN. It is interesting to note that, despite conflicting data, fracture-dislocations, and the degree of fragment displacement do not predict a higher incidence of AVN of the humeral head. The classification system uses five categories as follows: Stage 1 describes normal X-ray findings with pathology only recognized on MRI scans. Stage 4 demonstrates flattening of the humeral head with collapse. Stage 5 is the end stage, with degenerative changes that extend to the glenoid.
- **Osteonecrosis of the Talus:** The most frequent cause is trauma that results in displaced talus neck fractures. When an ankle or subtalar joint dislocation coexists, the likelihood of AVN rises. The vascular supply to the talus body is restricted due to its predominantly cartilaginous surface. For describing the course of the disease, the Hawkins classification works best. The Hawkins sign, a pathognomonic subchondral lucency, will disappear on plain radiographs in 6 to 8 weeks if osteonecrosis occurs.
- **Osteonecrosis of the Lunate:** More widely recognized as Keinbock disease, it is characterized by osteonecrosis and vascular insufficiency that lead to the collapse of the lunate. AVN may be caused by anatomical factors such as the presence of both dorsal and palmar blood supplies, biomechanical factors related to ulna variance, and a history of repetitive trauma. Four stages are used in the Lichtman staging of Keinbock disease. In stage 2, the first radiographic

characteristic that appears is lunate sclerosis without loss of height. The radiologic features of stage 3 disease are rotation of the palmar scaphoid and collapse of the lunate. The main characteristic of end-stage disease is degeneration of the intercarpal joints.

- **Osteonecrosis of the Scaphoid:** It is also referred to as Preiser disease, and its cause is unknown. Connective tissue disorders, steroid use, alcohol abuse, and trauma are risk factors. It usually affects the dominant hand of middle-aged men, though it can occur on both sides. Early in the course of the disease, scaphoid sclerosis is visible on a radiograph. Results from later stages show cystic alterations and fragmentation. MRI can identify variations in the T1/T2 signal across the scaphoid or just in the proximal pole. To evaluate advancement, the Herbert and Lanzetta classification scheme is employed. The four stages of the system start with modifications to the proximal pole of the scaphoid and end with carpal collapse.

9.4.8. Treatment/Management

9.4.8.1. Osteonecrosis of the Hip

The use of bisphosphonates in combination with alendronate therapy as a nonoperative treatment is debatable; however, in early cases of subchondral lucency, some trials have demonstrated the benefit of bisphosphonates in preventing a femoral head collapse and delaying the progression of the disease. However, its compliance may be jeopardized by the delayed onset of pain relief. In the end, many patients will require a total hip replacement; however, outcomes from joint salvaging techniques like core decompression vary. When osteonecrosis is still in its early stages and the lesions only affect a small portion of the femoral head's weight-bearing surface, core decompression is most beneficial. Biological agents that aid in bone repair or vascularized bone grafts may be used during the procedure. Early in the course of osteonecrosis, core decompression is a safe and efficient treatment. Its application in conjunction with autologous bone or bone marrow can raise the success rate. When the etiology is reversible, core decompression is recommended to lower intraosseous pressure and promote bone mending. Traditionally, the subchondral sclerotic area was drilled through using an 8 or 10-mm drill bit. As an alternative, the lesion can be decompressed by repeatedly drilling with a 3.2 mm guide wire.

In cases where the lesion can be moved away from the weight-bearing surface, rotational osteotomy may be recommended. Intertrochanteric varus osteotomy can be used to rotate diseases in the medial region, whereas intertrochanteric valgus and flexion-producing osteotomy can rotate diseases in the anterolateral region. Up to 90% of rotational osteotomies are successful, but they can increase the difficulty of subsequent total hip arthroplasty procedures. Total hip replacement is recommended for individuals with irreversible etiologies, large lesions, age greater than 40, advanced femoral head collapse, and degenerate acetabulum. The majority of prostheses for the femur and acetabulum are cementless; nevertheless, great care must be taken to prevent perforation when preparing the femoral canal. Results in terms of decreased pain and enhanced function are typically favorable. However, in young patients with osteonecrosis, a high rate of osteolysis and polyethylene wear has been reported. Hip arthrodesis would only be recommended for young patients who worked in physically demanding jobs.

9.4.8.2. Spontaneous Osteonecrosis of the Knee (SONK)

After a trial of protected weight-bearing and physical therapy with an emphasis on strengthening the quadriceps, most cases resolve. Bisphosphonates have been demonstrated to postpone postnecrotic remodeling and prevent joint surface collapse, which can reduce the need for surgery by 50%. Due to the higher prevalence of SONK in the elderly, a unicompartmental knee replacement offers a good functional outcome with a comparatively short recovery period. For larger lesions, however, a total knee replacement might be a better option. Following intraosseous decompression, smaller lesions have produced favorable surgical outcomes. A high tibial osteotomy may be necessary in cases involving malalignment. In certain patients with SONK in the precollapse stage, joint-preserving techniques like arthroscopy plus core decompression or osteochondral autograft transfer have effectively delayed knee replacement surgery.

9.4.8.3. Osteonecrosis of the Shoulder

The first line of treatment is nonoperative treatment, which includes physical therapy, pain management, and activity modification to limit manual labor and overhead activities. Stages determine the classification of operational management. Core decompression is the recommended course of treatment for early disease. In patients with moderate disease who have adequate epiphyseal bone stock and focal cartilage defects, hemiarthroplasty or humeral head resurfacing is advised. In cases of advanced disease, a total shoulder replacement is reserved.

9.4.8.4. Osteonecrosis of the Talus

An operation aimed at achieving stable fixation and operative anatomic reduction can reduce the incidence of talus osteonecrosis in talar neck fractures.

- **Keinböck Disease:** The objective of treating early-stage disease is to revascularize the lunate, either through direct bone grafting or indirect offloading techniques. Immobilization, including external fixation, is often attempted in stage 1 and stage 2 diseases. In stage 3, surgical options are available to address carpal collapse; however, in more advanced cases, joint sacrificing procedures such as wrist arthrodesis may be necessary.
- **Preiser Disease:** Treatment options in the early stages include bone grafting, radial wedge osteotomy, cortisone injections, and immobilization. In later stages, arthrodesis, proximal row carpectomy, scaphoid excision, or arthroscopic debridement may be necessary. Surgical intervention is often unavoidable.

9.4.9. Differential Diagnosis

- Bone marrow edema syndrome (aka, transient osteopenia)
- Complex regional pain syndrome (CRPS)
- Inflammatory synovitis
- Neoplastic bone conditions
- Osteoarthritis
- Osteochondrosis
- Osteomyelitis
- Osteoporosis
- Rheumatoid arthritis
- Septic arthritis
- Soft tissue trauma (e.g., labral tears, meniscal tears)
- Subchondral fractures

9.4.10. Prognosis

Osteonecrosis has a poor prognosis regardless of the initial management approach. As the illness worsens, the joint becomes irreparably damaged, and there is ongoing pain. Even worse cases of AVN can occur in the humeral head, where up to 81% of patients experience complete failure and require an arthroplasty. As a result, there is a high likelihood that osteonecrosis will worsen once it manifests in the patient.

Osteonecrosis of the hip can be halted from progressing with bone grafting and core decompression. However, total hip replacement is necessary in cases of advanced disease or when joint-preserving treatments fail, although this procedure carries a higher risk of complications. Early treatment of AVN involves shoulder hemiarthroplasty and core decompression, with favorable outcomes. Complete shoulder replacements, however, have higher rates of complications. End-stage AVN necessitates total shoulder arthroplasties, but the patient bears a risk of surgical complications. Immobilization is employed to treat AVN in the early stages of Preiser and Kienböck disease, but surgery is typically required in the end. In younger patients, surgical talus repair has been demonstrated to significantly enhance outcomes for AVN management.

9.4.11. Complications

Neurovascular compromise, prosthesis malfunctions, and surgical site infections are common postoperative complications for osteonecrosis. High failure rates occur when surgical intervention alone is insufficient to halt the progression of the disease. For instance, in 90% of patients treated for AVN of the hip, core decompression failed to halt the disease's progression. When performing an osteotomy of the radius in a patient with Kienböck disease, failure to consider the individual anatomy of the patient may result in excessive positive ulnar variance and postoperative ulnar pain. Complication rates are also significantly influenced by patient comorbidities. For example, sickle cell disease patients undergoing total joint replacement for acute kidney injury (AKI) had a higher overall mortality rate, as well as longer hospital stays, a higher risk of AKI, implant failure, pulmonary embolism, deep vein thrombosis, and myocardial infarction.

9.4.12. Deterrence and Patient Education

Osteonecrosis frequently begins even prior to a patient's onset of symptoms. If treatment is not received, it usually advances to end-stage disease. Patients with late-stage disease typically experience severe pain, debilitation, and even joint collapse, though symptoms can vary. Because patient presentations for this disease can vary greatly, it's critical to lower the risk factors. Avoiding excessive alcohol intake, quitting smoking, and reducing corticosteroid dosage to the lowest required are strategies to reduce risks. Joint damage is reduced by other lifestyle changes like eating a balanced diet and maintaining a healthy weight. Avoiding repetitive activities that strain joints is a good idea for manual laborers. Workers should, if at all possible, take regular breaks. Finally, take initiative. Patients with early-stage disease should seek routine well-being assessments from their primary care physician as they frequently do not exhibit symptoms.

9.4.13. Pearls and Other Issues

Osteonecrosis has a number of recognized risk factors, but the precise etiology is still unknown. It is more likely that a variety of circumstances and events work together to destroy bone cells. Intervention ranges from preservation techniques to more extensive salvage operations, depending on the stage of the disease's progression. Better outcomes are reported from treating the disease in its early stages, but this can be challenging because osteonecrosis is frequently asymptomatic in its early stages. The use of glucocorticoids is linked to most non-traumatic cases.

9.4.14. Enhancing Healthcare Team Outcomes

Orthopedic surgeons often face a diagnostic conundrum when dealing with osteonecrosis. Difficulties with diagnosis often lead to advanced cases of the disease presenting later than expected, increasing patient morbidity and frequently making it impossible to salvage the joint. Even though an orthopedic surgeon is nearly always involved in the care of patients with osteonecrosis, it is crucial to educate other medical professionals, including general practitioners, emergency room doctors, nurses, and physiotherapists, who come into contact with these patients at the hospital entrance. With each member contributing from their area of expertise, communicating openly with the rest of the team, and documenting all interactions with the patient so that the appropriate caregiver can be contacted if changes in the patient's regimen or rehabilitation are necessary, a well-functioning interprofessional healthcare team approach to patient care in these cases is made possible. The greatest patient outcomes will come from this interprofessional approach.

A Closer Look

Köhler Disease

Repetitive trauma during bone development is the cause of Kohler's Disease, which affects young children between the ages of 3 and 7 and results in damage to the navicular bone (the bone in the midfoot). Children who have Kohler's disease often complain of foot pain and may exhibit mild limping. Kohler's disease is one of a series of related conditions known as "osteochondroses," which are characterized by abnormalities in the growth of a bone and the joint that surrounds it. For six weeks, patients with Kohler's disease must be immobilized and rest in a camwalker boot in order for their symptoms to go away. Following immobilization, physical therapy treatment will aid in restoring function and mobility, which will accelerate the child's recovery.

Causes

Uncertainty surrounds the cause of Kohler's disease. It is believed that a temporary or permanent disruption of the blood supply to the developing navicular bone is the cause of Kohler's disease. Avascular necrosis, or the death of bone tissue in the absence of blood flow, results in the collapse of the bone. Repetitive stress on the bone is assumed to be the cause of a decrease in blood supply.

Diagnosis

To confirm a diagnosis, X-rays of the foot will be taken if Kohler's disease is suspected. The navicular bone in the midfoot is damaged, as seen by the typically abnormal X-rays.

Symptoms

Kohlers disease is characterized by:

- Pain usually over the midfoot
- Swelling
- Limping

Treatment

- Rest and pain relievers
- Sometimes a cast

The average duration of Kohler's bone disease is two years. It is necessary to take it easy, rest, and avoid bearing too much weight at once. Treatment-free resolution and no long-term effects are typically observed in this disease. A walking plaster cast placed below the knee for a few weeks may be helpful in severe cases. If a cast is walking, crutches are frequently not required.

9.5. Summary

- The most prevalent hip pathology in pre-adolescents and adolescents is slipped capital femoral epiphysis (SCFE), also known as slipped upper femoral epiphysis (SUFE).
- Most SCFE cases are idiopathic. Often, no previous trauma or injury occurs before symptoms start.
- Anteroposterior (AP) and frog-leg lateral views on bilateral hip radiographs should have been the initial step in the evaluation of patients with suspected SCFE. Bilateral radiographs are necessary in order to facilitate comparison. On plain radiographs, Klien's line is a radiographic finding that is utilized to identify SCFE.
- The development of femoral head osteonecrosis, chondrolysis, femoroacetabular impingement, labral tears, infection, chronic pain, and femoral growth arrest due to premature closure of the physis are among the complications associated with SCFE.
- Legg-Calvé-Perthes disease (LCPD), a childhood hip disorder, is caused by a disruption in blood flow to the head of the femur. The bone ceases to grow and perishes (osteonecrosis or avascular necrosis (AVN)) due to the diminished blood supply.
- Childhood hip disorders, such as Perthes disease, are caused by a disturbance in blood circulation to the head of the femur. The bone ceases to grow and perishes (osteonecrosis or AVN) due to the diminished blood supply.
- Perthes' disease is a prevalent hip disorder in young children, with an incidence rate of 5.5 per 1,00,000 children annually.
- Osteonecrosis, a degenerative bone ailment, is characterized by the demise of the bone's cellular constituents as a consequence of a disruption in the subchondral blood supply. It is also known as ischemic bone necrosis, aseptic necrosis, and AVN.
- Osteonecrosis is brought about by a reduction in the blood supply to the subchondral region.
- Osteonecrosis predominantly affects the hip, although it can also impact the talus, knee, and humerus. Infrequently, it affects the smaller wrist bones, such as the lunate.
- Osteocytes cannot be phagocytosed; instead, they have undergone apoptosis. Consequently, the osteocytes have not been replenished. Osteosclerosis and inadequate bone remodeling have ensued as a result of this process.
- Osteonecrosis exhibits an unfavorable prognosis irrespective of the initial management approach. As the condition deteriorates, the joint becomes irreparably damaged, and there is persistent pain.
- Neurovascular compromise, prosthesis malfunctions, and surgical site infections are prevalent postoperative complications associated with osteonecrosis.
- Osteonecrosis frequently initiates even prior to the onset of symptoms in patients. If treatment has not been received, it typically progresses to end-stage disease.

References

1. Ballard, J., & Cosgrove, A. P., (2002). Anterior physeal separation. A sign indicating a high risk for avascular necrosis after slipped capital femoral epiphysis. *J. Bone Joint Surg. Br., 84*(8), 1176–1179.
2. Barrios, C., Blasco, M. A., Blasco, M. C., & Gascó, J., (2005). Posterior sloping angle of the capital femoral physis: A predictor of bilaterality in slipped capital femoral epiphysis. *J. Pediatr. Orthop., 25*(4), 445–449.
3. Billing, L., Bogren, H. G., Henrikson, B., & Wallin, J., (2004). Slipped capital femoral epiphysis. The mechanical function of the periosteum: New aspects and theory including bilaterality. *Acta Radiol. Suppl. (Stockholm)*, (431), 1–27.
4. Breaud, J., Rubio, A., Leroux, J., & Griffet, J., (2009). Residual hip growth after pinning of slipped capital femoral epiphysis. *J. Pediatr. Orthop. B, 18*(1), 7–9.
5. Castañeda, P., Macías, C., Rocha, A., Harfush, A., & Cassis, N., (2009). Functional outcome of stable grade III slipped capital femoral epiphysis treated with in situ pinning. *J. Pediatr. Orthop., 29*(5), 454–458.
6. Gholve, P. A., Cameron, D. B., & Millis, M. B., (2009). Slipped capital femoral epiphysis update. *Curr Opin Pediatr, 21*(1), 39–45.
7. Green, D. W., Mogekwu, N., Scher, D. M., Handler, S., Chalmers, P., & Widmann, R. F., (2009). A modification of Klein's line to improve sensitivity of the anterior-posterior radiograph in slipped capital femoral epiphysis. *J. Pediatr. Orthop., 29*(5), 449–453.
8. Green, D. W., Reynolds, R. A., Khan, S. N., & Tolo, V., (2005). The delay in diagnosis of slipped capital femoral epiphysis: A review of 102 patients. *HSS J., 1*(1), 103–106.
9. John, A. H., (2008). *Tachdjian's Paediatric Orthopaedics* (4th edn) Saunders: Elsevier, Philadelphia.
10. Joseph, B., Mulpuri, K., & Verghese, G., (2001). Perthes' disease in adolescent. *J. Bone Joint Surg Br., 83*, 715.
11. Joseph, B., Nair, N. S., Narasimha, R. K. L., et al., (2003). Optimal timing for containment surgery for Perthes' disease. *J. Paediatr. Orthop., 23*, 601.
12. Kennedy, J. G., Hresko, M. T., Kasser, J. R., Shrock, K. B., Zurakowski, D., Waters, P. M., et al., (2001). Osteonecrosis of the femoral head associated with slipped capital femoral epiphysis. *J. Pediatr. Orthop., 21*(2), 189–193.
13. Loder, R. T., Starnes, T., Dikos, G., & Aronsson, D. D., (2006). Demographic predictors of severity of stable slipped capital femoral epiphyses. *J. Bone Joint Surg. Am., 88*(1), 97–105.
14. Murray, A. W., & Wilson, N. I., (2008). Changing incidence of slipped capital femoral epiphysis: A relationship with obesity? *J. Bone Joint Surg. Br., 90*(1), 92–94.
15. Parsch, K., Weller, S., & Parsch, D., (2009). Open reduction and smooth Kirschner wire fixation for unstable slipped capital femoral epiphysis. *J. Pediatr. Orthop., 29*(1), 1–8.
16. Scharschmidt, T., Jacquet, R., Weiner, D., Lowder, E., Schrickel, T., & Landis, W. J., (2009). Gene expression in slipped capital femoral epiphysis. Evaluation with laser capture microdissection and quantitative reverse transcription-polymerase chain reaction. *J. Bone Joint Surg. Am., 91*(2), 366–377.

Chapter 10

NUTRITIONAL, ENDOCRINE, DEGENERATIVE, AND AUTOIMMUNE DISORDERS

Contents

10.1. Introduction

A condition is considered chronic if it has persisted for more than six months. Not all long-term illnesses result in disability. However, a person's capacity to move around and take care of themselves may be significantly impacted by many chronic or degenerative conditions. The following are common degenerative and chronic conditions that can cause disability:

- Multiple sclerosis;
- Arthritis;
- Parkinson's disease;
- Muscular dystrophy;
- Huntington's disease.

Orientation and Directional Terms

Term	Definition	Illustration
Osteomalacia	Osteomalacia describes a disorder of "bone softening" in adults that is usually due to prolonged deficiency of vitamin D. This deficiency results in abnormal osteoid mineralization.	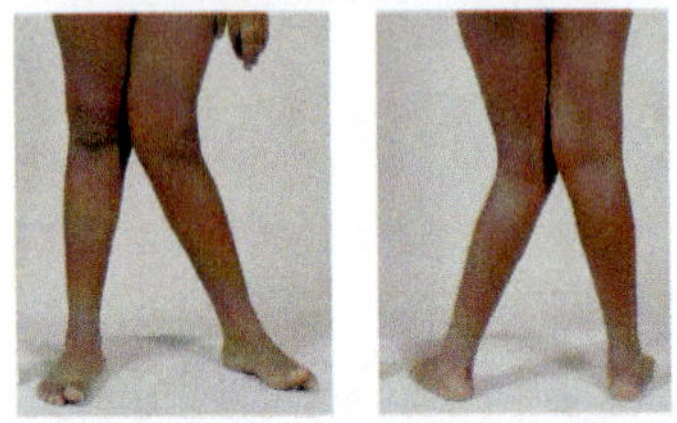
Hypocalcemia	Hypocalcemia, characterized by abnormally low calcium levels in the blood, can significantly impact a patient's health and well-being.	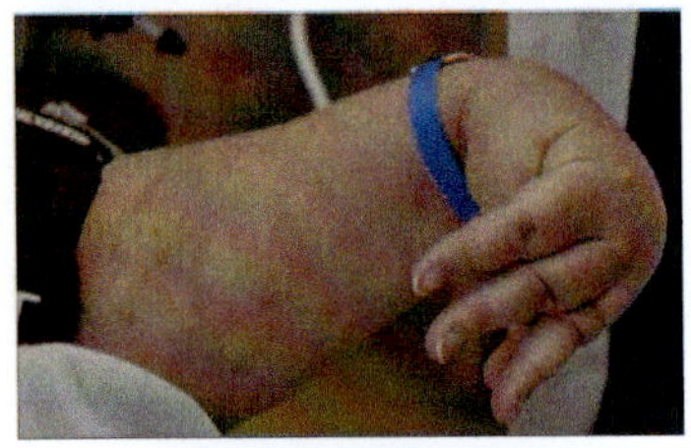
Calciferol	Calciferol is an alcoholic compound used as a supplement for vitamin D. Vitamin D maintains the health of bones. It is a fat-soluble vitamin that facilitates calcium and phosphorus absorption in the body. Our body requires exposure to sunlight to synthesize vitamin D.	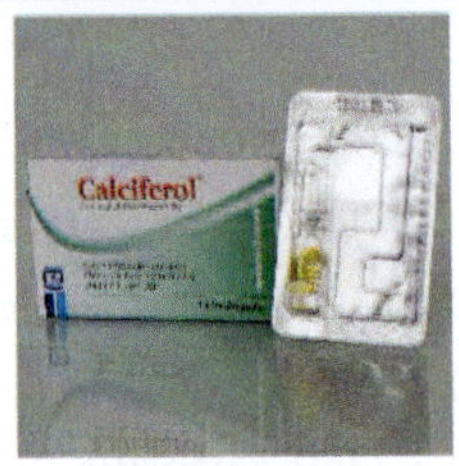
Paresthesias	Paresthesia is the sensation of tingling, numbness, or "pins and needles." This feeling is commonly experienced by everyone at some point in their lives. It is usually a harmless indication that a limb is "asleep" and requires a change in position or movement.	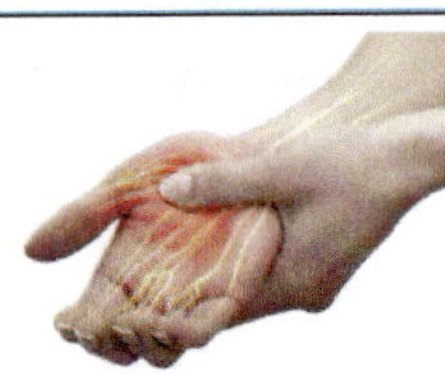
Pseudofractures	A pseudofracture, also known as a Looser zone, is a diagnostic finding in osteomalacia. Pseudofracture also rarely occurs in Paget's disease of bone, hyperparathyroidism, renal osteodystrophy, osteogenesis imperfecta, fibrous dysplasia, and hypophosphatasia.	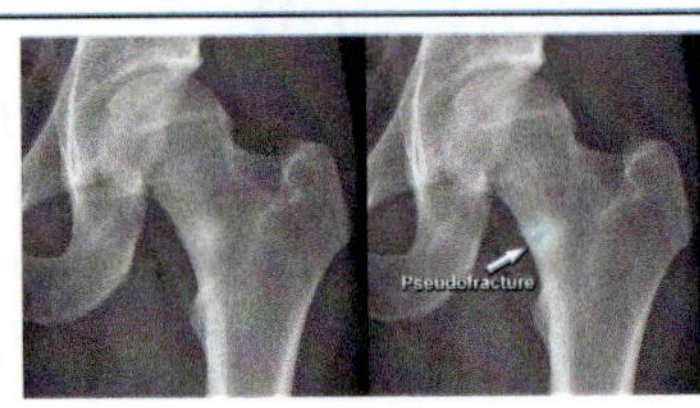

10.2. Rickets and Osteomalacia

Rickets is a disease that affects the development of the growth plates of bones in growing children. It is characterized by symptoms such as bone pain and leg bending. Rickets may also increase the likelihood of fractures (broken bones) in children. Osteomalacia, on the other hand, primarily affects adults but can also impact children. It is characterized by low levels of bone mineral, particularly calcium and phosphate. Osteomalacia can cause bone pain and increase the risk of fractures, similar to rickets. These two conditions are closely related, and it is common for a child with osteomalacia to also have rickets.

10.2.1. Pathogenesis

The bone is composed of a variety of cell types. The cells that form bones and deposit osteoid are called osteoblasts. Osteoclasts support the remodeling of bone. After that, calcium salts mineralize the osteoid. The mineralization defect in rickets causes osteoid to accumulate in the bone tissue beneath the growth plate (metaphysis). Over time, this results in weak bones and bowing.

10.2.2. Causes of Rickets/ Osteomalacia

Conditions resulting in hypophosphatemia and/ or hypocalcemia, either independently or as a result of vitamin D deficiency, are among the causes of rickets. Finding the cause is necessary to choose the best course of action.

10.2.2.1. Calcipenic Rickets

The hallmark of calcifenic (hypocalcemic) rickets is a deficiency in calcium or, more frequently, vitamin D. Diets of Indian children residing in the United Kingdom tend to be high in phytate and low in calcium. Table 10.1 provides the calcium content of common foods. If the calcium intake is extremely low, rickets can still occur even with adequate levels of vitamin D. Due to the fact that vitamin D promotes intestinal calcium absorption, this issue usually does not arise unless calcium intake is extremely low. The majority of children with rickets due to a calcium deficiency have normal serum levels of 25-hydroxyvitamin D (25(OH)D) and high concentrations of 1,25-dihydroxyvitamin D (1,25$(OH)_2$], indicating sufficient intake of vitamin D. These children may require more vitamin D, as indicated by their reaction to vitamin D replacement. As a result, children who are calcium deficient may require more vitamin D than is typical. Furthermore, even in the absence of a concurrent vitamin D deficiency, a low dietary calcium intake raises serum 1,25$(OH)_2$D concentrations, which shortens the half-life of 25(OH)D by likely increasing its catabolism. 25(OH)D concentrations are likewise in the vitamin D deficient range in most South Asian children with rickets.

Table 10.1. *Calcium Content of Various Foods*

Whole milk	1 cup (244 g)	276 mg
2% fat milk	1 cup (244 g)	285 mg
1% fat milk	1 cup (244 g)	290 mg
Yoghurt	227 g	275 mg
Brown or white bread	3 large slices	100 mg
Spinach, green vegetables	180–190 g	245–266 mg
Almonds	1/3 cup	100 mg
Fish	85 g	180–325 mg

Source: Study by Manisha, S., & Rakesh, S., (2012). titled "Rickets–Vitamin D deficiency and dependency" published in the Indian Journal of Endocrinology and Metabolism, 16(2), 164–176. doi: 10.4103/2230-8210.93732.

10.2.2.2. Phosphopenic Rickets

Renal phosphate wasting is a common cause of phosphopenic rickets. This can occur as a standalone condition or as a symptom of a more widespread renal tubular disorder such as Dent disease or Fanconi syndrome. Tumor-induced osteomalacia, autosomal dominant hypophosphatemic rickets, X-linked hypophosphatemic rickets (XLH), and hypophosphatemic rickets with hypercalciuria (autosomal recessive) are among the conditions that present with isolated phosphate loss. Nutrient deficiency is not a common cause. Measuring the concentrations of calcium, vitamin D, bicarbonate, glucose, amino acids, and bicarbonate in the urine can help differentiate between these causes. Rickets can also be classified as nutritional or non-nutritional. Among the 126 children with non-nutritional (refractory) rickets, 26% had renal failure, 71% had proximal RTA, 64% had hypophosphatemic rickets, and 16% had vitamin D dependent rickets (VDDR).

10.2.3. Vitamin D and Rickets

A deficit of vitamin D compromises skeletal health. It encourages intestinal calcium and phosphorus absorption, as well as enterocyte differentiation, promoting the mineralization of bone. Vitamin D also promotes bone resorption in hypophosphatemia or hypocalcemia, helping to maintain stable serum calcium and phosphorus levels. Hypophosphatemia and hypocalcemia can be caused by a deficiency or resistance to vitamin D. Hypophosphatemia and osteomalacia result from the stimulation of parathyroid hormone (PTH) in response to hypocalcemia. PTH acts on the kidney and bone to partially correct hypocalcemia, but it also increases phosphate excretion in the urine. Additionally, 25(OH)D is crucial for maintaining extraskeletal health. Vitamin D deficiency may be linked to certain immunological diseases such as multiple sclerosis, type 1 diabetes, rheumatoid arthritis, inflammatory bowel disease, mood disorders, and cancers like breast, prostate, and colon cancer. Low serum vitamin D levels in teenagers are associated with a higher risk of upper respiratory infections, metabolic syndrome, hypertension, and hyperglycemia.

10.2.4. Vitamin D Metabolism

Vitamin D, also known as calciferol, is a group of lipid-soluble compounds with a four-ringed cholesterol backbone. There are two main forms: vitamin D2 and vitamin D3. Vitamin D3, or cholecalciferol, is produced in the skin through the action of UV-B radiation. This form is found in animal products and some supplements. Vitamin D2, or ergocalciferol, is produced in plants when exposed to sunlight and is found in plant sources and some supplements. Only a small percentage of vitamin D comes from natural dietary sources. Dietary vitamin D is absorbed in the small intestine and transported to the liver where it is metabolized. It is then carried to target organs through the bloodstream. In the liver, vitamin D is converted to 25(OH) D before being filtered through the glomerulus and reabsorbed in the proximal tubules.

The most active form of calcidiol, $1{,}25(OH)_2D$ (calcitriol), is primarily hydroxylated in the kidney. The availability of 25(OH)D and the activity of the renal enzymes 1-α-hydroxylase and 24-α-hydroxylase determine the plasma $1{,}25(OH)_2D$ concentration. The main factors influencing the renal 1-α-hydroxylase enzyme are PTH, serum calcium and phosphate levels, and fibroblast growth factor 23 (FGF23). While high calcium, hyperphosphatemia, and $1{,}25(OH)_2D$ inhibit the enzyme, increased PTH, calcitonin, and hypophosphatemia stimulate it and improve $1{,}25(OH)_2D$ production. PTH synthesis and secretion are inhibited by $1{,}25(OH)_2D$, which provides negative feedback regulation of $1{,}25(OH)_2D$ production. Vitamin D receptors on the cell surface may also influence $1{,}25(OH)_2D$ synthesis; downregulating these receptors may be crucial in controlling vitamin D activation. FGF23, a recently identified phosphaturic hormone, prevents the kidneys from producing 1,25$(OH)_2$D by blocking 1-α-hydroxylase in the renal proximal tubule and concurrently upregulating 24-α-hydroxylase expression and 24,25$(OH)_2$D (an inactive metabolite) production. 1,25$(OH)_2$D initiates a feedback loop by stimulating FGF23. In order to maintain phosphate homeostasis, FGF23 reduces renal phosphate reabsorption and, as a result, offsets the increased gastrointestinal phosphate reabsorption caused by 1,25$(OH)_2$D (Table 10.2).

Table 10.2. *Vitamin D Content of Common Foods*

Cow's milk	3–401 U/L
Fortified infant formula	4,001 U/L
Butter	351 U/100 g
Egg yolk	20–251 U/yolk
Cod liver oil	1,360 IU/tsp
Fish	44–6,241 U/100 g
Yogurt	891 U/100 g
Cheese	12–441 U/100 g

Source: Manisha, S., & Rakesh, S., (2012). "Rickets–Vitamin D deficiency and dependency," Indian J. Endocrinol Metab., 16(2), 164–176. doi: 10.4103/2230-8210.93732.

When hypocalcemia occurs, the concentration of PTH in the serum rises, improving calcium tubular reabsorption as well as the kidney's 1-α-hydroxylase activity. Increased synthesis of 1,25$(OH)_2$D and intestinal calcium absorption follow from this. PTH also increases the activity of bone osteoclasts to release calcium stores from the bone and raise serum calcium levels. When a 24-hydroxylase hydroxylates a compound at position 24, it partially degrades both 1,25$(OH)_2$D and 25(OH)D. PTH decreases the activity of the 24-hydroxylase gene, allowing more active hormone to be formed, while 1,25$(OH)_2$D increases the gene's activity, encouraging its own inactivation. Prolactin, placental growth hormone, and estrogen may also regulate vitamin D metabolism to meet the increased calcium demands during pregnancy. Some other tissues can also produce 1,25$(OH)_2$D, but these tissues use the substance internally and do not circulate it. Activated macrophages in the lung and lymph nodes produce 1,25$(OH)_2$D extrarenally from 25(OH)D in a PTH-independent manner. Other extrarenal sites where the 1-α-hydroxylase enzyme is expressed include the gastrointestinal tract, skin, vasculature, mammary epithelial cells, and osteoblasts and osteoclasts.

10.2.5. Causes of Vitamin D Deficiency

Individuals may be deficient in vitamin D for any of the reasons discussed in subsections.

10.2.5.1. Reduced Cutaneous Synthesis

Vitamin D deficiency can occur in people who live without sun exposure.

10.2.5.2. Sun Exposure

Children may also experience dietary vitamin D deficiency. The incidence of this condition varies among ethnic groups based on skin pigmentation and supplement consumption. The recommended weekly exposure to sunlight for a Caucasian infant who is wearing diapers is 30 minutes, or two hours if the infant is fully clothed and not wearing a hat. Due to the protective pigmentation in their skin, Asians need to be exposed to the sun for about three times longer than Africans, who need to be exposed six times as long. The American Academy of Pediatrics (AAP) currently advises avoiding direct sunlight for infants under six months old, choosing outdoor activities for kids that limit their exposure to the sun, and applying sunscreen and protective clothes. For children with fair skin in lower latitudes, these guidelines are appropriate, especially during the summer. Nonetheless, more research is required to determine how UV-B exposure affects kids with darker skin who reside in northern latitudes. Vitamin D3 production in the skin is impeded in the winter months above 37° north latitude due to an 80–100% reduction in UV-B photons entering the Earth's atmosphere. UV-B and some UV-A light are absorbed by sunscreen, preventing them from penetrating the skin. The synthetic capacity of Vitamin D3 can be reduced by 95% and 98%, respectively, when using sunscreen with a sun protection factor (SPF) of 8 and SPF 15. For individuals with light skin, it is believed that 10 to 15 minutes of midday sun exposure (between 1,000 and 1,500 hours) in the spring, summer, and fall is sufficient for adequate vitamin D synthesis. After this level of exposure, it is advised to apply sunscreen with an SPF of 15 to avoid the harmful effects of long-term, excessive sun exposure. Full body clothing, as observed in certain cultures such as the Purdah law in the Muslim world, inhibits sufficient sun exposure. The amount of UV-B reaching the Earth's surface can be reduced by cloud cover, rising water vapor, and industrial pollution. Industrial pollution has also been linked to a higher incidence of vitamin D deficiency rickets. This is because skin-produced vitamin D is further broken down into inactive vitamin D metabolites, tachysterol, and lumisterol, following extended exposure to UV-B radiation.

10.2.5.3. Cold Climates

Vitamin D deficiency is also common in the latter part of winter due to reduced sun exposure. It has been reported that dark-skinned immigrants from warm climates to cold climates are prone to vitamin D deficiency. Even with sufficient sun exposure, Asian Indian immigrants to the US may still have a deficiency in vitamin D.

10.2.5.4. Extensive Burns

Even with sun exposure, vitamin D synthesis in the skin is lower than normal in patients with a history of severe burn injuries.

10.2.5.5. Nutritional Deficiency

Even with sufficient exposure to the sun, vitamin D deficiency can occur. It can happen to individuals who consume unfortified foods that lack vitamin D or if there is intestinal malabsorption of the vitamin. There are not many naturally occurring foods that contain vitamin D, and since most of them are meat or fish-based, they may not be well-received by societies that value vegetarianism. Nowadays, there are not many foods that are fortified with vitamin D. Regular fortification of vitamin D needs to be considered for milk and other food products.

10.2.5.6. Elderly People

As individuals age, their cutaneous vitamin D production and stores decrease. Older individuals often have lower vitamin D intakes. The elderly frequently experience achlorhydria, which reduces their ability to absorb calcium. Additionally, older people may spend more time indoors.

10.2.5.7. Maternal Vitamin D Deficiency

Age-related declines in cutaneous vitamin D production and stores occur. Older subjects typically consume lower levels of vitamin D. Achlorhydria restricts the body's ability to absorb calcium and is common in the elderly. Furthermore, elderly people might be kept indoors.

10.2.5.8. Prematurity

Premature babies don't get enough vitamin D from their mothers because they don't have enough time for transplacental transfer. Because of the fetal skeleton's calcification during the third trimester, which necessitates higher activation of 25(OH)D to $1,25(OH)_2D$ in the mother's kidneys and placenta, this is a crucial time for vitamin D transfer. Fetal vitamin D deficiency and, in extreme situations, fetal rickets can result from the mother's vitamin D deficiency during this time. Due to the fact that normal fetal tooth development depends on vitamin D, premature infants are more likely to have enamel defects in both primary and permanent teeth.

10.2.5.9. Exclusive Breastfeeding

Even in mothers who are deficient in vitamin D, breast milk has a low concentration of vitamin D (15–50 IU/L). Infants who are exclusively breastfed and consume an average of 750 mL of breast milk per day only absorb 10–40 IU of vitamin D per day. Most breastfed infants require at least 30 minutes of exposure to sunlight per week while wearing only a diaper in order to keep their 25(OH)D levels above 20 ng/mL. Because infant formulas are fortified (400 IU/L), vitamin D deficiency is rare in formula-fed infants. It may still happen, though, if the mother's vitamin D levels were low at the time of the baby's birth and if the formula's vitamin D level is inadequate.

10.2.5.10. Obesity

Obese people have low 25(OH)D levels because fat stores vitamin D. Therefore, those who are obese have higher vitamin D requirements.

10.2.5.11. Hospitalized Patients

Insufficient intake and insufficient sun exposure lead to vitamin D deficiency in these patients. Women undergoing osteoporosis treatment. When postmenopausal women are receiving osteoporosis therapy (bisphosphonates, raloxifene, calcitonin, or PTH), subclinical vitamin D deficiency is frequently observed.

10.2.5.12. Renal Diseases

10.2.5.12.1. Chronic Renal Disease

Due to reduced glomerular filtration, loss of the 1-α-hydroxylase enzyme as a result of structural renal damage, and suppression of enzyme activity as a result of hyperphosphatemia, patients with chronic kidney disease (CKD) produce less calcitriol $[1,25(OH)_2D]$. Hypocalcemia, hyperparathyroidism, and bone disease are the outcomes of this. Recent research has demonstrated the co-existence of 25(OH)D deficiency and $1,25(OH_2D$ deficiency in pre-dialysis and dialysis patients, particularly in female diabetics and patients receiving peritoneal dialysis.

10.2.5.12.2. Nephrotic Syndrome

The majority of calcidiol in serum is attached to DBP. Nephrotic syndrome patients lose DBP and may become vitamin D deficient.

10.2.5.12.3. Distal Renal Tubular Acidosis (dRTA)

In distal renal tubular acidosis (dRTA), acidosis, the cause of rickets, can also coexist with hypocalcemia. The presence of dRTA is suspected in conditions of hypokalemia, hyperchloremia, and normal anion gap metabolic acidosis.

10.2.5.12.4. Gastrointestinal Disease

Abnormal enterohepatic circulation can lead to decreased absorption of vitamin D and/or depletion of endogenous 25(OH)D stores when malabsorption is linked to diseases of the pancreas, small intestine, hepatobiliary tree with cholestatic liver disease, and extrahepatic biliary obstruction. Steatorrhea disrupts chylomicron-mediated absorption and fat emulsification, which leads to malabsorption of vitamin D. Individuals may only have low bone density, osteomalacia, or rickets. Cholestasis, exocrine pancreatic insufficiency (as in cystic fibrosis), food allergies, inflammatory bowel disease, and celiac disease are common examples.

10.2.5.12.5. Gastric Bypass

Calcium malabsorption causes secondary hyperparathyroidism (SHPT) in patients undergoing short-limb bypass despite normal 25(OH)D concentrations. Due to gastrointestinal acidity loss, proximal small bowel dysfunction that results in vitamin D malabsorption, a lack of sufficient absorbing surface, or a failure of intestinal mucosal cells to respond to vitamin D, patients who have undergone bariatric surgery or partial or total gastrectomy for peptic ulcer disease also experience vitamin D deficiency.

10.2.5.12.6. Liver Disease

Calcidiol [25(OH)D] is created in the liver through the hydroxylation of vitamin D. Therefore, 25(OH)D is lower in patients with severe parenchymal or obstructive liver disease. These individuals only show histological or biochemical signs of osteomalacia when there is also a concurrent nutritional deficit or disruption of the enterohepatic circulation.

10.2.5.12.7. Medications

Some anticonvulsants and antiretroviral medications used to treat HIV infection can cause vitamin D deficiency by increasing the catabolism of 25(OH)D and 1,25$(OH)_2$D. Patients taking phenytoin, phenobarbitone, carbamazepine, isoniazid, rifampicin, and theophylline experience decreased levels of calcidiol in the bloodstream because these medications induce P-450 enzyme activity, which metabolizes calcidiol into inactive vitamin D metabolites. Rickets may result from tenofovir. Medication used to treat HIV-related complications, such as pentamidine, recombinant growth hormone, and foscarnet, can cause abnormalities in calcium concentration. Patients on glucocorticoids have higher vitamin D requirements because glucocorticoids inhibit intestinal calcium absorption that is dependent on vitamin D. Ketoconazole and certain other antifungal medications raise the need for vitamin D as they inhibit 1-hydroxylation. For these patients, vitamin D supplements (400–4,000 IU/day) might be necessary.

10.2.6. Clinical Manifestations

The manifestations of rickets are initially seen at the distal forearm, knee, and costochondral junctions, which are the sites of rapid bone growth. Although skeletal dysplasias and rickets can have similar clinical features, skeletal dysplasias with metaphyseal involvement are usually diagnosed based on normal serum PTH and inorganic phosphorus concentrations in affected children.

10.2.6.1. Skeletal Findings

The skeletal abnormalities in phosphopenic and calcifenic rickets are comparable. Normal fontanelle closure occurs in the anterior by 18 months and in the posterior by 3 months. Nevertheless, the fontanelle closure is delayed in rickets patients. A few examples include parietal and frontal bossing, enlargement of the costochondral junction of the ribs (the "rachitic rosary"), Harrison sulcus from the diaphragm's muscular pull on the lower ribs, widening of the wrist and bowing of the distal radius and ulna, and progressive lateral bowing of the femur and tibia. It is evident that the ankle shows widening (double malleoli). The kind and location of deformities depend on the child's age and ability to support their own weight. The tibia and forearm bones exhibit abnormalities in infants. Toddlers' genu varum, or normal physiological bowing of the legs, is accentuated. Elderly children either have windswept deformity of the lower limbs (valgum on one side and genu varum on the other) or genu valgum. There could be scoliosis or kyphosis. The skeletal abnormalities in adults are uncommon, but in females, a triradiate pelvis may occur, which complicates a typical vaginal delivery (Figure 10.1).

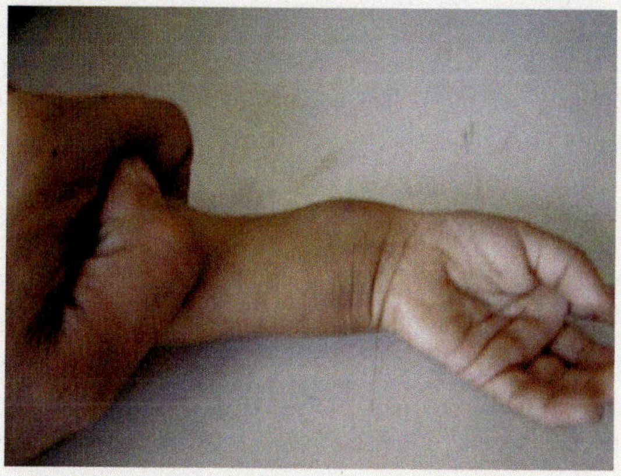

Figure 10.1. *Widening of the wrist.*

Source: By DRPEDS at English Wikipedia – Transferred from en.wikipedia to Commons., Public Domain, https://commons.wikimedia.org/w/index.php?curid=3064726.

10.2.6.2. Extraskeletal Findings

The child may exhibit no symptoms at all or show signs of pain, agitation, delayed motor milestones, and stunted growth. The result of visceroptosis is a pot belly. Children may walk with an analgesic gait or waddle. In the first year of life, hypocalcemic seizures are frequently presented. Children who have calcipenic rickets are more likely to contract infections. Dental enamel hypoplasia exists. Young infants with calcipenic rickets frequently have increased sweating, which may be brought on by bone pain. The most common symptoms of phosphopenic rickets are dental abscesses and malformations of the lower extremities. Children may exhibit paresthesias or irritability. Since the growth plate is fused in adults and adolescents, bony deformities are not visible. The majority of adult patients may therefore have no symptoms. Adult osteomalacia can occasionally begin subtly as aches and pains in the thighs and lumbar (lower back) area, then progress to the arms and ribs. In addition to being symmetrical and non-radiating, the affected bones are tender. Because of weak proximal muscles, it is difficult to stand up from a squatting position and climb stairs. Weight bearing can lead to the development of pathological fractures.

10.2.7. Laboratory Investigations

A patient exhibiting clinical signs of rickets is evaluated by taking their medical history, dietary habits, and history of liver or renal disease, as well as malabsorption. The following laboratory tests are used to help determine the etiology.

10.2.7.1. Radiographic Findings

At the growth plate of rapidly growing bones, children with rickets can exhibit specific changes. Specifically, the distal ulna in the upper limbs and the metaphyses above and below the knees in the lower limbs are where the changes are most noticeable. The widening of the epiphyseal plate is caused by unmineralized osteoid and loss of definition of the zone of provisional calcification at the epiphyseal/metaphyseal junction. The epiphyseal end of the metaphysis shows cupping and splaying, while cortical spurs and stippling begin to form. The epiphyseal bone centers are small, osteopenic, and may not be immediately visible. In both children and adults, the cortices are thin and the long bone shafts are osteopenic. The trabecular pattern appears similar to ground glass, with a coarse and fuzzy appearance.

There are abnormalities in the long bone shafts, and in cases of severe rickets, looser zones and pathological fractures (also known as Milkman's fractures) may be seen. Looser zones are a typical radiologic finding in osteomalacia. They are pseudofractures, narrow radiolucent lines, 2–4 mm wide, with sclerotic borders. They are symmetrical, bilateral, and positioned perpendicular to the cortical edges of the bones. They can be located on the pubic and ischial rami, at the femoral neck, on the medial aspect of the femoral shaft, or right beneath the lesser trochanter. In addition, the ulna, scapula, clavicle, ribs, and metatarsals may experience them. When a patient with osteomalacia has multiple, bilateral, symmetric pseudofractures, it is referred to as "Milkman syndrome.."

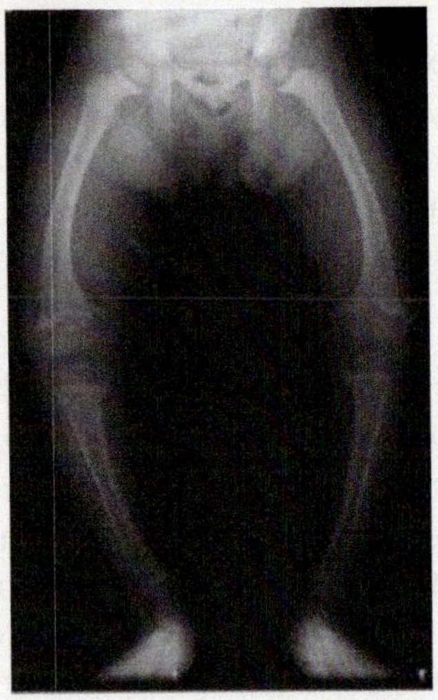

Figure 10.2. *X-ray of a two-year-old with rickets, with a marked bowing of the femurs and decreased bone density.*

Source: By The original uploader was Mrich at English Wikipedia. – Image created by Michael L. Richardson, M. D., (2004). de:Bild:Rachitis.jpg. Originally from en.wikipedia; description page is/was here., CC BY-SA 1.0, https://commons.wikimedia.org/w/index.php?curid=59299.

On bone scans, pseudofractures can also appear as hot spots. When looser zones are absent, osteopenia might be the sole observation, and osteomalacia might be mistaken for osteoporosis. Since looser zones frequently lie close to arteries, it has been hypothesized that they either represent stress fractures that have been repaired by the laying down of inadequately mineralized osteoid or that they represent bone erosion caused by artery pulsations. Biconcave vertebral bodies, or cod fish vertebrae, might exist. Long-term SHPT is less likely to cause skeletal alterations than the anomalies mentioned above. These consist of bone cysts, resorption of the distal ends of long bones like the humerus and clavicle, and subperiosteal resorption of the phalanges. Severe osteomalacia can cause pathologic fractures, tibial shortening and bowing, and coxa profunda hip deformity (Figure 10.2).

10.2.7.2. Bone Mineral Density (BMD)

Numerous investigations have revealed significantly lower bone density in the spine, hips, and forearms, as determined by dual-energy X-ray absorptiometry (DXA), in individuals suffering from osteomalacia associated with insufficient vitamin D. Reduced bone mineral density (BMD) does not, however, differentiate osteoporosis from osteomalacia, nor is it necessary for the diagnosis of osteomalacia. On the other hand, adults with XLH typically have normal or elevated BMD, particularly in the lumbar spine.

10.2.7.3. Bone Biopsy

The most reliable method for determining the diagnosis of osteomalacia/rickets is bone biopsy with tetracycline labeling. Because it is invasive and the diagnosis can typically be made using a combination of clinical and laboratory findings, it is rarely performed. Osteomalacia is characterized by the following histomorphometric features: extended mineralization lag time, widened osteoid seams, and increased osteoid volume. Since one of these findings may be present in other disorders, all of these features are required for the diagnosis. In patients with hyperparathyroidism, hyperthyroidism, and Paget's disease, there are wide osteoid seams that indicate high turnover. In contrast to osteomalacia, these disorders have an elevated rate of mineral apposition.

Alkaline phosphatase (ALP) is an excellent marker of disease activity because it participates in the mineralization of bone and growth plate cartilage. ALP levels are usually 500 IU/L in neonates and 1,000 IU/L in children up to nine years of age and decrease after puberty. Serum ALP concentrations are elevated in both hypocalcemic and hypophosphatemic rickets. ALP may be used to screen for rickets, with the caveat that rickets has sometimes been reported with normal ALP levels. When a high index of suspicion exists, a wrist or knee radiograph should be obtained. Serum phosphorus concentrations usually are low in both calcipenic and phosphopenic rickets. The serum calcium concentration is normal in phosphopenic rickets. Serum calcium levels are usually low in calcipenic rickets but may be normal in some stages of the disease due to a compensatory increase in PTH. The total reabsorption of phosphorus (TRP) and the maximal tubular reabsorption of phosphorus per glomerular filtration rate (TmP/GFR) usually are decreased in both types of rickets.

PTH levels in the blood are higher in cases of calcipenic rickets. PTH levels, on the other hand, are typically normal in cases of phosphopenic rickets. Since aminoaciduria is linked to hyperparathyroidism, familial hypophosphatemia rickets (FHR) does not exhibit it. Serum inorganic phosphorus (Pi) and PTH measurements are used in the diagnostic process to differentiate between phosphopenic and calcipenic rickets in cases of suspected rickets. In rickets linked to renal failure, serum creatinine levels are elevated and GFR levels may be low. The phosphate content is high here. In hypophosphatemic rickets with hypercalciuria, urine calcium levels are elevated, whereas in other types, they are reduced. Urine phosphorus, pH, glucose, serum creatinine, liver enzymes, and arterial blood gas are among the other lab tests. Urine amino acid, bicarbonate, glucose, and calcium concentrations can be measured to determine the causes of phosphopenic rickets in children.

Serum 25(OH)D measurements for children with calcipenic rickets aid in differentiating the most common type of rickets from those caused by vitamin D deficiency. The amount of vitamin D stored in the body is reflected in the serum concentration of 25(OH)D, which is low in vitamin D deficiency and normal or slightly elevated in the other forms. Calcipenic rickets can cause low, normal, or elevated $1,25(OH)_2D$ levels. $1,25(OH)_2D$ levels rise in response to increasing PTH levels at first, but because its substrate, 25(OH)D, is limited, they may then fall. In hypophosphatemic rickets and VDDR type II, $1,25(OH)_2D$ is elevated.

10.2.7.4. Vitamin D Levels

Measuring 25(OH)D levels is the most accurate way to determine vitamin D status. Serum calcium decreases as a result of decreased intestinal absorption of calcium brought on by a decline in 25(OH)D levels. As a result, there is an increase in serum PTH, which promotes the conversion of 25(OH)D to $1,25(OH)_2D$ and maintains calcium absorption. Therefore, the level of 25(OH) D that results in the greatest suppression of PTH and maximum calcium absorption is considered the optimal level. Clinical definitions of the ideal 25(OH)D concentration, such as the level required for fracture reduction, are also possible. The ideal 25(OH)D concentration for bone health is a matter of debate. Above 20 ng/mL, the Institute of Medicine (IOM) supports 25(OH)D concentrations. To reduce the risk of falls and fractures in older adults, the National Osteoporosis Foundation, the International Osteoporosis Foundation, and the American Geriatric Society recommend a minimum level of 30 ng/mL. Experts acknowledge that levels below 20 ng/mL are not ideal for maintaining bone health. It is unknown what the ideal serum 25(OH)D level is for maintaining extraskeletal health. Additionally, no safe upper serum level has been established. There is a higher chance of fractures and certain types of cancer (e.g., prostate, pancreatic), and mortality at concentrations higher than 30–48 ng/mL. While some advocate maintaining 25(OH)D levels between 30 and 50 ng/mL, the IOM systematic review supports keeping the serum 25(OH)D concentration between 20 and 40 ng/mL.

The current accepted criteria for determining the level of vitamin D in children and adolescents are as follows: 25(OH)D ≥ 20 ng/mL for vitamin D sufficiency, 25(OH)D ≤ 15 ng/mL for vitamin D insufficiency, and 25(OH)D ≥ 20 ng/mL for vitamin D deficiency. A level less than 5 ng/mL is considered a severe deficiency. These cut-offs may need to be adjusted if further pediatric research demonstrates the benefits of higher 25(OH)D levels. An individual is arbitrarily classified as having vitamin D excess if their 25(OH)D level is 100 ng/mL or higher; intoxication is defined as 150 ng/mL or higher.

10.2.7.5. Vitamin D Assays

The most accurate measure of vitamin D stores and status is the 25(OH)D level. The primary form of vitamin D in circulation is 25(OH)D, which has a half-life of 2–3 weeks. $1,25(OH)_2D$ is tightly regulated by PTH, calcium, and phosphate, and has a shorter half-life of approximately 4 hours. It circulates in much lower concentrations than 25(OH)D and does not decrease significantly until a severe case of vitamin D deficiency. Furthermore, renal function and its concentration have a stronger correlation than a vitamin D deficiency. Therefore, it is not helpful in determining vitamin D stores. Since both derivatives of 25(OH)D are physiologically active following 1-α-hydroxylation, the vitamin D assay ought to measure both of them. These include chemical assays [high-pressure liquid chromatography (HPLC) and mass spectrometry (MS)] and binding assays – immunoassays [i.e., radioimmunoassay (RIA), enzyme immunoassay (EIA), chemiluminescent immunoassay (CLIA)] and protein-binding assays [i.e., competitive protein-binding assays (CPBA) and automated chemiluminescence protein-binding assays (CLPBA)]. Assay variability is a significant issue. The gold standards for vitamin D assay are high-performance liquid chromatography/mass spectroscopy (HPLC) and LC-MS, which both yield higher vitamin D levels. The total value is reported by protein-binding assays and immunoassays. Vitamin D2 and D3 can both be reported by chemical assays.

10.2.8. Prevalence of Vitamin D Deficiency

In most developed countries nowadays, overt vitamin D deficiency is uncommon. It is characterized by hypocalcemia or hypophosphatemia, rickets, or osteomalacia. Subclinical vitamin D deficiency, however, is linked to fracture risk, osteoporosis, and an increased risk of falls. The prevalence of vitamin D deficiency varies with the definition used (<20 or <30 ng/mL). In the National Health and Nutrition Examination Survey (NHANES) 2000–2004, more than 30% of participants aged 12 years and older had 25(OH) D levels below 20 ng/mL. According to a study, vitamin D deficiency is highly common in India, accounting for 90% of cases in adults and 84% of cases in pregnant women. In the general population, low vitamin D levels are becoming more common. Between 1988 and 2004, the mean 25(OH)D concentration dropped from 30 to 24 ng/mL. Changes in body mass index (BMI), consumption of milk, use of sunscreen, and assay changes could all be to blame for this.

10.2.9. Optimal Intake

The range of estimates for vitamin D needs depends in part on sun exposure and the parameters used to classify a state as deficient. The IOM committee assumed minimal sun exposure when establishing the dietary reference intakes for vitamin D and identified a 25(OH)D level of at least 20 ng/mL as necessary to meet the needs of at least 97.5% of the population. The data used to determine the dietary reference intakes focused on the advantages of calcium and vitamin D for skeletal health rather than extraskeletal health.

10.2.9.1. Adults

According to the 2010 recommendations made by the Institute of Medicine (IOM), adults aged 18 to 70 years old should consume 600 IU of vitamin D per day. Higher intakes (RDA 800 IU) are necessary for high-risk groups, older adults (>71 years), and those confined indoors.

10.2.9.2. Infants

The Lawson Wilkins Pediatric Endocrine Society and the AAP advise that older children and adolescents, as well as all infants, including those who are exclusively breastfed, should begin taking 400 IU of vitamin D per day or more of the nutrient within a few days of birth. Formula-fed infants will also need supplementation to reach this goal unless they drink at least 1,000 mL of formula milk daily, as the majority of infant formulas contain at least 400 units/L of vitamin D. Giving the nursing mother high doses of vitamin D (4,000–6,400 IU/day) is another way to increase the vitamin D levels in infants who are exclusively breastfed. This intervention raises the amount of vitamin D in breast milk to a level where the baby can consume enough of it without the mother developing hypervitaminosis D. Moderately higher vitamin D dosages (e.g., a mother's blood levels of vitamin D of >30 ng/mL can usually be maintained by consuming 1,500–2,000 IU daily during pregnancy and lactation, which will also help the baby's vitamin D status at birth. However, these dosages might not produce enough vitamin D in breast milk to meet the baby's needs, so the baby might still need to take supplements.

10.2.9.3. Children

Initially, a daily intake of 200 IU was advised to ensure serum 25(OH)D levels greater than 11 ng/mL. However, these levels were found to be insufficient in preventing all cases of florid rickets, leading to the conclusion that the target serum level was inadequate. For children who do not consume at least one liter of vitamin D-fortified milk daily, the AAP then recommended a minimum daily intake of 400 units of vitamin D. The 2010 IOM guidelines increased the recommended daily allowance (RDA) for vitamin D in healthy children aged 1 to 18 years to 600 IU. The AAP has not yet revised the previous guidelines. Obese children, as well as those taking glucocorticoids, anticonvulsants, and HIV medications, may require higher dosages.

10.2.9.4. Pregnant and Lactating Mothers

It is advised to consume 600 IU of vitamin D. Some studies suggest that higher intakes may be necessary to maintain normal levels of 25(OH)D during pregnancy and lactation. In 2010, the IOM established the safe upper limit for vitamin D as 2,500 IU/day for ages 1–3 years, 3,000 IU/day for ages 4–8 years, and 4,000 IU/day for ages 9–71+ years (including pregnant or lactating women).

10.2.10. Screening for Vitamin D Deficiency

It is not necessary to screen every individual in the general public for serum 25(OH)D levels. Serum 25(OH)D levels should be measured in those who fall into the high-risk categories mentioned above. Afterward, supplementation with the estimated amount required to achieve the target 25(OH)D level should be administered three to four months later to confirm its attainment. It is crucial to screen for vitamin D deficiency in patients who report nonspecific musculoskeletal pain. Children with elevated levels of serum ALP (e.g., >500 IU/L in neonates or >1,000 IU/L in children up to nine years of age) should also undergo screening.

10.2.11. Preparations of Vitamin D

There are several vitamin D preparations available. Because vitamin D is inexpensive and efficient, it is used instead of its metabolites. Ergocalciferol and cholecalciferol are the two types of vitamin D supplements that are most often used. According to certain research, ergocalciferol (Vitamin D2) is not as effective as cholecalciferol (Vitamin D3) in raising serum 25(OH) D levels. There are 400, 800, 1,000, 2,000, 5,000, 10,000, and 60,000 unit capsules of vitamin D3. It can be obtained as an intramuscular injection (Arachital 6 lakhs units, which keeps vitamin D levels stable for a year) in certain nations. It can, however, cause excruciating pain. Vitamin D2 (ergocalciferol) is available for oral use in 400 and 50,000 unit capsules or in a liquid form (8,000 units/mL).

10.2.11.1. Vitamin D Metabolites

Treatment for vitamin D deficiency can involve the use of vitamin D metabolites, especially in cases where there is aberrant metabolism of the vitamin (liver or renal disease). The appropriate preparation and dosage are determined by the clinical condition:

- **Calcidiol:** Also known as 25(OH) D, is available in 800 and 2,000 IU capsules. It is ideal for patients with liver disease as it does not require hepatic 25-hydroxylation. Calcidiol has a faster onset of action and a shorter half-life (2–3 weeks) compared to Vitamins D3 and D2. Patients with severe liver disease and vitamin D deficiency can benefit from taking 2,000–8,000 IU/day of calcidiol. For those who do not respond to Vitamins D2 or D3 treatment, calcitriol may be considered.
- **Calcitriol [1,25(OH)$_2$D]:** It is supplied as an injection and in capsules weighing 0.05 and 0.5 mg. It is especially helpful for individuals with decreased calcitriol synthesis, such as those with type I and type II VDDR or CKD. Calcitriol is costly, does not increase vitamin D stores, and acts quickly. Its half-life is only six hours. Therefore, calcitriol is not recommended for nutritional deficiencies or stoss therapy. Due to the high incidence of hypercalcemia associated with it, it is important to closely monitor serum calcium levels. When 25(OH)D levels are used as a supplement, they do not represent a patient's clinical vitamin D status.
- **Doxercalciferol:** It is used to treat CKD-related SHPT. It is available in India as 0–2 mg capsules, making it the first pro-Vitamin D2 offered in the country.
- **Dihydrotachysterol (DHT):** It is a synthetic vitamin D analog that does not require renal hydroxylation. It is activated in the liver. Compared to vitamin D, DHT has a faster onset of action (two hours), a shorter half-life, and a stronger impact on the mineralization of bone salts. DHT is available in tablet form in doses of 0.125, 0.2, and 0.5 mg. It needs to undergo hepatic 25-hydroxylation before it can be used therapeutically.

Functionally, it is comparable to 1α-hydroxy vitamin D. DHT can only treat hypocalcemia caused by a vitamin D deficiency as it does not increase vitamin D stores. In conditions where calcitriol is used, DHT can be an alternative.

- **Paricalcitol:** Also known as 19-nor-1,25-dihydroxy vitamin D2, is an analog of 1,25-dihydroxyergocalciferol, the active form of vitamin D2. It can be administered intravenously in doses ranging from 0.04 to 0.24 μg/kg.

10.2.12. Treatment of Vitamin D Deficiency

10.2.12.1. Adults

The type and degree of the deficiency determine the dosage of vitamin D. Serum 25(OH) D concentrations in patients with normal absorptive capacity increase by approximately 1.0 ng/mL for every 100 units of added vitamin D3. It has been proven that vitamin D deficiency can be effectively treated with various dosage schedules. In a 2-month trial of oral vitamin D3 repletion in elderly women with hip fractures, serum 25(OH)D levels increased similarly in response to the same cumulative dose administered daily (1,500 units), weekly (10,500 units), or monthly (45,000 units). Although large annual doses of vitamin D3 raise serum 25(OH) D levels, they are not recommended due to the adverse effects of increased fractures and falls in the elderly. The following are different regimens that can be used:

- High-risk individuals with serum 25(OH)D concentrations less than 20 ng/mL should take 50,000 IU of vitamins D2 or D3 orally once a week for 6–8 weeks. After that, 800 units of vitamin D should be taken daily.
- If a high-risk individual has serum 25(OH)D levels between 20 and 30 ng/mL, initial supplementation with 600–800 units of vitamin D3 per day may be sufficient to maintain levels within the desired range.
- Pregnant women should not take weekly dosages of 50,000 units of vitamin D3 for 6–8 weeks. Instead, 600–800 units of vitamin D3 per day are considered a safer option. When treating vitamin D deficiency, urinary calcium excretion should be monitored, especially in women with a history of renal stones. This excretion increases during pregnancy.
- Vitamin D deficiency is typically corrected with high doses of 10,000–50,000 units per day in patients with malabsorption or gastrectomy. Hydroxylated vitamin D metabolites are a favorable choice due to their enhanced absorption.

These recommendations align with the practice guidelines of the endocrine society. To maintain a serum 25(OH)D concentration above 30 ng/mL in adults with vitamin D deficiency, the Endocrine Society guidelines suggest a daily maintenance dose of vitamins D2 or D3 at 1,500–2,000 IU.

For individuals aged 19 to 70, a minimum daily intake of 1,000 mg of total calcium is recommended. Women aged 51 to 70 and all adults aged 71 and above should aim for 1,200 mg per day. The upper limit (UL) of calcium intake for most adults is 2,000–2,500 mg per day. However, individuals with malabsorption may require a higher calcium dose of up to 4 g/ day. In cases of tetany or convulsions, parenteral calcium in the form of calcium gluconate becomes necessary. The recommended dose is 10–20 mg of elemental calcium per kg, administered intravenously slowly over 5–10 minutes as 1–2 mL/kg of 10% calcium gluconate. Boluses may need to be repeated. Additionally, until calcium levels normalize, calcitriol doses of 20–100 ng/kg/day in two or three divided doses may be necessary. Initially, high doses of calcium are required, followed by halving the doses for the next one to two weeks. Once vitamin D supplementation has been reduced to 400 IU/day and normal PTH and 25(OH)D levels are achieved, calcium supplementation is typically not necessary.

10.2.12.2. Children

Vitamin D2 (ergocalciferol) or vitamin D3 (cholecalciferol) are the most commonly used treatments for vitamin D deficiency. For the treatment of vitamin D deficiency rickets, a daily dose of 1,000 IU is advised for newborns under one month old, 1,000–5,000 IU for infants between one and twelve months old, and 5,000–10,000 IU for children aged one and up. The course of treatment is extended until radiographic healing is evident, at which point the daily vitamin D dosage is lowered to 400 IU. The recommended daily intake of calcium is roughly 1,000 mg (30–75 mg/kg of elemental calcium per day in three divided doses) in order to prevent the worsening of hypocalcemia known as "hungry bone" syndrome, which can occur after beginning vitamin D therapy. Within three months, the biochemical and radiological abnormalities resolve as a result of this. Medical therapy causes skeletal deformities to completely regress. Orthopedic intervention, however, may be necessary if deformities persist after the growth plates' radiologic appearance has stabilized. An alternative protocol is "stoss therapy," which consists of a high dose of oral vitamin D (6,00,000 IU) given on a single day, then maintained at 400–1,000 IU of vitamin D per day, or 50,000 IU of vitamin D2 weekly for 8 weeks orally (teenagers) followed by 400 IU/day. This dosage of vitamin D roughly equates to 5,000 IU per day for three months, which should be enough to start healing after three months. If poor compliance continues, high-dose vitamin D may need to be repeated sporadically, usually every three months. When there is a problem with compliance, trash therapy can help. Nevertheless, excessive vitamin D intake can result in hypercalcemia. Doses of 1,50,000 or 3,00,000 IU are equally effective with lesser side effects.

10.2.13. Adverse Effects of Vitamin D

Nephrocalcinosis, intraocular calcifications, hypercalcemia, and hypercalciuria are among the side effects of calcitriol therapy. Polyuria, pruritus, and azotemia are possible. Hypercalciuria and hypercalcemia are the first detectable effects of vitamin D toxicity, and they have only been noted at 25(OH)D concentrations greater than 88 ng/mL. Unaware of this, many patients take vitamin and mineral supplements that contain vitamin D. Before giving patients extra vitamin D, it is crucial to find out about any other dietary supplements they may be taking. Long-term sun exposure rarely results in vitamin D toxicity. For people with light skin, the concentrations of precursors to vitamin D that are produced in the skin reach equilibrium after about 20 minutes of UV exposure, and any additional vitamin D that is produced is broken down. Some sources estimate that when the entire body is exposed to sunlight, endogenous production amounts to about 10,000 IU per day.

Primary hyperparathyroidism coexists in certain vitamin D deficient patients, but this condition is not identified until vitamin D levels are restored. Given the potential for hypercalcemia and hypercalciuria in these patients, vitamin D replacement should be given with caution. On the other hand, calcium concentrations are typically normal or at the lower end of normal (rarely below normal) and PTH concentrations are slightly elevated in people with clinically significant vitamin D deficiency and SHPT. After consuming enough vitamin D, the PTH level ought to stabilize. Whereas urinary calcium in patients with primary hyperparathyroidism normalizes very quickly with vitamin D replacement, it is abnormally low in patients with vitamin D deficiency and SHPT and takes months to normalize.

10.2.14. Benefits of Vitamin D Repletion

10.2.14.1. Skeletal

Prospective, randomized, placebo-controlled studies on calcium and vitamin D in older individuals residing in the community have demonstrated the benefits of these supplements for skeletal health. The bone density of the lumbar spine and femoral neck increased at annualized rates of 4–5% per year. Additionally, vitamin D supplementation may help reduce the risk of fractures by improving muscle function and decreasing the likelihood of falls.

10.2.14.2. Extraskeletal Benefits

In addition to its impact on the skeletal system, vitamin D may also have positive effects on the immune and cardiovascular systems.

10.2.15. Monitoring

For healthy individuals, there is no need for serum 25(OH)D measurements before and after initiating vitamin D supplementation. However, patients receiving treatment for a deficiency should be closely monitored throughout the course of treatment. This includes regular physical examinations and biochemical assessments every two weeks. The biochemical evaluation should include measurements of serum calcium, phosphorus, ALP, PTH, and the calcium/creatinine ratio in urine. Radiographs should be taken after four weeks to assess improvement. Signs of response include clear radiographic improvement, normalized serum calcium and phosphorus levels, and a decline in ALP towards the reference range. After three months, when the growth plates should have returned to their normal appearance, the biochemistry and radiographs should be repeated. During maintenance therapy, patients may be assessed every three months. It is important to monitor renal function, such as the calcium/creatinine ratio and urine flow, as well as serum creatinine levels during each session. PTH levels should be tested after six months. Hand radiographs, renal ultrasonography, and ophthalmologic consultation (slit-lamp exam) should be conducted annually. Additionally, levels of 25(OH)D should be checked on a yearly basis.

10.2.16. Vitamin D Dependent Rickets

10.2.16.1. Vitamin D Dependent Rickets Type I

Pseudovitamin D-deficient rickets, or VDDR type I (VDDR-I), was first recognized in 1961. VDDR-I is a recessive disorder. Inactivating mutations in the CYP27B1 gene, located on 12 q13.3, cause 1-α-hydroxylase deficiency, which affects patients with VDDR-I. This deficiency results in abnormal calcium absorption and the inability to hydroxylate calcidiol to calcitriol. The hallmarks of VDDR-I include early onset skeletal disease (within the first year of life), severe hypocalcemia (sometimes with tetany), and moderate hypophosphatemia. Patients also exhibit enamel hypoplasia, hypotonia, motor retardation, muscle weakness, and stunted growth. As the condition progresses, patients experience radiographic symptoms of vitamin D deficiency rickets and osteomalacia, as confirmed by bone biopsy. Biochemical evaluation reveals elevated PTH, hypocalcemia, and increased phosphate and amino acid excretion in the urine. Low levels of calcitriol and normal serum levels of calcidiol are characteristic biochemical findings of VDDR-I. Treatment with 1,25$(OH)_2$D can reverse the biochemical and clinical signs of rickets. The dosage is determined based on body weight and disease severity. For severe rickets, the initial dosage is 1 mcg per day, which is maintained until the bones heal. Following that, the maintenance dose is adjusted based on the results of biochemical analyzes and ranges from 0.25 to 1 mcg/day. The objectives of the treatment are to prevent hypercalciuria, maintain PTH levels within normal ranges, and achieve normocalcemia.

10.2.16.2. Vitamin D Dependent Rickets Type II

Hereditary vitamin D resistant rickets, or VDDR type II (HVDRR), is an extremely rare autosomal recessive form of rickets with less than 50 known cases reported. It is associated with calcitriol end-organ resistance, typically caused by mutations in the gene that encodes the vitamin D receptor. The receptor defect hinders the action of calcitriol by interfering with the ability of the hormone-receptor complex to function. The following mutations or defects in the vitamin D receptor have been identified: (a) reduction in the number of 1,25$(OH)_2$D receptor binding sites; (b) failure of 1,25$(OH)_2$D binding to available receptors; (c) abnormal binding affinity of 1,25$(OH)_2$D to the receptor; (d) insufficient translocation of the 1,25$(OH)_2$D-receptor complex to the nucleus; and (e) decreased affinity of the 1,25$(OH)_2$D-receptor complex for the DNA-binding domain, resulting from changes in the structure of the receptor zinc-binding fingers.

The clinical spectrum of HVDRR is determined by the type of mutation within the vitamin D receptor and the level of residual vitamin D receptor activity. Upon birth, affected children typically appear normal, but within the first two years of life, they develop rickets. Alopecia, present in approximately two-thirds of cases, serves as an indicator of disease severity and is a distinct characteristic of the syndrome. The absence of vitamin D receptor activity in keratinocytes leads to alopecia. Other ectodermal anomalies may also be present, including oligodontia, epidermal cysts, and multiple milia.

To treat HVDRR, a therapeutic trial involving calcium and calcitriol supplements is employed. The response to treatment varies depending on the severity of the receptor defect. Initial therapy involves daily doses of 1,000 mg of calcium and 2 mcg of calcitriol. However, higher doses of calcium (up to 3 g/day) and calcitriol (up to 30–60 mcg/day) may be necessary. For patients who are resistant to standard treatment, long-term calcium infusion into a central vein can be considered, requiring maintenance over several months. Once radiographic healing is observed, oral calcium therapy may be sufficient.

During treatment, patients should be evaluated at least once a week. It is recommended to monitor serum levels of calcium, phosphorus, creatinine, ALP, 1,25$(OH)_2$D, PTH, and the calcium/creatinine ratio in urine. The dosage of calcitriol should be gradually increased until reaching serum concentrations up to 100 times the normal mean if there are no changes in the biochemical parameters. If there is no biochemical response after three to five months of treatment, therapy failure should be considered.

Even in nations with sufficient sun exposure, vitamin D deficiency is a significant contributor to rickets and osteomalacia. For those who are at risk, testing for vitamin D deficiency is advised. Treatment for the abnormalities and disrupted metabolism of the bones corrects them. Treatment for vitamin D deficiency enhances quality of life, and vitamin D has numerous extraskeletal benefits. Another vitamin D-related bone disease is called vitamin D-dependent rickets (VDDR), but it is inherited. Even though VDDR is rare, treatment requires recognition of the condition.

10.3. Hyperparathyroidism

The parathyroid glands are small structures, about the size of a grain of rice, located near the thyroid glands in the neck. When one or more of these glands become overactive, it leads to hyperparathyroidism. In cases where it is necessary, the parathyroid glands produce parathyroid hormone (PTH) to increase blood calcium levels. Excess PTH can be caused by:

- **Primary Hyperparathyroidism:** This which is often associated with enlargement (hyperplasia) of the parathyroid gland, the presence of a benign (non-cancerous) growth called an adenoma, or, in rare cases, a malignant (cancerous) tumor. The exact causes of enlargement are usually unknown, but there may be a genetic component.
- **Secondary Hyperparathyroidism:** This which occurs when the levels of minerals like phosphate and calcium are imbalanced due to certain medical conditions. This prompts the parathyroid glands to compensate. It can be triggered by conditions such as renal failure, deficiencies in calcium or vitamin D, or a combination of both.

10.3.1. Causes and Diagnoses

Primary hyperparathyroidism is caused by a single benign tumor called parathyroid adenoma in 80% of cases. Many of these adenomas are the cause of the majority of the residual. Rarely, parathyroid cancer could be the cause. Less than 1% of patients develop parathyroid carcinoma after multiglandular disease, which typically presents as hyperplasia of the four parathyroid glands (15–20% of patients). In rare cases, primary hyperparathyroidism develops, and most affected individuals have no family history. The risk of developing primary hyperparathyroidism is increased by radiation exposure. Exposure to lithium and thiazide diuretics is another risk factor. Numerous hereditary disorders, such as multiple endocrine neoplasia syndromes, familial hypocalcemia-jaw tumor syndrome, hyperparathyroidism-jaw tumor syndrome, and neonatal severe hyperparathyroidism, also increase the risk. DDT has been linked to parathyroid adenomas, but a direct correlation has not yet been proven.

The most common causes of secondary hyperparathyroidism are malabsorption, insufficient calcium intake, CKD, and vitamin D deficiency. Low blood calcium levels due to vitamin D deficiency, CKD, or other conditions are the most frequent causes of secondary hyperparathyroidism. Elevated levels of PTH and calcium in the blood are indicators of primary hyperparathyroidism. Prolonged secondary hyperparathyroidism often leads to tertiary hyperparathyroidism (Figure 10.3).

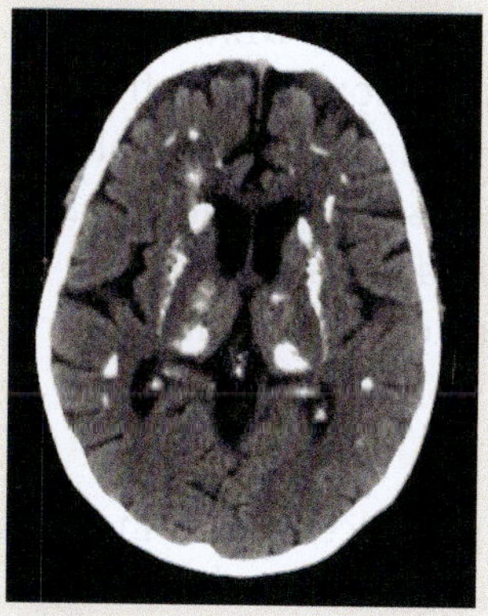

Figure 10.3. *Calcification in the brain due to hyperparathyroidism.*

Source: By James Heilman, MD – Own work, CC BY-SA 4.0, https://commons.wikimedia.org/w/index.php?curid=49082154.

The PTH immunoassay is considered the gold standard for diagnosis. The objective of the diagnostic process is to determine the type of hyperparathyroidism (primary, secondary, or tertiary) by measuring the levels of PTH, calcium, and phosphate in the serum after confirming elevated PTH levels. Primary hyperparathyroidism is characterized by low phosphate levels and elevated levels of calcium, vitamin D, and PTH. In secondary hyperparathyroidism, serum calcium and vitamin D levels are low, while phosphate and PTH levels are high. Tertiary hyperparathyroidism is characterized by low vitamin D levels and elevated serum PTH, calcium, and phosphate. Tertiary hyperparathyroidism can be distinguished from primary hyperparathyroidism by a history of chronic kidney failure and secondary hyperparathyroidism. Hyperparathyroidism can lead to normal anion gap metabolic acidosis by increasing renal bicarbonate loss and causing hyperchloremia. Increased ALP levels can be observed due to bone turnover. Additional tests can be performed to rule out other causes and complications of hyperparathyroidism. These tests may include genetic testing, a 24-hour urine calcium test for familial hypocalciuric hypercalcemia, and a DEXA scan to assess for osteoporosis, osteopenia, or fragility fractures. If there is concern for nephrolithiasis or nephrocalcinosis, additional tests such as a renal ultrasound or a CT scan without contrast can be conducted to evaluate for their presence.

10.3.2. Differential Diagnosis

Humoral hypercalcemia of malignancy, renal failure, malignant bone destruction (including multiple myeloma, metastatic breast cancer, and lymphoma), thiazide diuretics, lithium, immobilization, hyperthyroidism, milk alkali syndrome, multiple endocrine adenomatosis syndromes, and granulomatous diseases are among the differential diagnoses for hypercalcemia. Lab abnormalities similar to these can also be seen in familial benign hypocalciuric hypercalcemia. However, because there is little calcium in the urine, the calcium creatinine clearance ratio is usually less than 0.01.

10.3.2.1. Blood Tests

10.3.2.1.1. Intact PTH

Parathyroid hormone (PTH) levels in the presence of elevated calcium are either elevated or inappropriately normal in primary hyperparathyroidism. PTH levels in affected patients typically fluctuate significantly over time, and similar to calcium and calcium ion levels, multiple retests are necessary to identify any patterns. As of right now, only relatively intact and physiologically active PTH molecules are detected by the recognized PTH test, intact PTH. Earlier assays frequently found additional, dormant fragments. In patients with renal dysfunction, even intact PTH may be imprecise. If biotin has been consumed in the days preceding the blood test, intact PTH blood tests could be mistakenly low.

10.3.2.1.2. Calcium Levels

In instances of primary or tertiary hyperparathyroidism, elevated levels of PTH result in higher concentrations of calcium in the blood (hypercalcemia) due to:

- Increased bone resorption, allowing the flow of calcium from bone to blood;
- Reduced kidney clearance of calcium;
- Increased intestinal calcium absorption.

10.3.2.2. Serum Phosphate

Serum phosphate levels are abnormally low in primary hyperparathyroidism due to decreased phosphate reabsorption in the kidney tubules. However, this is the case in only roughly half of the cases. This is in contrast to tertiary hyperparathyroidism and secondary hyperparathyroidism, where kidney disease usually causes elevated serum phosphate levels.

10.3.2.3. Alkaline Phosphatase (ALP)

Because hyperparathyroidism causes a high turnover of bones, ALP levels are typically elevated. Levels in primary hyperparathyroidism may remain within the normal range, but considering the elevated plasma calcium levels, this is not considered normal.

10.3.2.4. Nuclear Medicine

In the field of nuclear medicine, a technetium sestamibi scan is utilized as a method to detect hyperparathyroidism (also known as parathyroid adenoma). Surgeons employ this technique to locate ectopic parathyroid adenomas, which are commonly found in the anterior mediastinum.

10.3.3. Epidemiology

In terms of epidemiology, the incidence of hyperparathyroidism in the developed world ranges from one to four per thousand individuals. The most prevalent form of hyperparathyroidism is primary hyperparathyroidism. Age and sex are two factors that increase the risk of primary hyperparathyroidism. It is typically diagnosed between the ages of 50 and 60, although cases before this age are not unheard of. Primary hyperparathyroidism affects women three times more frequently than men. The illness was first described in the 1700s and its connection to the parathyroid was discovered in the late 1800s. The first surgical treatment was performed in 1925. In 2010, there were 233 cases of primary hyperparathyroidism for every 1,00,000 women and 85 cases for every 1,00,000 men in the United States. Among women between the ages of 70 and 79, both White and Black women are the most affected. The two most common causes of secondary hyperparathyroidism are vitamin D deficiency and CKD. Within the United States, 15% of people have CKD, and approximately 50% of people worldwide suffer from vitamin D deficiency.

10.3.4. Signs and Symptoms

Approximately 75% of patients with primary hyperparathyroidism have no symptoms. Although the majority of primary patients do not exhibit any symptoms at the time of diagnosis, the term "asymptomatic" is not well defined and is limited to patients who do not exhibit any evident clinical sequelae, such as kidney stones, bone disease, or hypercalcemic crisis. These asymptomatic patients may have non-symptomatic conditions like depression, anxiety, gastrointestinal distress, and neuromuscular issues. A higher-than-normal level of calcium is found in the blood, which is often discovered incidentally during blood work for unrelated purposes. A lot of people only experience vague symptoms. Hypercalcemia frequently manifests as weakness, lethargy, nausea, constipation, vomiting, depression, bone pain, myalgias, joint pain, decreased appetite, nausea, vomiting, pancreatitis, abdominal pain, constipation, polyuria, polydipsia, kidney stones, vertigo, and osteopenia or osteoporosis. One possible sign of bone resorption is a history of acquired racquet nails, or brachyonychia. Rugger jersey spine is a pathognomic radiographic finding associated with hyperparathyroidism. Clinical examinations hardly ever reveal parathyroid adenomas. Most patients' symptoms are resolved when a parathyroid tumor is surgically removed. In cases of secondary hyperparathyroidism resulting from insufficient absorption of vitamin D, the parathyroid gland functions normally. However, bone resorption leads to clinical complications, which include bone syndromes such as osteomalacia, renal osteodystrophy, and rickets.

10.3.5. Development

There are two glands located superiorly and two inferiorly that make up the parathyroid. The parathyroid glands originate from the endoderm of the 3rd and 4th pharyngeal pouches and are situated on the posterior thyroid. To be more precise, the dorsal wing of the fourth pharyngeal pouch is where the superior parathyroid glands originate, and the inferior parathyroid glands come from the third. The parafollicular cells, or C-cells, are produced when the ultimopharyngeal bodies fuse with the posterolateral thyroid. The ultimopharyngeal body is derived from the ventral wing of the fourth pharyngeal pouch. In the seventh week of human embryo development, the parathyroid glands separate from the pharyngeal wall and attach to the posterior thyroid.

10.3.6. Mechanism

When blood ionized calcium (Ca^{2+}) concentrations rise above normal, parathyroid hormone secretion is increased; conversely, when Ca^{2+} levels fall, parathyroid hormone secretion is decreased. Normal parathyroid glands measure blood Ca^{2+} concentrations and secrete parathyroid hormone accordingly.

10.3.6.1. Regulation of PTH

The parathyroid G-protein coupled, calcium sensing receptors, which respond to changes in serum calcium levels, regulate the rapid production of PTH. Conversely, sustained changes in serum calcium levels affect mRNA-binding proteins, which modify the encoding of PTH mRNA. Additionally, there are calcium-independent mechanisms such as PTH transcription repression through 1α,25-dihydroxyvitamin D binding to the vitamin D receptor. Furthermore, 1α,25-dihydroxyvitamin D influences the expression of calcium-sensing receptors, which in turn affects PTH secretion.

10.3.6.2. Effects of PTH on Bones

PTH utilizes various methods to stimulate the release of calcium from the bones:

- PTH activates osteoblasts, leading to increased expression of RANKL and differentiation of osteoblasts into osteocytes.
- To promote osteoclast differentiation, PTH inhibits the secretion of osteoprotegerin.
- PTH also directly stimulates osteoclasts, resulting in the degradation of hydroxyapatite and organic material, leading to bone resorption. Subsequently, calcium is released from the bone into the bloodstream (Figure 10.4).

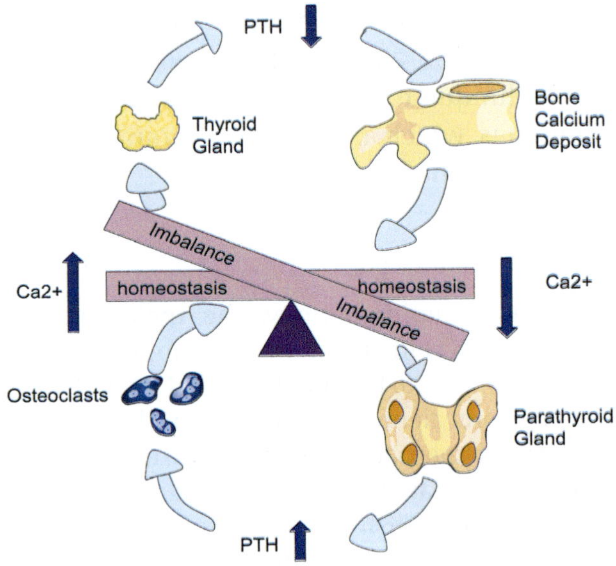

Figure 10.4. *Effects of PTH bone resorption.*

Source: By Mkaram19 – Own work, CC BY-SA 4.0, https://commons.wikimedia.org/w/index.php?curid=79526193.

10.3.6.3. Effects of PTH on the Kidneys

The ascending Loop of Henle and the proximal convoluted tubule are where calcium reabsorption takes place in the nephron. PTH increases calcium reabsorption in the nephron by acting on the collecting duct and distal convoluted tubule. PTH also lowers serum phosphate by inhibiting phosphate reabsorption in the proximal convoluted tubule. This results in a decrease in the production of insoluble calcium phosphate salts and an increase in ionized calcium in the serum.

10.3.6.4. Effects of PTH on the Small Intestines

The proximal convoluted tubule produces more 1-alpha-hydroxylase when PTH is present. Inactive 25-hydroxycholecalciferol is converted to active vitamin D (1,25 dihydroxycholecalciferol) by the activation of this enzyme. Calcium absorption via transcellular and paracellular pathways is made possible by active vitamin D. If the calcium level is unusually low, secondary hyperparathyroidism develops. In response, the normal glands continue to secrete a high amount of parathyroid hormone. This usually happens when there is hypocalcemia and low blood levels of 1,25-dihydroxyvitamin D_3. Insufficient consumption of vitamin D through diet or lack of sun exposure can lead to a deficiency of 1,25-dihydroxyvitamin D_3, as the body is unable to produce vitamin D from cholesterol on its own. Hypovitaminosis D that results is typically caused by a partial combination of these two factors. The liver changes vitamin D_3 (cholecalciferol) into 25-hydroxyvitamin D (calcidiol), which is then circulated to the kidneys where it is transformed into the active hormone 1,25-dihydroxyvitamin D_3. Therefore, CKD is a third cause of secondary hyperparathyroidism. Here, there is a compromise in the production of 1,25-dihydroxyvitamin D_3, which leads to hypocalcemia.

10.3.7. Treatment

Eliminating the adenoma or hyperactive parathyroid glands is the sole treatment option for primary hyperparathyroidism. In cases where a patient presents asymptomatically with slightly elevated blood calcium levels, normal kidney function, and normal bone density, monitoring may suffice. If surgery is not feasible, the drug cinacalcet can be utilized to lower PTH levels, although it does not provide a cure. Patients with significantly elevated blood calcium levels may require large intravenous doses of normal saline for treatment. The appropriateness of low vitamin D prior to surgery for patients with primary hyperparathyroidism is a subject of debate, but low vitamin D levels should be corrected in those with secondary hyperparathyroidism. Following a parathyroidectomy, efforts should be made to raise low vitamin D levels. Different treatments are required depending on the type of hyperparathyroidism.

10.3.7.1. Primary

For primary hyperparathyroidism, parathyroidectomy is a treatment option for symptomatic cases. It also improves bone mineral density (BMD) and reduces the risk of fragility fractures, osteoporosis, and nephrolithiasis. Furthermore, studies have demonstrated that parathyroidectomy for hyperparathyroidism can have benefits in terms of memory improvement, weakness alleviation, reduced exhaustion, and relief from depression. While all symptomatic patients with hyperparathyroidism should undergo a parathyroidectomy, there may be some asymptomatic patients who could also benefit from surgery.

Asymptomatic hyperparathyroidism with any of the following:

- 24-hour urine calcium excretion > 250 mg/day for females and > 300 mg/day for males.

- Blood calcium > 1 mg/dl over the upper reference limit of normal.
- > 30% of the patient's age-related normal creatinine clearance.
- Estimated glomerular filtration rate < 60 mL/min/1.73 m^2
- Bone density > 2.5 standard deviations below peak (i.e., T-score of −2.5)
- People age < 50
- Nephrolithiasis seen on imaging (ultrasound or CT)

Surgery can rarely result in hypoparathyroidism.

10.3.7.2. Secondary

The treatment for patients with secondary hyperparathyroidism should primarily focus on addressing the underlying cause of low calcium, which is typically vitamin D deficiency or chronic kidney failure. In these patients, elevated levels of parathyroid hormone (PTH) are an appropriate response to this condition. If the treatment is successful in addressing the underlying cause, PTH levels usually return to normal, unless there is an autonomous PTH secretion (tertiary hyperparathyroidism). One approach to manage hyperphosphatemia is to reduce phosphate intake through dietary restrictions. If dietary measures fail to lower phosphate levels below 5 μg/dL, phosphate binders may be used. Vitamin D supplementation can be beneficial in treating vitamin D deficiency. However, in patients with CKD who have hypercalcemia or elevated serum phosphate levels, vitamin D supplementation is not recommended.

10.3.7.3. Tertiary

In cases of tertiary hyperparathyroidism, parathyroidectomy is indicated when patients present with severe osteopenia, severe persistent hypercalcemia (>11.0 mg/dL), calciphylaxis, bone pain, or pathological fractures.

10.3.7.4. Calcimimetics

For patients with severe hypercalcemia and primary hyperparathyroidism who are not suitable candidates for parathyroidectomy, as well as those with secondary hyperparathyroidism receiving dialysis, treatment with a calcimimetic (such as cinacalcet) may be beneficial. While the use of calcimimetics in the treatment of secondary hyperparathyroidism can reduce the likelihood of requiring a parathyroidectomy, it does not alter the risk of premature mortality in individuals undergoing dialysis for CKD. Possible side effects of calcimimetic treatment include vomiting and low blood calcium levels.

10.4. Osteoporosis

Bones affected by osteoporosis become weak and brittle, easily breaking from simple stresses like coughing or bending over. The hip, wrist, or spine are the most common places for osteoporosis-related breaks. Living tissue, such as bone, is continually being broken down and replaced. When new bone is not growing to replace lost bone, the condition known as osteoporosis develops. Men and women of all races are affected by osteoporosis. The most vulnerable groups are, however, older women who have passed menopause and white and Asian women. Medication, a balanced diet, and weightlifting activities can strengthen bones that are already weak or stop bone loss.

10.4.1. Signs and Symptoms

The absence of symptoms and bone breakage are the typical indicators that a person has osteoporosis. Osteoporotic fractures are considered fragility fractures because they happen in circumstances where healthy individuals would not typically break a bone. Fragility fractures commonly affect the wrist, hip, ribs, and vertebral column. Examples of circumstances in which a person would not typically break a bone include falls from a height and routine daily tasks like coughing, lifting, and bending (Figure 10.5).

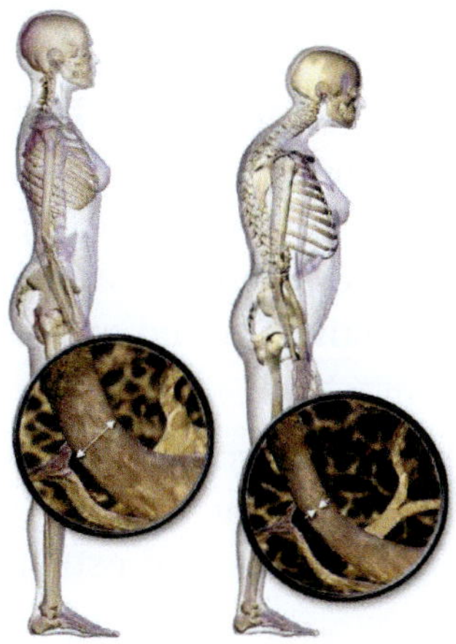

Figure 10.5. *Illustration depicting normal standing posture and osteoporosis.*

Source: By BruceBlaus. When using this image in external sources it can be cited as: Blausen.com staff (2014). & quot; Medical gallery of Blausen Medical 2014 " Wiki Journal of Medicine 1(2). doi: 10.15347/wjm/2014.010. ISSN 2002-4436. Own work, CC BY 3.0, https://commons.wikimedia.org/w/index.php?curid=27796967.

10.4.1.1. Fractures

Osteoporosis frequently presents itself as fractures, which can have disabling effects. Acute and chronic pain in elderly individuals is often associated with fractures related to osteoporosis, which can exacerbate their condition and increase the risk of premature death. These fractures may also be asymptomatic. The most common types of osteoporotic fractures occur in the wrist, spine, shoulder, and hip. Vertebral collapse (compression fracture) is characterized by sudden back pain. Radicular pain, or shooting pain from compressed nerve roots, is also commonly experienced, although symptoms such as cauda equina syndrome and spinal cord compression are less frequent. Multiple vertebral fractures lead to a stooped posture, loss of height, and chronic pain that restricts movement.

Fractures in long bones severely limit range of motion and may require surgical intervention. Prompt surgery is typically necessary for hip fractures due to the significant associated risks, including deep vein thrombosis and pulmonary embolism. Hip surgery is also linked to a higher mortality rate, with average rates of 23.3% in Europe, 17.9% in Asia, 21% in the US, and 24.9% in Australia. Fracture risk calculators assess an individual's risk of fracture based on various factors such as age, gender, weight, smoking and alcohol consumption, and BMD. Recognized calculators include FRAX, the Garvan FRC calculator, QFracture, and the open access FREM tool. It is also possible to adapt the FRAX tool to regularly collected health data. When osteoporosis leads to a broken bone, it is referred to as established osteoporosis. Osteoporosis is one aspect of frailty syndrome.

10.4.1.2. Risk of Falls

Growing older is associated with an elevated risk of falls. Falls can lead to skeletal injuries in various parts of the body, including the wrist, spine, hip, knee, foot, and ankle. Eye impairments caused by conditions such as glaucoma and macular degeneration, as well as issues with balance and movement abnormalities like Alzheimer's disease, dementia, and sarcopenia (age-related decrease in skeletal muscle), contribute to the risk of falls. Collapse, which is a temporary loss of posture, can occur with or without unconsciousness. Syncope, on the other hand, can have various causes, including cardiac arrhythmias (such as tachycardia), vasovagal syncope, orthostatic hypotension (abnormal drop in blood pressure upon standing), and seizures. To reduce the risk of falls in living areas, it is important to remove obstructions and loose carpets. Individuals who have previously experienced falls or have issues with balance or gait are particularly vulnerable.

10.4.1.3. Complications

In addition to increasing the risk of fractures and breaks, osteoporosis can lead to additional problems. Elderly individuals who experience osteoporosis-related bone fractures may face disability and a higher likelihood of death due to the injury. Osteoporosis can also result in increased disability, a decline in quality of life, and higher healthcare costs.

10.4.2. Risk Factors

The risk of developing osteoporosis can be increased by a variety of factors, such as age, race, lifestyle choices, and medical conditions and treatments.

10.4.2.1. Unchangeable Risks

There are certain risk factors for osteoporosis that are beyond the control, including:

- **Sex:** Women are more likely than men to develop osteoporosis.
- **Age:** The risk of osteoporosis increases as the person get older.
- **Race:** Asian and White individuals have the highest risk of osteoporosis.
- **Family History:** Having a parent or sibling with osteoporosis, especially if they have suffered a hip fracture, increases the risk.
- **Body Frame Size:** People with smaller body frames, both men and women, are typically at higher risk due to having less bone mass to rely on as they age.

10.4.2.2. Hormone Levels

Hormone levels also play a role in osteoporosis risk. Here are some examples:

- **Sexual Hormones:** Reduced sex hormone levels, such as estrogen in women during menopause, can weaken bones. Treatments for breast cancer that lower estrogen levels in women and prostate cancer treatments that lower testosterone levels in men can accelerate bone loss.
- **Thyroid Issues:** High levels of thyroid hormones can lead to bone loss. This can occur if the person take excessive medication for an underactive thyroid or if the thyroid is overactive.
- **Other Glands:** Hyperactive parathyroid and adrenal glands have also been linked to osteoporosis.

10.4.2.3. Dietary Factors

An increased risk of developing osteoporosis is seen in those with:

- **Low Calcium Intake:** Osteoporosis develops as a result of a lifetime deficiency in calcium. Insufficient consumption of calcium is linked to reduced bone mass, premature bone deterioration, and a higher likelihood of fractures.
- **Eating Disorders:** Both men and women's bones are weakened by severe dietary restriction and underweight.
- **Gastrointestinal Surgery:** Reducing the size of the stomach through surgery or removing a portion of the intestines reduces the surface area that is available for absorbing calcium and other nutrients. These surgical procedures cover weight loss as well as other gastrointestinal conditions.

10.4.2.4. Steroids and Other Medicines

Prednisone and cortisone are two examples of oral or injectable corticosteroid medications that can interfere with the process of rebuilding bone over time. Additionally linked to osteoporosis are drugs taken to treat or avoid:

- Seizures;
- Gastric reflux;
- Cancer;
- Transplant rejection.

10.4.2.5. Medical Problems

Those with certain medical conditions, such as the following, are more likely to develop osteoporosis.

- Celiac disease;
- Inflammatory bowel disease;
- Kidney or liver disease;
- Cancer;
- Multiple myeloma;
- Rheumatoid arthritis.

10.4.2.6. Lifestyle Choices

Osteoporosis risk can be elevated by certain unhealthy behaviors. Some instances are as follows:

- **Sedentary Lifestyle:** Compared to individuals who lead more active lives, those who spend a significant amount of time sitting down are more likely to develop osteoporosis. Engaging in weight-bearing activities, as well as those that promote proper posture and balance, can benefit the patient's bones. However, activities such as weightlifting, running, jumping, and dancing appear to be particularly advantageous.
- **Excessive Alcohol Consumption:** Consistently consuming more than two alcoholic beverages per day increases the risk of osteoporosis.
- **Tobacco Use:** Although the exact role of tobacco in osteoporosis is unknown, it has been demonstrated that tobacco use weakens bones.

10.4.3. Pathogenesis

An imbalance between bone resorption and bone formation is the underlying cause of osteoporosis in all cases. In healthy bone, the matrix undergoes constant remodeling, with up to 10% of the total bone mass being remodeled at any given time. According to Frost & Thomas (1963), this process occurs in bone multicellular units (BMUs). The transcription factor PU aids osteoclasts. One mechanism involves osteoblasts rebuilding the bone matrix while first degrading it. If osteoclasts break down the bone matrix at a faster rate than osteoblasts can generate new bone, low bone mass density can occur (Figure 10.6).

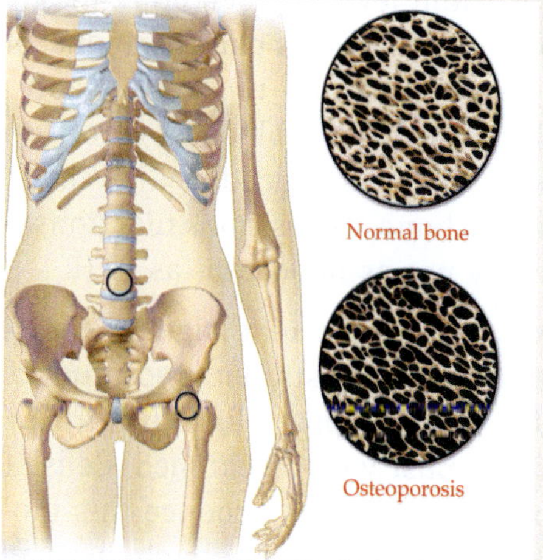

Figure 10.6. *Osteoporosis locations.*

Source: By BruceBlaus – Own work, CC BY-SA 4.0, https://commons.wikimedia.org/w/index.php?curid=46602308.

Osteoporosis is caused by three main mechanisms: excessive bone resorption, inadequate formation of new bone during remodeling (possibly as a result of mesenchymal stem cells biasing away from the osteoblast and toward the marrow adipocyte lineage), and inadequate peak bone mass (the skeleton develops insufficient mass and strength during growth). The formation of brittle bone tissue is caused by the interaction of these three processes. The rate of bone resorption is largely influenced by hormonal factors; low estrogen (e.g., due to menopause) both raises bone resorption and reduces the normal process of new bone formation in weight-bearing bones. Less estrogen than is typically required to stimulate the uterus and breast gland is required to suppress this process. In terms of controlling bone turnover, the α-form of the estrogen receptor seems to be the most significant. Apart from estrogen, calcium metabolism is a major factor in bone turnover. In addition, low levels of calcium and vitamin D can result in poor bone deposition. The parathyroid glands respond to low calcium levels by secreting parathyroid hormone, also known as parathormone, or PTH, which promotes bone resorption and keeps enough calcium in the blood. It is unclear how calcitonin, a hormone produced by the thyroid that raises bone deposition, functions and is most likely not as important as PTH.

Numerous molecular signals control the activation of osteoclasts, with receptor activator of nuclear factor kappa-B ligand (RANKL) being one of the most well-researched. Cells such as osteoblasts and others produce this molecule, including lymphocytes, which activate the nuclear factor κB (RANK) receptor activator. Osteoprotegerin (OPG) inhibits RANKL's capacity to enhance bone resorption by binding to it before it can bind to RANK. Tumor necrosis factor and its receptors are closely associated with RANKL, RANK, and OPG. Although its function is known, the role of the Wnt signaling pathway is not fully understood. Increased or decreased local production of eicosanoids and interleukins, which are believed to play a role in the regulation of bone turnover, may cause osteoporosis. Colony stimulating factor 1 receptor (CSF1R) activation controls osteoclast maturation and activity. The increase in TNF-α production linked to menopause causes stromal cells to produce CSF-1, which in turn activates CSF1R and encourages osteoclasts to reabsorb bone.

Trabecular bone, also known as cancellous bone, is the porous bone found at the ends of long bones and vertebrae. Conversely, cortical bone forms the resilient outer layer of bones and the inner portion of long bones. Due to the presence of osteoblasts and osteoclasts primarily on the bone surface, trabecular bone exhibits higher activity and undergoes more turnover and remodeling. Consequently, this leads to decreased bone density and disruptions in bone microarchitecture. Weaker trabecular bone spicules are prone to fracture and are subsequently replaced by weaker bone. Fractures commonly occur at sites with a higher ratio of trabecular bone to cortical bone, such as the wrist, hip, and spine. These areas heavily rely on trabecular bone for strength, rendering them more susceptible to degeneration when bone remodeling is irregular. The loss of cancellous or trabecular bone typically commences around ages 30–35, with women potentially experiencing up to a 50% loss and men around 30%.

10.4.4. Diagnosis

Osteoporosis can be diagnosed by measuring BMD and utilizing conventional radiography. DXA is the most frequently employed technique for measuring BMD. In addition to detecting abnormal BMD, investigations into potentially modifiable underlying causes are necessary to diagnose osteoporosis; blood tests may be employed for this purpose. Depending on the possibility of an underlying issue, investigations for cancer with bone metastases, multiple myeloma, Cushing's disease, and other previously mentioned causes may be conducted.

10.4.4.1. Conventional Radiography

Conventional radiography is beneficial for various purposes, including follow-up examinations in specific clinical settings such as soft tissue calcifications, secondary hyperparathyroidism, or osteomalacia in renal osteodystrophy. It can also be utilized in conjunction with CT or MRI to identify complications of osteopenia (reduced bone mass; pre-osteoporosis), such as fractures. However, radiography necessitates a significant amount of bone loss (approximately 30%) to be visible on X-ray images and is relatively insensitive to the early detection of diseases.

Increased radiolucency and cortical thinning are the two primary radiographic characteristics of generalized osteoporosis. Vertebral fractures are common consequences of osteoporosis, and spinal radiography can be extremely useful in diagnosing and monitoring these injuries. With plain-film X-rays, vertebral height can be objectively measured in several ways, including height loss combined with area reduction (especially when assessing vertical deformity in T4–L4) or a spinal fracture index that takes into account the number of affected vertebrae. Dowager's hump is caused by kyphosis of the thoracic spine, which is a result of involvement of multiple vertebral bodies.

10.4.4.2. Dual-Energy X-Ray

Dual-energy X-ray absorptiometry (DEXA scan) is considered the gold standard for diagnosing osteoporosis. Osteoporosis is diagnosed when a woman's BMD is equal to or less than 2.5 standard deviations below that of a young, healthy adult reference population (30–40 years old). This diagnosis can be expressed as a T-score. However, as individuals age, the prevalence of osteoporotic conditions increases due to the natural decline in bone density. The International Society for Clinical Densitometry holds the position that densitometric criteria alone should not be used to diagnose osteoporosis in men under 50. Furthermore, it recommends using Z-scores, which compare age groups to peak bone mass instead of T-scores, for premenopausal women. It also advises against using densitometric criteria alone to diagnose osteoporosis in these women.

10.4.4.3. Biomarkers

Chemical biomarkers are useful in detecting bone deterioration. Type-I collagen, a vital component of bones, is broken down by the enzyme cathepsin K. The resulting fragment, known as a neoepitope, can be identified by specific antibodies to assist in the diagnosis of osteoporosis. Osteoporosis biomarker C-telopeptides, a product of type I collagen breakdown, can be detected in elevated levels in urine.

10.4.4.4. Other Measuring Tools

Compared to DXA, quantitative computed tomography (QCT) provides distinct estimates of BMD for trabecular and cortical bone, as well as precise volumetric mineral density in milligrams per centimeter (mg/cm^3) instead of the relative Z-score of BMD. QCT has several advantages, including the ability to analyze a region of any size or shape, exclude irrelevant tissue such as fat, muscle, and air, be performed at axial and peripheral sites, be calculated from pre-existing CT scans without requiring a separate radiation dose, and not require knowledge of the patient's subpopulation to create a clinical score (e.g., the Z-score for every girl over a specific age range). However, QCT also has some drawbacks, such as requiring a higher radiation dose than DXA, bulky and costly CT scanners, and more operator-dependent results due to its less standardized practice compared to BMD. The introduction of peripheral QCT has addressed some of the limitations of DXA and QCT.

Quantitative ultrasonography offers numerous benefits for measuring osteoporosis. In comparison to DXA and QCT devices, this modality is less expensive, involves no ionizing radiation, and allows for quick and simple measurement. The calcaneus, which has a high percentage of trabecular bone that is replaced more frequently than cortical bone and provides early evidence of metabolic change, is the most frequently assessed skeletal site for quantitative ultrasound evaluation. The relative flatness and parallelism of the calcaneus also reduce repositioning errors. Additionally, this method can benefit not only adults but also children, neonates, and preterm infants. Some ultrasonography equipment can be applied to the tibia as well.

10.4.5. Screening

The U.S. Preventive Services Task Force (USPSTF) recommends that all women 65 years of age or older be screened by bone densitometry. They also advise screening younger women who have risk factors. Recommendations regarding the intervals between repeat screenings and the appropriate age to cease screening are not supported by enough evidence. It is unclear whether screening for osteoporosis in men is more harmful than beneficial. BMD testing is recommended by the International Society for Clinical Densitometry for men who are 70 years of age or older, or who are deemed to be at risk comparable to that of a 70-year-old. To help determine who is reasonable to test, a variety of tools are available.

10.4.6. Prevention

In many ways, preventing osteoporosis through lifestyle choices is the opposite of modifying the risk factors. It is generally advised to quit smoking and consume alcohol in moderation as a means of preventing osteoporosis because these two lifestyle factors have been related to the disease. Following a gluten-free diet reduces osteoporosis risk and boosts bone density in individuals with celiac disease. A minimum of one gram of calcium should be consumed each day, and it is advised to check vitamin D levels and take certain supplements if needed.

10.4.6.1. Nutrition

Research on the advantages of calcium and vitamin D supplementation is contradictory, presumably because most of the studies included participants with low dietary intakes. Another risk factor for osteoporotic fractures is vitamin K deficiency. Vitamin K is required for the gamma-glutamyl carboxylase (GGCX) gene.

Variations in bone metabolism and BMD may be caused by functional polymorphisms in the gene. Osteoporosis is also treated with vitamin K2, and individual differences in the response to vitamin K treatment may be explained by GGCX polymorphisms. Legumes, beans, dairy products, and leafy greens are dietary sources of calcium. Whether dairy products are a sufficient source of calcium to prevent fractures has been the subject of conflicting research.

For individuals 19 to 50 years of age, the National Academy of Sciences suggests consuming 1,000 mg of calcium, and for those over 50, 1,200 mg.

10.4.6.2. Physical Exercise

Exercise may help maintain bone health, but the evidence for this claim is weak. According to some research, exercise may help postmenopausal women maintain their bone density and may also slightly lower their risk of bone fractures (absolute difference: 4%). Exercise involving weight-bearing has been shown to induce an adaptive response in the skeleton. Weight-bearing exercise protects bone density by promoting osteoblast activity.

A position statement concluded that early weight-bearing activities and higher bone activity prevent adult bone fragility. Swimming and cycling do not qualify as weight-bearing exercises. Professional cycling racing has an adverse effect on bone density and does not help slow down bone loss with age. Exercise may help patients with vertebral fractures feel less pain and have a higher quality of life, according to low-quality research, and moderate-quality research suggests that exercise will probably help patients with vertebral fractures perform better physically.

10.4.6.3. Hormone Therapy

Osteoporosis is more common in women who have reached menopause because lower estrogen levels raise the risk of osteoporosis. Hormone replacement therapy may help lower this incidence.

10.4.7. Management

10.4.7.1. Lifestyle

Exercises that increase muscle strength and/or weight-bearing endurance can help individuals with osteoporosis develop stronger bones. For postmenopausal women, resistance training, weight-bearing exercises, and aerobics all help maintain or increase BMD. Postmenopausal women should consume vitamin D and calcium daily. Preventing falls can help avoid the consequences of osteoporosis. There is some evidence, particularly among residents of assisted living facilities, in favor of using hip protectors.

10.4.7.2. Pharmacologic Therapy

The US National Osteoporosis Foundation recommends pharmacologic treatment for patients who have experienced hip or spine fractures related to osteoporosis, those with a BMD of 2.5 standard deviations (SD) or more below the average for young individuals (T-score of -2.5 or lower), and those with a BMD between 1 and 2.5 SD below the average whose 10-year risk of hip fracture is 3% or higher according to FRAX. Bisphosphonates can help reduce the risk of future fractures in individuals who have already suffered a fracture due to osteoporosis, particularly when taken for a duration of three to four years. There is no evidence to suggest that bisphosphonates impact the overall risk of mortality. The use of bisphosphonates for secondary osteoporosis in children lacks sufficient evidence.

The comparative effectiveness of different bisphosphonates has not been directly studied, thus it remains unclear if one is superior to another. The reduction in fracture risk varies from 25% to 70% depending on the affected bone. Prolonged use of bisphosphonates may carry a minimal risk of atypical femoral fractures and osteonecrosis of the jaw.

Considering the limited benefits observed after three to five years of use and the potential adverse effects, it may be reasonable to discontinue treatment at this point. Some medical experts propose discontinuing oral medications after five years or intravenous medications after three years for low-risk individuals, while high-risk individuals could consider up to 10 years of oral medication or six years of intravenous treatment.

Preventing osteoporotic fractures is the primary objective in managing osteoporosis. However, for individuals who have already experienced a fracture, preventing a secondary fracture becomes a matter of greater urgency. This is due to the higher risk of developing another fracture in individuals who have already experienced one, which significantly increases morbidity and mortality. There were no noticeable differences observed among the five bisphosphonates in terms of preventing secondary fractures in the total number of fracture endpoints. Nevertheless, zoledronate demonstrated better efficacy in preventing nonvertebral non-hip fractures, while alendronate was found to be the most effective in secondary prevention of vertebral and hip fractures. It is concerning that many individuals do not receive appropriate pharmacological therapy following a low-impact fracture. There is no evidence to support the claim that taking risedronate or etidronate reduces the risk of fracture in individuals with osteoporosis who have never experienced a bone fracture.

While alendronate does not have an impact on other types of fractures, it does reduce the occurrence of spine fractures. Alarmingly, within a year, half of the individuals discontinue their medication. It is not necessary to reassess BMD while undergoing bisphosphonate treatment. There is tentative evidence suggesting that males with osteoporosis may benefit from such treatment.

Although fluoride supplements increase bone density, they do not appear to reduce the risk of fractures, suggesting that they are ineffective in treating postmenopausal osteoporosis. Treatment for postmenopausal osteoporosis in women has shown promise with teriparatide, a recombinant parathyroid hormone. Additionally, some data suggests that strontium ranelate helps postmenopausal women with osteoporosis reduce their risk of both vertebral and nonvertebral fractures. Although hormone replacement treatment is beneficial for osteoporosis, it is only advised for women who also experience menopausal symptoms. On its own, it is not advised for osteoporosis. Although raloxifene effectively reduces the risk of vertebral fractures, it does not affect nonvertebral fracture risk. Moreover, it raises the risk of blood clots and strokes while lowering the risk of breast cancer. Denosumab has been shown to be beneficial in preventing fractures in females, but not in males.

Testosterone has been demonstrated to increase bone quantity and quality in hypogonadal men, but as of 2008, no studies had assessed its impact on fracture risk in men with normal testosterone levels. Although it used to be advised, calcitonin is no longer advised because of the possible cancer risk and dubious impact on fracture risk. For postmenopausal women, alendronic acid/cholecalciferol is a treatment option for this condition.

Monoclonal antibody romosozumab, marketed under the brand Evenity, targets sclerostin. Romosozumab is the only medication therapy for osteoporosis that simultaneously inhibits bone resorption and has anabolic effects. It is typically reserved for patients with a very high risk of fractures. In postmenopausal women with osteoporosis, certain drugs such as alendronate, etidronate, risedronate, raloxifene, and strontium ranelate can help prevent osteoporotic fragility fractures. Preliminary research suggests that Chinese herbal remedies may have a positive impact on BMD.

10.4.8. Prognosis

The fracture itself rarely results in death, despite the fact that individuals with osteoporosis have an increased mortality rate due to fracture complications. Reduced mobility and an increased risk of various complications, including pneumonia, deep vein thrombosis, and/or pulmonary embolism, are two outcomes that can result from hip fractures. The six-month mortality rate after a hip fracture for individuals 50 years of age and older was found to be approximately 13.5%. Almost 13% of these individuals required complete assistance to mobilize following their hip fracture. Although they have less of an effect on death, vertebral fractures can cause deformity and excruciating, difficult-to-control chronic pain of neurogenic origin. Even though they are uncommon, multiple vertebral fractures can cause kyphosis, a severe hunchback that can make breathing difficult due to the pressure on internal organs. Osteoporotic fractures are linked to a lower health-related quality of life in addition to an increased risk of death and other complications. Millions of fractures occur each year as a result of the condition, most often to the wrist, hip, and lumbar vertebrae. Men are also prone to fragility fractures of the ribs.

10.5. Osteoarthritis

The most prevalent type of arthritis, affecting millions of people globally, is osteoarthritis. It occurs as the cartilage that cushions the ends of the bones ages and becomes less effective. While osteoarthritis can affect any joint, the hands, knees, hips, and spine are the most commonly affected. Although joint damage cannot be reversed, symptoms of osteoarthritis are typically manageable. Maintaining a healthy weight, engaging in regular exercise, and taking certain medications may help to slow the progression of the disease and improve joint function and pain (Figure 10.7).

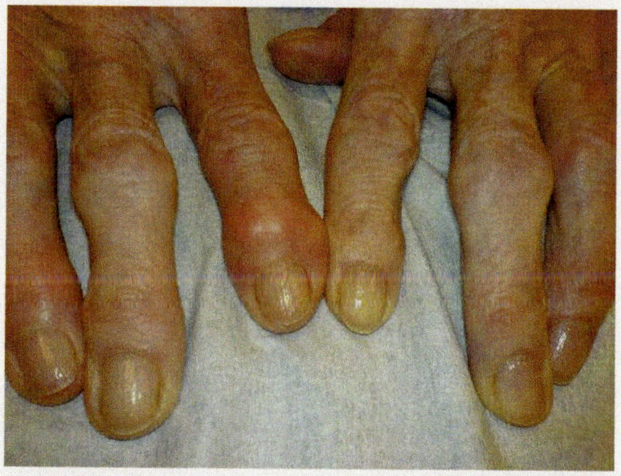

Figure 10.7. *The formation of hard knobs at the middle finger joints (known as Bouchard's nodes) and at the farthest joints of the fingers (known as Heberden's nodes) is a common feature of osteoarthritis in the hands.*

Source: By Drahreg01 – Own work, CC BY-SA 3.0, https://commons.wikimedia.org/w/index.php?curid=1358952.

10.5.1. Etiology

Age, gender, obesity, anatomical factors, muscle weakness, and joint injury (from sports or occupation) are risk factors for osteoarthritis (OA). Primary osteoarthritis (OA) is the most prevalent subtype of the condition. It is identified when there is no underlying trauma or illness, but it is linked to the risk factors mentioned earlier. When a joint abnormality already exists, secondary OA develops. Trauma or injury, congenital joint disorders, infectious arthritis, inflammatory arthritis, avascular necrosis (AVN), Paget disease, osteopetrosis, osteochondritis dissecans, metabolic disorders (hemochromatosis, Wilson's disease), hemoglobinopathy, Ehlers-Danlos syndrome, or Marfan syndrome are among the predisposing conditions.

10.5.2. Epidemiology

About 33.3% to 33.6% of people worldwide suffer from OA. It is the 11th most crippling disease globally, affecting 43 million people with moderate to severe disability. Only 60% of adults over 65 in the United States are thought to have symptoms, even though 80% of them have radiographic evidence of OA. This is because the frequency of radiographic OA is at least twice that of symptomatic OA. Thus, radiographic alterations do not establish OA as the reason for the patient's joint pain. At a total cost of almost $15 billion in 2011, almost 1 million hospitalizations were due to OA, making it the second most expensive disease in the US.

10.5.3. Pathophysiology

OA affects the entire joint, leaving no tissue unaffected. The aforementioned risk factors, mechanical stress, and aberrant joint mechanics interact to cause osteoarthritis (OA). Pro-inflammatory markers and proteases are produced as a result of the combination, which ultimately mediates joint destruction. It is unknown what exact sequence of events leads to the total disintegration of the joint. In most cases, surface fibrillation, irregularity, and focal erosions appear at the articular cartilage level, where OA first manifests. These erosions eventually reach the bone and keep getting bigger, affecting a larger area of the joint surface. After cartilage damage, the collagen matrix is harmed microscopically, which leads chondrocytes to multiply and group together. A phenotypic shift to hypertrophic chondrocytes results in ossification and the formation of osteophytes from cartilage outgrowths. The chondrocytes experience apoptosis as more of the collagen matrix is destroyed. Subchondral bone thickening is caused by improperly mineralized collagen; bone cysts are rare in advanced disease. In erosive OA, bony erosions are even more uncommon. Similar to inflammatory arthritis, there is some degree of synovial inflammation and hypertrophy, but this is not the primary cause of the condition. Menisci, ligaments, and joint capsules are examples of soft-tissue structures that are impacted. Both calcium phosphate and calcium pyrophosphate dihydrate crystals are found in end-stage OA. Although their exact function is unknown, they are assumed to play a part in synovial inflammation.

10.5.4. History and Physical Details

There are significant individual differences in how osteoarthritis (OA) manifests and advances. Joint pain, stiffness, and restricted movement are the three main symptoms of OA. Additionally, patients may exhibit balance problems and muscle weakness. Pain, usually associated with activity, subsides with rest. As the disease progresses, patients experience more persistent pain that hinders daily activities and eventually severely limits their functional ability. Instability (patients complain that the joint is "giving way" or "buckling," a sign of muscle weakness) and bony swelling are other potential manifestations. Osteoarthritis (OA) commonly affects the hips, knees, first metatarsophalangeal joints, proximal and distal interphalangeal joints (DIPs), lower cervical and lumbar spine joints, and first carpometacarpal (CMC) joints. In its presentation, OA can be either polyarticular or monoarticular. Different stages of the disease can manifest in different joints. Examination results for OA often reveal non-inflammatory effusions, crepitus, bony enlargement, and restricted range of motion. Pain may be present with passive motion and tenderness at the joint lines. Classic physical examination findings in hand OA include Heberden's nodes, which are posterior swellings of DIP joints, Bouchard's nodes, which are posterior swellings of PIP joints, and "squaring" at the base of the thumb, which affects the first CMC joints.

10.5.5. Evaluation

Every patient should undergo a comprehensive physical examination, which includes a focused musculoskeletal exam and a detailed medical history. Some of the results are outlined above. When one of the following criteria is met, a confident diagnosis of osteoarthritis (OA) can be made:

- Pain that worsens with activity and improves with rest;
- The patient is older than 45;
- Morning stiffness that lasts less than 30 minutes;
- Bony joint enlargement; and
- A restriction in range of motion.

Among other soft tissue abnormalities, a differential diagnosis should include rheumatoid arthritis, psoriatic arthritis, crystalline arthritis, hemochromatosis, bursitis, AVN, tendinitis, and radiculopathy. Blood tests that are typically normal in OA include CBC, ESR, rheumatoid factor, and ANA, though they may be ordered to rule out inflammatory arthritis. A diagnosis of osteoarthritis (OA) is consistent with a white blood cell count of less than 2,000/microL, primarily mononuclear (non-inflammatory) cells, if synovial fluid is obtained. Radiographic findings, such as marginal osteophytes, joint space narrowing, subchondral sclerosis, and cysts, can be seen on X-rays of the affected joint. However, these findings are not correlated with the severity of the disease and may not be present at the beginning of the illness. Although MRI is not usually recommended for OA diagnosis, it can identify OA earlier than standard radiographs. Additionally, osteophytes, synovial effusion, and inflammation that may be connected to OA can all be found with ultrasound. For OA, there are various classification schemes. They typically consist of the following: radiographic appearance, age at onset, presumed etiology (primary vs. secondary), as well as advancement rate. The most popular classification scheme is that used by the American College of Rheumatology (ACR). It is currently impossible to predict which patients will experience an early disease arrest and which will advance to severe OA.

10.5.6. Treatment/Management

Reducing pain and functional loss are the two main objectives of osteoarthritis (OA) treatment. Both pharmacologic and non-pharmacologic therapies are integral components of a comprehensive management strategy for this disease. Patients with milder symptoms can typically be managed with pharmacologic therapies alone, while more advanced cases necessitate a combination of both approaches. The key elements of non-pharmacologic therapy include: (i) avoiding activities that exacerbate joint symptoms or lead to excessive strain; (ii) engaging in strengthening exercises; (iii) achieving weight loss; and (iv) utilizing occupational therapy interventions such as braces, splints, canes, or crutches to alleviate joint stress. Weight loss is particularly crucial for overweight or obese individuals, as even a modest reduction in weight can result in a significant decrease in load across the knee joint. Formal physical therapy can greatly benefit patients by providing guidance on appropriate exercises and assisting with the correct utilization of assistive devices like canes. Physicians should routinely recommend exercise regimens that incorporate both resistance and aerobic training, as numerous studies have demonstrated their efficacy in reducing pain and improving physical function. Mechanical correction of joint malalignment can be achieved through the use of orthotics or realignment knee braces.

For OA, there are oral, topical, and/or intraarticular pharmacological options. The most common and least expensive pharmacologic treatments for OA are acetaminophen and oral NSAIDs, which are typically chosen as the first line of treatment. NSAIDs are typically prescribed topically or orally, and they should be started on an as-needed basis rather than on a set schedule at first. Because oral NSAIDs can be toxic to the gastrointestinal tract and cause adverse effects in the kidneys, heart, and lungs, their long-term use should be closely monitored. Topical NSAIDs frequently cause localized skin irritation, but they are less effective than their oral counterparts and have fewer gastrointestinal and other systemic side effects.

Another useful treatment for OA is intraarticular joint injections, particularly when there is severe pain. The response to glucocorticoid injections varies, and repeated injections are still a topic of debate. Injections of hyaluronic acid are an additional option, although there is debate regarding their superiority over placebo. Notably, oral glucocorticoids play no part. Duloxetine is only moderately effective in treating osteoarthritis (OA); in patients who do not respond adequately to these treatments and who may not be candidates for surgery or who refuse it completely, opioids may be used. It is crucial to remember that every patient responds to treatment differently, and choosing the right agents often involves a lot of trial and error.

Surgery is the last resort for patients with knee or hip OA who have not responded to several non-pharmacologic and pharmaceutical treatment modalities. Both hip and knee replacements have very low failure rates and can offer greater functionality and pain relief. When predicting the outcome of surgery, timing is crucial. When compared to individuals who undergo surgery earlier in the course of the disease, very poor functional status and significant muscle weakness may not result in improved postoperative functional status.

10.5.7. Differential Diagnosis

Differentials include:

- Rheumatoid arthritis;
- Psoriatic arthritis;
- Crystalline arthritis;
- Bursitis;
- Tendinitis;
- Hemochromatosis;
- Avascular necrosis;
- Radiculopathy;
- Other soft-tissue conditions.

10.5.8. Prognosis

The prognosis for individuals with osteoarthritis is contingent upon the joints impacted, as well as the degree of symptomatology and functional impairment. Osteoarthritis does not affect some patients significantly, but it can severely disable others. In certain circumstances, surgery to replace a damaged joint may be the most suitable option.

10.5.9. Complications

Osteoarthritis is a degenerative condition that worsens over time and often causes persistent pain. Joint stiffness and pain can become severe enough to hinder daily tasks. Osteoarthritis pain and disability can lead to depression and sleep disturbances.

10.5.10. Postoperative and Rehabilitation Care

Lifestyle changes, particularly engaging in exercise and weight reduction, are recommended.

10.5.11. Deterrence and Patient Education

The clinical team must explain the pathophysiology and etiology of the arthritic process, as well as the intervention plan, which will vary depending on the patient's age, the degree of dysfunction, the number of affected joints, the expectations for future activities, and the available therapeutic options. Emphasizing adherence to prescribed medication, weight loss, and exercise/physical therapy regimens is crucial.

10.5.12. Enhancing Healthcare Team Outcomes

A chronic, progressive condition that affects millions of people as they age is osteoarthritis. A group of medical specialists, including an internist, radiologist, endocrinologist, orthopedic surgeon, and rheumatologist, collaboratively manages this incurable condition. The interprofessional healthcare team also includes essential members such as a physical therapist, pharmacist, and nurse. Effective communication and collaboration among all healthcare disciplines are crucial to achieving optimal outcomes. Osteoarthritis patients should be educated about the natural course of the disease and the available treatment options. For obese patients, consulting a dietitian and participating in an exercise regimen is recommended. Research suggests that engaging in water-based activities can help reduce symptoms and improve joint function, making it advisable to see a physical therapist. Additionally, many patients may benefit from using a walking aid. Patients experiencing pain should educate themselves about different medications and supplements, as well as potential side effects. Patient education is essential in reducing the morbidity associated with this disorder.

10.5.12.1. Evidence-Based Outcomes

Patients with osteoarthritis have varying prognoses depending on the joint, number, and severity of affected joints. Osteoarthritis has no known cure, and the current approaches to treating it focus on symptom relief. Obesity, advanced age, multiple joint involvement, and the presence of varus deformity are factors linked to the disease's rapid progression. Joint replacement patients typically have good prognoses, with success rates exceeding 80%. Nevertheless, most prosthetic joints require replacement surgery after 10 to 15 years due to wear and tear. Preoperative approaches are crucial for patients because surgical complications can be grave and incapacitating.

10.6. Rheumatoid Arthritis

Among the inflammatory types of arthritis is rheumatoid arthritis (RA). It is a chronic illness that can lead to pain and stiffness in various body joints. Although it can affect any joint, the small joints of the hands and feet are where it usually begins. Rheumatoid arthritis often affects both sides of the body, affecting, for example, both hands and both knees. According to the Centers for Disease Control and Prevention, approximately 11.5 million adults in the U.S. suffer from rheumatoid arthritis, and 71 out of every 1,00,000 individuals receive an RA diagnosis each year. The risk of RA is two to three times higher in women than in men. Even though symptoms typically appear between the ages of 30 and 60, younger people can also be affected (Figure 10.8).

Similar symptoms in children and teenagers are frequently associated with juvenile arthritis, another autoimmune condition. Juvenile arthritis comes in a variety of forms, but almost all of them differ from adult rheumatoid arthritis. For this reason, juvenile idiopathic arthritis (JIA) is the new common term for juvenile rheumatoid arthritis (JRA), which is no longer commonly used. Rheumatoid arthritis damages joints over time and can lead to severe disability if left untreated. Thankfully, modern drugs frequently stop joint damage from worsening.

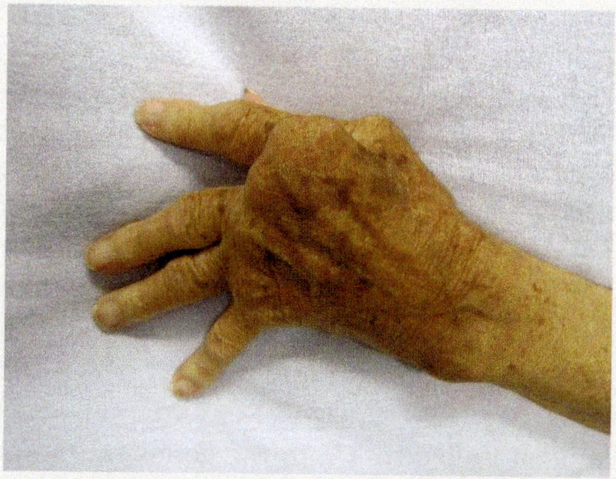

Figure 10.8. *A hand severely affected by rheumatoid arthritis. This degree of swelling and deformation does not typically occur with current treatment.*

Source: By James Heilman, MD – Own work, CC BY-SA 3.0, https://commons.wikimedia.org/w/index.php?curid=11110471

Thanks to these advancements in treatment, the severe joint deformity commonly associated with RA—such as bent, crooked fingers and knuckles—is becoming less common. While there is not a cure for RA, joint destruction and other complications can typically be avoided with early diagnosis and appropriate treatment. When rheumatoid arthritis fails to respond to medication, orthopedic procedures can significantly enhance function, mobility, and overall quality of life in severely affected joints.

10.6.1. Etiology

The development of rheumatoid arthritis (RA) is largely influenced by genetic factors, with genetics playing a significant role in the etiology of the disease. The interaction between an individual's genotype and environmental factors is believed to contribute to the development of RA. A study conducted in the UK involving 91 pairs of identical twins and 112 pairs of fraternal twins found a higher concordance rate in identical twins (15%) compared to fraternal twins (5%). The heritability of RA is estimated to be between 40% and 65% for seropositive RA and 20% for seronegative RA. Specific HLA-DRB1 alleles, such as HLA-DRB1*04, HLA-DRB1*01, and HLA-DRB1*10, have been linked to an increased risk of developing RA. These alleles contain a shared epitope (SE) – a conserved sequence of 5 amino acids in the third hypervariable region of the DRB1 chain, which is associated with an increased risk of developing RA. Variants in other genes, such as PAD14, PTPN22, CTLA4, IL-2RA, STAT4, TRAF1, CCR6, and IRF5, have also been linked to RA. In the genes MIR146A, PTPN22, PSORS1C1, and SNPs, single nucleotide polymorphisms (SNPs) are linked to severe illness. Various ethnic groups have different genetic polymorphisms that are associated with RA. Heritable alterations without modifying the DNA sequence are referred to as epigenetic changes. These changes can occur in the DNA or the chromatin and include histone modification, non-coding RNA-mediated regulation, and DNA methylation. RA-FLS (fibroblast-like synoviocytes) are more likely to be invasive than synoviocytes from osteoarthritis (OA) patients because they overexpress the tyrosine phosphatase SHP-2, which is encoded by the PTPN11 gene. The enhancer region within the PTPN11 intron has two hypermethylated sites, leading to aberrant epigenetic regulation of the gene and modification of RA-FLS function.

The largest environmental risk factor for rheumatoid arthritis is cigarette smoking. Research has indicated that there is an interaction between smoking and the shared epitope (SE) in individuals who have tested positive for the anti-citrullinated protein antibody (anti-CCP), which increases the risk of RA. Seropositive RA is more closely associated with other environmental triggers. Other environmental triggers may also play a role in triggering RA. These include *P. gingivalis*, asbestos, silica, and textile dust. This suggests that an autoimmune inflammatory response in the joints is subsequently induced by external exposure to different antigens in regions of the host that are not in close proximity to the joints. The GI tract, oropharynx, and lungs are some of these distant locations. Alterations in the composition and function of the intestinal microbiome have also been linked to rheumatoid arthritis. Dysbiosis, or an imbalance in the gut microbiome, leads to changes in its composition in individuals with rheumatoid arthritis. Specifically, patients with RA have a less diverse gut microbiome compared to individuals without the disease. The genera *Actinobacteria, Collinsella, Eggerthalla*, and *Faecalibacterium* are found in higher levels. Collinsella has been associated with increased severity of rheumatoid arthritis and alters the permeability of the gut mucosa.

10.6.2. Epidemiology

According to the Global Burden of Disease 2010 Study, the prevalence of RA is approximately 0.24% worldwide. In North America, Australia, and other areas with

European ancestry, as well as Western and Northern Europe, RA is more common. In East Asia and Africa, the prevalence is even lower than in Central and South America. About 40 cases of RA per 1,00,000 people are reported each year in the US and other Western Northern European countries. Based on epidemiological data, women are more likely than men to develop RA, with a lifetime risk of 3% for women and 1% for men. The risk of RA also increases with age, peaking between 65 and 80 years of age. During that time, urban areas had a higher prevalence of RA (0.69%) than rural areas (0.54%). RA was more common during that time (0.49%) in high-income nations than in low-income nations (0.35%). Asia and South America had lower rates of RA prevalence than North America and Europe. There is a dearth of data from Africa, and what little there is depends greatly on the nation; in sub-Saharan Africa, RA is less common than in North Africa. Comparatively speaking to the rest of Asia, RA is far less common in East Asia. A meta-analysis of 67 studies found that the global period prevalence increased by 9.75% between 1980 and 2019.

As previously mentioned, there is a genetic predisposition to rheumatoid arthritis (RA), which was found to be approximately 40% in a sizable Swedish study conducted in 2013. Additionally, the study found that early-onset and seropositive RA have higher heritabilities. Their report states that the risk of RA with a first-degree relative who tests positive for RA is three times higher than the risk with a second-degree relative who tests positive for RA, which is two times higher. It is now possible to identify several distinct genetic predispositions that could account for this discovery. The shared epitope in the HLA-DRB1 region is the strongest genetic predisposition for RA.

Cigarette smoking is the modifiable risk factor most strongly associated with RA. Nutrition and diet have been demonstrated to be important environmental factors that can trigger RA. The typical "western" diet, which is high in fat, low in fiber, and high in calories, raises the risk of RA. Long-chain omega-3 polyunsaturated fatty acid consumption is linked to a lower risk of RA. Another well-established risk factor for RA is obesity. Patients with a BMI of more than 30 kg/m^2 have a 30% increased risk of RA, while those with a BMI of 25 to 29.9 kg/m^2 have a 15% increased risk.

10.6.3. Pathophysiology

Certain genetically predisposed individuals may experience rheumatoid arthritis (RA) as a result of environmental factors. One notable example is the development of ACPA-positive RA in patients who smoke and possess the HLA-DRB1 shared epitope gene. While RF and ACPA antibodies are the most well-known autoantibodies in RA, there are a few others that are relatively specific to the disease. When antibodies are present, the term seropositive RA is used to describe rheumatoid arthritis. RF antibodies refer to any isotype of antibody that binds to the Fc region of IgG. RA patients commonly exhibit antibodies against citrullinated proteins. Anti-perinuclear factor antibodies were first discovered in RA patients in 1964, and anti-keratin antibodies were identified through various assays in 1979. These antibodies were later found to have high specificity for RA in the 1990s, specifically targeting the citrullinated peptide filaggrin. Citrullinated peptides serve as the epitope recognized by these antibodies. To detect these antibodies in a clinical setting, an ELISA test utilizing cyclic citrullinated peptide (CCP) was developed. These antibodies are referred to as anti-cyclic citrullinated peptide antibodies (ACPA). Citrulline is produced when peptidyl arginine deiminase (PAD) post-translationally modifies arginine. This reaction occurs in areas of inflammation and tissue damage, such as the lungs of smokers. Citrulline-containing epitopes are preferentially presented by the HLA-DRB1 shared epitope. ACPA can be of the IgG, IgM, or IgA isotypes. ACPA has the ability to bind to citrullinated residues on self-proteins such as vimentin, fibronectin, fibrinogen, histones, and type 2 collagen.

The lung, gums, and gastrointestinal tract are examples of locations far from the synovial joints where the immune response in RA begins. These tissues produce modified proteins through biochemical processes such as citrullination. It is believed that the mechanism underlying environment-triggered RA results from the repeated activation of innate immunity. Taking the lungs as an example, smoking causes alveolar macrophages to express peptidyl arginine deiminase (PAD), leading to the conversion of arginine to citrulline in the airway. This process generates a neoantigen, which triggers an immune response and the production of antibodies against citrullinated proteins (ACPAs). Anti-modified protein antibodies (AMPA) are an immune response that patients are genetically predisposed to develop against modified proteins. The reaction of PAD with arginine results in citrullination. The PAD2 and PAD4 isoforms have the strongest associations with RA. Anti-PAD4 antibodies are highly specific for RA, present in RA patients, and linked to ACPA positivity. *Porphyromonas gingivalis*, a bacteria that causes inflammation, is associated with the inflammatory response in gingivitis and other mucosal areas. Leukocytes that produce PAD4 are recruited. *P. gingivalis* also produces a PAD-like enzyme. The resident proteins that these enzymes citrullinate have the potential to function as autoantigens. Anti-acetylated protein antibodies have recently been linked to RA, mostly in seropositive patients (affecting about 40% of RA patients). The enzymatic process of acetylation, which is thought to be mediated by bacteria and may be connected to both microbiome dysbiosis and RA, transforms lysine into acetyllysine. The precise mechanism is still unknown at this point. As a result, autoantibodies made by acetylation, carbamylation, and citrullination can target a variety of altered proteins.

Prior to the onset of clinical arthritis, autoantibodies are present. Long before RA reaches its clinical stage, or what is known as pre-symptomatic or pre-clinical RA, autoimmune disease begins to develop at the molecular and cellular level. Although the patients are asymptomatic, certain immunologic and biochemical abnormalities have been discovered during this phase. Serum levels of RF and ACPA can be detected up to 10 years prior to the manifestation of clinical symptoms. Both the serum cytokine levels and ACPA concentration rise with time. Many patients acquire autoantibodies without manifesting the illness. Some patients will eventually develop immune-mediated inflammation primarily centered in the synovium instead of autoimmunity. The synovium's plasma cells generate these autoantibodies. Immune cells, including innate (monocytes, dendritic cells, mast cells) and adaptive (T-helper 1, Th1), Th17, B cells, and plasma cells, infiltrate the synovium in RA patients. Activation of synovial fibroblast-like synovial cells (FSC) occurs. Instead of being found in the synovium, neutrophils migrate from the blood into the synovial fluid.

Within the synovial compartment, cytokines and chemokines such as granulocyte-monocyte colony-stimulating factor (GM-CSF), interleukin-6 (IL-6), and tumor necrosis factor (TNF) activate endothelial cells and attract immune cells. In rheumatoid synovium, the fibroblast-like synoviocytes (FLS) adopt an invasive phenotype. Rheumatoid arthritis is characterized by bone erosions, which are caused by osteoclast generation stimulated by

RANKL produced by inflammatory cells and FLS. It is noteworthy that synovial biopsies were essentially unremarkable in seropositive patients with arthralgia. It is hypothesized that for a disease to manifest clinically, a second environmental trigger is required. Once this is confirmed, a damaging inflammatory process begins. Joint damage increases as a result of the migration of FLS from one joint to another.

Every component of the immune system is involved, including innate immunity and adaptive immunity, which encompass the immune responses of the cellular (T cell) and humoral (B cell) tissues. Macrophages, which produce TNF, IL-6, IL-1, GM-CSF, IL-15, IL-18, IL-32, and chemokines that promote tissue inflammation, are part of the innate immune response. Other components of innate immunity include endothelial cells, which facilitate the migration of immune and inflammatory cells, such as neutrophils, into the synovial fluid. These cells then produce pro-inflammatory substances, such as prostaglandins, proteases, and reactive oxygen intermediates, which degrade cartilage. Proinflammatory cytokines, PDGF, and chemokines stimulate resident fibroblast-like synoviocytes (FLS) to proliferate with invasive features and generate Matrix MetalloProteinases (MMP) and A Disintegrin and Metalloproteinase with Thrombospondin motifs (ADAMTS). TNF, IL-1, and IL-17 activate chondrocytes, which then produce matrix enzymes that damage cartilage. Vasoactive amines, leukotrienes, proteases, and TNF are produced by resident mast cells. RANKL plays a critical role in causing bone erosions by activating osteoclasts. The complement system is another component of innate immunity. It is triggered by immune complexes containing RF and ACPA, which results in the pro-inflammatory chemicals C3a and C5a, which attract and activate neutrophils as well as activate mast cells and macrophages.

T lymphocytes and B cells, which respond to antigenic stimuli, are components of adaptive immunity. One major antigen that initiates autoimmunity in RA is modified proteins, such as citrullinated proteins. These altered proteins activate T cells at mucosal sites, which in turn cause B cells to produce AMPA, including ACPA. This immune reaction in certain patients progresses to an immune-mediated inflammation of the synovium. The subsynovial region of the synovium is populated by T and B cells that reside there. From a histological standpoint, the mononuclear cell infiltrate bears resemblance to a lymphoid organ. Dendritic cells serve as a bridge between innate and adaptive immunity by presenting antigens to T cells that are specific to those antigens. Upon interaction with T lymphocytes, antigen-specific B cells become activated and differentiate into plasma cells that produce ACPA and RF. Through binding to their antigens, these autoantibodies form immune complexes that can amplify the inflammatory response via complement activation. Activated T cells can differentiate into type 1 (Th1) and type 17 (Th17) helper T cells. Th17 cells secrete IL-17, a cytokine that promotes inflammation and attracts neutrophils and other T cells.

The synovium generates significant amounts of cytokines, which play a crucial role in intensifying a prolonged inflammatory response that leads to cartilage loss and bone erosion. Chronic inflammation also influences associated comorbidities, including an increased risk of cardiovascular disease.

10.6.4. Histopathology

New synovial blood vessel growth is one of the first histopathologic findings in RA. This leads to the transmigration of lymphocytes and polymorphonuclear leukocytes into the synovial fluid. The highly catabolic synovium necessitates angiogenesis, which is facilitated by proinflammatory cytokines such as tumor necrosis factor (TNF). Cytokines induce the production of adhesion molecules by endothelial cells during angiogenesis, thereby promoting cell migration into the synovium. Despite angiogenesis, the hypoxic environment of RA synovial fluid stimulates the synthesis of MMPs and cyclooxygenase (COX) 2-derived nociceptive eicosanoids. Consequently, the synovium becomes further inflamed. Monocytes proliferate, and the synovial membrane thickens with small villous projections into the joint space during the early stages of the disease due to the influx of inflammatory cells into the synovial membrane.

The histopathology of rheumatoid synovium reveals extensive activation and proliferation of FLS, as well as the accumulation of T cells, including Th1, Th17, and Treg cells, in the subsynovial region. Additionally, B cells proliferate and undergo plasma cell differentiation. Lymph nodes and other secondary lymphoid tissues may resemble synovial tissue in appearance. The subsynovial tissue also contains fibroblasts, mast cells, dendritic cells, and macrophages. Rheumatoid synovial tissue develops an invasive nature, causing minor erosions by eroding into the bone. Small vessel vasculitis occurs first in rheumatoid nodules, and then there is a chronic inflammatory granulomatous phase. Rheumatoid arthritis frequently results in the development of rheumatoid nodules, which affect the dermis or subcutis in peri-articular areas. This condition, known as accelerated rheumatoid nodulosis, is related to methotrexate therapy when it occurs in multiples. It can be anywhere in size from a few millimeters to several centimeters. In gross terms, it resembles a white, fibrous lesion with yellowish patches that are indicative of collagenous necrobiosis. Histologically, the condition can appear identical to granuloma annulare. The dermis and hypodermis exhibit irregular geographic-like necrobiosis, encircled by well-developed palisade-like histiocytes, occasionally accompanied by neutrophils and lymphocytes. Mast cells and giant cells may occasionally be seen. Within the core of the necrobiotic areas are collagen and fibrin. Plasma cells have infiltrated the surrounding dermis and hypodermis perivascularly. Rheumatoid nodules can very rarely develop in the lungs.

10.6.5. History and Physical Details

The most frequent and prominent symptoms are edema and joint pain, which typically begin slowly over several weeks to months. The small joints of the hands and feet usually experience joint involvement first, followed by the larger joints. Stiffness, especially in the morning, is a defining feature. Palindromic rheumatism is characterized by an episodic pattern of symptoms that can occasionally be observed, although most of the time, symptoms have a slow and subtle onset. Palindromic rheumatism is considered a distinct phenotype of RA because not all patients with it progress to develop RA, and because they respond to hydroxychloroquine. As previously mentioned, RA primarily affects small peripheral joints, such as the hands. The cervical spine is the only part of the spine where the axial joints may be affected due to the presence of synovial joints. The lumbar spine, on the other hand, is not affected. Some patients may present with monoarticular and extraarticular involvement (lungs), even though multiple small joint involvements are a common feature. Patients with RA will experience joint damage, deformities, disability, and an increased risk of death if they are not treated with disease-modifying anti-rheumatic medications (DMARDs). RA is a chronic, progressive disease.

Upon physical examination, the affected joint will hurt when moved or pressure is applied, regardless of the presence of joint swelling. It will be possible to palpate thickening of the synovium and a boggy feel. Wrist involvement may present with typical signs and symptoms of carpal tunnel syndrome (CTS), although joint erythema and warmth are typically absent. Physical examination will reveal decreased grip strength if multiple joints are involved. In advanced chronic disease, physical findings such as the bowstring sign, swan neck deformity, Boutonniere deformity, ulnar deviation, and metacarpophalangeal joint subluxation can be observed. Later-stage RA is also characterized by decreased range of motion in the knees, elbows, and shoulders. Along with other toe abnormalities, hallux valgus is a common foot condition. The most prevalent extraarticular manifestation of RA is rheumatoid nodules, which can develop over the patella, Achilles tendons, hand and foot joints, and pressure points like the olecranon, although they are most frequently found in these areas.

Among all RA patients, 5 to 16% develop interstitial lung disease (ILD), which is linked to higher mortality rates and RA-specific autoantibodies. Prior to developing joint inflammation with positive RF and ACPA, certain patients may exhibit ILD. Anti-carbamylated protein antibodies (anti-CarP), anti-malondialdehyde-acetaldehyde antibodies (anti-MAA), and ACPA are associated with rheumatoid arthritis (RA)-associated interstitial lung disease (ILD). In patients with RA, the MUC5B promoter variant rs35705950 has been linked to ILD. This variant represents a gain of function and encodes mucin 5B. When comparing RA-ILD to unaffected controls, the odds ratio was 3.8 (95% CI 2.8–5.2), and when comparing RA ILD to RA without ILD, the odds ratio was 3.1 (95% CI 1.8–5.4).

Ophthalmological manifestations encompass dry mouth and eyes that are associated with secondary Sjogren syndrome. Furthermore, with the advent of novel RA therapies, inflammatory eye diseases such as scleritis and episcleritis have become less prevalent. Similarly, the occurrence of Felty syndrome—characterized by long-standing seropositive RA (including RF and ANA), leukopenia, and splenomegaly—is diminishing. These patients may exhibit an increased susceptibility to bacterial infection in addition to chronic non-healing ulcers. Another potential presenting symptom of RA is vasculitis affecting medium- and small-sized blood vessels. Nevertheless, the incidence of vasculitis in RA patients is minimal. Individuals afflicted with rheumatoid vasculitis may present with asymmetric polyneuropathy or mononeuritis multiplex.

10.6.6. Evaluation

Thrombocytosis and anemia of chronic disease are frequently identified through laboratory testing. If the rare Felty syndrome is present, neutropenia may also be observed. Rheumatoid factor (RF) is found in 80%–90% of rheumatoid arthritis (RA) patients, with a sensitivity of 69% and a specificity of 85%. Anti-citrullinated protein antibody (ACPA) is detected in 70%–80% of patients with a sensitivity of 67% and a specificity of 95%. Seropositive RA patients are defined as those who have either RF, ACPA, or both. Approximately 10% of RA patients are seronegative, meaning they have neither ACPA nor RF. It is important to note that the presence of rheumatoid factor alone does not confirm a diagnosis of rheumatoid arthritis, as it can also be found in other connective tissue disorders such as granulomatosis with polyangiitis, Sjogren syndrome, scleroderma, and systemic lupus erythematosus. However, if both RF and ACPA are positive, the sensitivity and specificity of the diagnosis significantly increase. It is also worth mentioning that RF and ACPA can be present for months or even years before clinical arthritis symptoms manifest.

Joint involvement with advanced disease will exhibit periarticular osteopenia, narrowing of the joint space, and marginal bony erosions on plain radiographs. Bone and cartilage deterioration are considered pathognomonic, if not entirely specific, findings for RA. However, these results are consistent with advanced illness. Prior to the appearance of radiographic evidence of bone erosion, magnetic resonance imaging (MRI) and ultrasonography can be beneficial in the early stages of the disease. A decrease in signal from the bone marrow on T1-weighted and gadolinium-enhanced images indicates bone marrow edema. Furthermore, MRIs can reveal synovial thickening, which has been shown to predict the eventual occurrence of bony erosions. The clinical utility of MRI and whether it should be included in the diagnostic criteria for RA are still unknown.

RA presents a range of clinical manifestations, and early diagnosis can be challenging due to the absence of a universally accepted test for the disease. Previously, a patient was diagnosed with RA if they met at least four of the following criteria for a minimum of six weeks: symmetric arthritis, arthritis of the hands, elevated acute phase reactants, elevated rheumatoid factor, morning stiffness, and radiologic evidence of RA. While these criteria did not specifically address RA, they did differentiate between inflammatory and non-inflammatory arthritis. However, a significant drawback was their insensitivity to early-stage RA. The diagnostic criteria were revised with the development of serologic markers. Below is a summary of the 2010 ACR and the European League Against Rheumatism (ACR/EULAR) diagnostic criteria for RA, which consist of four distinct domains:

2010 ACR/EULAR classification criteria for RA:

- Number and size of involved joints:
  - 2 to 10 large joints = 1 point (shoulders, elbows, hips, knees, and ankles).
  - 1 to 3 small joints = 2 points (metacarpophalangeal joints, proximal interphalangeal joints, second through fifth metatarsophalangeal joints, thumb interphalangeal joints, and wrists).
  - 4 to 10 small joints = 3 points.
  - Greater than 10 joints (including at least 1 small joint) = 5 points.
- Serological testing for rheumatoid factor or anti-citrullinated peptide/protein antibody:
  - Low positive = 2 points.
  - High positive = 3 points.
- Elevated acute phase reactant (erythrocyte sedimentation rate [ESR] or C-reactive protein [CRP]) = 1 point.
- Symptom duration of at least six weeks = 1 point.

The patient is classified as having RA if their total score is greater than or equal to 6. These diagnostic and classification criteria are primarily applied in clinical trials and other studies involving RA patients. It is important to note that any swollen or tender joint found during an examination is considered to have joint involvement. Imaging studies can also be used to determine the presence of synovitis or joint involvement. The 2010 ACR/EULAR criteria do not include the DIPs, first CMC joints, and first metatarsophalangeal joints. Additionally, these criteria should only be used for patients whose joint involvement cannot be adequately explained by other inflammatory conditions such as psoriasis or systemic lupus erythematosus. Specific testing is required to rule out these illnesses. The new criteria have been observed to have a higher specificity and negative predictive value, maintain the same sensitivity as the previous criteria for diagnosing RA, and better predict the probability of RA.

10.6.7. Treatment/Management

Early diagnosis and initiation of treatment are crucial for patients with rheumatoid arthritis (RA) to prevent irreversible joint damage. The International Task Force Guidelines, published in 2014, provide the following recommendations for the treatment of RA:

- The main objectives of treatment are achieving long-term clinical remission and optimizing the quality of life, with no signs or symptoms linked to inflammatory disease activity.
- In cases where clinical remission cannot be achieved, low disease activity can be considered as an alternative.
- Patients with moderate to severe disease activity should have their disease activity evaluated monthly.
- Patients with little disease activity or in clinical remission should have their disease activity evaluated every three to six months.

To assist clinicians in assessing the disease activity of RA patients, several clinical assessment tools have been developed. The ACR revised its recommendation in 2019 and suggested the use of the following evaluation tools, as they meet the minimal evaluation requirements set by the ACR. In clinical practice, the combination of DAS28, CDAI, and RAPID3 is user-friendly and incorporates input from both patients and providers, as well as laboratory tests:

- Clinical disease activity index (CDAI);
- Disease activity score (DAS);
- Disease activity score 28 Joints (DAS28-ESR/CRP);
- Patient-derived DAS28;
- Hospital Universitario La Princesa index (HUPI);
- Multi-biomarker disease activity score (MBDA score, VECTRA DA);
- Rheumatoid arthritis disease activity index (RADAI);
- Rheumatoid arthritis disease activity index 5 (RADAI-5);
- Routine assessment of patient index data 3 (RAPID3);
- Routine assessment of patient index data 5 (RAPID5);
- Simplified disease activity index (SDAI).

Usually used to treat rheumatoid arthritis (RA), disease-modifying antirheumatic medications (DMARDs) include methotrexate, leflunomide, hydroxychloroquine, and sulfasalazine. Examples of anti-TNF-alpha inhibitors are etanercept, infliximab, adalimumab, golimumab, and certolizumab pegol. Abatacept (CTLA4-Ig), tocilizumab, sarilumab, and rituximab are examples of additional biologic DMARDs, including T-cell costimulation inhibitors, interleukin (IL) 6 inhibitors, and anti-CD20 B-cell depleting monoclonal antibodies. Targeted synthetic DMARDs, such as tofacitinib, baricitinib, and upadacitinib, are examples of Janus kinases (JAK) inhibitors.

In patients with a serious active infection, DMARD therapy, including biologic agents and targeted synthetic agents (tofacitinib), should be temporarily stopped. Once the infection has cleared up and the antimicrobial treatment has been finished, they can be resumed. It is crucial to keep in mind that screening for tuberculosis and hepatitis B and C should be done for all patients beginning treatment for RA. Patients with liver disease should not take methotrexate. Patients with latent tuberculosis should wait at least one month after finishing their current course of treatment before starting targeted and biologic treatments. Conventional DMARD therapy should be administered to patients who are unable to take or finish treatment for latent tuberculosis. Biologic agents should be avoided in patients with underlying skin cancer and lymphoproliferative disorders, except for rituximab, where there is evidence of benefit from B-cell suppression. The American College of Radiology (ACR) advises patients to have vaccinations against pneumococcal disease, hepatitis, influenza, human papillomavirus (HPV), herpes zoster virus (HZV), and COVID-19 prior to beginning RA therapy.

10.6.7.1. Non-Steroidal Anti-Inflammatory Drugs (NSAIDs)

NSAIDs are frequently used to treat joint pain and inflammation symptoms, but they do not alter the course of any disease. There are approximately 20 such medications that are all effective at maximum dosages. The toxicities and adverse effects vary somewhat. Although NSAIDs vary in their effects on the cardiovascular system, there is a Black Box warning for cardiovascular disease. Hematologic, renal, and gastrointestinal toxicity are additional risks associated with NSAIDs. The patient, their comorbidities, and the provider's experience with the particular medication all play a role in determining which NSAID is prescribed. Although they are not commonly used, non-acetylated salicylates, sometimes known as salalate, have a favorable safety profile with minimal GI, renal, or hematologic side effects. Guidelines exist regarding NSAID use in relation to gastrointestinal and cardiovascular comorbidities in patients.

- **Efficacy:** Indomethacin, piroxicam.
- **Convenience (1–2 Doses per Day):** Meloxicam, naproxen, celecoxib, nabumetone.
- **Overall Safety:** Nabumetone.
- **GI Safety:** Celecoxib, nabumetone.
- **Renal Safety:** Possible nabumetone.
- **Hematologic Safety (No Antiplatelet Effect):** Celecoxib, meloxicam, nabumetone.

10.6.7.2. Corticosteroids

Patients with RA frequently use corticosteroids. In a number of circumstances, corticosteroids should be taken into account. Corticosteroids can be used as bridge therapy in a newly diagnosed patient with very active RA until DMARD therapy is started. Early corticosteroid use in RA patients has been shown in some studies to improve outcomes and have disease-modifying effects, including slowing radiographic progression. A different study found no evidence of corticosteroid bridge therapy's long-term advantages. For mild RA flare-ups, short courses of corticosteroids may be helpful. For single-joint flares, intra-articular corticosteroids may be used. To keep their disease under control, about 50% of RA patients need to take low-dose corticosteroids (prednisone 2.5–7.5 mg daily). Prolonged use of corticosteroids is linked to various side effects, such as increased risk of infections, weight gain, and osteoporosis.

10.6.7.3. Nonbiologic DMARDs

Methotrexate, hydroxychloroquine (HCQ), azathioprine (AZA), leflunomide, sulfasalazine, and cyclosporine are among the medications in this category. The first medication of choice for patients with rheumatoid arthritis (RA) is methotrexate. The suggested treatment plan involves initiating methotrexate at a dose of 10–15 mg per week, gradually increasing it by 5 mg per month, and aiming for a weekly dose of 20–25 mg. Patients who do not respond well to oral administration or who experience intolerance may consider subcutaneous administration. Methotrexate's bioavailability was found to be enhanced in patients receiving 15 mg per week or more of the drug when the dose was split (10 mg in the morning and 10 mg in the evening each week), and they still experienced some disease activity. It has been demonstrated that triple therapy—methotrexate, hydroxychloroquine, and sulfasalazine—is an effective treatment plan for RA. However, triple therapy is not well tolerated, and a significant number of patients discontinue this course of treatment.

10.6.7.4. TNF Inhibitors

Etanercept, infliximab, adalimumab, certolizumab, and golimumab are among the TNF inhibitors. The ACR advises against the use of TNF inhibitors prior to attempting a nonbiologic DMARD. However, research suggests that administering TNF inhibitors is preferable to administering another nonbiologic DMARD to patients who have not responded to methotrexate therapy. Reactivation of latent tuberculosis and opportunistic infections are the most concerning side effects of these agents. Although the use of methotrexate in combination with these agents has been shown to reduce this complication, there is some concern regarding the development of antibodies against these agents, which may eventually decrease their effectiveness. These agents should not be used in cases of acute infection, advanced heart failure, demyelinating disease, or recent cancer.

10.6.7.5. Rituximab

If patients have uncontrolled RA and have not responded to TNF inhibitors, a biologic DMARD called rituximab may be added to the treatment regimen. When administered intravenously, rituximab depletes CD20+ B-cells and reduces the immune response to vaccines in recipients. Patients who are seropositive and receiving methotrexate also respond better to rituximab. It is a preferred agent in patients with underlying lymphoproliferative disorders, as mentioned above.

10.6.7.6. Abatacept

By binding to CD80 and CD86, abatacept inhibits T-cell activation. It is administered subcutaneously once a week or as a monthly intravenous infusion. Patients with uncontrolled RA who have not responded well to TNF inhibitor and methotrexate therapy can benefit from the proven efficacy of abatacept, which can provide relief for a duration ranging from six months to five years.

10.6.7.7. Interleukin 6 Inhibitors

For adults with moderate-to-severe active RA who have not responded well to TNF inhibitor therapy, tocilizumab, an IL-6 receptor inhibitor, may offer benefits. Tocilizumab treatment leads to clinically significant improvement in these patients. Sarilumab, another medication in this class, has been shown to enhance clinical outcomes in patients with uncontrolled RA who are already receiving TNF inhibitor therapy.

10.6.7.8. Janus Kinase (JAK) Inhibitors

JAK is a family of tyrosine kinases involved in intracellular signal transduction in immune cells and hematopoiesis. Oral JAK inhibitors, such as tofacitinib, are approved as second-line treatments for RA as they reduce cytokine synthesis.

ACR and EULAR treatment guidelines:

- Regardless of the degree of disease activity, patients who have not yet started disease-modifying antirheumatic drug (DMARD) therapy for early RA should do so, according to the treatment guidelines of the American College of Physicians.
- Methotrexate monotherapy is the recommended treatment for patients with early disease and low disease activity.

- In patients who are intolerant to methotrexate or for whom it is contraindicated, leflunomide or sulfasalazine is the initial line of treatment.
- Therapy should be changed if DMARD monotherapy is ineffective at controlling disease activity (regardless of concurrent glucocorticoid use). At this point, methotrexate can either be continued or stopped. Tumor necrosis factor (TNF) inhibitors, non-tumor necrosis factor biologic agents, or dual traditional/nonbiologic DMARD therapy are suggested as additional therapeutic options following the failure of DMARD monotherapy.
- Regardless of the degree of disease activity, methotrexate is the recommended drug for initial monotherapy in patients with established RA who have never used a DMARD.
- Regardless of concurrent glucocorticoid use, dual DMARD therapy, a TNF inhibitor, a non-TNF biologic agent, or tofacitinib therapy can be added if monotherapy with DMARD fails to control disease activity in established RA.
- DMARD therapy should be added in addition to TNF inhibitor therapy if disease activity is still high while on the monotherapy.
- In the event that methotrexate is used in conjunction with a non-TNF biologic agent but disease activity is still high after using a TNF inhibitor.
- Once anti-TNF and non-TNF agents have been tried, if disease activity is still high, try another non-TNF biologic agent before tofacitinib.
- If still uncontrolled despite the above trials, use tofacitinib.
- Low-dose glucocorticoid therapy should be added for a brief time if disease activity is still high after trying the combination therapies mentioned above.
- Patients with congestive heart failure should not take TNF inhibitors.
- Instead of TNF inhibitors, patients with hepatitis C who have not received treatment or are not receiving treatment should receive nonbiologic DMARD therapy.

10.6.7.9. Safety Considerations with Biologic and Targeted Synthetic DMARDs

- **Serious Infections:** Two to three times as many infections are linked to all biologic and targeted synthetic DMARDs. Refrain from using live vaccines, hold all agents while an infection is active, and wait for surgical procedures. It is important to check for latent tuberculosis in all patients who have opportunistic infections, such as TB and fungal infections.
- **Herpes Zoster:** JAK inhibitors.
- **Neutropenia:** IL-6 inhibitors, JAK inhibitors, rituximab.
- **Elevated LFTs, Elevated Cholesterol:** IL-6 inhibitors, JAK inhibitors.
- **Thrombosis:** JAK inhibitors.
- **CHF:** TNH inhibitors.

- **Cardiovascular Events:** JAK inhibitors (Black Box warning).
- **Demyelinating Diseases:** TNF inhibitors.

10.6.8. Staging

Stages of RA as Defined by the ACR:

- **Stage 1:** No destructive changes on X-rays
- **Stage 2:** X-ray evidence of subchondral bone destruction and periarticular osteoporosis is present, but there is no joint deformity.
- **Stage 3:** X-ray evidence shows periarticular osteoporosis, joint deformity, and destruction of bone and cartilage.
- **Stage 4:** Presence of stage 3 characteristics in addition to fibrous or bony ankylosis.

10.6.9. Prognosis

Rheumatoid arthritis is a progressive disease that increases morbidity and mortality and has no known cure. Every person will go through several exacerbations and, in the absence of treatment, generally have poor outcomes with increased mortality and disability. In terms of swollen joint count and tender joint count, early treatment (within six months of symptom onset) has demonstrated improved functional capacity and decreased disease activity. Nonetheless, patients who received treatment early on or later (after six months of symptoms) had similar mortality rates, and both groups showed a significant improvement over those who did not receive treatment. Within 10 years of receiving a diagnosis, about 40% of RA patients will experience a functional disability that limits their capacity to work and perform everyday tasks. The development of additional chronic illnesses or complications in RA patients has a significant impact on their prognosis. The association between RA and atherosclerotic cardiovascular disease, which accelerates coronary artery disease (CAD), is the most prominent example of this correlation. RA raises the risk of lung conditions, cancer, and cardiovascular disease, all of which raise the chance of early death for these patients.

10.6.10. Complications

Multiple organ systems are affected by complications of RA, which have been shown to negatively impact clinical outcomes for patients with RA. It is crucial to closely monitor patients for the development of these issues and promptly adjust treatment plans as needed. In RA patients, there is a risk of recurrent serious opportunistic infections, necessitating the temporary discontinuation of DMARD therapy until the infection is resolved. The higher incidence of infections in RA patients is believed to be attributed to both the use of DMARD therapy and the underlying immune dysfunction caused by the disease itself.

10.6.10.1. Complications and Comorbidities Associated with Uncontrolled Systemic Inflammation

- Prolonged inflammation of the joints leading to radiographic damage, progressive deformity, and functional impairment.
- Seropositive RA is known to cause Felty syndrome and anemia of chronic illness.
- Up to 10% of RA patients with pulmonary disease may develop secondary Sjögren syndrome, which is linked to the disease. Other uncommon to rare side effects include Felty's syndrome and inflammatory eye disease. Although rare, rheumatoid vasculitis can have

severe consequences if it occurs, with clinical presentation ranging from severe systemic involvement similar to polyarteritis nodosa to focal digital involvement.

- RA is also associated with bronchiolitis, interstitial lung disease, and pleuritis. Pulmonary injury is a rare adverse effect of methotrexate and anti-TNF agents used in the treatment of RA. Additionally, individuals with RA have a higher incidence of pulmonary embolism. Approximately 5%–16% of RA patients develop interstitial lung disease (ILD), which is associated with increased mortality and RA-specific autoantibodies. Some patients may exhibit ILD before experiencing joint inflammation with positive RF and ACPA. RA-associated ILD is linked to anti-carbamylated protein antibodies (anti-CarP), anti-MAA, and ACPA. The MUC5B promoter variant rs35705950, which encodes mucin 5B, is associated with ILD in RA patients. The odds ratio for RA-ILD compared to unaffected controls is 3.8 (95% CI: 2.8–5.2), and the odds ratio for RA-ILD compared to RA without ILD is 3.1 (95% CI: 1.8–5.4).
- There is a strong correlation between RA and CAD. RA serves as an independent risk factor for the development and progression of CAD. Accelerated atherosclerosis in RA patients is the primary contributor to morbidity and mortality, leading to CAD and peripheral vascular disease. Chronic inflammation is believed to be the underlying cause of the increased insulin resistance and diabetes mellitus observed in RA. Treatment with specific DMARDs, such as methotrexate, hydroxychloroquine, and TNF antagonists, significantly improves glucose control in these patients. Both conventional and biologic DMARDs are associated with a lower risk of cardiovascular events. Methotrexate, when combined with biologic agents, further reduces the risk of cardiovascular events. TNF inhibitors and abatacept appear to have the most significant impact on cardiovascular disease.
- Along with a higher incidence of non-Hodgkin lymphoma, patients with RA are also at a higher risk of developing lymphoma. These patients experience an accelerated clinical course of RA, with diffuse B-cell lymphoma frequently being the most prevalent subtype. Patients with RA are more likely to develop non-Hodgkin's lymphoma, although this condition primarily affects those whose RA is persistently active. It doesn't seem that using biologic DMARDs raises the risk of lymphoma.

10.6.10.2. Complications and Comorbidities Associated with RA Disease and Treatment

- Premature death.
- Serious infections.
- Osteopenia and osteoporosis are side effects of the underlying condition that can also be induced by medication (glucocorticoids). Patients with RA have a 60–100%

higher risk of fracture compared to the general population. The same patient characteristics that increase the risk of osteoporosis also elevate the risk of this complication in RA patients: postmenopausal status, low BMI, and advanced age.

- As previously mentioned, even after controlling for other risk factors of thromboembolic disease, patients with RA still face an increased risk of venous thromboembolic disease. Numerous studies have demonstrated that patients undergoing JAK inhibitor and TNF inhibitor therapy have an elevated risk of thromboembolic disease. However, there is no consensus regarding this association. Some research suggests that rather than being a side effect of the agents, the increased thromboembolic disease associated with their use may be a result of heightened disease activity.

10.6.10.3. Other Complications

One important complication of RA is depression. It is observed in patients with chronic active diseases and severe physical dysfunction. According to a 2013 meta-analysis, patients with RA had a prevalence of depression ranging from 17% to 39%.

10.6.11. Deterrence and Patient Education

Because of its significant genetic component, rheumatoid arthritis (RA) cannot be completely prevented. However, it is important to consider modifiable risk factors such as quitting smoking and maintaining a balanced diet. It is recommended that individuals at risk for RA follow a healthy diet, engage in regular exercise, and maintain a healthy body weight.

10.6.12. Enhancing Healthcare Team Outcomes

Rheumatoid arthritis, a chronic illness with no known cure, affects multiple organs. Therefore, comprehensive care is best provided by an interprofessional team. Patient education plays a key role and should be provided by primary care physicians, rheumatologists, nurses, and pharmacists. The nurse should inform the patient about the symptoms and indicators of various organ systems, as well as when to seek medical attention. To improve joint function, the patient should initiate an exercise regimen. Occupational therapy consultation can assist the patient in managing activities of daily living. The pharmacist should educate the patient about the various medications used to treat rheumatoid arthritis, including possible side effects. They should also monitor for drug interactions and communicate any necessary therapy modifications to the team.

Clinicians and nurses should advise patients to quit smoking, maintain a healthy weight, receive necessary immunizations, and adhere to a nutritious diet during each clinic visit. Ensuring that the patient has adequate support networks and a habitable home should be a priority for the social worker. Encouraging the patient to participate in support groups is crucial. The involvement of a mental health nurse and counselor is necessary to assist patients in coping with their disease, as many of them experience depression due to progressive disability, chronic pain, and a diminished quality of life. An all-encompassing interprofessional team can provide a multimodal approach to treating RA and improving patient outcomes. Relapses and remissions are common in RA. Some patients may have conditions that only mildly affect their quality of life, while others may have more severe conditions. Patients with multiple joint involvements, a high titer of autoantibodies, HLA-DRB1 genotypes, female gender, initial presentation with multiple joint involvements, and extra-articular involvement typically experience worse outcomes. Additionally, the medications used to treat rheumatoid arthritis often have significant side effects that are poorly tolerated. Many patients may experience adverse cardiac events that ultimately lead to death as the disease progresses. Patients with rheumatoid arthritis have an overall mortality rate three times higher than that of the general population. A comprehensive interprofessional team approach is essential in the management and monitoring of patients with RA to achieve better clinical outcomes.

A Closer Look

Living with Rheumatoid Arthritis

RA has no known cure. However, it is crucial to reduce discomfort and inflammation in order to maintain joint health. Collaborate with the healthcare provider to develop a comprehensive treatment plan that combines medication and physical therapy. Make necessary lifestyle adjustments to improve the patient's quality of life. These adjustments include:

- Balancing activity and rest. Alternate between periods of activity and rest to minimize joint stress, alleviate symptoms, and protect the joints.
- Utilizing assistive devices. Walkers, crutches, and canes can help maintain mobility and improve balance by reducing stress on specific joints.
- Using adaptive equipment. Reachers and grabbers can reduce strain and increase your reach, while dressing aids can make getting dressed easier.
- Managing medication use. Certain medications for RA carry risks. Work with the healthcare provider to develop a strategy to minimize these risks.
- Seeking support. Find a support group that can assist the patient in managing the effects of RA.

10.7. Summary

- Rickets is an ailment that afflicts the maturing youth, impacting the development of bone growth plates. Two indications of rickets are bone discomfort and leg curvature. Furthermore, it may heighten the likelihood of a child experiencing a fracture, or a broken bone. Osteomalacia is a condition that predominantly affects adults, although it can also manifest in children. It is characterized by diminished levels of bone mineral, specifically calcium and phosphate.
- The bone is comprised of a variety of cellular types. The cells that constitute bones and deposit osteoid are referred to as osteoblasts. Osteoclasts facilitate the remodeling of bone.
- Conditions that lead to hypophosphatemia and/or hypocalcemia, either independently or as a consequence of vitamin D deficiency, are among the etiologies of rickets.
- The manifestations of rickets are initially observed at the distal forearm, knee, and costochondral junctions, which are the locations of rapid bone growth.
- A patient who presents with clinical signs of rickets is assessed by obtaining their medical history, dietary habits, and history of liver or renal disease, as well as malabsorption.
- The parathyroid glands are small structures that are situated in close proximity to the thyroid glands in the neck. When one or more of these glands become excessively active, hyperparathyroidism ensues.
- In 80% of cases, primary hyperparathyroidism is caused by a solitary benign tumor known as a parathyroid adenoma. Many of these adenomas have been found to be the underlying cause of the majority of the remaining cases.
- Bones affected by osteoporosis become weakened and fragile, easily fractured from minor stresses such as coughing or bending over. The hip, wrist, or spine are the most common sites for fractures related to osteoporosis.
- The risk of developing osteoporosis can be heightened by various factors, such as advanced age, ethnicity, lifestyle choices, and medical conditions and treatments.
- The most prevalent form of arthritis, impacting millions of individuals worldwide, is osteoarthritis. It occurs as the cartilage that cushions the ends of the bones ages and loses its effectiveness. While osteoarthritis can affect any joint, the hands, knees, hips, and spine are the most frequently affected.
- Among the inflammatory forms of arthritis is rheumatoid arthritis (RA). It is a chronic ailment that can result in pain and stiffness in various joints of the body. Although it has the potential to affect any joint, it typically originates in the small joints of the hands and feet.
- Early diagnosis and initiation of treatment are imperative for RA patients in order to prevent irreversible joint damage.
- Rheumatoid arthritis is a progressive condition that has the potential to increase morbidity and mortality and currently lacks a known cure. Each individual experiences multiple exacerbations and, in the absence of treatment, generally experiences unfavorable outcomes with increased mortality and disability.

References

1. Compston, J. E., McClung, M. R., & Leslie, W. D., (2019). Osteoporosis. *Lancet, 393*(10169), 364–376. PMID: 30696576 pubmed.ncbi.nlm.nih.gov/30696576/.
2. De Paula, F. J. A., Black, D. M., & Rosen, C. J., (2020). Osteoporosis: Basic and clinical aspects; Chap 30. In: Melmed, S., Auchus, R. J., Goldfine, A. B., Loenig, R. J., et al., (eds.), *Williams Textbook of Endocrinology* (14th edn.). Philadelphia, PA: Elsevier.
3. Hollenberg, A., & Wiersinga, W. M., (2020). Hyperthyroid disorders; Chap 12. In: Melmed, S., Auchus, R. J., Goldfine, A. B., Koenig, R. J., & Rosen, C. J., (eds.), *Williams Textbook of Endocrinology* (14th edn.). Philadelphia, PA: Elsevier.
4. Kemmler, W., Bebenek, M., Kohl, M., & Von, S. S., (2015). Exercise, and fractures in postmenopausal women. Final results of the controlled Erlangen Fitness and Osteoporosis Prevention Study (EFOPS). *Osteoporos Int., 26*(10), 2491–2499. PMID: 25963237 pubmed.ncbi.nlm.nih.gov/25963237/.
5. LeBoff, M. S., Greenspan, S. L., Insogna, K. L., et al., (2022). The clinician's guide to prevention and treatment of osteoporosis. *Osteoporos Int., 33*(10), 2049–2102. PMID: 35478046 pubmed.ncbi.nlm.nih.gov/35478046/.
6. Qaseem, A., Forciea, M. A., McLean, R. M., et al., (2017). Treatment of low bone density or osteoporosis to prevent fractures in men and women: A clinical practice guideline update from the American College of Physicians. *Ann Intern Med., 166*(11), 818–839. PMID: 28492856 pubmed.ncbi.nlm.nih.gov/28492856/.
7. Thakker, R. V., (2020). The parathyroid glands, hypercalcemia, and hypocalcemia; Chap 232. In: Goldman, L., & Schafer, A. I., (eds.), *Goldman-Cecil Medicine* (26th edn.) Philadelphia, PA: Elsevier.

Chapter

MISCELLANEOUS CONDITIONS 11

Contents

11.1. Introduction

The primary constituents of bone, which is a living, growing tissue, are collagen and calcium. The skeleton, or hard framework made of bones, supports and shields the body's soft organs. In the human body, there are two kinds of bones. The outer layer of bones is made up of dense, compact cortical bones. The inner layer of bones is made up of spongy, honeycomb-shaped trabecular or cancellous bones. The bones enable movement and support the body in addition to shielding the organs from harm. Furthermore, bones serve as a storehouse for minerals like calcium. A person's bone strength and flexibility may be impacted by an illness or condition. Numerous factors, including as genetics, the environment, diet, and infections, can contribute to these conditions.

Orientation and Directional Terms

Term	Definition	Illustration
Cortical bones	Cortical (or compact) bone makes up approximately 80% of the total skeletal tissue mass. It has a high matrix mass per unit volume and low porosity.	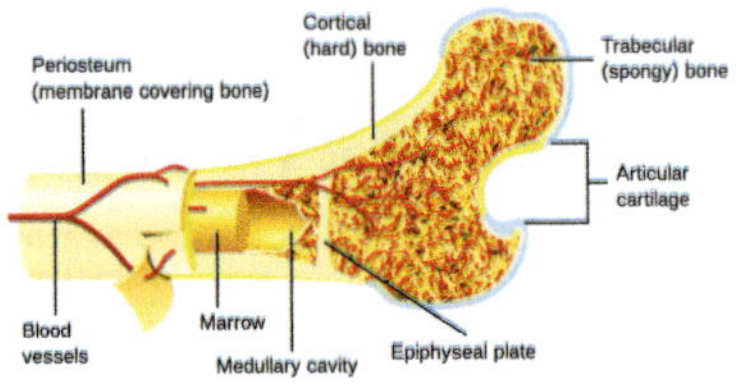
Congenital anomalies	Congenital anomalies comprise a wide range of abnormalities of body structure or function that are present at birth and are of prenatal origin.	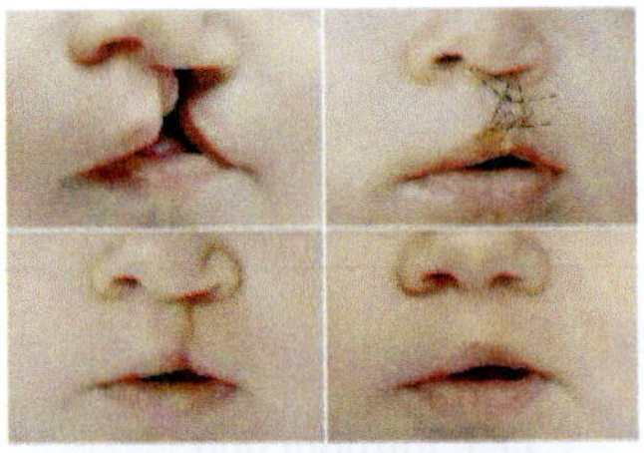
Mallet finger	Mallet finger is an injury to the thin tendon that straightens the end joint of a finger or thumb.	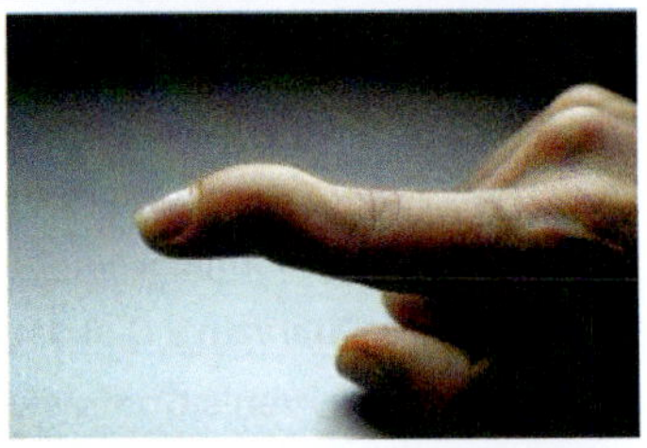
Boutonniere deformities	Boutonniere deformity describes a medical condition in which the finger is flexed at the proximal interphalangeal joint (PIP), and there is hyperextension at the distal interphalangeal joint (DIP).	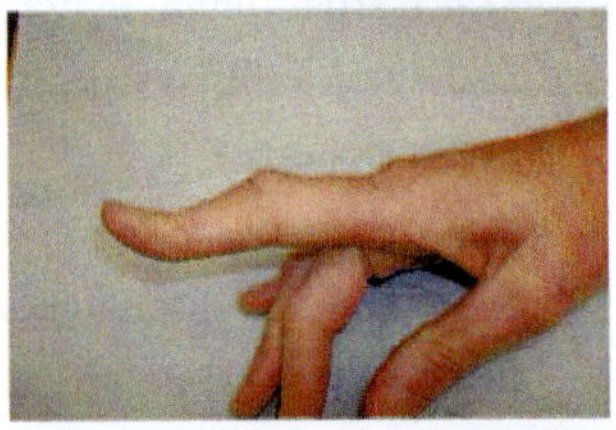
Inflammatory arthritides	Inflammatory arthritis includes a group of arthritis accompanied by joint pain, swelling, warmth, tenderness in the joints, and morning stiffness that lasts for an hour.	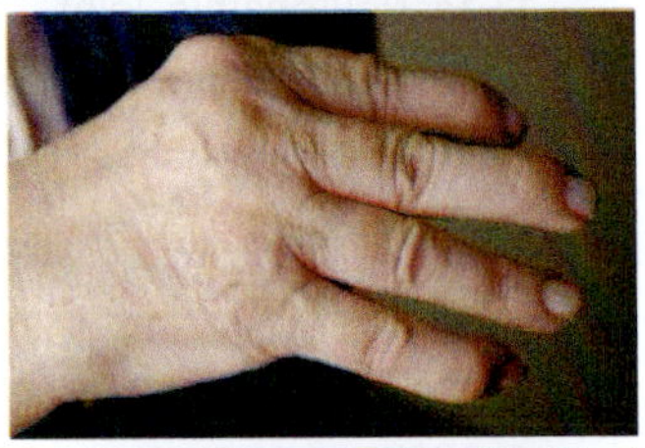
Microtrauma	Microtrauma refers to any of the numerous potential minor injuries to the body. During microtrauma, muscle fibers may experience microtears.	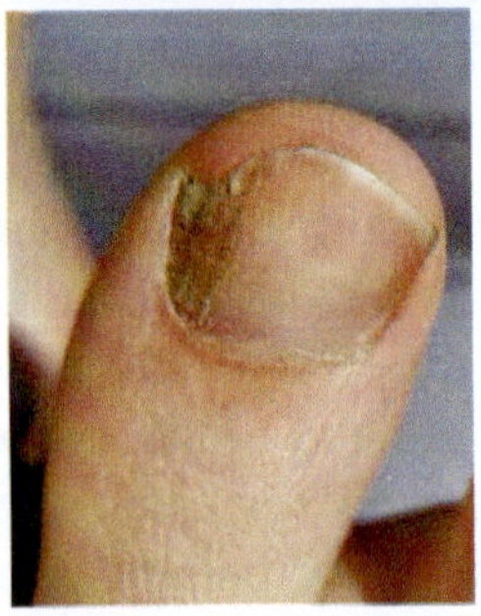

11.2. Congenital and Developmental Anomalies

Anomalies of a structural or functional nature that develop during intrauterine life are referred to as congenital disorders. These conditions, which are also known as birth defects, congenital anomalies, or congenital malformations, develop during pregnancy and can be detected prior to, during, or after birth. There are hundreds of thousands of deaths linked to congenital disorders, which affect an estimated 6% of babies born worldwide. Stillbirths and aborted pregnancies are not frequently included in statistics, so the actual number of cases may be much higher. Treatment options for certain congenital disorders, like clubfoot, hernias, and cleft lip and palate, include both surgical and non-surgical procedures. Some can have long-lasting effects, such as Down syndrome, heart defects, and neural tube defects. One of the primary causes of the worldwide disease burden is congenital disorders, which disproportionately affect low- and middle-income nations. Additionally, there are fewer facilities in these areas to treat conditions like clubfoot, which can have more severe and enduring effects.

11.2.1. Types of Congenital Anomalies

There are two main categories of congenital anomalies.

- **Structural Congenital Anomalies:** An issue pertaining to the structure of body parts is associated with structural congenital anomalies. These might consist of:
  - Cleft lip or cleft palate;
  - Heart defects, such as missing or misshaped valves;
  - Atypical limbs, such as a clubfoot;
  - Abnormalities of the growth and development of the brain and spinal cord, as well as neural tube defects like spina bifida.
- **Functional or Developmental Congenital Anomalies:** Congenital abnormalities that are developmental or functional are associated with issues related to the normal operation of a bodily system or part. These issues may consist of:
  - **Nervous System or Brain Problems:** These include behavioral issues, speech or language difficulties, movement issues, seizures, and intellectual and developmental disabilities. The neurological system can be affected by congenital abnormalities such as Down syndrome, Prader-Willi syndrome, and Fragile X syndrome.
  - **Sensory Problems:** Examples include visual issues like blindness or deafness and hearing loss.
  - **Metabolic Disorders:** These include conditions that impair the body's capacity to eliminate waste products or dangerous chemicals, as well as issues with specific chemical reactions that occur within the body. The two most prevalent metabolic conditions are hypothyroidism and phenylketonuria.
  - **Degenerative Disorders:** These are conditions that cause one or more aspects of health to gradually deteriorate, even though they may not be

evident at birth. Degenerative disorders include muscular dystrophy and X-linked adrenoleukodystrophy, the latter of which was the subject of the film "Lorenzo's Oil" and causes issues with the nervous system and adrenal glands.

Some congenital anomalies cause issues with multiple body systems or functions, resulting in both structural and functional issues.

11.2.2. Causes

It is estimated that about half of congenital disorders have no known cause. Nevertheless, chromosomal abnormalities, environmental teratogens, multifactorial inheritance, single gene defects, and micronutrient deficiencies are among the known causes.

Genetic causes can be linked to mutations or inherited genes. Being consanguineous, or having blood ties to one's parents, raises the likelihood of congenital defects and almost doubles the risk of early childhood and neonatal mortality, intellectual disability, and other illnesses. An additional factor raising the likelihood of chromosomal abnormalities, such as Down syndrome, is advanced maternal age.

Congenital disorders are known to become more common as a result of certain diseases, such as the Zika virus, syphilis, and rubella. Certain anomalies, like hemophilia C and cystic fibrosis, are more common in particular ethnic groups.

Nearly all congenital disorders—94%—occur in low- and middle-income nations. Potential reasons encompass inadequate screening and prenatal care, inadequate availability of nutrient-dense foods for expectant mothers, alcohol or tobacco use or contact, and heightened susceptibility to infections or environmental pollutants.

Among other things, screening, immunization, fortifying staple foods with nutrients like iodine and folic acid, and receiving proper prenatal care can all help prevent some congenital disorders.

11.2.3. Prevention

Preventive public health initiatives aim to reduce the prevalence of specific congenital disorders by eliminating risk factors and enhancing protective factors. Key interventions and strategies include:

- Ensuring that teenage girls and mothers maintain a healthy weight and consume a balanced diet that includes a variety of fruits and vegetables.
- Ensuring that mothers and teenage girls receive sufficient vitamins and minerals from their diet, particularly folic acid.
- Encouraging mothers to abstain from dangerous substances, particularly alcohol and tobacco.
- Advising pregnant women (and occasionally women of childbearing age) to avoid traveling to areas where infections known to be linked to congenital disorders are on the rise.
- Minimizing or eliminating pregnant women's exposure to harmful substances in the environment, such as heavy metals or pesticides.
- Managing diabetes before and during pregnancy through diet, exercise, counseling, and the use of insulin when necessary.
- Ensuring that any medication or medical radiation exposure, such as that from imaging scans, for

expectant mothers is appropriate and supported by a thorough evaluation of the risks and benefits to their health.

- Immunization, particularly for children and women, is crucial for protection against the rubella virus.
- Expanding and improving the education provided to medical professionals and other stakeholders who support the prevention of congenital disorders; and.
- Examination for infections, particularly syphilis, varicella, and rubella, as well as treatment consideration.

11.2.4. Screening, Treatment, and Care

11.2.4.1. Screening

Preconception and periconceptional care encompasses medical genetic screening and counseling in addition to standard reproductive health practices. The three time slots indicated above are suitable for screening.

- **Preconception Screening:** This can help determine who is more likely to develop a particular disorder or to pass that disorder on to their offspring. In nations where consanguineous marriage is prevalent, screening—which includes obtaining family histories and carrier screening—is especially important.
- **Peri-Conception Screening:** Screening results should be used to determine the appropriate course of care based on the individual's risk, as maternal characteristics may increase it. In addition to checking for alcohol or tobacco use or other risks, this may involve screening for young or elderly mothers. When screening for severe fetal anomalies in the second trimester, ultrasound can be used to check for Down syndrome and significant structural abnormalities. Screening of maternal blood can be done for many chromosomal abnormalities using free fetal DNA, or for placental markers to help predict the risk of chromosomal abnormalities or neural tube defects. For women who are at high risk for infections and chromosomal abnormalities, diagnostic procedures like amniocentesis and chorionic villus sampling can be administered.
- **Neonatal Screening:** Newborn screening is a crucial first step in the detection process. Enabling early referral and the start of medical or surgical treatment lowers the death and morbidity rate from congenital disorders.

Early detection of hearing loss offers the chance for early intervention as well as improved speech, language, and communication abilities. Early congenital cataract screening in infants increases the chance of sight by facilitating early referral and surgical correction.

Certain metabolic, hematologic, and endocrine disorders—many of which may not have symptoms right away—may be checked for in newborns. The conditions that are screened for differ depending on the cost and prevalence of each country. Even in low- and middle-income nations, newborn screening is becoming more and more common.

11.2.4.2. Treatment and Care

Some congenital disorders can be effectively managed through medical or surgical treatments. However, access to such interventions can vary depending on the country and the level of the healthcare system. Fortunately, advanced care is now more accessible in low- and middle-income countries. Surgery, accompanied by proper follow-up care, can greatly reduce the risk of death (such as in the case of congenital heart defects) or complications (such as with conditions like congenital talipes or cleft lip/palate) associated with structural congenital disorders. Unfortunately, the importance of this aspect of treatment in decreasing mortality and morbidity is often underestimated. Early detection through screening, referral, and management at specialized centers, particularly for issues like cardiac defects, is crucial in improving outcomes for individuals with congenital disorders at all levels of the healthcare system.

The quality of life can be enhanced by medical treatment for specific endocrine, hematological, and metabolic disorders. Congenital hypothyroidism is a prime example, where prompt diagnosis and treatment enable full physical and mental development to healthy adulthood, while a delayed diagnosis or lack of access to a straightforward treatment increases the risk of severe intellectual disability. Certain congenital disorders may necessitate long-term care for children, including speech, occupational, and physical therapy, as well as community and family support.

11.2.5. Impact

An estimated 2,95,000 newborns worldwide pass away before turning 4 weeks old every year as a result of congenital conditions and related complications. Health issues and disabilities that last a lifetime can result from congenital abnormalities. With timely surgery or other treatment, more than half of the disability-adjusted life years (DALYs) lost annually as a result of congenital disorders could be avoided. For instance, clubfoot affects 1,00,000 newborns annually, a condition that is easily treated. However, if left untreated, this illness can result in severe and irreversible disability. Social stigma and discrimination are common outcomes of congenital disorders, and they can cause embarrassment, isolation, and other reductions in community interaction. These illnesses also come at a high financial cost; long-term disability has a big effect on people's lives, families, healthcare systems, and communities. These effects are greater in low- and middle-income nations where it may be more difficult to live with an impairment due to a lack of accessibility and availability of support services.

11.3. Mallet Finger

Mallet finger is an injury to the tendon that straightens the tip of the finger (or thumb). It is also referred to as drop finger or baseball finger.

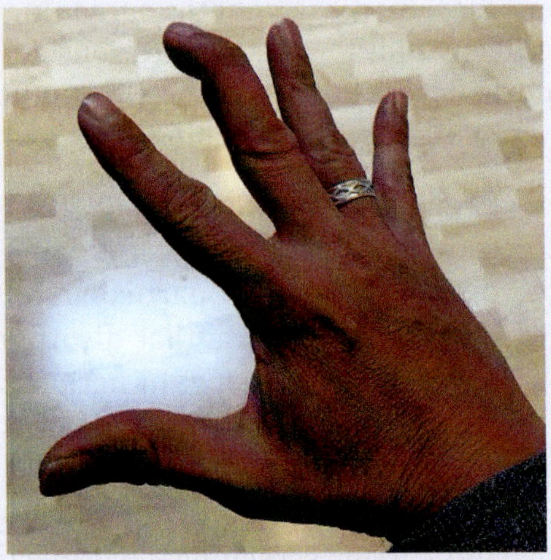

Figure 11.1. *Mallet finger of the middle finger. The tip of the finger bends downwards while the other fingers stay straight.*

Source: By Clappstar – Own work, CC BY-SA 4.0, https://commons.wikimedia.org/w/index.php?curid=66805162.

Tendons provide stability and motion by connecting the muscles to the bones. The tendon may tear or detach from the finger bone due to an injury. It is possible to injure both the tendon and the finger bone simultaneously. Symptoms of mallet finger include pain, drooping at the tip, difficulty in extending the finger, and a bruised or swollen appearance (Figure 11.1). In sports such as baseball, basketball, or football, mallet finger is a common injury that occurs when attempting to catch a hard ball, resulting in impact on the extended fingertip. Typically, the injury affects a finger on the dominant hand.

11.3.1. Etiology

Ruptures of the distal extensor tendon occur in mallet finger injuries. The rupture occurs when the distal phalanx of a finger is forced into flexion while being actively extended, for example in ball sports, if a ball hits the fingertip of an extended finger.

- The extrinsic extensor tendon originates in the forearm, passes over the metacarpophalangeal joint, and then attaches to the distal phalanx via an indirect attachment to the proximal phalanx. These tendons enable the digits to extend.
- An interruption of the extensor tendon results in a mallet finger injury. When a distal phalanx avulsion fracture is caused by a tendon injury, it is referred to as a mallet fracture.
- Nonoperative treatments are supported by the available data, but prompt treatment is necessary to prevent unfavorable outcomes.

11.3.2. Epidemiology

Mallet finger injuries and other injuries involving the terminal extensor tendon are common. Terminal extensor tendon injuries account for 5.6% of hand and wrist injuries.

Mallet finger injuries have the following characteristics:

- Typically occur at work or during sporting events.
- Are frequently seen in males between the ages of five and thirty, and occasionally in older women. The average age of men who sustain finger injuries from mallets is 34 years, while women have an average age of 41.
- Are more common in ball sports when the ball hits an extended fingertip, causing the extensor tendon to be disrupted and forcing the distal interphalangeal joint (DIP) into a flexed position.
- Lower impact injuries, such as an elderly person jamming their finger while performing daily tasks like tucking in bedsheets or pulling up socks, can also result in terminal extensor tendon injuries.
- The most commonly affected fingers are usually the middle or long finger, as well as the ring finger of the dominant hand.

11.3.3. Causes

An injury to the extensor tendon, which straightens the DIP just before the fingernail, is the underlying cause of this condition. There are two types of mallet fingers. The first type is a tendon rupture, which is an injury to the extensor tendon itself. This can occur suddenly from cutting or jamming the finger, or it can develop gradually due to arthritis progressively stretching the tendon. The second type is a fracture at the insertion point of the extensor tendon, which prevents the tendon from exerting force on the entire bone. While the tendon remains intact, the bone to which it is attached fractures. In children, the fracture may occur at the growth plate of the distal phalanx.

Mallet fingers can be caused by an object, such as a ball, striking the fingertip or thumb. The impact can result in a mallet finger with either a fractured bone or a ruptured tendon. Due to its frequent occurrence when catching a baseball without gloves, this condition is sometimes referred to as "baseball finger." Excessive bending of the small joint during use, such as when lifting heavy objects that put pressure on the joint, can also lead to this condition. Occasionally, even a small amount of force applied at an incorrect angle can cause a tendon to rupture. Examples include scrubbing dishes vigorously or accidentally knocking something over while putting clothes in a drawer.

A deep cut on the back of the finger from a knife or other sharp object can also cause a mallet finger. This incision has the potential to penetrate the bone and split the extensor tendon from the bone.

11.3.4. Signs and Symptoms

The fingertip of a mallet finger droops and is incapable of straightening on its own. Initially, it often appears to be just a "jammed finger." The finger might hurt, swell, or become bruised. On the back of the finger, there may be a bump that is visible just below the nail. Blood may accumulate under the nail, and the nail itself may split at the base. This most commonly occurs in mallet fingers with broken bones. An "open" mallet finger begins with a sharp cut or laceration that penetrates the tendon and reaches the bone, affecting the last joint of the finger. Some individuals may occasionally exhibit mild drooping of the last joint in all of their fingers. This is not caused by injuries, but rather by the pliability or looseness of their tissues.

11.3.5. Treatment

11.3.5.1. Diagnosis

Medical attention should be sought within the first few days following the injury, particularly if there is blood under the nail or if the nail is broken off at the base. This could indicate an open (compound) fracture or a nail bed injury. Even slight bruising or swelling in an injury could indicate a fracture. Images from an ultrasound or X-ray can be used to determine whether the finger deformity is the result of a fracture. If there are numerous fracture fragments, CT scans might be prescribed. Only the bone's tip at the attachment site may be fractured. However, occasionally the fracture affects the joint's structural integrity. Children may have a fracture in the growing portion of the bone. These wounds have the potential to cause long-term infection or abnormal distal phalanx growth. Mallet fingers with exposed bone or a cut tendon need to be treated immediately to prevent infection (Figure 11.2).

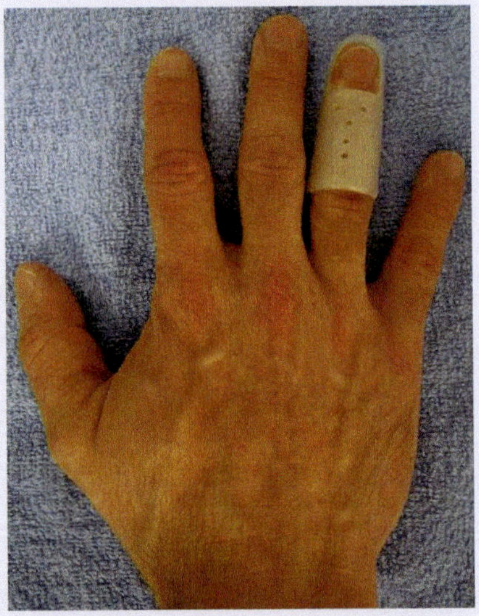

Figure 11.2. *An example of a splint for mallet finger.*

Source: By James Heilman, MD – Own work, CC BY-SA 3.0, https://commons.wikimedia.org/w/index.php?curid=12789324.

A mallet finger can cause pain and functional impairment if not promptly treated. Persistent pain and recurrent injuries are often attributed to joint issues, which can result from a misaligned joint fracture. Gradual development of arthritis is also possible. Proper alignment of bone fragments allows new bone growth to fill the gap, resulting in a persistent droop. However, this condition may not cause pain and only become problematic during specific activities.

11.3.5.2. Nonsurgical Treatment

In many cases, nonsurgical treatment is sufficient for mallet finger injuries. Non-removable finger splinting can be used as a comprehensive treatment until the tendon heals or the fracture is sealed by bone. If there is no cut or laceration, applying ice can help reduce swelling. Elevating the hand with fingers pointing upward is also recommended. To temporarily immobilize the finger, tape the bottom or top of the finger across the joint using a tongue depressor or a clean popsicle stick. The tape should be loose enough to allow proper blood flow and sensation to the fingertip. There are various options for mallet finger splints and casts that provide effective and comfortable support for all activities during the healing process, which can take weeks or months depending on the diagnosis and subsided swelling. It is important to keep the finger straight until the small joint is fully healed. This is the typical course of action when a tendon ruptures due to a jam. A splint is usually worn continuously for approximately eight weeks. Even a brief flexion of the joint after removing the splint can impede healing and prolong the recovery period. It is crucial to keep the skin dry under the splint. After the tendon or bone has healed, the splint is worn only during sleep and physical activity for a few more weeks or months to prevent re-injury.

The patient's desire for the injury to be merely a sprain may result in a delay in the commencement of treatment. Despite potentially less satisfactory outcomes, splinting can still be effective if initiated several weeks after the injury. The hand therapist or surgeon will provide the patient with instructions on how to properly wear the splint. They will also demonstrate exercises that will allow to maintain movement in the middle joint while keeping the end joint immobile. Once the mallet finger has healed, the surgeon or hand therapist will teach exercises for the small end joint, which tends to become extremely stiff from the splinting. With this treatment, the finger typically regains its normal appearance and function, although it may have a slight droop, be bumpy, or have a permanently different shape.

11.3.5.3. Surgical Treatment

If there is a significant bone fragment or misalignment of the joint following a mallet finger injury, surgery may be necessary. In such cases, joint realignment can be achieved using wires or tiny screws. Surgery may also be considered if using a splint is challenging or has not been successful in the past. Surgical options may involve fusing the joint to maintain straightness, suturing the tendon together or creating a new tendon, or inserting a wire into the finger to keep it straight. The hand surgeon will recommend the most appropriate course of action tailored to the specific situation.

11.3.6. Complications

After nonsurgical or surgical treatment of mallet fractures, the following complications may arise:

- Residual extensor lag (observed during physical examination).
- Swan neck deformities (characterized by hyperextension of the proximal interphalangeal joint and abnormal flexion of the DIP due to disruption of the volar plate

caused by the disrupted extensor tendon).

11.4. Boutonniere Deformity

A medical condition known as boutonnière deformity causes the finger to be hyperextended at the DIP and flexed at the proximal interphalangeal joint (PIP). This is typically brought on by acute trauma and results from a rupture of the PIP central slip. The impacted digit's extensor function is harmed as a result. An additional cause of a boutonniere deformity is laceration injuries to the dorsal capsule and central slip. In addition, burn injuries can result in boutonniere deformities. Tension ischemia may be the cause of tendon rupture. In general, boutonniere deformities are often associated with inflammatory arthritis, including rheumatoid arthritis (Figure 11.3).

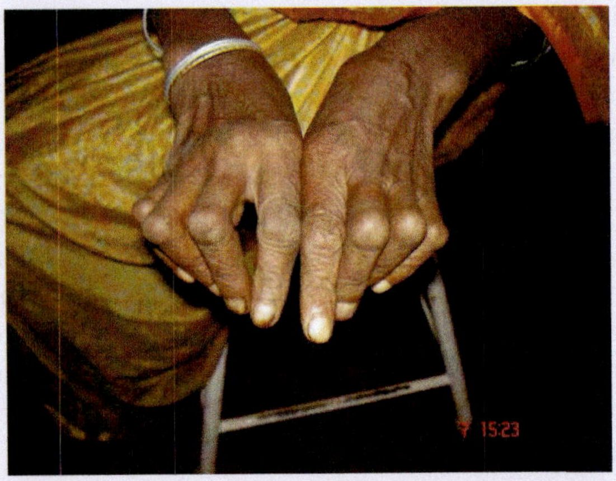

Figure 11.3. *Hand deformity in a patient with rheumatoid arthritis showing boutonniere deformity.*

Source: By Prashanthns – Own work, CC BY-SA 3.0, https://commons.wikimedia.org/w/index.php?curid=9567754.

11.4.1. Etiology

The primary cause of this PIP joint flexion deformity is injury to the extensor tendon. The lateral aspects of the tendon split off, causing disruption to the extensor tendon. The proximal phalanx's head then pokes through the damaged tendon elements. This deformity got its name, most likely because, during surgical exploration, it resembled a buttonhole. Sports-related boutonniere deformities are most frequently caused by injuries sustained in basketball and football.

11.4.2. Epidemiology

Although jam-injuries are a diverse group of trauma-related injuries, one well-known consequence of jam-injuries is the development of boutonniere deformities as a result of central slip injuries. A boutonniere deformity affects at least one digit in up to half or 50% of rheumatoid arthritis patients.

11.4.3. Pathophysiology

A digit's central slip of the extensor tendon and the triangle ligament are damaged, leading to a boutonniere deformity. The lateral bands will voluntarily displace as a result of this ligament and tendon disruption. As a result, the finger is forced to flex, which limits the range of motion of the dip joint. The oblique retinacular ligament progressively contracts over time. The ligament contracture will progressively exacerbate the joint's hyperextension deformity. If burn damage or rheumatoid arthritis (RA) is the secondary cause, the pathophysiology is different. Inflammatory cells gather in the joint's synovial fluid when an inflammatory arthritide, like RA, is present, forming a layer of fibrous tissue. This causes injury to ligaments and cartilage as well as erosion of the bone. Pain and loss of function are caused by the joints' gradual deformation.

11.4.4. History and Physical Details

The mechanism of injury to the affected digit should be ascertained by obtaining a comprehensive history and physical examination.

Depending on the cause of the injury, there are different treatment options. Early detection of the injury can help to avoid long-term problems and deformities from these injuries. The onset of a deformity may take several weeks. A deformity can take several weeks to manifest. In the setting of a laceration injury, the area needs to be thoroughly cleaned and examined in a "bloodless field" for tendon integrity. Frequently, a central slip injury is occult in the context of jam injuries. The Elson test, which includes the following steps, can be used to evaluate tendon integrity:

- The injured finger is placed over the edge of a table or other surface by the patient. At the level of the PIP joint, the fingers are flexed along the surface edge.
- At the level of the middle phalanx, the examiner applies pressure to the digit.
- The patient is told to spread their finger at the PIP joint (against the pressure vector).
- When the DIP is observed to hyperextend at the DIP joint, the test is deemed positive.

If boutonniere deformity is caused by rheumatoid arthritis, a complete medical history should be obtained, encompassing the length of symptoms, medications taken in the past and present, pain threshold, and extent of disability.

11.4.5. Evaluation

It is recommended to obtain radiographs to assess for any associated fractures. It is crucial to identify any cortical disruption of the bones that articulate with the central slip of the tendon. Lateral radiographs can be used to evaluate the degree of hyperextension.

11.4.6. Treatment/Management

The goal of treatment is to restore full range of motion to the affected finger. Both nonsurgical and surgical treatment options are available. Nonsurgical treatment, such as splinting, involves immobilizing the affected joint to allow for flexion or extension of the proximal interphalangeal (PIP) joint. This immobilization facilitates tendon healing and prevents spontaneous separation. Splints are typically worn for three to six weeks, depending on the severity of the injury and the patient's age. Patients are often advised to continue wearing the splint at night for a few additional weeks. Exercises to improve strength and flexibility of the affected digit should also be incorporated into the management plan. In cases where the injury occurred during sports participation, the injured area may require additional splinting or taping for protection upon resuming activity. Surgical correction may be necessary if there is significant displacement of a bone fragment or if the tendon is completely severed. This option may also be considered if conservative measures, such as splinting, do not yield satisfactory results. Surgical correction of extensor injuries typically involves the use of wires or screws for large avulsions. Delayed treatment beyond three weeks can make correction more challenging.

The treatment options for a boutonniere deformity, if it is a long-term side effect of rheumatoid arthritis, include glucocorticoids, biologic response modifiers, disease-modifying anti-rheumatic drugs (DMARDs), nonsteroidal anti-inflammatory drugs (NSAIDs), and analgesics. DMARDs are used to slow the progression of rheumatoid arthritis and are often used in combination therapy. Although they have different mechanisms of action, DMARDs function similarly in affecting the disease process. Biologic response modifiers, which are genetically altered, obstruct immune system signals that cause tissue damage, with many of these drugs targeting the function of tumor necrosis factor. Glucocorticoids are anti-inflammatory and anti-autoimmune drugs that are frequently used in conjunction with DMARDs. NSAIDs do not slow down the disease progression but can help manage pain, swelling, and inflammation. Analgesics are solely used for pain management.

If nonsurgical treatments are ineffective, joint replacement surgery may be necessary. Another surgical technique is joint fusion, which involves joining the joint surfaces of the affected digits. Joint fusion offers the benefits of reducing pain, improving joint stability, and halting the progression of joint deformity. Patients are advised to keep the proximal interphalangeal joint straight for several weeks after surgery by wearing a brace or splint. Physical or occupational therapy is often required after bracing.

11.4.7. Differential Diagnosis

This entails the following aspects:

- The PIP joint is dislocated. The traditional cause of this is trauma, and the deformity is often more noticeable.
- Burn injuries can result in skin contracture at the proximal finger.
- Less common causes of contractures include epidermolysis bullosa, Hansen's disease, and other illnesses.

11.4.8. Prognosis

The primary goal of successful treatment outcomes is to prevent the development of a boutonniere deformity. Serial digital casting has proven to be a reasonably effective method. Complete recovery in terms of range of motion is rare and depends on the severity of the injury.

11.4.9. Complications

Complications with or without treatment include:

- Chronic joint stiffness;
- Reinjury/redislocation;
- Post-traumatic arthritis;
- Chronic swelling;
- Decreased range of motion.

11.4.10. Deterrence and Patient Education

As patients rarely return to their baseline functionality and prognoses and outcomes often vary, the doctor plays a crucial role in managing expectations. Patients should be informed about various consequences, including early arthritis, limited chronic range of motion, and a tendency to re-injure themselves. When a patient experiences a jammed finger, a doctor specializing in treating athletes, especially those prone to finger injuries like football and basketball players, should advise them to seek medical attention as soon as possible. It is important to inform patients that delaying treatment may have long-term effects that could prevent them from participating in sports in the future.

11.4.11. Enhancing Healthcare Team Outcomes

For the complex diagnosis and treatment of boutonniere deformity, an interdisciplinary team consisting of a primary care physician, nurse practitioner, physical therapist, orthopedic surgeon, and hand surgeon is necessary. The goal of treatment is to regain full range of motion in the affected finger. Both surgical and nonsurgical options are available for treatment. If nonsurgical treatments are ineffective, surgical joint replacement may be required. Another surgical procedure, known as joint fusion, involves joining the joint surfaces of the two affected digits. Joint fusion offers three advantages: it reduces pain, improves joint stability, and prevents further joint deformity. Following surgery, patients are advised to wear a brace or splint for a few weeks to keep the proximal interphalangeal joint straight. Splinting is often followed by physical or occupational therapy. In the case of boutonniere deformity, the results are confidential. While recovery is possible, improved range of motion and function may not occur quickly.

11.5. Trigger Finger/Thumb

A disorder known as trigger finger affects the tendons that flex the fingers and thumb. When this happens, the fingers usually feel as though they are locking or catching when the person bend and straighten them. Additional symptoms could be thumb and finger pain and stiffness. Another name for the illness is stenosing tenosynovitis. The thumb and ring finger are the most frequently impacted fingers, though any digit may be impacted. Trigger thumb is the appropriate term for the condition when it affects the thumb (Figure 11.4).

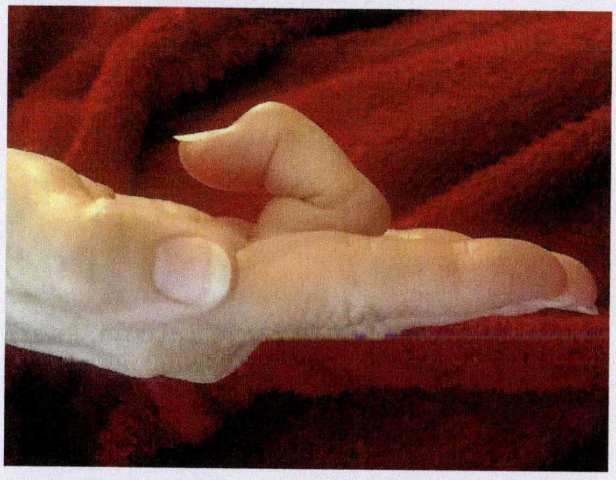

Figure 11.4. *Side view of trigger finger in the right middle finger.*

Source: By RCraig09 – Own work, CC BY-SA 4.0, https://commons.wikimedia.org/w/index.php?curid=131823404.

11.5.1. Etiology

Trigger finger has a multifactorial etiology. Adult patients with trigger finger have been linked to certain comorbid conditions, such as diabetes, rheumatoid arthritis, CTS, amyloidosis, gout, and thyroid disease. Traumatic forces cause the tendon and its sheath to hypertrophy and narrow, making it difficult for the tendon to move freely within the sheath. As a result, locking and catching occur. The etiology in children seems to be developmental, with the thumb's flexor tendon and tendon sheath not being the right size. The size of the tendon and the A1 pulley sheath differ as a result of the proliferation of fibroblasts. Even though idiopathic causes account for most cases at this age, congenital metabolic (e.g., Hurler syndrome) as well as inflammatory diseases (e.g., rheumatoid arthritis in children).

11.5.2. Epidemiology

The incidence of trigger finger is bimodal, peaking before the age of eight years and again in patients in their 40s and 50s. In general, adults are more likely to have trigger fingers. Trigger finger is most common in the thumb and equally affects boys and girls in childhood. Trigger finger affects women far more frequently in adulthood, and usually affects their dominant hand.

11.5.3. Pathophysiology

Microtrauma causes the flexor tendon-sheath complex to become inflamed and injured, whether it is caused by compression forces or repetitive use.

The A1 pulley experiences the most force and is therefore the one that is impacted the most frequently. Over time, inflammation causes the tendon to stick inside its sheath, giving the patient the impression that the tendon is locking. Patients typically have no trouble flexing their fingers because the flexor tendon apparatus is stronger than the extensor tendon apparatus.

When a patient tries to extend their fingers, they will experience locking because the inflammation causes the flexor tendon to become trapped in the flexor sheath.

11.5.4. Histopathology

This disease presents with a clinical diagnosis. However, histopathology has revealed the coexistence of hypertrophy, inflammation, and fibro-cartilaginous metaplasia at the tendon-pulley interface.

11.5.5. History and Physical Details

Patients commonly experience discomfort or limited function in the affected digit. Some may notice increasing discomfort on the palmar side of the digit when flexing it, accompanied by swelling or the presence of a lump. A painful clicking sensation is often reported. In certain cases, patients may have difficulty straightening the finger or moving it from a bent position. Symptoms can manifest gradually or suddenly. Patients may also experience stiffness or pain in the dominant hand if the trigger finger affects their ability to work. During a physical examination, a tender lump may be palpated at the distal end of the palmar crease. The affected digit may be flexed and exhibit limited smooth movement, causing pain and snapping sensations when attempting to extend it.

11.5.6. Evaluation

Trigger finger is clinically diagnosed when a patient's finger locks during flexion, clicks painfully, and catches upon extension. It is also suspected when there is an inflammatory nodule at the base of the affected finger. Ultrasound can be utilized to evaluate this condition. It can reveal inflammation and irregularities in the underlying flexor tendon, as well as thickening of the pulley. However, it may not reliably predict the exact location. Dynamic ultrasound can be employed to demonstrate the catching and clicking that occurs during tendon sliding. Simple radiographs can be used to rule out other conditions, such as an occult fracture. CT and MRI scans are generally not necessary.

11.5.7. Treatment/Management

The two classes of trigger finger management are as follows:

- **Non-Surgical:** Trigger finger is typically treated nonoperatively, especially if it is uncomplicated and symptoms have only been present for a short period of time. This treatment approach often involves steroid injections and the use of splints.
  - **Steroid Injection:** These are frequently an effective initial line of treatment for individuals with trigger finger. Compared to surgery, it is a less invasive, less expensive, and simpler approach.
    The efficacy of steroid administration depends on its delivery into the tendon sheath. Although recurrence of symptoms is possible, many patients may find relief with a steroid injection. Infections, skin discolorations, hypopigmentation, and tissue atrophy can be potential side effects of steroid injections. Prolonged symptom sufferers have a lower chance of recovery.
  - **Splinting:** It is based on the concept of reducing inflammation, which restricts tendon gliding. A MCP blocking splint is used, with the finger

positioned at 10° to 15° of flexion for 6 to 10 weeks. However, individuals with severe or prolonged symptoms are unlikely to benefit from this approach.

- **Surgical:** The gold standard for surgically treating trigger finger is an open release of the A1 pulley. Surgical intervention should be considered when necessary.
  - Splinting and/or injection therapy did not result in any improvement.
  - Irreducibly locked trigger finger.
  - Childhood trigger thumb: it is thought that if the deformity is not surgically released at this age, infants may develop a fixed flexion deformity of the interphalangeal (IP) joint. The results of conservative treatment for trigger finger in children are unpredictable because the condition can have more varied causes than just a thicker A1 pulley (Figure 11.5).

Performing a percutaneous release of the A1 pulley can be considered as a different approach to managing the condition. However, it is important to have a thorough understanding of specific landmarks before attempting this technique. While studies have shown that the percutaneous method is effective and safe for treating the thumb, some healthcare providers advise against using it due to the risk of damaging the digital nerves that run over the A1 pulley. Potential issues include incomplete release of the pulley and harm to the flexor tendons and digital nerves.

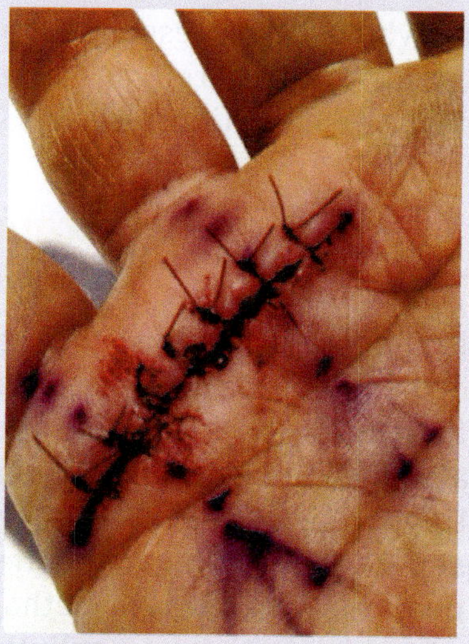

Figure 11.5. *Post-operative photo of trigger finger release surgery in a diabetic patient.*

Source: By Jonathan Eisen – https://plus.google.com/103101121348859087349/posts/V492nruyUTK, CC BY-SA 3.0, https://commons.wikimedia.org/w/index.php?curid=26134710.

11.5.8. Differential Diagnosis

- Abnormal sesamoids;
- Acromegaly;
- Ganglion cyst on the wrist;
- Ganglion involving the tendon sheath;
- Infection within the tendon sheaths;
- Presence of loose body in MCP joint;
- Subluxation of extensor digitorum communis.

11.5.9. Prognosis

Treatment improves the prognosis. The majority of patients respond well to corticosteroid injections. When the underlying ailment is treated, a small percentage of cases resolve on their own. However, it may take months to fully recover, even with steroid injections. Patients with diabetes often require surgery as they respond less favorably to corticosteroids.

For patients who have not responded to steroid injections, trigger finger release surgery is a viable and successful option.

11.5.10. Enhancing Healthcare Team Outcomes

An interdisciplinary team consisting of a hand surgeon, orthopedic surgeon, plastic surgeon, nurse practitioner, physical therapist, and primary care physician is optimal for diagnosing and treating trigger finger. Trigger finger is diagnosed clinically. The initial treatment typically involves non-surgical methods such as corticosteroid injections or splinting. It is important to inform patients that they may experience significant pain for a few days following a steroid injection. After receiving a steroid injection, patients should be advised to avoid strenuous activity for a few weeks to reduce the risk of tendon rupture.

When non-surgical treatments prove to be ineffective, surgical intervention is recommended. However, it is important to note that surgery is not always successful and complications can arise. Additionally, surgery may not be suitable for treating trigger finger. Therefore, it is crucial to educate the patient about non-surgical techniques before considering surgery. It is common to encounter damage to the digital nerves and incomplete release with the surgical approach. Open communication among team members is essential in providing the patient with realistic expectations, which ultimately enhances satisfaction with the treatment.

11.6. De Quervain's Disease

De Quervain's Disease, also known as de Quervain's tendinosis or de Quervain's tendinitis, is characterized by painful inflammation of the thumb tendons. Healthcare professionals may use either of these names to refer to the same condition. Tendons are strong and flexible tissues that connect muscles to bones, resembling ropes. They enable the movement of bones when muscles contract or are squeezed. The thumb and wrist are connected by two tendons, which normally pass through a sheath, a tissue tunnel, with ease. However, when the sheath surrounding the thumb tendons becomes swollen or thickened, it can lead to De Quervain's tenosynovitis.

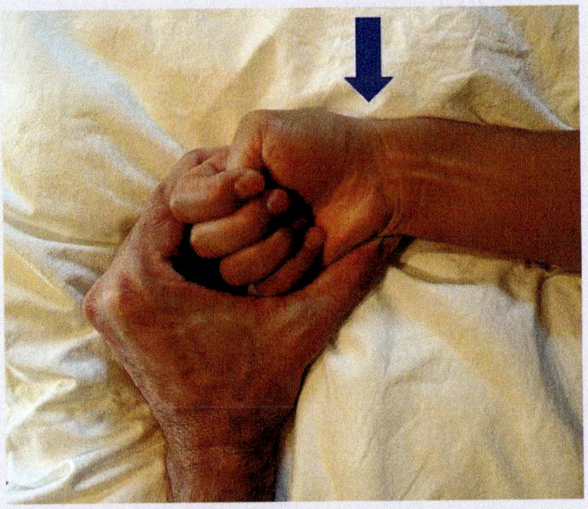

Figure 11.6. *The modified Eichoff maneuver, commonly referred to as the Finkelstein's test. The arrow mark indicates where the pain is worsened in de Quervain syndrome.*

Source: By James Heilman, MD – Own work, CC BY-SA 4.0, https://commons.wikimedia.org/w/index.php?curid=70126883.

This swelling causes increased friction when using the thumb and wrist, resulting in pain and difficulty with certain motions. Individuals with De Quervain's tenosynovitis often experience radiating pain in the forearm near the base of the thumb (Figure 11.6).

11.6.1. Etiology

De Quervain tenosynovitis has been associated with myxoid degeneration characterized by fibrous tissue deposits and increased vascularity, rather than acute inflammation of the synovial lining. However, the exact cause of this condition remains unknown. The abductor pollicis longus and extensor pollicis brevis tendons become entrapped and painful due to thickening of the tendon sheath caused by these deposits. Repetitive wrist motions, such as radial wrist deviation, simultaneous extension, and thumb radial abduction, are linked to this condition. Mothers of newborns who frequently lift their babies while their wrists shift from ulnar to radial deviation and their thumbs are considered the classic patient population. Acute wrist injuries, increased frictional forces on the wrist from forceful wrist and thumb movements, pathogenic causes, inflammatory illnesses, and anatomical variations in the first dorsal compartment are some potential etiologies for the disease.

11.6.2. Epidemiology

According to one study, the highest prevalence of de Quervain tenosynovitis occurs in individuals in their forties and fifties, with a prevalence estimate of 0.5% in men and 1.3% in women. Another study reported a prevalence of 0.13% for men and 0.36% for women. People with a history of medial or lateral epicondylitis may be more susceptible to the condition. When the child is lifted less frequently, spontaneous resolution usually occurs, as is often the case with bilateral involvement reported in new mothers or child care providers. There are two main risk factors for the disease: pregnancy and physical labor.

11.6.3. Pathophysiology

The extensor retinaculum separates the extensor tendons of the wrist into six compartments. The tendons of the abductor pollicis longus and extensor pollicis brevis are located in the first dorsal compartment of the wrist, which is separated from the other five dorsal compartments by a synovial sheath. These tendons are prone to entrapment as they pass through a fibrous tunnel that spans 2 cm and crosses the radial styloid, beneath the transverse fibers of the extensor retinaculum. This risk is heightened in cases involving acute trauma or repetitive motion. The thickening of the tendon sheath leads to a reduction in the size of the first compartment, resulting in stenosing tenosynovitis of the wrist.

The increased stress on the tendon sheaths causes the formation of fibrocartilage, which thickens the tendons. The tendon sheaths exhibit neovascularization. Myxoid degeneration is also observed in the tendons in this condition. The first dorsal compartment often contains a septum between the two tendons, which limits the volume of the first compartment and has significant implications for both nonoperative and operative treatment.

11.6.4. History and Physical Details

Patients commonly present with radial-sided wrist pain that exacerbates during thumb and wrist movements. This condition may result in pain and difficulty in opening jar lids. Typically, tenderness is observed over the radial styloid. Wrist swelling, when present, tends to occur near the radial styloid. The typical patient population includes third-trimester pregnant women or breastfeeding mothers who frequently hold their children. Various provocative clinical tests have been described for diagnosing de Quervain tenosynovitis. In the Finkelstein test, the patient is required to flex their thumb palmarly while the examiner ulnarly deviates their wrist. A positive test is indicated by sharp pain along the radial wrist in the first dorsal compartment. The Eichhoff test involves wrist deviation towards the ulna while clenching the thumb with the other fingers. A positive test elicits a sharp shooting pain over the radial aspect of the wrist. Another provocative clinical test described for this condition is the WHAT test, which involves wrist hyperflexion and thumb abduction.

11.6.5. Evaluation

De Quervain tenosynovitis is diagnosed based on the typical history and physical examination findings. Plain radiographs can help rule out other potential causes of radial wrist pain, such as thumb carpometacarpal (CMC) joint osteoarthritis, but they do not confirm the diagnosis. Wrist ultrasonography aids in identifying the septum in the first dorsal compartment, and its visualization enhances the success rates of corticosteroid injections. If surgical management is chosen, preoperative identification of the septum via ultrasonography is beneficial as effective pain relief requires the release of both subcompartments.

11.6.6. Treatment/Management

De Quervain tenosynovitis has the potential to resolve spontaneously and may not necessitate medical intervention. The most common nonsurgical treatment options for patients with persistent symptoms include corticosteroid injections, systemic anti-inflammatories, and splinting. Splinting with a thumb spica brace may provide short-term relief, but compliance is often low and failure and recurrence rates are frequently high. For patients who prefer to avoid intervention, splinting could serve as a temporary solution. Wrist immobilization may only benefit patients experiencing mild pain. Additionally, prolonged immobilization in a rigid splint or thumb spica cast may be detrimental as it can exacerbate the myxoid degeneration of the involved tendons. Therefore, immobilization in a semi-rigid splint that can be removed may be more advantageous. Reports indicate that one or two corticosteroid injections can provide nearly complete relief in 52–90% of patients. The tendons can be palpated in the tendon sheath, which is located 1 cm proximal to the radial styloid, where the injection is administered. To minimize the risk of subcutaneous atrophy and hypopigmentation, efforts should be made to palpably infiltrate both the extensor pollicis brevis and abductor pollicis longus sheaths as deeply as possible within the fibro-osseous tunnel. It has been reported that utilizing ultrasound guidance during injection allows for adequate injection and visualization of the multiple septae and sheaths that may be present in the first dorsal extensor compartment. When the corticosteroid injection is performed under ultrasound guidance, the success rate of the procedure increases. Approximately 50% of patients report that a single injection alleviates their symptoms. A second injection may benefit around 40 to 45% of patients. Potential side effects of steroid injections include hypopigmentation, fat atrophy, and dermal atrophy, which are typically associated with subcutaneous injection rather than tendon sheath injection. These side effects may improve or resolve over time. Additionally, receiving multiple injections within a short period may weaken the tendons, leading to thinning and eventual rupture.

There is a lack of consensus or high-quality evidence regarding the effectiveness of other nonoperative treatment modalities, such as acupuncture, therapeutic ultrasound therapy, and laser therapy. Surgery may be necessary if corticosteroid injections fail to relieve symptoms or if symptoms recur. Typically, surgery is performed in an outpatient setting. Local, regional, or general anesthesia may be used, and a tourniquet is commonly employed to control intraoperative bleeding and facilitate identification of important anatomical structures. The procedure involves making a transverse skin incision approximately 2 cm in length across the first dorsal compartment. Blunt dissection is used to expose the ligament covering the first dorsal compartment, taking care to avoid damage to the branches of the superficial radial sensory nerve. The dorsal margin of the sheath is then incised. If subsheaths are present, they are identified and excised. After releasing all subcompartments, the skin is closed, a thick, soft dressing is applied, and early mobilization is initiated.

Usually, post-operative care is minimal. Often, a basic dressing or wrap is used in place of more involved wound care. It is recommended that patients start using it early for light activities and daily living tasks. Patients are usually discharged to resume their regular activities after the sutures are removed, which usually takes two weeks. For several months following surgery, patients may have mild swelling and soreness at the surgical site. Although rare, surgical complications can still happen. The most common conditions are local soft tissue infection and wound dehiscence, which are usually treated with nonoperative measures like oral antibiotics and local wound care, respectively. Sharp transection, traction injuries, and scarring-related compression can all cause injuries to the superficial radial nerve that covers the first dorsal compartment. Severe sensitivity, pain, and paresthesias may follow from this. Although it can occasionally resolve on its own, surgical intervention for neurolysis or neuroma treatment is infrequently necessary. Patients may also have wrist flexion and extension as well as subluxation of the first dorsal compartment tendons after the release. When the tendons rub or sublux over the radial styloid, this could be uncomfortable. This could be related to the tendon sheath being excessively released during surgery. Another complication associated with the operative management of this condition is hypertrophic scarring.

11.6.7. Differential Diagnosis

The differential diagnoses that can mimic this condition include:

- Osteoarthritis of the first carpometacarpal joint;
- Scaphoid fracture;
- Radial styloid fracture;
- Sensory branch of radial nerve neuritis (Wartenberg's syndrome);
- Intersection syndrome;
- Trigger thumb.

11.6.8. Prognosis

The majority of patients respond well to nonoperative management. Many patients find that corticosteroid injections, whether or not they involve immobilization, are effective. Most patients experience pain relief when the first dorsal compartment is released, even in cases where the nonoperative command is unsuccessful. For these patients, the prognosis is therefore typically favorable. The presence of a septum in the first compartment, female sex, hypothyroidism, and mental illness are some risk factors for nonoperative treatment failure.

11.6.9. Complications

Complications related to surgery include:

- Injury to the superficial radial nerve;
- The abductor pollicis longus and extensor pollicis brevis are trapped;
- Subluxation of the tendons.

11.6.10. Deterrence and Patient Education

Patients should be informed about the risk factors, available treatments, and potential side effects of the disease. If multiple steroid injections are necessary, it is recommended to space them out by a few weeks to minimize the risk of side effects.

11.6.11. Enhancing Healthcare Team Outcomes

Tenosynovitis de Quervain is a common condition that may be seen by various specialists, including emergency room doctors, orthopedic surgeons, hand surgeons, or primary care physicians. Nurses in rehabilitation facilities and workers' compensation clinics may also encounter this disorder. Additionally, patients may seek assistance from pharmacists for pain relief. Early diagnosis is crucial in preventing the morbidity associated with this condition. Patients who seek treatment achieve excellent results, while those who do not receive treatment often experience ongoing pain leading to disability. Although surgery yields the best outcomes, complications can occur. Cortisone injections are effective but may result in recurrences. Moreover, recovery from cortisone injections can take three to nine months. To prevent symptom recurrence, all patients should avoid repetitive actions. Some patients may require a change in employment, while others may benefit from long-term hand rehabilitation exercises.

11.7. Dupuytren's Contracture

Dupuytren's disease affects the palmar fascia, which is a layer of fibrous tissue located above the tendons, nerves, blood vessels, and bones in the palm and fingers, and beneath the skin. Over time, this fascia thickens and contracts, causing the fingers to feel pulled inward and towards the palm. This can result in Dupuytren's contracture, which is when the fingers are unable or have difficulty fully straightening. For some people, this can lead to problems carrying out daily tasks due to issues with hand function. However, there are nonsurgical and surgical treatment options available to help improve motion in the affected fingers and slow the progression of the disease (Figure 11.7).

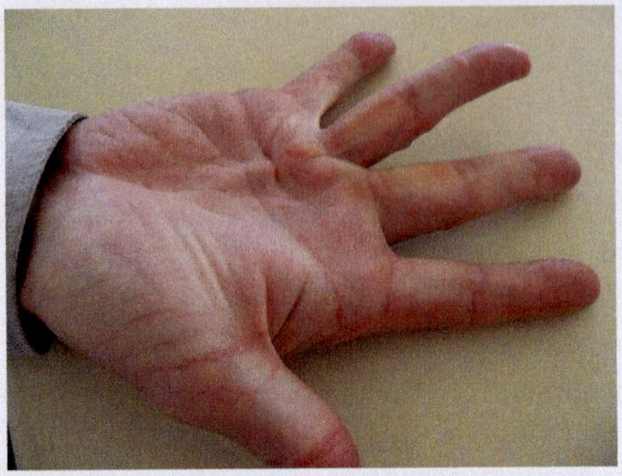

Figure 11.7. *Dupuytren's contracture of the ring finger.*

Source: By Frank C. Müller, CC BY-SA 4.0, https://commons.wikimedia.org/w/index.php?curid=647743.

11.7.1. Etiology

Dupuytren disease is a genetic disorder that is mostly caused by various factors, and it is often inherited in an autosomal dominant manner. While conditions such as diabetes, seizure disorders, alcoholism, smoking, HIV, and vascular disease are associated with it, there is no evidence linking it to occupation or hobbies. Additionally, the disease can result in ectopic manifestations beyond the hand, which can be observed in Ledderhose disease (plantar fascia) at a rate of 10% to 30%, Peyronie disease (Dartos fascia of the penis) at a rate of 2% to 8%, and Garrod disease (dorsal knuckle pads) at a rate of 40% to 50%.

11.7.2. Epidemiology

This particular condition is most commonly seen in individuals of Northern European or Scandinavian ancestry. In a study conducted in Denmark in 2015, it was estimated that the condition's overall heritability is 80%. This condition is less prevalent in populations from Southern Europe and South America, and even rarer in African and Asian populations. Males are affected at a ratio of 2:1 compared to females, and the disease tends to be more severe in men. If the disease manifests at an earlier age, it is usually associated with a more severe progression. In Asian populations, the palm is more commonly affected than the digits, which can result in the condition going unnoticed.

11.7.3. Pathophysiology

Dupuytren's disease is a condition that affects the hand and is caused by the abnormal growth of myofibroblasts, which produce type III collagen. This growth is triggered by various cytokines such as interleukin-1, transforming growth factor beta-1, transforming growth factor beta-2, epidermal growth factor (EGF), platelet-derived growth factor, and connective tissue growth factor. The disease progresses through three phases – proliferative, involution, and residual.

During the proliferative phase, there is a high concentration of fibroblasts and immature myofibroblasts in a whorled pattern. In the involution phase, fibroblasts align along the hand's longitudinal axis, and in the residual phase, there are relatively acellular cords that cause contracture deformity. The condition may stabilize or even reverse in at least 50–70% of cases and does not always worsen. The disease causes hand deformities due to the abnormal fascial bands changing into pathological cords. Central cords are caused by pretendinous bands and lead to metacarpal phalangeal (MCP) joint contracture and skin pitting. Natiomotor cords cause webspace contractures, and the disease process can cause proximal interphalangeal (PIP) contracture, with spiral cords being the most significant component. Spiral cords are sourced from four primary structures – the pretendinous band, spiral band, lateral digital sheath, and Grayson ligament. Surgeons should be aware that the neurovascular bundle in the digit is displaced centrally, superficially, and proximally due to the spiral cord. Importantly, the Cleland ligament or the transverse ligament of the palmar aponeurosis are not affected by Dupuytren's disease.

Risk factors for increased severity and recurrence of the disease after treatment include the presence of Garrod pads, Ledderhose, or Peyronies diseases, male gender, bilateral disease, involvement of siblings or parents, and onset before age 50. Dupuytren's disease is also influenced by genetic factors.

11.7.4. Histopathology

Histologic examination of Dupuytren nodules reveals the presence of myofibroblasts and fibroblasts. The long axis of the cell in myofibroblasts is aligned with contractile actin microfilaments. Myofibroblasts attach to one another through fibronectin and extracellular fibrils. The extracellular matrix is primarily composed of type III collagen. Approximately 10% of the cells in Dupuytren nodules are immune cells, mostly macrophages and lymphocytes. Nodules are highly cellular and packed with myofibroblasts, whereas cords are primarily made up of fibroblasts and have relatively few cells. Proinflammatory cytokines such as tumor necrosis factor (TNF), interleukin-6 (IL-6), and IL-8 are secreted by macrophages and lymphocytes. Dense T-cell infiltrates have been found in Dupuytren nodules, indicating that the condition may be an autoimmune T cell-mediated illness. A recent study revealed an activated T-cell infiltrate near blood vessels within Dupuytren nodules, supporting this notion. Furthermore, *in vitro* research has revealed cells expressing T-cell receptors that are restricted. These findings suggest that microvascular alterations in the hand caused by an autoantigen may be the source of a local immune response.

11.7.5. History and Physical

Dupuytren's disease begins with a small lump in the palm, typically near the distal palmar crease. These lumps eventually develop into tight cords, initially causing only palpable cords in the palm. As the cords thicken and shorten, they lead to fixed flexion contractures of the fingers at the MCP and PIP joints. This results in limited hand movement and noticeable cords extending into the affected digits. Nodules, cords, and finger contractures are characteristic features of Dupuytren's disease. Pain is uncommon, with the 4th and 5th digits commonly affected. Even if the condition affects both hands, the severity may differ. Nodule palpation is usually painless unless the ulnar nerve is compressed, and the nodules may become tender with tenosynovitis.

Physical findings:

- Blanching of the skin when the finger is extended;
- Proximal to the nodules, the cords are painless;
- Pits and grooves may be present;
- Tenderness may be felt in the knuckle pads covering the PIP joints;
- If there is involvement of the plantar fascia, the disease is more severe (Ledderhose disease).
- During the Hueston tabletop test, the patient will be asked to place their palm flat on the examination table. If the patient is unable to straighten their fingers due to a flexion contracture deformity, the test result will be positive.

11.7.6. Evaluation

Although they are not necessary, hand X-rays can be taken to check for bony abnormalities like arthritis that could cause a loss of range of motion. It is also advised to do a laboratory study to rule out diabetes. Nodules and thickened palmar fascia may be seen on an ultrasound

11.7.7. Treatment/Management

The way a disease affects a patient's quality of life determines what treatments are indicated. Many patients who have a positive tabletop test, 30° MCP contracture, or 15° to 20° PIP contracture will choose to receive treatment. Conservative care, collagenase injection, needle aponeurotomy, and/or surgical resection and fasciectomy are available as treatment options.

11.7.7.1. Conservative Management

Those individuals with a painless and stable illness, without any functional impairment, should be closely monitored. It is advisable to conduct regular follow-ups every six months to assess the progression of the disorder. In the initial stages of the disease, the application of heat and ultrasonic waves during physical and occupational therapy sessions can be beneficial. Additionally, some patients may find it advantageous to utilize a brace or splint to stretch their fingers. Maintaining a good range of motion in the fingers is crucial to prevent adhesions. Injectable corticosteroids may provide relief for certain patients, particularly those experiencing painful nodules. However, it is important to note that not all patients respond positively to steroid injections, as recurrence rates of up to 50% have been reported. Furthermore, corticosteroid injections carry the risk of tendon rupture, pigmentation changes, and fat atrophy.

Other treatment options that have been explored include tamoxifen, imiquimod, 5-fluorouracil, anti-tumor necrosis factor agents, and botulinum toxin. However, none of these treatments have been proven to be universally effective or superior. Radiation therapy may be considered as a potential treatment option only in the early stages of the illness, but it is accompanied by a lengthy list of side effects.

11.7.7.2. Needle Aponeurectomy

Usually, mild contractures are the only indications for needle aponeurotomy. The minimally invasive procedure is frequently carried out in an office environment. The cord is severed with a needle. After manipulating the digit, the patient is fitted with a night extension splint. Contractures of the metacarpal-phalangeal joint have improved the most. This procedure has the advantage of being minimally invasive and possibly yielding immediate results. Iatrogenic damage to tendons and nerves, as well as a 58% recurrence rate, are drawbacks.

11.7.7.3. Collagenase Injection

A minimally invasive treatment derived from *Clostridium histolyticum* is collagenase injections. A metalloprotease enzyme is injected, lysing collagen while protecting Type IV collagen, which is required for the basement membrane of blood vessels and nerves. About 0.25 mL for MCP and 0.20 mL for PIP contractures are usually administered subcutaneously, directly into the cord, using a needle. After the injection, the affected digit is worked on under local anesthesia for 24 to 48 hours. For six months, night extension splinting is kept in place. Injections of collagenase have been demonstrated to reduce contractures by 75%, with a recurrence rate of only 35%. Injection-related complications include pulley rupture, complex regional pain syndrome (CRPS), edema, skin tearing, and tendon rupture.

11.7.7.4. Surgery

A partial or complete surgical fasciectomy is possible. The limited removal of diseased tissue inside a ray is known as a partial palmar fasciectomy. In order to identify neurovascular structures before coming into contact with the spiral cord, dissection is typically done from the proximal to the distal region. Each patient's incisions are made in a unique Brunner zigzag pattern. A V-Y incision and Z-plasty can also be used to lengthen contracted skin. Care must be taken to preserve the neurovascular bundles. The neurovascular bundles need to be preserved with caution. The rate of recurrence is 30% at one to two years, 15% at three to five years, and less than 10% at 10 years.

Although it is rarely done, total palmar fasciectomy is an alternative that involves removing all of the palmar and digital fascia, including healthy tissue. It is recommended for persistent digital cords, diseases that infiltrate the body, or recurrence following partial surgery. Skin necrosis, hematomas (the most frequent complication), flare reactions, neurovascular injury, digital ischemia, swelling, and infection are among the complications following a fasciectomy. Recurrence is common with all treatment modalities, regardless of the treatment, and at five years, it approaches 20–50%.

11.7.8. Differential Diagnosis

It is important to distinguish Dupuytren disease from other hand conditions such as soft tissue tumors, ulnar neuropathy, ganglion cysts, stenosing flexor tenosynovitis, and flexor tendonitis. Unlike Dupuytren disease, stenosing tenosynovitis is characterized by a painful triggering finger that becomes immobile after flexion. Moreover, a nodule close to the MCP joint, known as the A1 pulley, may be palpable to the examiner. In such cases, it is crucial to differentiate between a soft tissue tumor and a moveable cyst originating from the metacarpal-phalangeal joint that nodules the flexor tendon.

11.7.9. Prognosis

Dupuytren contracture can have different levels of severity and can cause various negative effects. Contractures in the PIP and MCP joints can make daily activities, employment, and lifestyle choices difficult. In addition, some patients may experience pain from the nodules. In some cases, Dupuytren contracture may also be associated with Peyronie's disease or knuckle pad involvement, which may indicate a serious underlying condition.

11.7.10. Complications

Necrosis of the wound margin, hematoma, nerve damage, digital ischemia, infection, swelling, recurrence, and postoperative flare-ups are among the side effects of surgical treatment. Digital ischemia may result from stretch injuries to vessels in digits with a history of prolonged flexion contracture, or it may be the direct result of damage to the digit's vascular supply. As previously mentioned, the neurovascular bundles are displaced centrally and palmarly by the spiral cord, making them more vulnerable to damage.

Pain with diffuse swelling, hyperesthesia, redness, and stiffness are symptoms of a Dupuytren flare-up. Steroids, cervical sympathetic block, therapy, and A1 pulley release are used to treat this complication. CRPS is not more likely to occur following carpal tunnel release surgery in conjunction with fasciectomy.

11.7.11. Postoperative and Rehabilitation Care

Patients who undergo hand surgery need to enroll in hand therapy, which plays a crucial role in maintaining their hand range of motion. To prevent contractures, physical therapy must be continued for at least three months. Although the full benefits of surgery take time to appear, they usually become apparent after six to eight weeks. Postoperative hand rehabilitation techniques involve the use of dynamic and static splints, scar and edema management, and routine range-of-motion exercises. The inflammatory phase of wound healing, which typically occurs three to five days after surgery, should be followed by these therapeutic interventions. Effective postoperative management is essential because it accounts for up to 50% of overall surgical outcomes.

11.7.12. Enhancing Healthcare Team Outcomes

An interprofessional team, consisting of the patient's primary care physician, hand therapist, dermatologist, and orthopedic/hand surgeon, is responsible for managing Dupuytren contracture. There are various treatment options available to treat the condition. Open methods are more comprehensive in removing damaged tissue and enable direct visualization of vital neurovascular structures. However, injection-based therapy is less invasive, but has a higher chance of causing harm to nearby structures and might not entirely release contractures. Although all treatments have some chance of recurrence, non-operative and injection-based options have the highest rate. The treating surgeon and the patient's primary care physician usually keep an eye on these patients. The patient's primary care physician can help them control their blood sugar, cut back on alcohol, and quit smoking. Treatment should only be offered to symptomatic patients who have limitations in their range of motion since all treatments have potential side effects. To achieve better results, the healthcare team must have close communication with each other. Hand therapists play a crucial role in helping patients regain their range of motion when treating this illness.

11.8. Carpal Tunnel Syndrome (CTS)

Carpal tunnel syndrome (CTS) is a medical condition that causes hand and wrist pain, tingling, numbness, and weakness. It occurs when the median nerve, which runs through a gap in the wrist bones called the carpal tunnel, is irritated or under pressure. This nerve is responsible for providing sensation to most of the fingers and hands, as well as facilitating forearm movement. When it gets compressed or damaged, it can cause abnormal sensations or weakness in the hand and wrist. If a person experience any of these symptoms, it's important to see a doctor as soon as possible. Treatment for CTS is usually effective, but delaying treatment can lead to permanent nerve damage (Figure 11.8).

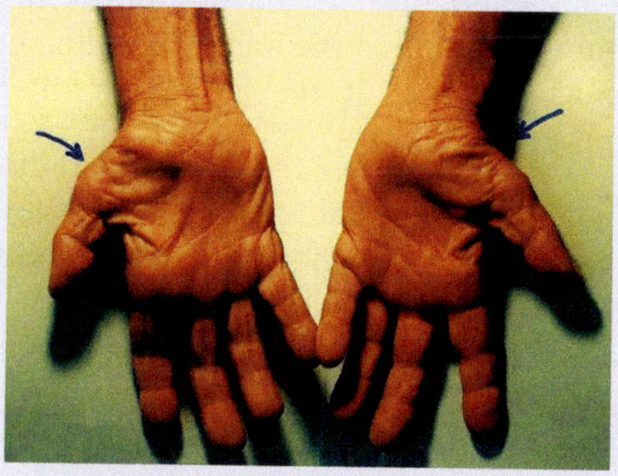

Figure 11.8. *Untreated carpal tunnel syndrome.*

Source: By Dr. Harry Gouvas, MD, PhD – I Dr. Harry Gouvas, MD, PhD created this work entirely by myself., Public Domain, https://commons.wikimedia.org/w/index.php?curid=16376968.

11.8.1. Etiology

The carpal tunnel is a narrow passage in the wrist formed by the transverse carpal ligament at its upper boundary and the carpal bones at its lower boundary. The carpal tunnel houses the median nerve and nine flexor tendons. CTS can develop due to ischemia damage to the median nerve, high blood pressure or mechanical trauma. The pressure within the carpal tunnel ranges from 2 to 10 mmHg under normal conditions. However, when the wrist is extended or flexed, the pressure can rise up to 8 to 10 times higher than usual. Repeated compression of a nerve can cause demyelination at the site of compression. The development of endoneurial edema results from a disturbance in blood flow to the endoneurial capillary system.

Although the exact cause of elevated CTS is still unknown, several factors can increase the risk of developing CTS. These factors include modifications to the carpal tunnel, changes to the body's fluid equilibrium, or the presence of direct neuropathic factors. Among the risk factors linked to CTS are the following:

- Dislocation or subluxation of the carpus;
- Fractures or skewed consolidation of the distal radius;
- Wrist arthrosis, inflammatory arthritis, and infectious arthritis;
- Acromegaly;
- Cysts or tumors within the tunnel;
- Pregnancy;
- Menopause;
- Obesity;
- Kidney failure;
- Hypothyroidism;
- Use of oral contraceptives;
- Congestive heart failure;
- Diabetes;
- Alcoholism;
- Vitamin deficiency or toxicity;
- Exposure to toxins.

Any value above 0.7 on the square wrist test, which calculates the ratio of wrist thickness to wrist width, suggests a higher risk of developing CTS.

11.8.2. Epidemiology

Carpal tunnel syndrome (CTS) affects 1 to 5% of the general population, with a higher prevalence in females than in males, with a ratio of 3:1. Obese individuals are at twice the risk of developing CTS. The condition commonly occurs in adults between the ages of 40 and 60, and it is rare in children.

11.8.3. Pathophysiology

Multifactorial conditions such as CTS usually occur as a result of a combination of environmental, social, occupational, and patient-specific factors. Therefore, finding a single, specific cause is typically difficult unless there is a definite physical finding that directly explains the patient's symptoms.

The pathology linked to CTS usually occurs due to a combination of traction and compression, which often affects the median nerve. The compressive factor can cause a cycle of elevated intracranial pressure, blockage of general venous outflow, accumulation of localized edema, and disruption of the intraneural microcirculation of the median nerve. When lesions form on the myelin sheath and axon, nerve function is hampered, leading to inflammation and a loss of the normal physiological protective and supportive functions of the surrounding connective tissues.

The altered structural integrity of the nerve exacerbates the dysfunctional environment, which can be aggravated by repeated wrist motions and traction, resulting in additional nerve damage. Inflammation can also occur in any of the nine flexor tendons that cross the carpal tunnel, compressing the median nerve. Autonomic nerve fibers carried within the median nerve may also become affected, although sensory fibers are frequently impacted before motor fibers.

11.8.4. History and Physical Details

Numbness, tingling, and pain in the thumb and in the radial, middle, and outer regions of the fourth digits are common complaints from patients with CTS. These symptoms usually get worse at night and can appear anywhere from as localized as the wrist, as widespread as the hand, as radiating to the forearm, or as high as the elbow and reaching the shoulder. Initially, the symptoms are sporadic and connected to certain activities like driving, reading newspapers, and painting. CTS is characterized by symptoms that worsen at night, especially if the patient finds relief by shaking their hand or wrist. Advanced disease is indicated by progression to permanent sensory loss, muscle weakness, clumsiness, and difficulties with activities like buttoning clothes and opening doorknobs. Although CTS often affects both hands, it usually affects the dominant hand first. If the numbness in the fifth finger spreads to the hand's dorsum, neck, or thenar eminence, it may indicate a different diagnosis.

During a physical examination, it may become evident that there is sensory loss or weakness in the median nerve distribution. The palmar sensory cutaneous nerve usually avoids the carpal tunnel rather than passing through it, which means that sensory loss typically spares the thenar eminence. Other potential findings include reduced strength in thumb opposition and abduction, as well as atrophy of the thenar eminence. There are several different provocative tests available to try and replicate CTS symptoms, each with different levels of specificity and sensitivity. To obtain a more thorough evaluation, it is recommended to combine these test results with the patient's clinical history.

The carpal compression test is the most reliable provocative maneuver, in which consistent pressure is applied directly over the carpal tunnel for 30 seconds. If paresthesias or pain occur within the median nerve distribution during this test, it is considered positive. The test has an 83% specificity and 64% sensitivity.

In the Phalen test, also known as the reverse prayer, the patient fully flexes their wrists by bringing both dorsal surfaces together, bending their elbows, and maintaining this position for one minute. A positive result is indicated by paresthesias and pain in the fingers innervated by the median nerve. The test has a 68% sensitivity and a 73% specificity.

In the Tinel test, a medical practitioner stimulates the median nerve by applying pressure directly over the carpal tunnel. If the test results show symptoms, it is considered positive. The Tinel test has a 50% sensitivity and a 77% specificity.

11.8.5. Evaluation

Patients with mild CTS typically do not need further diagnostic testing, as a clinical diagnosis is sufficient. However, electrodiagnostic (EDX) testing, such as nerve conduction studies, should be conducted on patients who display unusual symptoms, pain that disrupts sleep, persistent numbness or weakness in the hand, or any impairment in hand function (excluding pregnant women). Electromyography (EMG) may also be used to aid in surgical decision-making and rule out other diagnoses. EMG can detect residual axonal integrity even when no sensory or motor components are elicited. Abnormalities in EDX tests linked to specific symptoms and indicators are the gold standard for CTS diagnosis. EDX testing can also evaluate the severity of nerve damage and provide information on prognosis, as clinical symptoms may not always accurately reflect the true extent of median nerve damage. CTS has three standard severity levels: mild, moderate, and severe. Electrophysiological testing indicates only sensory abnormalities in patients with mild CTS, while both motor and sensory abnormalities are present in patients with moderate CTS. Imaging is only necessary when there is a possibility of a structural abnormality. Further investigation may be required for potential anatomical anomalies such as tumors or ganglion cysts. Magnetic resonance imaging or ultrasound are the preferred modalities for this type of imaging.

11.8.6. Treatment/Management

Conservative therapy is the preferred treatment for mild cases of CTS. This includes using wrist splints at night to keep the wrist in a neutral position. Wrist splints are the first choice for treatment and if the patient's symptoms improve, it is best to continue using them. However, if there is no improvement, it may be worth considering combining splinting with other therapeutic methods.

Glucocorticoid injections can also provide immediate relief, but their long-term outcomes are not different from splinting. An effective first-line alternative to wrist splinting is a glucocorticoid injection. Methylprednisolone is injected into the carpal tunnel using ultrasound guidance or anatomic landmarks at a dose of 20–40 mg combined with 1% lidocaine. The period of anticipated relief usually lasts for three months. It is recommended to limit injections to no more than every six months for each wrist. If the patient does not respond to one or two injections, it is advisable to evaluate them for surgical intervention. It's important to note that there are potential side effects of glucocorticoid injections, such as exacerbation of median nerve compression, inadvertent injection into the ulnar or median nerves, and the possibility of digital flexor tendon rupture.

If initial conservative therapy fails, splinting along with a glucocorticoid injection may be considered as an additional option for treatment. However, for those who do not prefer injections, a short course of oral prednisone therapy may be helpful. This treatment usually involves taking 20 mg of prednisone once daily for 10 to 14 days. It is important to note that prolonged use of oral glucocorticoids can have negative side effects and should be avoided. Referring to a specialized hand therapist can be beneficial as they can provide methods like ultrasound therapy, exercises for gliding nerves and tendons, and carpal bone mobilization. According to the American Academy of Orthopedic Surgeons, there is no evidence that oral medications are more effective than placebos in treating CTS. It has also been found that diuretics and nonsteroidal anti-inflammatory drugs are not effective in treating CTS.

In cases where patients with CTS are not responding to conservative treatments or have severe CTS, surgical intervention may be necessary. Electrophysiological testing is required to confirm the severity of CTS before carpal tunnel release surgery can be performed, either openly or endoscopically. This minimally invasive procedure involves making a small incision in the transverse carpal ligament to release pressure on the median nerve. Patients are usually discharged from the hospital the same day, which saves them from spending a night there. In general, surgery has better long-term results than conservative treatment, with initial success rates exceeding 90%. However, long-term outcomes are a little less encouraging, with an approximate success rate of 60% at the five-year mark.

11.8.7. Differential Diagnosis

When assessing a patient who may have CTS, it is important to take into account several different musculoskeletal and nervous system disorders that can present similarly:

- Brachial plexopathy;
- Cervical myofascial pain;
- Cervical spondylosis;
- Compartment syndrome;
- Ischemic stroke;
- Mononeuritis multiplex;
- Multiple sclerosis;
- Median neuropathy in the forearm;
- Motor neuron disease;
- Diabetic neuropathy;
- Cervical radiculopathy;
- Overuse injury;
- Traumatic brachial plexopathy;
- Radiation-induced brachial plexopathy;
- Neuropathies;
- Tendonitis;
- Tenosynovitis;
- Thoracic outlet syndrome.

11.8.8. Prognosis

Carpal tunnel syndrome (CTS) can cause permanent damage to the median nerve, which can worsen over time. Even after surgery, about a third of patients may experience some degree of recurrence of the syndrome after five years. Conservative treatment can be effective for 70%–90% of mild-to-moderate CTS cases. However, some patients may require surgery as the condition progresses. Patients with CTS who have a wrist fracture or diabetes as a secondary cause tend to have a worse prognosis than those without any underlying conditions. Patients with normal electrophysiological studies have worse surgical outcomes and more complications compared to patients with abnormalities on these tests. The presence of axonal loss detected during electrophysiological testing is an indication of a poor prognosis.

11.8.9. Complications

Complications related to CTS can occur due to the illness itself or the treatments used to manage it. CTS can cause irreversible damage to the median nerve, leading to long-term disability and impairment. Muscles located at the base of the thumb can become weak and atrophied, causing reduced dexterity. People with this condition may also experience chronic pain in their hands and wrists, which may eventually lead to the development of CRPS. The most common outcome of carpal tunnel surgery is the development of a neuroma in the palmar cutaneous branch of the median nerve. Patients may also experience incomplete resolution of symptoms, joint stiffness, dysesthesias, and hypertrophic scars.

11.8.10. Postoperative and Rehabilitation Care

In the process of treating CTS, splinting and good hand ergonomics are important components. To lessen pain and reduce swelling, therapists use paraffin wax, iontophoresis, and ultrasound. Research has produced conflicting findings about how well these modalities work to improve outcomes. To fully evaluate the efficacy of these interventions, more excellent research is needed. Based on available data, the use of trigger point release, massage, and nerve-gliding exercises has demonstrated significant improvements in nerve conduction, pain reduction, and muscle strength. The physical or occupational therapist who is treating the patient should consider implementing these strategies.

11.8.11. Deterrence and Patient Education

When the median nerve in the wrist is compressed, CTS occurs. Experts speculate that a combination of genetic predisposition, specific medical conditions, and environmental factors collectively contribute to the onset of CTS, although the exact cause of nerve compression is still unknown. CTS symptoms affect the first three fingers and the area of the ring finger closest to the thumb. These symptoms include pain, tingling, numbness, and possibly weakness. They may appear in one or both hands and can even spread up the arm. Consequently, individuals with CTS may experience clumsiness and difficulty performing simple tasks such as turning knobs and buttoning clothes.

Compared to men, women are more likely to experience CTS. Additionally, individuals working in occupations that involve repetitive hand movements or the use of vibrating equipment have a higher risk of developing CTS. Pregnancy, rheumatoid arthritis, diabetes, obesity, hypothyroidism, and other conditions also increase the likelihood of developing CTS. Mild CTS symptoms can be diagnosed by a healthcare professional without the need for additional testing. However, individuals experiencing unusual or severe symptoms should undergo EDX testing. These electrical nerve tests provide medical professionals with information about the proper transmission of electrical signals along the median nerve and the appropriate response of hand and wrist muscles to these signals. Initial treatments for CTS usually consist of injecting steroids directly into the wrist or wearing a wrist splint at night. Patients may occasionally be prescribed oral steroids. Splints are especially beneficial during pregnancy because the symptoms usually go away after giving birth. Getting treatment from a hand therapist with specialized training may also be helpful. For patients with severe symptoms or those who do not improve with conservative treatment, medical professionals advise surgery. By releasing the ligament covering the carpal tunnel, more room is created during the surgical procedure.

11.8.12. Enhancing Healthcare Team Outcomes

Carpal tunnel syndrome (CTS) is a common type of nerve entrapment neuropathy that requires the attention of various medical specialists. If not treated promptly, the symptoms of CTS can become debilitating. To diagnose and treat CTS effectively, clinicians from different specialties such as obstetrics, orthopedics, neurology, primary care, endocrinology, and physical or occupational therapy are required. Combining different therapies may be more effective than using individual treatments. Therefore, medical professionals should communicate and educate patients about the advantages, disadvantages, and effectiveness of various CTS treatment options, while also helping them set realistic expectations for their treatment outcomes. To help patients regain normal function, effective communication and teamwork among healthcare professionals are crucial. The cooperative interprofessional team approach plays a critical role in achieving better results for CTS patients.

11.9. Tennis Elbow

Tennis elbow, also known as lateral epicondylitis, is caused by the overuse of the elbow's muscles and tendons. It is commonly associated with repetitive arm and wrist movements. However, it's a misconception that only tennis players suffer from this condition. People in professions that involve repetitive motions, such as butchers, carpenters, painters, and plumbers, are also at risk of developing tennis elbow. The cause of tennis elbow is often unknown.

Tennis elbow usually affects the area on the outer part of the elbow where the hard, cord-like tissues of the forearm muscles attach. This area consists of tendons. Pain may spread to the wrist and forearm. Tennis elbow can be treated with physical therapy, medication, and rest. However, if these treatments don't work, or if they interfere with daily life, surgery or an injection may be required (Figure 11.9).

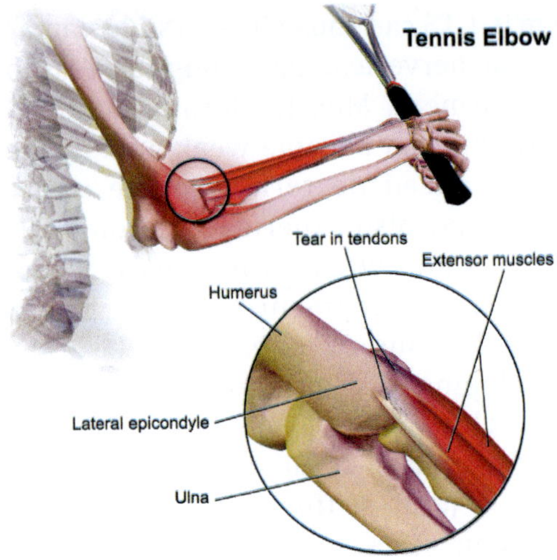

Figure 11.9. *Location of tennis elbow.*

Source: By BruceBlaus – Own work, CC BY-SA 4.0, https://commons.wikimedia.org/w/index.php?curid=44923322.

11.9.1. Etiology

Tennis elbow is a common overuse injury that occurs due to repetitive strain caused by repetitive gripping of objects or wrist extension. Although it is historically associated with tennis players, it can be caused by any activity that involves constant wrist extension, radial deviation, and forearm supination. Athletes participating in sports such as badminton, squash, and other related activities can also experience this injury. Inadequate equipment or mechanics can often cause this condition in athletes.

11.9.2. Epidemiology

Tennis elbow is the most common cause of elbow pain in patients with generalized elbow pain. The condition affects both men and women equally, and the annual incidence in the US ranges from 1% to 3%. Even though tennis players account for only 10% of patients, the condition is commonly referred to as tennis elbow. Half of all tennis players experience elbow pain, and 75% of them have true tennis elbow. This condition is more common in people over 40 years of age. Risk factors for developing tennis elbow in the general population include smoking, obesity, vigorous activity (managing physical loads over 20 kg), and repetitive movement for at least two hours a day.

Tennis elbow has a favorable natural course, with 80%–90% of patients experiencing spontaneous recovery within one to two years.

11.9.3. Pathophysiology

The primary cause of this condition is a degenerative process that results from overuse of both the common extensor tendon and the extensor carpi radialis brevis (ECRB). The histological findings typically include granulation tissue, micro-rupture, vascular hyperplasia, an abundance of fibroblasts, unstructured collagen, and a noticeable absence of the typical inflammatory cells (neutrophils, lymphocytes, and macrophages) in the tissue, along with degenerative changes. The term "angiofibroblastic dysplasia" was originally used to describe the microscopic features and appearance of the condition in several histologic studies. Ultrasound evaluation often reveals thickening and heterogeneity of the common extensor tendon, calcifications, intra-substance tears, and marked irregularity of the lateral epicondyle.

11.9.4. Histopathology

Many studies detailing the histologic appearance of pathologic ECRB specimens describe any combination of the following features:

- Hypertrophic or abundant fibroblasts;
- Collagen disorganization;
- Vascular hyperplasia;
- Lack of inflammatory cells.

11.9.5. History and Physical Details

Patients often report experiencing pain that starts slowly, but upon further inquiry, they frequently describe a history of overuse rather than a specific traumatic incident that caused the pain. Typically, the pain starts one to three days following an unfamiliar activity that requires frequent wrist extension. This could be due to the use of new equipment or an unusual training situation, like an athlete working out for an unusually long or intense period of time. Acute strains or injuries resulting from activities like lifting a large object or hitting a forceful backhand stroke in a game of tennis can also cause this condition. This sudden trauma may trigger a longer-term process (i.e., an overuse injury that is both acute and chronic). The pain usually occurs over the lateral elbow and worsens with movement, but gets better with rest. The pain can range in intensity from mild (which flares up with aggravating activities like tennis or using a hand tool repeatedly) to severe (where simple actions like picking up and holding a coffee cup or a sign with a coffee cup on it will trigger the pain).

When examined, the lateral epicondyle is typically the site of greatest tenderness, although it can also occasionally be found in a focal, distal location 1–2 cm from the lateral epicondyle itself. The connecting muscle may be noticeably tense, and the tendon as a whole may feel somewhat uncomfortable when palpated. Resisted wrist extension will exacerbate the patient's pain or cause it to recur, particularly if the elbow is extended and the forearm is pronated. Further evidence for the diagnosis comes from the particularly painful response to resistive extension of the middle finger while the elbow is extended, which is due to the increased stress placed on the tendon. Most importantly, there should not be any tingling or numbness in the affected areas. Although these conditions can coexist, these symptoms indicate an alternative process, such as radial nerve entrapment.

11.9.6. Evaluation

Imaging is often unnecessary for diagnosing lateral epicondylitis. However, if the patient's medical history and physical examination suggest the possibility of additional injuries or conditions, the healthcare provider may order an elbow radiography series (anteroposterior (AP) and lateral). Other conditions that may require imaging include bursitis, fractures, tumors, and concurrent degenerative joint changes. If nonoperative management techniques fail to improve the patient's condition, the physician may consider requesting an MRI or ultrasound to assess for tears, stress fractures, or osteochondral defects.

11.9.7. Treatment/Management

11.9.7.1. Nonoperative Management

Resting from the offending activity is the first line of treatment for lateral epicondylitis, depending on the severity of the pain. After exertion, the patient can apply ice and take oral or topical NSAIDs to help manage pain. To release tension at the lateral epicondyle, forearm counterforce straps are recommended. These should be worn when engaging in activities. However, it's important to note that the use of counterforce straps is somewhat debatable since direct mechanical compression on the area itself can cause pain over the area of maximal tenderness. To relieve the strain on the wrist extensors, a cock-up wrist splint is one type of brace that may be prescribed. Occupational or physical therapy that focuses on forearm strengthening and stretching, followed by a progression to eccentric muscle strengthening of the common extensor tendon, is beneficial. If conservative pain management fails, consider more sophisticated or invasive methods such as topical nitrates, botulinum toxin, autologous platelet-rich plasma, and dextrose prolotherapy (Figure 11.10).

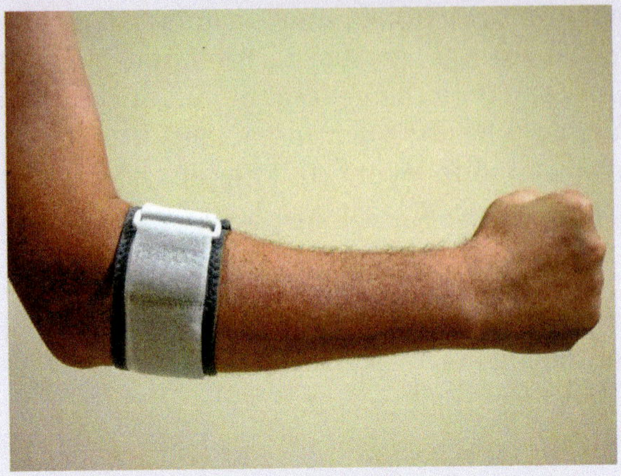

Figure 11.10. *Counterforce orthosis reduces the elongation within the musculotendinous fibers.*

Source: By Yahia. Mokhtar – Own work, CC BY-SA 4.0, https://commons.wikimedia.org/w/index.php?curid=46061040.

11.9.7.2. Surgical Management

When it comes to treating lateral epicondylitis, surgery should only be considered as a last resort. It is recommended to try extended non-operative care for a period of 6 to 12 months before considering surgical treatment. Most surgeons prefer to perform different levels of tendinous origin release at the lateral epicondyle and/or ECR debridement. If the surgeon decides not to detach the ECRB, then it is important to perform a generous debridement of the pathologic tissue at the ECRB origin, along with confirmation of debridement of the bony bed of tissue at the lateral epicondyle that is healthy and bleeding. This will promote the potential for healing.

11.9.8. Differential Diagnosis

The following conditions are included in the differential diagnosis of lateral epicondylitis, but they are not the only ones:

- Elbow bursitis;

- Cervical radiculopathy;
- Posterolateral elbow plica;
- Posterolateral rotatory instability (PLRI);
- Radial nerve entrapment;
- Radial tunnel syndrome;
- Palpation 3 to 4 cm distal and anterior to the lateral epicondyle;
- Pain with resisted third-finger extension;
- Pain with resisted forearm supination;
- Occult fracture(s);
- Capitellar osteochondritis dissecans;
- Triceps tendinitis;
- Radiocapitellar osteoarthritis;
- Shingles.

11.9.9. Prognosis

Lateral epicondylitis is a condition that usually has a favorable prognosis. If patients receive conservative treatments such as rest, ice, and anti-inflammatory medications, they will experience relief from pain within a year in most cases. However, if the initial treatment does not work, patients may benefit from physical and occupational therapy. It is important to note that patients who abandon their treatment plan often experience a return of their symptoms.

11.9.10. Complications

After normal activity is resumed, lateral epicondylitis can recur, and other complications may arise, such as tendon rupture from repeated steroid injections and poor response to conservative treatment.

Postoperative complications may include the following:

- Failing to address concomitant pathology.
- Patients should be informed about the risks and benefits of surgery, which can include infection, blood loss, neurovascular injury, continued pain, stiffness, or continued or worsening overall dysfunction. Patients may report worse outcomes and lack of improvement if the primary cause of symptoms is not addressed.
- In as many as 5% of patients receiving treatment for lateral epicondylitis, radial nerve entrapment may go unnoticed or untreated clinically.
- Iatrogenic LUCL injury can occur iatrogenically, and the risk is elevated if the surgical dissection goes past the radial head equator.
- If there is significant LUCL compromise or extension, postoperative iatrogenic posterolateral rotatory instability (PLRI) may develop.
- Iatrogenic neurovascular injury.
- Radial nerve injury.
- Heterotopic ossification.
- Reduce risk by irrigating heavily with salt water after debridement and decortication.
- Infection.

11.9.11. Deterrence and Patient Education

To prevent strain and overuse of the elbow and forearm, it's important to advise patients on the optimal biomechanical movements and preventive measures for the elbow joint. The following advice topics should be considered:

- Avoid end range of motion extremes in both extension and flexion.
- Repetitive wrist and hand movements should be avoided. If they can't be avoided, take frequent breaks.
- When lifting weights or performing other heavy tasks, avoid extending the arm to its maximum length. Instead, bend the elbow slightly.
- Hold heavy tools with two hands. When playing tennis, use the backhand with two hands.
- Limit repetitive grasping and gripping motions.
- If a movement causes pain to return, avoid it and report it to the clinician's office.

11.9.12. Pearls and Other Issues

Patients can typically have follow-up appointments as necessary after diagnosis, patient education, and a prescription for conservative treatment. In chronic cases, additional follow-up may be required to assess more advanced therapies. In up to 15% of cases, radial tunnel syndrome and posterior interosseous nerve entrapment may coexist. If radicular symptoms are present, it is important to consider this diagnosis as a potential coexisting condition or alternate diagnosis. Corticosteroid injections have shown short-term benefits (less than six weeks), but are ineffective in the long run.

Topical nitrates are believed to enhance local blood flow, which aids in tendon healing. Extracorporeal shockwave therapy has been suggested as a potential long-term treatment for this condition. However, thus far, this therapy has not yielded any significant improvements. Platelet-rich plasma and dextrose prolotherapy are pro-inflammatory agents that aim to irritate or inflame the tendon and initiate a healing response, although the evidence supporting this claim has been conflicting. In terms of evidence, platelet-rich plasma appears to be more promising than dextrose prolotherapy. Interestingly, compared to corticosteroid injections, patients with chronic pain caused by this condition report lower pain levels and higher functional levels.

11.9.13. Enhancing Healthcare Team Outcomes

Tennis elbow is a common condition that can occur from playing sports such as golf or racket sports. It is important for patients to be educated about this condition since elbow pain is a common complaint among patients who visit their primary care physician. It is recommended to stretch before engaging in any vigorous physical activity, and resting the hand is also important when pain starts. Physicians should emphasize the importance of increasing muscular strength and conditioning, and using the right equipment. Most tennis elbow patients recover within three to eighteen months with rest, and surgery is rarely necessary.

11.10. Golfer's Elbow

Golfer's elbow is a medical condition that causes pain in the inner side of the elbow where the tendons of the forearm muscles connect to the bony bump. This pain can spread down to the forearm and wrist. It is similar to tennis elbow which affects the outer part of the elbow. Golfer's elbow can occur in anyone who repeatedly engages in wrist movements or finger gripping activities, not just golfers. The good news is that with proper treatment and rest, people with golfer's elbow can resume their normal activities, including golf, without any significant interruption.

11.10.1. Etiology

Medial epicondylitis is a condition that can be caused by playing certain sports such as golf, American football, tennis, bowling, weightlifting, javelin throwing, archery, and other racquet sports. This condition is often seen in pitchers and athletes who throw objects overhead due to high energy valgus forces during the late cocking and acceleration phase. Golfers can also develop this condition during the peak of their backswing up to the moment before the ball hits the ground. However, over 90% of cases are not related to sports. Forceful and repetitive labor-intensive occupations such as construction, plumbing, and carpentry are also known to cause medial epicondylitis.

11.10.2. Epidemiology

According to a study, medial epicondylitis is less common than lateral epicondylitis, accounting for only 10–20% of cases. Its prevalence is about 0.4% of the population. This condition is most commonly seen in people aged 45–64, and it affects women more frequently than men. Some occupations have a higher prevalence of medial epicondylitis, ranging from 3.8% to 8.2%. More cases are found in the dominant arm. Athletes who have incorrect technique, equipment, or functional risk factors such as low strength, low endurance, or limited flexibility are at a higher risk of developing this condition. Heavy physical labor, excessive repetition, smoking, comorbidities, high body mass index (BMI), and high psychosocial work demands are all risk factors associated with certain occupations. General risk factors for this condition include type 2 diabetes mellitus and cigarette use. Women who are obese are also at higher risk. Cases of medial epicondylitis are not usually related to exercise, leisure, or recreational activities, and they are less common in people with higher education levels.

11.10.3. Pathophysiology

Medial epicondylitis, also known as overuse tendinopathy, is caused by repetitive and persistent loading of the wrist flexors and pronator teres muscles, leading to angiofibroblastic changes. This repetitive strain causes microtears in the tendon, which results in tendonosis.

All muscles, except for the palmaris longus, are equally affected, and there is no inflammation of bones. The collagen fibers in the tendon remodel due to repetitive microtears, leading to an increase in the amount of mucoid ground substance. Calcification or focal necrosis may occur, leading to a decrease in collagen strength and an increase in tendon fragility. Scar tissue formation and tendon thickening may also occur. Although less common, acute trauma can also cause medial epicondylitis due to a sudden, forceful contraction of the muscles.

11.10.4. History and Physical Details

Patients may report a history of gripping, valgus stress, or acute traumatic blows to the elbow. They may feel a sharp pain starting at the epicondyle that travels down into the wrist and forearm on the medial or ulnar side of the elbow. The pain is usually subtle despite the possibility of acute injuries. Activities such as throwing, gripping, and forearm motion can exacerbate the pain.

Athletes may experience this when performing tennis strokes with the forearm, golf swing, and overhead throwing. The pain tends to go away when there is no movement. Patients may experience elbow stiffness, weakness, numbness, or tingling, which are most commonly reported in the ulnar nerve distribution. Grip strength weakness may also be present in more persistent cases. Approximately 20% of patients may have symptoms related to the ulnar nerve.

In acute cases, abnormalities may be observed on inspection, while chronic cases are less likely to show erythema, warmth, or swelling upon examination. The area 5 to 10 millimeters distal and anterior to the medial epicondyle will be tender for the patient, particularly in the vicinity of the conjoined tendon and the pronator teres and flexor carpi radialis muscles. Pain is felt when the wrist is resistively forced to flex or pronate. The affected arm of the patient might be weak, but the range of motion is generally normal.

The test for golfer's elbow (medial epicondylitis) has two components: an active and a passive part. During the active component, the patient resists wrist flexion with the arm extended and palm facing up. The passive component involves extending the wrist with the elbow straight. If the patient experiences pain during this maneuver, the test is positive. It is essential to perform Tinel's test to check for ulnar neuropathy and to stress the ulnar collateral ligament, particularly in athletes who throw regularly.

11.10.5. Evaluation

The main way to diagnose medial epicondylitis is through clinical examination. Radiographs are useful in ruling out other causes of elbow pain as they usually show normal results. Around 20–30% of patients may exhibit signs of calcific tendinopathy or periostitis. If the child's growth plates are still open and the diagnosis is unclear, a radiographic comparison with the unaffected arm may be necessary. Ultrasound is a quick, easy, and affordable method to evaluate the muscle and tendon and differentiate it from other causes. It has a high positive and negative predictive value, sensitivity, and specificity for diagnosing medial epicondylitis. It also allows for dynamic evaluation and can detect hypoechoic tissue in areas of chronic degeneration (Figure 11.11).

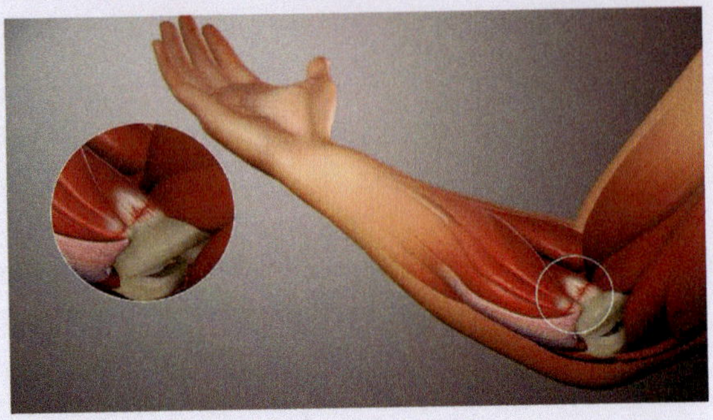

Figure 11.11. *Still shot from a 3D medical animation illustrating golfer's elbow affecting the medial epicondyle on the lower inside of the joint.*

Source: By www.scientificanimations.com – http://www.scientificanimations.com/wiki-images/, CC BY-SA 4.0, https://commons.wikimedia.org/w/index.php?curid=50860430.

Medial epicondylitis is diagnosed using a magnetic resonance imaging (MRI) test, which is also used to rule out other potential causes of medial elbow pain such as ulnar collateral ligament tears or strains, osteochondritis dissecans, or other soft tissue injuries. Computed tomography (CT) and bone scans can also help eliminate additional causes. If there is concern about involvement of the ulnar nerve, electromyograms, and nerve conduction studies may be necessary.

11.10.6. Treatment/Management

Though less common and more difficult to treat than lateral epicondylitis, the majority of medial epicondylitis cases are treated without surgery. The first course of action should be to cease the offending behaviors, which may require a reduction in their volume, frequency, or intensity. It is important to note that this may not always be feasible, especially for a professional athlete or worker who cannot afford to take time off. Acetaminophen and non-steroidal anti-inflammatory drugs (NSAIDs) are two analgesics that may provide relief. Opioids should not be used. Ice is beneficial, especially after exertion. Treatment for tendinopathies with topical nitroglycerin patches has shown promise.

Physical therapy is the primary treatment option for medial epicondylitis. The goal is to achieve complete and painless wrist and elbow motion. Eccentric activity should be the main focus of strength training. A variety of techniques such as electrical stimulation, iontophoresis, phonophoresis, dry needling, extracorporeal shockwave therapy, and ultrasonography may be helpful. Soft tissue and manipulation techniques lead to a better and faster recovery from medial epicondylitis symptoms by allowing for more intense stretching and strengthening.

Using a cock-up wrist splint at night can be helpful in unloading the tendon and reducing discomfort. Kinesiology taping applied to the elbows can also be beneficial. For more severe cases, palpation-guided corticosteroid injections or ultrasound can be employed. Platelet-rich plasma injections have been shown to reduce pain and improve function in cases of refractory epicondylitis. Botox injections have also been investigated as an off-label treatment and have shown promise in cases that are refractory. Prolotherapy may offer relief in cases that are refractory. Before surgical referral, an ultrasound-guided percutaneous tenotomy attempt may be made.

However, surgical management is typically not necessary as only 2.8% of patients require intervention. In refractory cases, debridement of pathologic tissue and release of the common flexor tendon at the epicondyle can be done surgically. The mini-open muscle resection procedure involves removing degenerative tissue of the flexor carpis radialis. Another surgical approach called facial elevation and tendon origin resection (FETOR) is also available.

11.10.7. Differential Diagnosis

The diagnosis of medial epicondylitis can be quite complex, as it can be caused by a range of different conditions. These could include nerve problems, such as C6 or C7 radiculopathy, cubital tunnel syndrome, ulnar or median neuropathy, ulnar neuritis, anterior interosseous nerve entrapment, or tardy ulnar nerve palsy.

It could also be caused by ligamentous injury, such as ulnar or medial collateral ligament instability, sprain, or tear, or osseous problems like medial epicondyle avulsion fracture or osteophytes. Intra-articular problems like adhesive capsulitis (AC), arthrofibrosis, or loose bodies, myofascial problems like flexor or pronator strain, tendinopathy (lateral epicondylitis, triceps tendonitis), synovitis, valgus extension overload, or dermatological issues (e.g., zoster herpes) could also be the cause.

11.10.8. Staging

There is no widely recognized staging protocol for medial epicondylitis.

11.10.9. Prognosis

Medial epicondylitis has a good prognosis. After undergoing physical therapy and making changes to their activities, most patients are able to return to their jobs or sports.

11.10.10. Complications

However, persistent pain is the most common complication of this condition. Other possible complications include CTS, lateral epicondylitis, rotator cuff tendinitis, ulnar neuropathy, or injury to the ulnar collateral ligament. Surgical management can also lead to complications such as injury to the ulnar nerve, infection, and medial antebrachial cutaneous nerve neuropathy.

11.10.11. Postoperative and Rehabilitation Care

Rehabilitation and post-operative care are determined by the surgeon's preference. Typically, post-operative care involves an early phase aimed at reducing pain and swelling, followed by progressive range of motion exercises, eccentric strengthening exercises, and stretching. The goal of the later phase is to resume activity.

11.10.12. Consultations

For simple cases of medial epicondylitis, a pediatrician or primary care physician can provide treatment. However, in cases of refractory symptoms, it is recommended to seek advice from an orthopedic surgeon or sports medicine specialist.

11.10.13. Deterrence and Patient Education

There are no evidence-based recommendations for preventing medial epicondylitis. The best strategy to prevent tendinitis and tendinopathy is to avoid performing the offending activity or activities too often. Maintaining physical therapy may help prevent the recurrence of medial epicondylitis in individuals who have had it in the past and have recovered.

11.10.14. Pearls and Other Issues

- Medial elbow pain is frequently caused by medial epicondylitis.
- It is linked to either an activity (plumbing, carpentry, or construction) or a job (racquet sports, golf, and throwing).
- Patients typically experience worsening medial elbow pain when their wrists flex or pronate.
- Bracing, injections, physical therapy, and non-opiate analgesia are some of the conservative management techniques used.
- Refractory cases requiring surgical release are rare.

11.10.15. Enhancing Healthcare Team Outcomes

Medial epicondylitis is a common condition that is treated by various medical professionals such as sports physicians, orthopedic nurses, emergency room doctors, primary care physicians, and orthopedic surgeons. The diagnosis is usually straightforward, but the course of treatment may vary depending on the severity of the ailment. In most cases, the offending behavior is temporarily stopped, and patients benefit from physical therapy. Nighttime splinting with a cock-up wrist splint can be helpful, as well as using a counterforce brace to reduce pain by unloading the tendon. Kinesiology taping applied to the elbows may also be beneficial. Other therapies, such as palpation-guided corticosteroid injections or ultrasound, are available. In severe cases, surgery may be the final option. Although relapse of the condition is not uncommon, most patients have good outcomes overall.

11.11. Supraspinatus Tendinitis

Supraspinatus tendinopathy is a common and painful condition that usually affects individuals over middle age. It is a leading cause of shoulder pain and affects the supraspinatus tendon, which is located in the subacromial space as part of the rotator cuff muscles. Overusing the supraspinatus tendon is thought to be the main cause of this condition. Repetitive stress and strain from sports or work-related activities can lead to degeneration of the supraspinatus tendon, resulting in tendinopathy. The tendon is prone to impingement under the acromion, passing between the acromion and the humeral head.

11.11.1. Etiology

The supraspinatus tendon muscle unit experiences the most stress forces during shoulder abduction. When the humeral head is in the abduction and forward flexion positions, it functions to lower it. This depression maintains the deltoid's mechanical advantage and, therefore, its power by keeping the humeral head centered on the glenoid. The tendon itself enters the greater tuberosity at its most anterior and superior points. The biggest dimensions of the triangular insertion footprint are 6.9 mm from medial to lateral and 12.6 mm from anterior to posterior. The short tendonous insertion that is closest to the tuberosity beneath the acromion is the point of susceptibility.

11.11.2. Pathophysiology

There are different possible causes of tendinitis in the rotator cuff, which can be classified as impingement or external mechanisms. It is important to understand the distinction between them since they lead to different rotator cuff pathologies and clinical presentations.

11.11.3. History and Physical Details

It is not always the case that rotator cuff dysfunction isolates the superior aspect of the shoulder. The most frequent reason for presenting with a rotator cuff injury is pain, and the most common sites of pain for all newcomers are anterior or lateral. A knowledgeable clinician should be able to identify the various possible origins of shoulder pain. Anterior pain, for instance, could indicate pathologies of the proximal biceps tendon; anterolateral, or straight, lateral pain, could indicate subacromial impingement or dysfunction of the rotator cuff; and posterior shoulder pain could indicate degenerative conditions of the shoulder or pain referred from the neck. Individuals who have subacromial impingement frequently report pain during overhead activities and may also report weakness. In one study, pain was a factor in the presentations of over 98% of the patients. Patients may experience weakness, deep shoulder aching, sleep disturbances, and pain with overhead activities.

To examine the shoulder, look for any obvious asymmetry in both the shoulder and the scapula. Scapular winging and dyskinesia should be assessed. In the event of rotator cuff pathology, there might or might not be wasting around the scapula. Request that the patient flex their arm forward in order to conduct a focused examination of the supraspinatus. Rotator cuff pathology may be indicated by pain during liftoff or pain at 90° to 120° of active elevation. Additionally, pain during the active, slow de-elevation of the arm could be a sign of cuff pathology. It is important to take precautions to rule out AC as a diagnosis. Both active and passive (supine) range of motion should be assessed in this case by the clinician. In cases of solitary supraspinatus tendinitis, also known as rotator cuff syndrome or dysfunction, passive range of motion should be complete in all planes.

Patients with tendonitis or isolated rotator cuff dysfunction should have normal neurovascular exams. When an evaluator notices focal weakness outside of the shoulder, decreased pulse with overhead arm positioning, or radicular or dermatomal sensory abnormalities, they should be on the lookout for alternative or concurrent diagnoses such as brachial plexopathy, thoracic outlet syndrome, cervical radiculopathy, or peripheral nerve compression. The Hawkins test, which involves flexing the arm 90° forward and passively rotating the arm significantly internally, may also replicate acromial contact with the inflamed bursa or tendon that is causing pain. In addition, the Jobe (or empty can) test requires the patient to hold their arm in the thumbs-down position, abduct it 90°, and flex it 30° forward. This position's pain and/or weakness could be signs of supraspinatus pathology. To further question the cuff, one can assess the patient in the same way by administering a thumbs up (or full can) test. The diagnosis of supraspinatus tendonitis, external shoulder impingement, or subacromial bursitis may result from a series of favorable tests. A complete supraspinatus tear may be more likely to be the cause of weakness that is frank or painless, but this finding does not rule out the diagnosis.

11.11.4. Evaluation

Assessing patients with shoulder pain can vary depending on the case, with some easily diagnosed through examination. However, those presenting with severe swelling, redness, deformation, or profound weakness might require a more thorough investigation. Initial shoulder imaging, including radiographic views, can help identify potential issues. The Dutch Orthopedic Association has set guidelines for managing subacromial pain syndrome, recommending early anti-inflammatories, injections for persistent cases, and MRI for cases lasting longer than six weeks. MRI can provide detailed information on tendon tears and inflammation, aiding in treatment decision-making. These guidelines can be helpful in providing a structured approach to patient care.

An MRI of the shoulder without contrast is the most appropriate study to characterize soft tissues in cases where the diagnosis is uncertain. This is typically recommended for patients who experience severe symptoms, are misdiagnosed, or have not responded to conservative treatment for longer than six weeks. Instability and overuse symptoms, such as secondary impingement, are usually associated with swimmers or overhead athletes. There are cases of athletes experiencing scapular dyskinesia, lax shoulders, and frequent training. For this population, physical therapy, rest, and a gradual return to activities are the cornerstones of treatment. It can be distinguished from degenerative shoulder pathologies and is more common in younger, more athletic individuals.

11.11.5. Treatment/Management

The first course of treatment for supraspinatus tendinopathy is conservative, involving stretching exercises, applying heat and cold, and avoiding activities that could worsen the condition. Painkillers and non-steroidal anti-inflammatory drugs (NSAIDs) are given initially to reduce pain and inflammation. This will alleviate discomfort and swelling. Strengthening the tendons and muscles that make up the supraspinatus is the next step in treatment. Weakness in the tendons makes it difficult to move the arm, so a physiotherapist will create exercises to help strengthen them. The physiotherapist will also design exercises to help the patient extend their shoulder range of motion, as this condition severely limits shoulder movement. Research shows that therapeutic exercises are useful for strengthening and remodeling degenerated supraspinatus tendons. Another treatment option is bracing.

Once the patient can move their arm with less difficulty and strength has begun to return, they can gradually resume daily activities. However, it is not recommended to resume regular activities until the condition has fully healed and recovered, which can take anywhere from a few weeks to four weeks. If the patient plays sports or has a job that requires a lot of overhead movement, it could take an additional two weeks. Tendinopathies are a common issue in musculoskeletal medicine, and the physician will recommend the appropriate course of action following a careful physical examination and, if necessary, diagnostic testing.

11.11.6. Differential Diagnosis

Acromioclavicular arthritis, glenohumeral arthritis, bicipital tendonitis, calcific tendonitis, AC, and subacromial impingement should all be considered in the differential diagnosis. Be aware that several of these can happen concurrently and frequently arise as a continuum of supraspinatus tendonitis.

11.11.7. Complications

Supraspinatus tendonitis can lead to the development of a rotator cuff tear. It was initially believed that untreated impingement, along with tendon hemorrhage and tendonitis, caused rotator cuff tears. If an individual experiences repeated episodes, they may require surgery where rotator cuff attrition can be identified. In these cases, there is more than a 50% chance that subclinical rotator cuff tendinopathy could progress to clinical symptoms.

11.11.8. Deterrence and Patient Education

It may be useful to educate patients on safe overhead work practices to prevent shoulder injuries. However, it's doubtful that this effort would completely eliminate the disease process, considering how common it is. Instead, patients should be taught about the importance of non-operative measures, the possibility of the disease progressing, and the range of treatment options available to them. This will empower them to take an active role in their own care.

11.11.9. Enhancing Healthcare Team Outcomes

Managing a patient with supraspinatus tendonitis can be challenging, particularly in complex cases. It requires collaborative teamwork among healthcare professionals, including imaging colleagues, nursing staff, and physical therapists. Clear communication among all team members regarding their respective responsibilities is necessary to provide the best possible care for the patient. According to available data, a therapy-based approach that avoids surgery may be the best course of action for this patient. The care team should focus on providing education, a clear plan of care, and goals. A specialized nurse with orthopedic expertise can assist with the examination, arrange physical therapy, and support any necessary surgical procedures. If medication is being used, the physician and nurse can collaborate with a pharmacist to ensure that the dosage is appropriate and there are no drug interactions. It is essential for the patient's recovery that all members of the care team communicate any acute changes in function, as these patients may experience significant rotator cuff failure in the future.

11.12. Adhesive Capsulitis (AC)

Frozen shoulder, also known as adhesive capsulitis (AC), is a condition that causes pain and stiffness in the shoulder. Over time, the shoulder becomes extremely difficult to move. Although a frozen shoulder can improve after a period of worsening symptoms, it may take up to three years to fully recover. Physical therapy is the main recommended treatment for frozen shoulder, with an emphasis on shoulder flexibility. Frozen shoulder is most commonly experienced by people between the ages of 40 and 60, and women are more likely than men to be affected by it. Moreover, individuals with diabetes and thyroid disorders are at a higher risk of developing frozen shoulder. However, anyone can experience it at any time, and it may occur following surgery or an injury.

11.12.1. Etiology

The exact cause of frozen shoulder is still unknown. Nonetheless, a few likely risk factors have been found:

- Diabetes mellitus (with a prevalence of up to 20%);
- Stroke;
- Thyroid disorder;
- Shoulder injury;
- Dupuytren disease;
- Parkinson disease;
- Cancer;
- Complex regional pain syndrome (CRPS).

11.12.2. Epidemiology

Adhesive capsulitis (AC) affects up to 5% of cases. It is more common in the non-dominant shoulder and more prevalent in women than men.

11.12.3. Pathophysiology

Frozen shoulder is often described as the fibrotic, inflammatory contracture of the rotator interval, capsule, and ligaments. However, there is still much to learn about this condition. According to arthroscopic observations, the most widely accepted pathology involves cytokine-mediated synovial inflammation with fibroblastic proliferation. Adhesions caused by increased collagen around the rotator interval and the formation of nodular bands are also common findings. The first structure to be impacted is usually the coracohumeral ligament, which is responsible for restricting external rotation of the arm in early frozen shoulder. In later stages, the glenohumeral joint capsule thickens and contracts, further limiting range of motion in all directions.

11.12.4. Histopathology

Histopathology studies of the glenohumeral capsule have shown an increase in fibroblasts, myofibroblasts, and inflammatory cells such as mast cells, B lymphocytes, and macrophages.

11.12.5. History and Physical Details

Individuals with early AC typically experience sudden, unilateral anterior shoulder pain. Passive and active range of motion is restricted, affecting external rotation first and then shoulder abduction. Depending on the stage and severity, the condition can interfere with daily activities, work, and leisure. Frozen shoulder can cause limited reaching, especially during overhead (e.g., hanging clothes) or side-reaching (e.g., fastening a seatbelt) activities. Patients also experience limited shoulder rotation, making it difficult to dress, brush their hair, and maintain personal hygiene. Neck pain is a common complication of frozen shoulder due to the overuse of cervical muscles to compensate for the loss of shoulder motion.

Patients often have difficulty complying with a full series of physical examinations due to the pain and stiffness associated with frozen shoulder. However, physical findings are crucial for a proper diagnosis. Two physical examinations, which involve tests of combined motion and touching the scapula from behind the neck and behind the back, are frequently used to diagnose AC. The most pathognomonic characteristic of AC is the loss of passive range of motion. In practical terms, a review of active motion may be omitted if there is a significant limitation of passive range of motion. However, in patients who present with a progressive restriction of range of motion at follow-ups, the diagnosis of AC should be reexamined because an imperceptible limitation of shoulder motion may exist in the early stages.

Patients with a frozen shoulder typically exhibit marked limitations in both their active and passive range of motion, particularly in external rotation and abduction. Limited range of motion not only suggests that a frozen shoulder has developed, but it can also be a "red flag" for an underlying cancer or fracture.

11.12.6. Evaluation

A diagnosis of frozen shoulder is made by taking a patient's medical history, performing a physical examination, and using imaging techniques to rule out other conditions rather than confirming the presence of AC. It is difficult to definitively confirm the diagnosis of AC with a single test, either lab or imaging. Diagnostic imaging is only useful for ruling out other diseases that may coexist, such as glenohumeral joint osteoarthritis and rotator cuff tendon tears. Musculoskeletal ultrasonography (MUS) is the primary imaging technique used for shoulder pathology, but there are currently no specific ultrasonography findings available for the diagnosis of AC. However, thickening of the coracohumeral ligament and fluid accumulation around the long head of the biceps tendon are two features that may be found in AC patients. While these findings are common in shoulders with AC, biceps peri-tendinous effusion is unique to AC, but may be present in other shoulder pathologies. Ultrasonography is less helpful in diagnosing instability or SLAP lesions. Routine radiographs of the shoulder are recommended to rule out other causes, such as tumors or osteoarthritis in the glenohumeral and acromioclavicular regions. The glenohumeral joint capsule and coracohumeral ligament may appear thicker on an MRI, and an MRI arthrography could reveal a decrease in the joint space volume.

The "lidocaine test" is a diagnostic tool used to identify subacromial conditions that are unclear through clinical examination. The test involves injecting local anesthetics into the subacromial space to observe the patient's response. Patients with AC will experience passive movement limitation even after the injection. Conversely, patients with subacromial impingement syndrome (such as rotator cuff or bursa pathology) will typically experience an improvement in passive range of motion after the injection. The injection can be administered with ease under ultrasonography guidance.

11.12.7. Treatment/Management

Pharmacological management and physical therapy comprise the majority of non-operative treatment options for AC.

11.12.7.1. Early Frozen Shoulder

Early AC is often treated as subacromial pathology. The early "freezing" stage of AC can be classified as inflammatory. However, as the condition progresses, range of motion restriction becomes more predominant, and inflammation-related pain becomes less severe. Therefore, the inflammation becomes less pronounced in later stages. It is important to take the disease stage into account when developing a treatment plan. Accurate identification of the clinical stage can aid in more specialized treatment planning. During the "freezing" stage, the main goals of treatment should be patient education, pain management, and inflammation reduction. Acetaminophen or nonsteroidal anti-inflammatory drugs (NSAIDs) are potential first treatments for AC. Although there is little evidence to support the use of NSAIDs in the treatment of frozen shoulder, they may be prescribed to treat the condition if it is causing nighttime pain. However, opioid analgesics might be necessary in extreme circumstances.

To manage pain and regain normal shoulder mobility, physical therapy is essential. Manual therapies that use mild stretching and soft tissue mobilization are effective in this regard. In terms of physical modalities, no agent has proven to be better than another. The patient may receive a prescription, such as cryotherapy, transcutaneous electrical nerve stimulation (TENS) unit, or therapeutic ultrasound. Therapeutic exercise should be the main focus of physical therapy management. During the initial stage of frozen shoulder, some patients may not tolerate mobilization exercises due to extreme pain. However, to slow down range of motion restriction, supervised therapeutic exercise should be performed. Additionally, the patients should receive a daily home exercise program.

For patients with moderate-to-severe pain who do not respond to non-operative treatments, intra-articular corticosteroid injection should be taken into consideration. For accurate needle placement, fluoroscopic or ultrasonographic guidance should be used when administering the injection. After an injection, rehabilitation exercises ought to be recommended.

11.12.7.2. Developed Frozen Shoulder

The illness of frozen shoulder progresses through the "frozen" and "thawing" phases after the inflammation-induced painful period ends. In the advanced stages, the goal of treatment should be to restore the limited range of motion. Physical therapists should provide a comprehensive set of exercises for mobilization to restore joint mobility, especially for subacromial pathologies. For patients who do not respond well to non-operative treatments, invasive therapies such as blocking the suprascapular nerve or the interscalene brachial plexus may be considered. In cases where non-operative treatment fails to yield improvement after six months, patients may consider more aggressive treatments like arthroscopic capsular release (especially in the rotator interval), manipulation under anesthesia, and capsular hydrodilatation, which involves stretching the joint capsule by applying pressure from a saline injection.

11.12.8. Differential Diagnosis

Adhesive capsulitis (AC), commonly known as frozen shoulder, can be challenging to diagnose as its symptoms are similar to rotator cuff tendinopathy and subacromial pathology, mainly in the early (freezing) stage. Early diagnosis of AC may be delayed as it may present with similar symptoms to other shoulder conditions. Patients typically experience pain, and there may be a less noticeable range of motion in the case of rotator cuff pathology and shoulder impingement. However, frozen shoulder can be differentiated from other shoulder conditions in a few ways. Patients with frozen shoulder often report a history of overuse activity or a spontaneous onset without any known cause, while patients with rotator cuff pathology and shoulder impingement usually report performing repetitive overhead movements or lifting heavy objects as causes. If there is a history of cancer, extra care should be taken while diagnosing and treating the condition.

Typical illnesses that resemble early adhesive capsulitis include:

- Rotator cuff tendinopathy and subacromial pathology;
- Post-stroke subluxation of the shoulder;
- Referred pain (cervical spine or malignancy, e.g., Pancoast tumor).

As the frozen shoulder progresses, severe restriction of motion becomes more evident, making diagnosis easier. However, it's important to consider the possibility of glenohumeral joint arthritis, which can be ruled out by allowing the shoulder to move freely after a lidocaine injection to the joint. The age of onset can also provide useful information for diagnosis. Patients under 40 are less likely to develop frozen shoulder, while those over 70 are more likely to experience glenohumeral osteoarthritis or rotator cuff tears rather than AC.

11.12.9. Staging

AC refers to adhesive capsulitis, which is a condition where passive shoulder motion becomes progressively restricted. Typically, the development of this condition is classified into three overlapping phases, but it is recommended to use a simpler two-stage scheme: early and developed frozen shoulder, for practical purposes.

- Freezing (2 to 9 months): Early;
- Frozen (4 to 12 months): Developed;
- Thawing (12 to 42 months): Developed.
- **Freezing:** An initial painful phase that worsens at night and gradually restricts range of motion in the glenohumeral joint.
- **Frozen:** The second phase was less painful than the "Freezing" stage, but it still included stiffness and a persistent limitation in glenohumeral joint motion.
- **Thawing:** The third stage, or recovery phase, during which range of motion gradually returns.

11.12.10. Prognosis

AC length ranges from 1 to 3.5 years with a mean of 30 months. After five years, 15% of patients experience symptoms in the opposite shoulder.

11.12.11. Complications

- Residual pain;
- Residual stiffness;
- Fracture of the humerus;
- Rupture of the biceps tendon after shoulder manipulation.

11.12.12. Consultations

- Physical therapy;
- Pain specialist;
- Orthopedic surgeon.

11.12.13. Enhancing Healthcare Team Outcomes

A team of medical experts that includes an orthopedic surgeon, a rehabilitation specialist, a nurse practitioner, a pharmacist, and a pain consultant are typically involved in managing frozen shoulder. The pharmacist is also responsible for instructing the patient on how to manage their pain. Patients receiving corticosteroids require close monitoring for any adverse drug reactions. Physical therapy is the key to recovery for most patients. Supervised home physical therapy may be beneficial for some patients. Finally, patients must be informed that while recovery is possible, it will be gradual and may take years.

11.12.13.1. Outcomes

Most individuals with frozen shoulder eventually recover, although it may take anywhere from one to three years. Regular physical therapy and arm exercises will usually result in a gradual improvement in symptoms. At present, data does not suggest that people with diabetes experience worse outcomes than individuals without the disease. However, about 10% of patients may still experience shoulder stiffness and impairment. After undergoing arthroscopic surgery, symptoms typically improve gradually, but the recovery process is slow. To ensure complete recovery, postoperative physical therapy is necessary.

11.13. Calcaneal Spur

A bone spur, also known as a heel spur, protrudes from the bottom of the heel where the heel bone joins the plantar fascia, the ligament that runs from the heel to the ball of the foot. Approximately 15% of people suffer from heel spurs, which gradually increase in size over time. Many individuals are unaware of their heel spur until they experience heel pain and seek treatment. Non-surgical treatments can help alleviate symptoms, but surgical removal is also a viable option for treating heel spurs.

11.13.1. Signs and Symptoms

One of the most common symptoms of heel spur is pain around the affected area. This pain usually intensifies after prolonged periods of rest, and some patients report that their heel pain is worse when they wake up in the morning. Patients may find it uncomfortable to put weight on the injured heel, and the problem may worsen if the patient engage in activities such as running, walking or lifting heavy weights.

11.13.2. Causes

Calcaneal spurs are often caused by plantar fasciitis, a condition that results from stress on the plantar fascia ligament. This stress can lead to the formation of a heel spur where the plantar fascia connects to the heel bone.

Several factors can contribute to plantar heel pain, including foot alignment with the lower leg and ankle, foot mobility, muscle strength and endurance. External factors such as the type of shoe worn, the kind of floor walked on, and the length of time spent standing or exercising on the feet can also impact plantar heel pain. Improper foot and heel care can lead to the formation of calcaneal spurs. Heel spurs are most prevalent in people who are obese, have flat feet, or frequently wear high-heeled shoes. Flat feet may result from minimal ankle dorsiflexion during the stance phase of the gait cycle, which increases tension on the plantar fascia.

11.13.3. Diagnosis

A lateral foot X-ray can be used in conjunction with a physical examination to identify spur outgrowths (Figure 11.12).

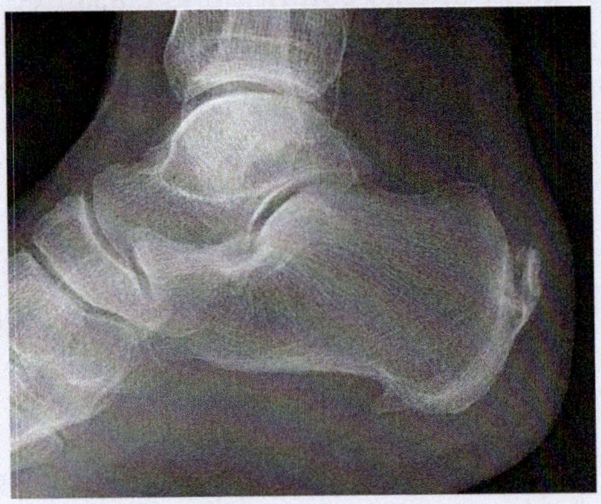

Figure 11.12. *A radiograph showing osteophytes on the posterior and inferior aspects of the calcaneus.*

Source: By Mikael Häggström – Own work, CC0, https://commons.wikimedia.org/w/index.php?curid=55092349.

11.13.4. Treatment

Frequently regarded as a repetitive stress injury, modifying one's lifestyle is typically the first step in a management plan. For example, focusing on working out one's calves and feet can be beneficial. Strong muscles in the lower legs and calves can prevent the formation of heel spurs by relieving pressure on the bone. Instant pain relief can be achieved by applying ice to the affected area. Additionally, there are various ways to relieve plantar heel pain. Many foot diseases are associated with plantar heel pain. Corticosteroid injections have proven to reduce pain for up to a month after the injection, which may have an impact on the development of calcaneal spurs. However, corticosteroid injections have side effects such as peripheral nerve injury, plantar fascia rupture, and post-injection flare. Although calcaneal taping, dry needling, and laser therapy are used to manage plantar heel pain, there is no concrete evidence to support their clinical application in pain management.

11.13.5. Prognosis

Studies tracking patients with plantar fasciitis and calcaneal spur found that 20%–75% had no symptoms within a year or less.

11.14. Neuropathic Joint

Injuries to a neuropathic extremity can lead to a severe joint condition called Charcot neuropathic osteoarthropathy. This condition can cause foot fractures and dislocations, which can be very debilitating. It is important to accurately diagnose and treat acute Charcot to prevent irreversible foot deformities and enable a stable, plantigrade foot that is suitable for walking.

11.14.1. Etiology

Charcot neuropathic osteoarthropathy is a condition that affects people with various peripheral neuropathies and causes bone and joint fragmentation in the foot and ankle. This condition is typically triggered by trauma, diabetes, neuropathy, and metabolic abnormalities of the bone. The inflammatory response can cause abnormal plantar pressures that put the foot's bony architecture permanently at risk for ulceration, osteomyelitis, and amputation. Diabetic neuropathy is the most common cause of Charcot. This debilitating condition affects patients with established peripheral neuropathy in their lower extremities. There are numerous complex etiologies for this condition, which can also be caused by leprosy, poliomyelitis, syphilis, syringomyelia, spinal cord injury, and chronic alcoholism.

11.14.2. Epidemiology

It is estimated that Charcot affects between 0.1% and 0.9% of people with diabetes, and 63% of patients with Charcot neuropathic osteoarthropathy experience foot ulcerations.

11.14.3. Pathophysiology

There are two widely accepted theories that explain the pathophysiology of Charcot. These are the neuro-traumatic and neurovascular theories. According to the neuro-traumatic theory, repeated microtrauma causes joint destruction and neuropathy. On the other hand, the neurovascular theory believes that increased peripheral blood flow leads to osteolysis and demineralization.

Certain inflammatory markers have been found to be linked to the emergence of an acute Charcot foot. One of these markers is the cytokine nuclear factor-kB ligand (RANKL), which plays a critical role in the development of Charcot by promoting the growth of osteoclastogenesis. Normally, calcitonin gene-related peptide (CGRP) inhibits the synthesis of RANKL at the nerve terminal. However, CGRP is not active in the neuropathic foot, which means there is no inhibition to the synthesis of RANKL.

Osteoprotegerin (OPG) typically moderates the RANKL osteoclastic relationship by serving as a decoy receptor for RANKL binding. However, this correlation between RANKL and OPG is broken in the Charcot foot. The uncontrolled synthesis of RANKL is responsible for the increased bone turnover and accumulation observed in the Charcot limb. CGRP may also play a role in maintaining the integrity of the joint capsule. Its absence in the Charcot foot may result in the joint destruction and dislocation that characterize the condition.

11.14.4. Histopathology

Histological features such as irregular cartilage thinning, subchondral cysts, sclerotic bone, and ghost chondrocytes can resemble degenerative joint disease. It is important to differentiate between osteomyelitis and acute Charcot joint inflammation through histology and bone biopsies. Osteomyelitis is characterized by bone necrosis, reactive new bone formation, and the presence of plasma cells, lymphocytes, and neutrophils. Additionally, there may be capillary proliferation and fibrosis.

11.14.5. History and Physical Details

In order to accurately diagnose Charcot, there must be a high suspicion for it. Charcot is marked by an erythematous foot that has swelling and redness. It often occurs unilaterally and presents with an abrupt onset of symptoms that may be caused by repeated micro-trauma (walking) or macro-trauma (ankle sprain). Initially, Charcot can be misdiagnosed as cellulitis or deep vein thrombosis because of their similar clinical appearances – a red, hot, swollen foot with skeletal lysis on radiographs – and frequently unilateral presentation. Osteomyelitis and Charcot can be mistaken for one another, but these entities can happen at the same time even though they are different and distinct processes. Additionally, there is evidence that Charcot can be caused by osteomyelitis because osteomyelitis causes the body to release cytokines, which trigger an inflammatory cascade.

If the infected bone was surgically removed, the chance of osteomyelitis developing into Charcot is increased even more. This is because trauma in the form of osteomyelitis and surgery both encourage an inflammatory response that opens the door for Charcot to appear.

Surgery can cause trauma and alter the shape of the foot, which can lead to changes in the way the patient walk and put pressure on the foot. This can trigger inflammation, especially if you've had an amputation or other foot surgery that changes the pressure points on the foot. Even slight changes in pressure can cause small injuries that set off a chain reaction of inflammation, leading to a condition called acute Charcot.

11.14.6. Evaluation

11.14.6.1. Stages of Charcot

There are two popular classification schemes available for mapping the phases of Charcot, namely the Sanders and Frykberg classification and the Eichenholtz classification. The Eichenholtz classification describes the three stages of disease progression based on clinical and radiographic findings. On the other hand, the Sanders/Frykberg classification is used for typing and classifying the five common anatomical locations of Charcot in the foot.

11.14.6.2. Eichenholtz

Stage 0 Pre-Charcot/Prodromal:

- Clinically: swollen, red, and heated foot. Absolutely no deformity.
- Radiographically, there have not been any changes. Normal radiograph.

Stage I Development/Destruction:

- Clinically: no pain, elevated temperature, erythema, and foot edema.
- Radiographically, the presence of fracture-dislocation, subchondral bone fragmentation, subluxation of the joint, and bony debris at the joints can be observed.

Stage II Coalescence:

- Clinically: Less inflammatory markers.
- A worsening of features in stage 1. Bone fragments are being taken in while forming new bone, and larger fragments are coalescing together with endogenous sclerosis. There is also increased stability.

Stage III Consolidation:

- Inflammation resolution and bone remodeling can cause changes to foot architecture and create new pressure points that increase the risk of ulceration.
- Radiographically: Remodeling of affected bones and joints

Sanders and Frykberg:

- Metatarsophalangeal to interphalangeal joints: 15%;
- Tarsometatarsal joints: 40%;
- Naviculocuneiform joint, navicular-cuneiform, talonavicular and calcaneocuboid joints: 30%;
- Ankle and subtalar joints: 10%;
- Calcaneus: 5%.

11.14.7. Treatment/Management

The objective of treating Charcot foot is to reduce the deformity of the foot over time, so that a stable and functional foot that is suitable for walking can eventually develop. During the acute phase, it is crucial to immobilize the foot and limit weight-bearing to prevent any permanent deformities. This can be achieved through non-operative methods such as fully non-weight-bearing or protective weight-bearing devices. Assistive technologies such as wheelchairs and crutches can help with non-weight-bearing. For weight-bearing protection, total contact casts (TCC) can be used in combination with a controlled ankle motion (CAM) walker. TCC (Total Contact Casting) is a method that allows a person to walk while reducing and distributing pressure on the foot. According to the Eichenholtz classification, the hyperemic phase can linger for weeks. If the rate of healing is not outpaced by stress, the foot may heal the fractures in a stable position with the use of these protective measures.

There are various pharmacological treatments available to regulate osteoclastic activity in Charcot foot, such as bisphosphonates and calcitonin supplements. Bisphosphonates can be beneficial in the acute phase of the condition as they inhibit osteoclastic reabsorption. Calcitonin also acts as an antiresorptive agent. Other options include pamidronate or zoledronic acid, which target osteoclast precursors in newly formed bone matrix.

Surgery is another treatment option, but the timing of intervention in acute or chronic Charcot phase is still debated. In the acute phase, there is increased inflammation and cytokines that lead to edema and bone resorption. The goal of Charcot foot reconstruction is to surgically off-load the affected area to prevent ulceration and deformity progression. Surgeons may use techniques such as exostectomy, tenotomy, or fusion with external and internal fixation. Additional hardware may be used to reinforce the soft bone and create a stable structure. Minimally invasive intramedullary techniques may also be employed, depending on the surgeon's expertise.

Optimizing medical conditions such as smoking cessation, controlling HbA1c to below 7%–8%, and recognizing micro- or macro-vascular disease can lessen potential complications post-operatively.

11.14.8. Differential Diagnosis

Given that both conditions can have similar radiological and clinical appearances, osteomyelitis is the most significant differential diagnosis for Charcot. Important differentials include cellulitis, septic arthritis, gout, pseudogout, foot/ankle sprains or fractures, and deep vein thrombosis. Around 25% of the time, Charcot is misdiagnosed, which can delay the correct diagnosis by up to seven months.

11.14.9. Treatment Planning

The process of diagnosing and validating a clinically suspected Charcot foot requires diagnostic imaging, including initial radiographs. The disease's progression through the Eichenholtz stages is then tracked using serial radiographs of the foot or ankle. In order to visualize the extent of the bone destruction for pre-operative planning, a CT scan might be necessary before surgery. Nuclear imaging of labeled white blood cells has a high sensitivity and specificity when used to distinguish between Charcot and osteomyelitis (Figure 11.13).

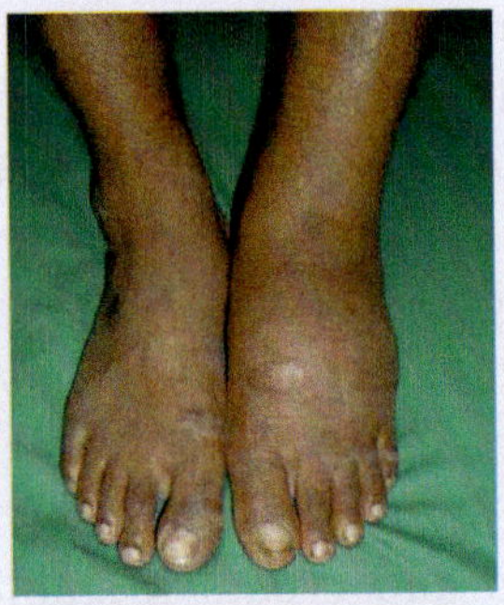

Figure 11.13. *A 45-year-old man with diabetes mellitus presented with diffusely swollen, warm, and non-tender left foot due to Charcot arthropathy. There are no changes to the skin itself.*

Source: By J. Terrence Jose Jerome – Divergent Lisfranc's Dislocation and Fracture in the Charcot Foot: A case report. Foot and Ankle Online Journal (FAOJ), 1(6), 3., CC BY 3.0, https://commons.wikimedia.org/w/index.php?curid=8685599.

11.14.10. Complications

- Foot deformities include hammertoes, ankle equinus contracture, flatfoot, and rocker-bottom feet.
- Boney prominences, which may result in infection, ulceration, or even death in certain situations.
- Recurrence of Charcot joint
- From the first diagnosis of acute Charcot, the five-year mortality rate is 13%, which is similar to diabetics without Charcot.

11.14.11. Deterrence and Patient Education

Patients should be made aware of the gravity of their illness and the potentially fatal consequences that may arise from not strictly adhering to the treatment plan. In cases of Charcot joint deformity, a rigid and deformed foot may necessitate multiple phases of reconstructive surgery. Conversely, a Charcot joint-induced rocker bottom deformity can rapidly progress into a neuropathic ulceration accompanied by an underlying bone infection, which may ultimately require amputation. The likelihood of a major lower extremity amputation increases by 15 to 40 times when a foot exhibits a rocker bottom deformity. The five-year mortality rate following a major amputation in diabetic patients ranges from 30% to 80%. Furthermore, diabetics who undergo major amputations have higher mortality rates after one and five years compared to those with breast and colon cancer. Basic preventive measures encompass avoiding injuries, ensuring appropriate glucose control, and conducting daily self-foot checks.

11.14.12. Pearls and Other Issues

Charcot osteoarthropathy is a rare but serious complication of peripheral neuropathy that can mimic various other common diabetic foot conditions. It is important to make an accurate diagnosis of Charcot osteoarthropathy as it can lead to permanent foot deformity, increasing the risk of ulceration and amputation. Treatment during the acute phase involves immobilizing the affected limb and avoiding weight-bearing to prevent any further damage. However, achieving complete immobilization and non-weight bearing is not always possible, and non-adherence may arise due to factors such as the length of time needed for non-weight bearing, physical incapacity, and work-related constraints. In such cases, offloading ambulating devices can be used as an alternative treatment option. These devices include knee scooters, total contact casts, and CAM walkers with offloading insoles.

11.14.13. Enhancing Healthcare Team Outcomes

Interprofessional collaboration is crucial for managing Charcot joints because misdiagnosis or nontreatment can exacerbate the condition and lead to amputation. The two primary goals of treatment are to prevent the neuropathic joint from deteriorating and prevent amputation. Immobilization may be helpful in the acute phase, and later on, the patient may be instructed to reduce weight-bearing. For most patients, an ambulatory device can be beneficial. Protected weight-bearing can be achieved by combining total contact casts (TCC) with a CAM walker. TCC is an effective method that redistributes and reduces pressure on the plantar foot while allowing ambulation. According to the Eichenholtz classification, the hyperemic phase can last for several weeks. If the stress does not exceed the rate of healing, the foot can heal fractures in a stable position with the use of these protective measures. Additionally, there are pharmaceutical interventions such as bisphosphonates and calcitonin supplements that can regulate osteoclastic activity. Lastly, patients must wear appropriate footwear both indoors and outside and receive education on foot safety. Unfortunately, there is always a risk of amputation once Charcot joint develops.

11.15. Congenital Torticollis or Wry Neck

Torticollis is a condition where the muscles in the baby's neck become twisted, causing their head to tilt to one side. This can make their neck appear to be at an unusual angle, with their chin slanted to one side and the top of their head to the other.

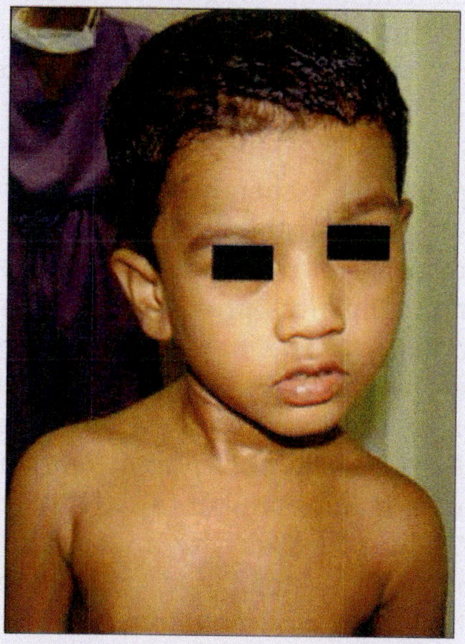

Figure 11.14. *Preoperative clinical photograph of a child with congenital muscular torticollis affecting the right sternocleidomastoid muscle.*

Source: Kumar, N., & Srijon, M., (2013). "Congenital muscular torticollis," Ann Maxillofac Surg., 3(2), 198–200. doi: 10.4103/2231-0746.119222.

Torticollis is also known as wryneck, and its name derives from the Latin words "tortus," meaning twisted, and "collum," meaning neck. It is a common condition in babies and children and can be either congenital, present from birth, or acquired later in infancy or childhood.

Congenital torticollis is the most common type. The baby is unlikely to experience any pain, and may not notice it until they gain more control of their movements, usually a few weeks after birth (Figure 11.14).

Acquired torticollis can develop in babies during their first four to six months of life or later. It can occur suddenly or gradually. This condition can be either harmless or indicate a serious underlying health problem.

11.15.1. Etiology

The exact cause of congenital torticollis is unknown, and there are multiple theories. However, none of them are supported by evidence. The most commonly mentioned conditions include intrauterine malposition (pelvic position), ischemia, and birth trauma. Intrauterine malformation is the most likely reason for congenital torticollis. It is more likely to occur during first pregnancies, decreased amniotic fluid volume, or uterine compression syndrome, which are associated with limited intrauterine space. Other causes of congenital torticollis include positional deformation, vertebral anomalies, unilateral atlantooccipital fusion, Klippel-Feil syndrome, unilateral absence of sternocleidomastoid, and pterygium colli. Congenital muscular torticollis is the most common type of torticollis in children and is linked to anomalies in the sternocleidomastoid muscle.

The muscles in the neck work together in a complex system. There are two levels of muscles: the deep muscles near the spine and the superficial muscles near the surface. The most commonly targeted muscle is the sternocleidomastoid, which is located at the front of the neck and is visible and palpable. Its fibers have an upward and outward direction, and it attaches to the sternum (breastbone), clavicle (collarbone), occipital region (back of the head) and mastoid process (bony bump behind the ear). It is responsible for tilting the head to one side, flexing the head forward, and rotating the head to the opposite side. If this muscle is injured, the head and neck will tilt towards the side of the injury and rotate to the opposite side. This condition is usually diagnosed in newborns or infants.

11.15.2. Epidemiology

Congenital torticollis, a condition where the neck muscles of a newborn are twisted or contracted, has a worldwide incidence rate of between 0.3% and 1.9%. According to some studies, it is the third most common congenital orthopedic anomaly, affecting 1 in every 250 newborns, with a higher incidence rate in male newborns and first pregnancies. The incidence of congenital torticollis is 2% in traumatic births and 0.3% in non-traumatic births. During delivery, around 19% and 56% of pelvic presentations require the use of forceps and suction cups, respectively, which can increase the risk of traumatic birth and congenital torticollis. Children born to first-time mothers have a higher incidence rate of 53% and are more likely to experience traumatic childbirth. The condition typically appears in newborns between the ages of two to three weeks and can last for up to a year. It usually affects only one side of the neck, but in rare cases, it can affect both sides. In 50% of cases, a visible and palpable swelling called sternomastoid tumor is present.

Congenital muscular torticollis is categorized into three types:

- **Postural (20%):** The baby prefers a certain posture, but there is no muscle tension or restriction of passive range of motion.
- **Muscular (30%):** There is a limit to the baby's passive range of motion due to muscle tightness in the sternocleidomastoid muscle.
- **Sternocleidomastoid Mass (50%):**

The baby has restricted passive range of motion and thickening of the sternocleidomastoid muscle.

11.15.3. Pathophysiology

In cases of congenital muscular torticollis, a palpable mass can be felt in the sternocleidomastoid muscle. This mass is mainly made up of fibrous tissue. Typically, it disappears during infancy and is replaced by a fibrous band. Muscle biopsies and MRI analyzes of the mass suggest that there might be muscle damage, most likely caused by compression and stretching. It's also possible that the compression of the venous neck during childbirth resulted in reduced blood flow, leading to compartmental syndrome. Histological examinations of material taken at delivery revealed fibrosis, degeneration of the muscle fibers, and edema, indicating the presence of compartment syndrome.

11.15.4. Histopathology

Congenital torticollis is primarily characterized by endomysial fibrosis, which results in collagen deposition and fibroblast accumulation around the muscle fibers, ultimately causing muscle atrophy. Examining the area closely reveals no necrosis or hemorrhages. Under a microscope, degenerative skeletal muscle fiber, scar-like collagen, and a diffuse proliferation of uniform fibroblasts and myofibroblasts are visible. It exhibits positive staining for actin and vimentin.

11.15.5. History and Physical Details

A comprehensive clinical history, the presence or absence of a history of oligohydramnios, a history of trauma during delivery or pelvic presentation, and a careful physical examination with special attention to sternocleidomastoid palpation should all be included in the evaluation of a newborn. Reduced range of motion and a painless swelling across the side of the neck are among the findings; these are visible in newborns between two and three weeks old. Infants typically present with their heads tilted and flexed to the side of the lesion if the mass is small or missed during the neonatal period. Around 50% of cases have a diagnosis confirmed before two months; most cases are reported by parents; some cases correlate with plagiocephaly, though the correlation may differ based on the type of nodule found. It might develop for two months until it reaches about the size of an almond, at which point it might start to regress and eventually vanish completely by the eighth month of life.

The sternocleidomastoid muscle gets thicker and more compressed in older children, which leads to restricted neck movement in rotating and tilting. This rotation can cause positional plagiocephaly, which is a flattening of the head. This condition might also be linked to other musculoskeletal issues like brachial plexus palsy, developmental dysplasia of the hip, and positional musculoskeletal deformities including metatarsus adductus and calcaneovalgus feet. Infants with congenital torticollis tend to sleep on the affected side, leading to unilateral muscle shortening. This position applies uneven pressure on the developing facial bones and skull, which can result in cheekbone remodeling, leading to facial hemihypoplasia or plagiocephaly. These changes also affect proper breastfeeding positioning, making it harder for the baby to suckle. As a child grows and develops motor skills, language, and balance in various postures like sitting and crawling, compensations from disparate systems may arise, which can affect orthostatic postures such as scoliosis.

11.15.6. Evaluation

The simplest and most efficient way to diagnose is through a physical examination. Physical therapists can perform an arthrodial goniometer assessment to measure the passive cervical range of motion. Other representative assessment methods for congenital torticollis include an active range of motion assessment and a global assessment. Assessing the nervous system and the auditory system is essential to ruling out other differential diagnoses. To ascertain whether the pupil fixes and follows objects, it is imperative to evaluate the following aspects of visual function: pupillary response to light, red reflex presence, and eye alignment. The oculomotor muscles (lateral rectus or superior oblique) may frequently be weak; torticollis arises as a compensatory mechanism to enhance vision. If a physical examination reveals no signs of muscle contracture and intact joint amplitudes, then ophthalmology should be consulted regarding this suspicion.

In patients with congenital torticollis, the observed incidence of hip dysplasia is about 15%. According to other studies, one in five babies has hip dysplasia associated with it. A higher incidence of hip dysplasia is correlated with several risk factors, including female sex, first childbirth, a family history of hip dysplasia, the presence of other deformities like congenital torticollis, pelvic presentation at birth, cesarean delivery, and large fetus. Although it is usually unilateral, this condition can also be bilateral. Hip dysplasia must be diagnosed as soon as possible. The prognosis is improved by early detection and effective treatment of this asymptomatic condition in newborns. Delayed diagnosis can lead to consequences such as mental impairment, degenerative arthritis, chronic pain, and lameness.

As a result, proper screening for hip dysplasia is crucial for identifying the condition's clinical symptoms and ensuring an early diagnosis. If in doubt, consult a specialist. Both major and minor clinical signs are systematically used in the clinical diagnosis. Hip abduction limitation and the Ortolani/Barlow sign are major indicators. The asymmetry of the folds (thighs and inguinal) and the Galeazzi sign are the minor indicators. Planning a course of treatment for congenital torticolis requires careful assessment. Clinical signs of congenital torticollis include:

- Fibrosis, or the sternocleidomastoid muscle shortening.
- A significant reduction in the range of motion of the neck, coupled with a tilt of the head in the frontal plane and rotation in the transverse plane towards the opposite side.
- During the first three months of life, there was a noticeable tumor-like mass on the sternocleidomastoid muscle, which resulted in limited neck mobility and a fixed, tilted neck position.
- Modification of cranial morphology associated with plagiocephaly can be corrected by repositioning the ear and flattening the affected areas of the skull.
- Compensation positions for the affected side in the cervical, thoracic, trunk, extremities, shoulder elevation, or trunk inclination.

Most diagnoses are made clinically; complementary diagnostic tests are rarely used to make a diagnosis. Around 50% of cases have a diagnosis made before two months; most cases are identified by the parents and may be associated with plagiocephaly. Particularly during the neonatal stage, ultrasonography is the most often used imaging modality. To rule out nonmuscular causes of torticollis, magnetic resonance imaging (MRI) can be helpful. In addition to long-term monitoring and post-treatment evaluation, ultrasound is useful in evaluating neck masses and pseudo-tumors. The edema is firm, soft to the touch, and movable beneath the skin. Severity affects the age at which a presentation occurs; postural is the earlier form. Between the ages of 4 and 8 months, the tumor usually goes away.

In cases where the etiology is unclear based on the imaging modalities, histopathologic studies are rarely required. Fine-needle aspiration cytology (FNAC) specimens are an option in the early stages of the condition. Because biopsy or surgical specimens are taken later in the disease, their findings are less comprehensive. Since at least 15% of infants have associated hip dysplasia, routine hip examinations, as well as ultrasound scans by 4 to 6 weeks of age, or plain radiographs of the hips by 4 to 6 months of age, are advised.

11.15.7. Treatment/Management

There is no established therapy for congenital torticollis, and there are multiple approaches to its treatment. Experts in various fields, such as physical therapy and osteopathy, recommend techniques for treating infant torticollis. With proper care, 90–95% of children show improvement before their first birthday, and 97% of patients improve if treatment begins before six months of age. Since it affects the child's normal motor development, a palpable sternocleidomastoid mass is a crucial sign that intervention for congenital torticollis should begin by the child's second month of life.

The main objectives are to develop symmetry in the face, head, and neck, prevent contractures, and achieve an age-appropriate active and passive range of motion. Close monitoring and passive range stretching are the primary components of initial treatment. It is recommended that parents position the child at specific times, such as during feedings, by rotating the chin towards the shoulder on the affected side. When awake and supervised, infants can practice prone motor skills by being placed on their stomach. Manual stretches, including flexion, extension, and lateral rotation, should be performed in sets of 15 at least three times a week, with each stretch lasting approximately one second and a 10-second break in between. Stretching methods are the most important and scientifically supported treatment approach if there is a fibrous component.

The purpose of the collar for tubular orthosis in cases of torticollis is to maintain a neutral posture on the affected side of the neck. The child can wear it during waking hours and it is recommended for children older than four months.

Other resources, such as the adjunctive use of botulinum toxin injection in the sternocleidomastoid and other nearby muscles, may be utilized in cases where physical therapy is ineffective. Physical therapy is an important part of the follow-up at every stage, but surgery is the last resort in other, more severe cases.

Surgery: If after six months of manual stretching there is no improvement and there are defects in passive rotation and lateral bending of more than 15°, or if there is a tumor in the sternocleidomastoid, surgery may be indicated. "Z" lengthening, radical sternocleidomastoid resection, and unipolar/bipolar sternocleidomastoid muscle lengthening are all part of the procedure.

11.15.8. Differential Diagnosis

Differential diagnosis is necessary to rule out the following pathologies:

- Vertebral anomalies like hemivertebrae and Klippel-Feil Syndrome;
- Unilateral congenital absence of the SCM muscle;
- Congenital scoliosis;
- Ocular torticollis;
- Sandifer syndrome;
- Arnold Chiari malformation;

- Neurological diseases;
- Visual disturbances;
- Syringomyelia;
- Cervical spine tumor;
- Brain tumor.

Torticollis and other structural abnormalities are frequently correlated with fusion and segmentation osseous abnormalities. Radiology is able to distinguish between these and torticollis. Neurogenic causes include tumors of the central nervous system (CNS) and torticollis of the eyes. In these cases, the cause of torticollis is not sternocleidomastoid abnormalities; rather, it is underlying visual or neurological issues. A typical neck examination with a full range of motion is conducted here as well. The underlying cause of torticollis must be identified and treated in order to be corrected.

11.15.9. Prognosis

The majority of cases are benign and resolve spontaneously or with manual stretching. Additionally, craniofacial asymmetry is improved, especially in cases that receive early treatment.

11.15.10. Complications

Situations where treatment is either unavailable or delayed can lead to permanent anatomic abnormalities. Apart from functional impairment, it can be disfiguring and raise cosmetic concerns. The ability to distinguish between a benign condition such as positional plagiocephaly and craniosynostosis is crucial, as the former is frequently linked to the latter. The distinction between the two may require close inspection of the sutures and imaging, such as an ultrasound or radiograph. In order to stop the skull from remodeling, parents of children with plagiocephaly should be advised to change positions often. For the purpose of improving neck motion, physical therapy referrals are crucial. Should the contracted sternocleidomastoid muscle not be released, craniofacial asymmetry could develop over time. To stop the progression of facial asymmetry, efforts should be made to treat torticollis.

11.15.11. Enhancing Healthcare Team Outcomes

An interdisciplinary team is the most effective in managing congenital torticollis in order to prevent high postural morbidity. Most patients are initially recognized by the parent who takes the child or infant to the primary care physician. To improve the prognosis, congenital torticollis must be identified as soon as possible. Prompt noninvasive correction is initiated upon early diagnosis, thereby averting long-term deformity complications. Parents should be informed about the illness, how they can help manage it, and how long the condition will last. Healthcare professionals need to understand the connection between congenital torticollis, how it affects a child's gross motor development, and that most kids outgrow any motor delays caused by the disorder by the time they are three to five years old. The child should be monitored by a pediatric nurse until the congenital torticollis completely resolves. Most kids who receive appropriate therapy from a cooperative interprofessional team have positive results.

11.16. Spondylolisthesis

A disorder of the spine called spondylolisthesis affects the lower vertebrae (spinal bones). One of the lower vertebrae slips forward onto the bone directly beneath it as a result of this disease. Although it is a painful condition, most cases can be treated. Therapeutic and surgical methods can be applied. By using the appropriate exercise methods, this illness can be prevented.

11.16.1. Etiology

Spondylolisthesis is typically assigned one of the following five main etiologies: degenerative, isthmic, traumatic, dysplastic, or pathologic. Degenerative spondylolisthesis occurs when there are degenerative changes in the spine without a pars interarticularis defect. It is usually associated with the degeneration of the facet joints and discs, which leads to instability and forward movement of one vertebral body in relation to the other. Isthmic spondylolisthesis is caused by inherent pars interarticularis defects. Although the exact cause is unknown, it is believed that microtrauma from repeated lumbar extension during adolescence, particularly from sports like football, wrestling, and gymnastics, may contribute to its development. Traumatic spondylolisthesis is most commonly caused by fractures of the pars interarticularis or the facet joint structure. Congenital dysplastic spondylolisthesis occurs due to an abnormal alignment of the facet joints caused by a variation in their orientation. In dysplastic spondylolisthesis, the facet joints are oriented more sagittally than the usual coronal orientation. Pathologic spondylolisthesis may result from a focal process, such as an infection, neoplasm, or iatrogenic origin, or it may be caused by systemic factors, such as bone or connective tissue disorders. Additional risk factors for spondylolisthesis include scoliosis, occult spina bifida at the S1 level, and having a first-degree relative with spondylolisthesis.

11.16.2. Epidemiology

With the exception of trauma, spondylolisthesis most frequently affects the lower lumbar spine, but it can also occur in the cervical and thoracic spines. Degenerative spondylolisthesis is more prevalent in women than in men and primarily affects adults. Obesity increases the risk of developing this condition. Although it is more common in adolescents and young adults, isthmic spondylolisthesis may go undiagnosed until symptoms manifest in adulthood. Males are more likely to have isthmic spondylolisthesis. In children, dysplastic spondylolisthesis is more common, with females being affected more frequently than males. Current estimates for prevalence are 6 to 7% for isthmic spondylolisthesis by the age of 18 years, and up to 18% of adult patients undergoing MRI of the lumbar spine. Grade I spondylolisthesis accounts for 75% of all cases. The L5–S1 level is where spondylolisthesis most frequently manifests itself, with the anterior translation of the L5 vertebral body on the S1 vertebral body. The second most typical site of spondylolisthesis is the L4–5 level.

11.16.3. Pathophysiology

A weakening of the structures that maintain the alignment of the vertebral bodies can lead to spondylolisthesis. When one vertebra moves in relation to its neighboring vertebrae, mechanical motion may cause local pain, or compression of the exiting nerve roots or spinal cord may cause radicular or myelopathic pain. During puberty, pediatric patients are more likely to experience an increase in spondylolisthesis grade. It is less common for older patients with lower grades I or II spondylolistheses to eventually advance to higher grades.

11.16.4. History and Physical Details

In cases of lumbar spondylolisthesis, patients typically experience intermittent and localized low back pain. Conversely, for cervical spondylolisthesis, they commonly experience localized neck pain. The pain worsens when flexing and extending the affected segment due to motion-induced mechanical pain. Direct palpation of the affected segment may also exacerbate the pain. Radicular pain can occur as a result of compression on the exiting nerve roots due to narrowing of the nerve foramina caused by one vertebra slipping on the other. Additionally, associated disc protrusion, lateral recess narrowing, or central stenosis can impinge on the traversing nerve root, which is the root to the level below. Occasionally, pain may improve when in certain positions, such as lying supine. This improvement is attributed to the reduction in instability of spondylolisthesis with a supine posture, which alleviates pressure on the bony elements and opens the neural foramen or spinal canal. Other symptoms of lumbar spondylolisthesis include pain in the buttocks, numbness or weakness in the leg(s), difficulty walking, and in rare cases, loss of bowel or bladder control.

11.16.5. Evaluation

The standard for diagnosing spondylolisthesis is AP and lateral plain films, along with lateral flexion-extension plain films. Instability can be indicated by aberrant alignment of one vertebral body relative to the next or by potential flexion and extension motion.

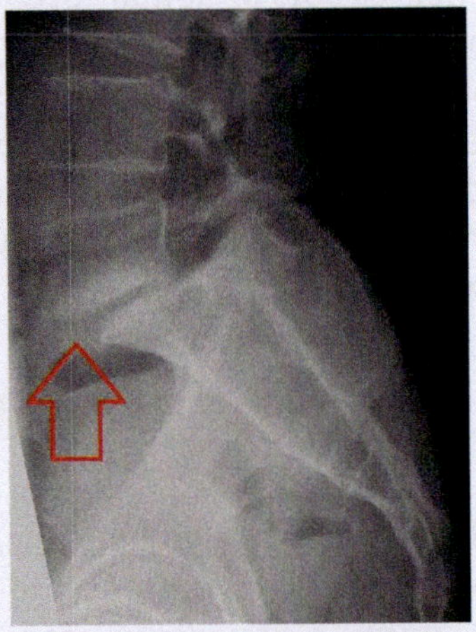

Figure 11.15. *X-ray of the lateral lumbar spine with a grade III anterolisthesis at the L5–S1 level.*

Source: By Lucien Monfils – Own work, CC BY-SA 3.0, https://commons.wikimedia.org/w/index.php?curid=4332075.

One possible pars defect in isthmic spondylolisthesis is known as the "Scotty dog collar." The hyperdensity where the cartoon dog's collar would be indicates the pars interarticularis fracture in the Scotty dog collar. For the most accurate diagnosis of spondylolisthesis, computed tomography (CT) of the spine offers the highest sensitivity and specificity. Sagittal reconstructions are a better way to see spondylolisthesis than axial CT imaging. While associated soft tissue and disc abnormalities can be seen on a spine MRI, it can be more difficult to see bony detail and a possible pars defect (Figure 11.15).

11.16.6. Treatment/Management

Conservative therapy, which includes nonsteroidal anti-inflammatory drugs (NSAIDs), heat, mild exercise, traction, bracing, and/or bed rest, is usually the first line of treatment for grade I and II spondylolisthesis. Younger patients with low-grade spondylolisthesis will require surgery if conservative treatment is not successful in 10 to 15% of cases. There are no set standards for surgical care. A variety of surgical techniques are used in treatment, such as interbody fusion, fusion with or without instrumentation, and decompression. Individuals who are unstable are more likely to need surgery. If possible, some surgeons advise reducing the spondylolisthesis because it can improve spinopelvic sagittal alignment, lessen the chance of future degenerative spinal changes, and lessen foraminal narrowing. In cases of impacted spondylolisthesis and higher grades, the reduction may be riskier and more difficult.

11.16.7. Differential Diagnosis

- Degenerative lumbar disc disease;
- Lumbar disc problems;
- Lumbosacral disc injuries;
- Lumbosacral discogenic pain syndrome;
- Lumbosacral facet syndrome;
- Lumbosacral radiculopathy;
- Lumbosacral spine acute bony injuries;

- Lumbosacral spondylosis;
- Myofascial pain in athletes.

11.16.8. Pearls and Other Issues

The most widely used method for grading spondylolisthesis is Meyerding's classification. It is based on the percentage of anterior translation in relation to the adjacent level. Grade I spondylolisthesis represents 1 to 25% slippage, grade II indicates up to 50% slippage, grade III indicates up to 75% slippage, and grade IV indicates 76%–100% slippage. Spondyloptosis, also known as grade V spondylolisthesis, occurs when there is more than 100% slippage. Subtypes of isthmic spondylolisthesis include subtype A (stress fractures of the pars), subtype B (elongation of the pars without overt fracture), and subtype C (acute fracture of the pars). Subtypes of pathologic spondylolisthesis include subtype A (systemic causes) and subtype B (focal processes).

11.16.9. Enhancing Healthcare Team Outcomes

To achieve optimal care for patients with degenerative spondylolisthesis, a specialized team consisting of an orthopedic nurse, physical therapist, and orthopedic or neurosurgeon is essential. Chiropractors may also be involved in the initial diagnosis.

The treating clinician will develop a management plan and involve other team members as necessary. Surgical cases will require collaboration with nursing staff and physical therapists for pre-, intra-, and post-operative care, while non-operative cases will involve physical therapists in monitoring progress. Prioritizing weight loss is important for the team, as it can alleviate symptoms and improve quality of life. Working together in an interprofessional setting is crucial for achieving the best possible outcomes for patients.

11.17. Bursa and Bursitis

The tiny, fluid-filled sacs, or bursae, that cushion the bones, tendons, and muscles next to the joints are impacted by the painful illness known as bursitis. Inflamed bursae give rise to bursitis. The shoulder, elbow, and hip are the most typical sites for bursitis.

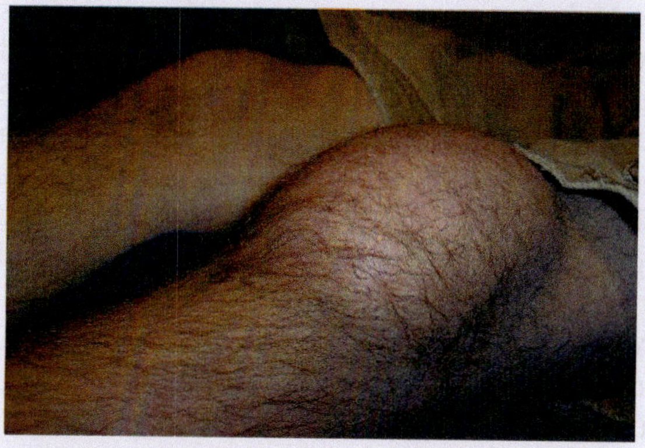

Figure 11.16. *Aseptic prepatellar bursitis.*

Source: By Atropos235 – Own work, CC BY-SA 2.5, https://commons.wikimedia.org/w/index.php?curid=4079323.

Bursitis can also occur at the base of the big toe, near the heel, and by the knee. Near joints that undergo repetitive motion regularly, bursitis frequently develops. Resting the afflicted joint and shielding it from additional damage are usual forms of treatment. After receiving the right care, bursitis pain usually disappears in a few weeks, but flare-ups are frequent (Figure 11.16).

11.17.1. Etiology

The clinician must be aware of the numerous causes of bursitis. The most common etiology is prolonged pressure, where the bursa is stressed between a hard surface and a bony prominence. Examples of prolonged pressure that can lead to bursitis include individuals who work on their knees without sufficient padding or students who regularly rest their elbows on their desks. Additionally, bursitis can result from repetitive motions that irritate the bursa. Direct pressure applied to the bursa is the second most common cause of bursitis. Since the inciting incident may have appeared harmless at the time, patients often cannot recall it. Traumatic bursitis patients may experience septic bursitis, typically caused by the bursa's direct penetration through the skin. Septic bursitis can also occur due to hematogenous spread, although this is uncommon due to the bursa's limited blood supply. The majority of septic bursitis cases are caused by Staphylococcus aureus. Bursitis can also be caused by autoimmune diseases, systemic inflammatory diseases, and arthropathies such as gout, scleroderma, osteoarthritis, rheumatoid arthritis, and systemic lupus erythematosus. Finally, bursitis may have an idiopathic cause, and invasive procedures have the potential to cause septic bursitis in particular.

11.17.2. Epidemiology

Generally speaking, bursitis affects both males and females equally. However, pes anserine and trochanteric bursitis have shown a documented predilection towards women. Additionally, individuals who are obese are more likely to experience these types of bursitis. The occupational distribution of certain professions, such as plumbers, gardeners, mechanics, and construction workers, among others, leads to a higher prevalence of olecranon bursitis in men. Various slang terms have been coined to reflect these epidemiologic connections, as certain occupational stressors increase the risk of developing bursitis. For instance, prepatellar bursitis is commonly known as housemaid's knee, while olecranon bursitis is occasionally referred to as student's elbow.

Similarly, ischial bursitis is known as weaver's bottom, and infrapatellar bursitis is frequently called clergyman's knee. Dancers and figure skaters often experience bursitis of the subcutaneous calcaneal bursa due to wearing boots that are too small or poorly fitting. Prolonged pressure on the injured bursa is typically the cause of bursitis in each of these cases. While bursitis can affect individuals of all ages, the elderly may be more vulnerable due to the presence of osteoarthritis and other chronic diseases that can increase the risk of bursitis. Immunocompromised individuals, such as those with diabetes, certain rheumatologic diseases, alcoholism, or HIV, are also more susceptible to developing septic bursitis.

11.17.3. Pathophysiology

As a synovial lining that collapses on itself until a subsequent trigger causes it to become irritated and fill with synovial fluid, the bursa itself is a potential space. When the inflamed bursa is compressed against bone, muscle, tendon, ligaments, or skin, the patient feels pain. Despite the name, not every case of bursitis is linked to an obvious inflammatory response. That being said, increased levels of inflammatory mediators, including cyclooxygenases (COXs), tumor necrosis factor-alpha, and particular interleukins, have been found when the subacromial bursa of patients with subacromial bursitis has been examined.

11.17.4. History and Physical Details

There are two types of bursitis: acute and chronic, and each has a distinct symptom presentation. A thorough medical history and knowledge of the patient's daily activities will enable the clinician to distinguish between the two forms of bursitis and other possible diagnoses. Whereas inflammatory arthropathies, overuse, repetitive pressure, or microtraumas are more likely causes of chronic bursitis, acute bursitis usually results from trauma, infection, or crystalline joint disease. When a bursa is palpated, patients with acute bursitis typically exhibit pain. Pain may cause the involved joint's range of motion to be restricted. Pain is also elicited by active motion involving the affected bursa; however, the degree of pain varies based on the bursa's location and the biomechanics of moving the surrounding tissues, muscles, and bones. For example, many patients will feel pain when moving actively but not when moving passively. There is little to no pain when the surrounding muscles are not contracted, which prevents the bursa from being compressed. Certain types of acute bursitis cause pain when the afflicted joint is flexed, but not when it is extended. Prepactellar and olecranon bursitis are frequently associated with these symptoms.

Chronic bursitis is often painless, in contrast to the physical examination findings in acute bursitis. The bursa has significantly swollen and thickened due to its ability to expand and hold extra fluid. Assessing the skin is crucial in determining whether bursitis is acute or chronic. It is important to evaluate the skin for warmth, erythema, and trauma. One study discovered that a temperature increase of just 2.2°C between the skin covering the affected bursa and the unaffected contralateral bursa was highly sensitive and specific for septic bursitis. This temperature difference is both highly sensitive and specific. Even in cases of acute bursitis, deep bursitis may not cause any noticeable changes in the skin or tenderness when palpating the surrounding structures. Lastly, the onset of bursitis can sometimes be associated with musculoskeletal imbalances or specific anatomical variations. Trochanteric bursitis, often caused by gluteus minimus or medius tendinopathy, can be exacerbated by decreased core strength and persistent back pain. Pes anserine bursitis can be caused by mechanical factors such as pes planus and genu valgum.

11.17.5. Evaluation

Certain forms of bursitis can be diagnosed clinically and without the need for additional research; nonetheless, imaging is useful in both diagnosing and treating bursitis. When there is diagnostic uncertainty, imaging can help to clarify the differential diagnosis or even offer a precise diagnosis. When there is a history of trauma or there is a concern for a foreign body or fracture causing swelling or pain, plain film imaging of the affected joint or bursa should be taken into consideration. Both MRI and ultrasound, which have the added advantage of providing real-time images within a joint or region surrounding the bursa and can be used to monitor changes with active and passive movement, can be used to assess the deeper bursa.

Ultrasound is beneficial in distinguishing between cellulitis and infectious bursitis by detecting cobblestoning of the fat over a bursa. Color Doppler can also be used to identify signs of infection, such as hyperemia of the bursa and surrounding tissues. Aspiration of the swollen bursa is recommended in cases of suspected septic bursitis or bursitis caused by crystalline disease. The aspirated fluid should be analyzed for cell count, Gram stain, culture, glucose levels, and crystal presence. A white blood cell count of less than $500/mm^3$ in the aspirated fluid indicates noninfectious and non-crystalline bursitis.

11.17.6. Treatment/Management

Most cases of bursitis will resolve on their own. However, there are several modalities available to alleviate the patient's pain and ensure full functionality of the affected area. Conservative treatment aims to relieve symptoms through the application of compression, elevation, ice, and rest. Patients should receive ergonomic education to prevent exacerbating movements. For individuals whose job involves prolonged pressure on the elbows or knees, cushioning certain superficial bursae can be beneficial. Patients with ischial bursitis can benefit from using a foam donut, and core-strengthening stretches and exercises can help improve and reduce symptoms.

In cases of bursitis, it is advisable to wear properly fitting shoes that relieve pressure on the Achilles tendon. Acetaminophen and/or NSAIDs are the first-line treatments for pain relief. Corticosteroid injections, sometimes combined with a local anesthetic, can provide relief for deeper bursae. However, for superficial bursae, local corticosteroid injections are not recommended due to the higher risk of iatrogenic septic bursitis, local tendon damage, skin atrophy, and draining sinus tracts. Corticosteroid injections also carry the risk of alleviating pain to the point where a different condition, such as a rotator cuff tear, goes undiagnosed, delaying the necessary surgical repair. The use of corticosteroid injections for chronic bursitis is generally not well supported by available data, and a recent study found no benefit from this treatment. Physical therapy and range-of-motion exercises can enhance the strength of the muscles supporting the bursa surrounding the affected area. This is particularly crucial in cases of subacromial bursitis, as immobilization can lead to frozen shoulder, retraction, and atrophy.

The doctor must treat the underlying inflammatory condition when treating bursitis brought on by systemic inflammatory diseases. The first-line treatment for septic bursitis is to use systemic antibiotics that are active against gram-positive bacteria. Oral antibiotics are usually sufficient to treat most patients with septic bursitis as an outpatient; hospitalization is necessary only in cases where systemic or whole-joint involvement is suspected or the patient shows signs of instability. The bursa may be surgically removed in certain uncooperative cases; this is typically accomplished through endoscopic or arthroscopic techniques.

11.17.7. Differential Diagnosis

Numerous other pathologic conditions can be mistaken for bursitis or even occur simultaneously in the same spot. The differential diagnosis of joint pain is broad and includes a wide range of conditions. Osteoarthritis, rheumatoid arthritis, and other inflammatory conditions can be mistaken for many forms of bursitis. Furthermore, the differential is highly dependent on where the suspected bursitis is located. Shoulder impingement, labral tears, and rotator cuff tears are among the differential diagnoses for a patient with shoulder pain. These conditions frequently coexist, and one of them may have actually caused bursitis. Gout can also mimic bursitis, particularly at the prepatellar, infrapatellar, and olecranon bursas, as these joints are frequently the site of gouty tophi formation or pseudogout pain. Given that the bursa is located close to the sciatic nerve and that patients may experience lancinating pain, insidious bursitis is sometimes mistaken for sciatica. To differentiate ischial bursitis from sciatica, the pain will be more noticeable when sitting.

It is also possible to confuse ischial bursitis with other conditions that cause sacroiliitis, such as ankylosing spondylitis or an inflammatory enthesopathy. It is necessary to distinguish trochanteric bursitis from iliotibial band syndrome; in the former case, tenderness is more distal in contrast to the proximal location of the trochanteric bursa. Similar symptoms can be seen in iliopsoas bursitis as in arthritis, synovitis, labral tears, overuse injuries from running, and avascular necrosis (AVN) of the femoral head. Bursitis of the medial collateral ligament and pes anserine bursitis can mimic MCL tears or strains, meniscal injuries, or even fractures of the tibial plateau. Since an effusion is uncommon in cases of knee bursitis, this can aid the clinician in distinguishing the condition from the other conditions mentioned. When retrocalcaneal bursitis is first evaluated, it may mimic plantar fasciitis, enthesopathy, Achilles tendinitis, or pain from bone spurs. Similar to numerous other types of bursitis, these conditions might exist together or have been the cause of one another initially. Finally, a septic bursa may be mistaken for a septic joint or even for a straightforward case of cellulitis affecting the skin covering the bursa. It is critical that the clinician makes this distinction between these infectious processes because there may be significant differences in how they should be managed. If an infected joint is missed, the patient may experience severe morbidity and death.

11.17.8. Prognosis

Most patients with bursitis have a good prognosis; it is not a fatal condition. The majority of them are treated as outpatients. Recurrences are common in patients who do not avoid the trigger or continue with the same activity.

11.17.9. Enhancing Healthcare Team Outcomes

In clinical practice, bursitis is a highly prevalent condition that is managed by a diverse team of healthcare professionals. This interprofessional team typically includes an orthopedic surgeon, rheumatologist, primary care physician, sports physician, emergency department physician, and nurse practitioner. Their collective expertise ensures comprehensive management of the condition and consistent treatment outcomes. Following a diagnosis, supportive care is usually the recommended approach. In the majority of cases, non-infectious bursitis resolves on its own within a few weeks. However, if the bursa fluid is infected, consultation with an orthopedic surgeon and infectious disease specialist is necessary. Physical therapy may be beneficial for some patients in restoring functionality post-treatment. It is important to educate patients about the importance of avoiding activities that initially caused their bursitis.

For patients who do not respond to conservative treatments, injectable steroid pain relievers may be required. Range of motion exercises, aimed at strengthening the muscles surrounding the bursa, should be taught by physical therapists and orthopedic specialty nurses. Throughout the follow-up period, close monitoring of the patient's symptoms is essential, involving the nurse practitioner, primary care physician, and nurse. Surgery should only be considered as a last resort when all other options have been exhausted.

11.17.9.1. Outcomes

For the most part, patients with bursitis have positive outcomes.

A Closer Look

Spondylosis

Spondylosis is a disorder characterized by abnormal wear on the cervical vertebrae and the cartilage that lines the neck. It frequently causes persistent neck pain.

Over time, spinal wear can lead to spondylosis, affecting the joints between the bones of the cervical spine and the disks or cushions between the neck vertebrae.

These changes have the potential to gradually compress or exert pressure on one or more nerve roots. In more severe cases, the spinal cord may also be affected, impacting both the arms and legs.

These changes can be initiated by the daily grind, with individuals who lead active lifestyles at work or in sports being more susceptible to experiencing them.

Symptoms of spondylosis often appear gradually over time, but they can also manifest suddenly or worsen suddenly. Symptoms include:

- Pain that may be mild, or it can be deep and so severe that the person is unable to move
- Pain over the shoulder blade
- Pain that spreads to the upper arm, forearm, or fingers (in rare cases)

Other common symptoms are:

- Neck stiffness that gets worse over time
- Numbness or abnormal sensations in the shoulders, arms, or legs (in rare cases)
- Headaches, especially in the back of the head
- **Diagnosis of Spondylosis:** The initial step that the healthcare provider will take is to conduct a physical examination. The individual may be requested to tilt their head to the side and forward as the physician gently applies pressure to the top of their head. During this test, an increase in pain or numbness is typically an indication of spinal nerve compression. Weakness or loss of feeling may suggest damage to the spinal cord or specific nerve roots. An X-ray of the neck or spine may be conducted to check for arthritis or other changes in the spine.
- **Treatment:** Depending on patient's needs, the healthcare provider can suggest a range of treatments for cervical spondylosis pain relief. These may include:
- **Medicines:** Taking muscle relaxants, opioid painkillers, and nonsteroidal anti-inflammatory drugs like aspirin or ibuprofen may be helpful.
- **Physical Therapy:** Strengthening and stretching techniques can be learned from a physical therapist, which may alleviate the symptoms.

- **Ice or Heat:** Follow the advice of the physician or physical therapist and use an ice pack to cool the neck or a warming pad to apply heat.
- **Collar:** Wearing a soft collar around the neck for short periods of time may improve the symptoms. However, wearing it for an extended period may weaken the neck.
- **Injections:** A medical professional can administer steroid medication and painkillers through injections next to the spinal cord or into the painful neck joint.
- **Surgery:** It is not required in the majority of cases. However, if deemed necessary, surgeons can perform various operations to alleviate pressure on the spinal cord or the nerves exiting the spine. The area surrounding the point of nerve exit can be surgically cleared of bone, as well as bone from other vertebral bodies. Following one of these procedures, it may be necessary to fuse the spinal bones. The surgery will be performed under anesthesia, ensuring that the person will not experience any discomfort.
- **Prevention:** While cervical spondylosis may not be entirely preventable, reduce the risk by taking the following measures:
  - Stay physically active.
  - Use good posture.
  - When working out or participating in sports, always use the proper gear and form to avoid neck injuries.
  - Avoid trauma to the neck

11.18. Summary

- Anomalies of a structural or functional nature that have developed during intrauterine life are commonly known as congenital disorders. These conditions, which are also referred to as birth defects, congenital anomalies, or congenital malformations, have developed during pregnancy and could have been detected prior to, during, or after birth.
- Mallet finger is an injury to the tendon that straightens the tip of one's finger (or thumb). It is alternatively referred to as drop finger or baseball finger. Tendons have the function of providing stability and motion by connecting muscles to bones.
- A medical condition referred to as boutonnière deformity causes the finger to be hyperextended at the DIP and flexed at the proximal interphalangeal joint (PIP). This is typically induced by acute trauma and results from a rupture of the PIP central slip.
- A condition referred to as trigger finger impacts the tendons responsible for flexing the fingers and thumb. In such cases, the fingers typically undergo a sensation of locking or catching during bending and straightening movements. Additional symptoms may encompass discomfort and rigidity in the thumb and fingers.
- The thumb tendons become painfully inflamed in a condition also known as de Quervain's tendinosis or de Quervain's tendinitis.
- The palmar fascia, the fibrous layer of tissue that lies above the tendons, nerves, blood vessels, and bones in the palm and fingers and beneath the skin, has been affected by Dupuytren's disease. The fascia has thickened and contracted (shortened) in patients with Dupuytren's disease over time.
- Carpal tunnel syndrome (CTS) is a medical condition that has resulted in hand and wrist pain, tingling, numbness, and weakness.
- Overuse of the muscles and tendons in the elbow can lead to a condition called tennis elbow, which is also known as lateral epicondylitis. This condition often arises due to repetitive motions of the arm and wrist.
- Golfer's elbow is a condition that causes pain at the point where the tendons of the forearm muscles connect to the bony bump on the inner side of the elbow. This pain can radiate down into the forearm and wrist.
- Supraspinatus tendinopathy is a prevalent and incapacitating condition that usually manifests after middle age. It is a primary cause of shoulder pain and affects the supraspinatus tendon, which is a component of the rotator cuff muscles located in the subacromial space.
- Adhesive capsulitis (AC), commonly referred to as frozen shoulder, is a painful and rigid condition of the shoulder. The shoulder becomes progressively more challenging to move over time.
- A heel spur, also known as a bone spur, is a bony growth that protrudes from the heel bone where it joins the plantar fascia ligament. The plantar fascia is a ligament that runs from the heel to the ball of the foot. Heel spurs are a relatively common condition, affecting approximately 15% of individuals.

- Neuropathic trauma can cause Charcot neuroarthropathy, leading to foot fractures and dislocations.
- Torticollis in babies twists the neck muscles and tilts the head to one side, causing the neck to appear at an unusual angle, with the chin slanted to one side and the top of the head to the other.
- A condition of the spine known as spondylolisthesis affects the lower vertebrae (spinal bones). One of the lower vertebrae has slipped forward onto the bone directly beneath it as a result of this ailment.
- The minuscule, fluid-filled sacs, or bursae, that provide cushioning for the bones, tendons, and muscles adjacent to the joints have been affected by the painful condition referred to as bursitis. Inflamed bursae have given rise to bursitis. The shoulder, elbow, and hip are the most common sites for bursitis.

References

1. Binstead, J. T., Tafti, D., & Hatcher, J. D., (2021). Boutonnière deformity. In: *StatPearls* [Internet]. Treasure Island (FL): StatPearls Publishing. https://www.ncbi.nlm.nih.gov/books/NBK470323/ (accessed on 20 March 2024).
2. Botero, S. S., Diaz, J. J., Benaïda, A., Collon, S., Facca, S., & Liverneaux, P. A., (2016). Review of acute traumatic closed mallet finger injuries in adults. *Archives of Plastic Surgery, 43*(2), 134.
3. Brotzman, S. B., & Manske, R. C., (2011). *Clinical Orthopedic Rehabilitation: An Evidence-Based Approach*. Elsevier Health Sciences,
4. De Jong, J. P., Nguyen, J. T., Sonnema, A. J., Nguyen, E. C., Amadio, P. C., & Moran, S. L., (2014). The incidence of acute traumatic tendon injuries in the hand and wrist: A 10-year population-based study. *Clinics in Orthopedic Surgery, 6*(2), 196–202.
5. Freiberg, A., (2007). Management of proximal interphalangeal joint injuries. *Can. J. Plast. Surg., 15*(4), 199–203. https://pubmed.ncbi.nlm.nih.gov/16843790/ (accessed on 20 March 2024).
6. Johnson, C., Swanson, M., & Manolopoulos, K., (2019). A case report: Treatment of a zone III extensor tendon injury using a single relative motion with dorsal hood orthosis and a modified short arc motion protocol. *Journal of Hand Therapy*.
7. Kim, J. P., Go, J. H., Hwang, C. H., & Shin, W. J., (2014). Restoration of the central slip in congenital form of boutonnière deformity: Case report. *J. Hand. Surg. Am., 39*(10), 1978–1981. https://pubmed.ncbi.nlm.nih.gov/25042044/ (accessed on 20 March 2024).
8. Kothari, M. J., (2016). *Carpal Tunnel Syndrome: Clinical Manifestations and Diagnosis.* http://www.uptodate.com/contents/carpal-tunnel-syndrome-clinical-manifestations-and-diagnosis?source=machineLearning&search=carpal+tunnel+weakness&selectedTitle=2%7E150&sectionRank=2&anchor=H2#H2 (accessed on 20 March 2024).
9. Lin, J. S., & Samora, J. B., (2018). Surgical and nonsurgical management of mallet finger: A systematic review. *The Journal of Hand Surgery, 43*(2), 146–163.
10. Madsen, J. M., (2004). "Prepatellar bursitis." In: Greenberg, M. I., (ed.). *Greenberg's Text-Atlas of Emergency Medicine* (p. 922). Lippincott Williams & Wilkins. ISBN 9780781745864.

11. McKeon, K. E., & Lee, D. H., (2015). Posttraumatic boutonnière and swan neck deformities. *J. Am. Acad. Orthop. Surg., 23*(10), 623–632. https://pubmed.ncbi.nlm.nih.gov/26320165/ (accessed on 20 March 2024).
12. Papadopoulos, D. V., Bednar, M. S., Davidson, A., & Schmidt, C. C., (2021). Hand Surgery. In: McMahon, P. J., & Skinner, H. B., (eds.), *Current Diagnosis & Treatment in Orthopedics,* (6th edn.). McGraw Hill.
13. Smit, J. M., Beets, M. R., Zeebregts, C. J., Rood, A., & Welters, C. F., (2010). Treatment options for mallet finger: A review. *Plastic and Reconstructive Surgery, 126*(5), 1624–1629.
14. Thillemann, J. K., Thillemann, T. M., Kristensen, P. K., Foldager-Jensen, A. D., & Munk, B., (2020). Splinting versus extension-block pinning of bony mallet finger: A randomized clinical trial. *Journal of Hand Surgery (European Volume)*, 1753193420917567.
15. Yee, J., & Waseem, M., (2019). Mallet finger injuries. In: *StatPearls* [Internet]. StatPearls Publishing. Available from: https://www.ncbi.nlm.nih.gov/books/NBK459373/ (accessed on 20 March 2024).

INDEX

C

D

J

K

L

M

N

O

T

U

V

W

X

Printed and bound by CPI Group (UK) Ltd, Croydon, CR0 4YY
18/09/2026
14965065-0004